Early Detection of Neurological Disorders Using Machine Learning Systems

Sudip Paul
North-Eastern Hill University Shillong, India

Pallab Bhattacharya
National Institute of Pharmaceutical Education and Research (NIPER) Ahmedabad, India

Arindam Bit
National Institute of Technology Raipur, India

A volume in the Advances in Medical Technologies and Clinical Practice (AMTCP) Book Series

IGI Global
DISSEMINATOR OF KNOWLEDGE

Published in the United States of America by
IGI Global
Medical Information Science Reference (an imprint of IGI Global)
701 E. Chocolate Avenue
Hershey PA, USA 17033
Tel: 717-533-8845
Fax: 717-533-8661
E-mail: cust@igi-global.com
Web site: http://www.igi-global.com

Library of Congress Cataloging-in-Publication Data

Names: Paul, Sudip, 1984- editor. | Bhattacharya, Pallab, 1978- editor. | Bit, Arindam, 1985- editor.
Title: Early detection of neurological disorders using machine learning systems / Sudip Paul, Pallab Bhattacharya, and Arindam Bit, editors.
Description: Hershey, PA : Medical Information Science Reference, [2020] | Includes bibliographical references.
Identifiers: LCCN 2018055807| ISBN 9781522585671 (hardcover) | ISBN 9781522585688 (ebook)
Subjects: | MESH: Nervous System Diseases--diagnosis | Machine Learning | Diagnosis, Computer-Assisted | Big Data
Classification: LCC RC348 | NLM WL 141 | DDC 616.8/0475--dc23 LC record available at https://lccn.loc.gov/2018055807

This book is published in the IGI Global book series Advances in Medical Technologies and Clinical Practice (AMTCP) (ISSN: 2327-9354; eISSN: 2327-9370)

British Cataloguing in Publication Data
A Cataloguing in Publication record for this book is available from the British Library.

All work contributed to this book is new, previously-unpublished material. The views expressed in this book are those of the authors, but not necessarily of the publisher.

For electronic access to this publication, please contact: eresources@igi-global.com.

Advances in Medical Technologies and Clinical Practice (AMTCP) Book Series

Srikanta Patnaik
SOA University, India
Priti Das
S.C.B. Medical College, India

ISSN:2327-9354
EISSN:2327-9370

Mission

Medical technological innovation continues to provide avenues of research for faster and safer diagnosis and treatments for patients. Practitioners must stay up to date with these latest advancements to provide the best care for nursing and clinical practices.

The **Advances in Medical Technologies and Clinical Practice (AMTCP) Book Series** brings together the most recent research on the latest technology used in areas of nursing informatics, clinical technology, biomedicine, diagnostic technologies, and more. Researchers, students, and practitioners in this field will benefit from this fundamental coverage on the use of technology in clinical practices.

Coverage

- Clinical Nutrition
- Nutrition
- Patient-Centered Care
- Telemedicine
- Medical Imaging
- E-Health
- Diagnostic Technologies
- Clinical Data Mining
- Biometrics
- Clinical High-Performance Computing

IGI Global is currently accepting manuscripts for publication within this series. To submit a proposal for a volume in this series, please contact our Acquisition Editors at Acquisitions@igi-global.com or visit: http://www.igi-global.com/publish/.

The Advances in Medical Technologies and Clinical Practice (AMTCP) Book Series (ISSN 2327-9354) is published by IGI Global, 701 E. Chocolate Avenue, Hershey, PA 17033-1240, USA, www.igi-global.com. This series is composed of titles available for purchase individually; each title is edited to be contextually exclusive from any other title within the series. For pricing and ordering information please visit http://www.igi-global.com/book-series/advances-medical-technologies-clinical-practice/73682. Postmaster: Send all address changes to above address.

Titles in this Series

For a list of additional titles in this series, please visit: www.igi-global.com/book-series

Computational Methods and Algorithms for Medicine and Optimized Clinical Practice
Kwok Tai Chui (City University of Hong Kong, Hong Kong) and Miltiadis D. Lytras (Effat University, Saudi Arabia)
Medical Information Science Reference • copyright 2019 • 290pp • H/C (ISBN: 9781522582441) • US $245.00 (our price)

Advanced Classification Techniques for Healthcare Analysis
Chinmay Chakraborty (Birla Institute of Technology Mesra, India)
Medical Information Science Reference • copyright 2019 • 424pp • H/C (ISBN: 9781522577966) • US $285.00 (our price)

Tele-Audiology and the Optimization of Hearing Healthcare Delivery
Elaine Saunders (Blamey Saunders Hears, Australia)
Medical Information Science Reference • copyright 2019 • 274pp • H/C (ISBN: 9781522581918) • US $225.00 (our price)

Design and Implementation of Healthcare Biometric Systems
Dakshina Ranjan Kisku (National Institute of Technology Durgapur, India) Phalguni Gupta (National Institute of Technical Teachers Training and Research, India) and Jamuna Kanta Sing (Jadavpur University, India)
Medical Information Science Reference • copyright 2019 • 300pp • H/C (ISBN: 9781522575252) • US $265.00 (our price)

Computer Applications in Drug Discovery and Development
A. Puratchikody (Anna University, India) S. Lakshmana Prabu (Anna University, India) and A. Umamaheswari (Anna University, India)
Medical Information Science Reference • copyright 2019 • 332pp • H/C (ISBN: 9781522573265) • US $255.00 (our price)

Computational Techniques for Dental Image Analysis
K. Kamalanand (Anna University, India) B. Thayumanavan (Sathyabama University Dental College and Hospital, India) and P. Mannar Jawahar (Anna University, India)
Medical Information Science Reference • copyright 2019 • 334pp • H/C (ISBN: 9781522562436) • US $225.00 (our price)

IGI Global
DISSEMINATOR OF KNOWLEDGE

701 East Chocolate Avenue, Hershey, PA 17033, USA
Tel: 717-533-8845 x100 • Fax: 717-533-8661
E-Mail: cust@igi-global.com • www.igi-global.com

Table of Contents

Preface xiv

Chapter 1
Mapping the Intellectual Structure of the Field Neurological Disorders: A Bibliometric Analysis....... 1
S. Ravikumar, North-Eastern Hill University Shillong, India

Chapter 2
Neurofeedback: Retrain the Brain 13
Meena Gupta, North-Eastern Hill University Shillong, India
Dinesh Bhatia, North-Eastern Hill University Shillong, India

Chapter 3
Neurological Disorders, Rehabilitation, and Associated Technologies: An Overview 26
Sateesh Reddy Avutu, North-Eastern Hill University Shillong, India
Dinesh Bhatia, North-Eastern Hill University Shillong, India

Chapter 4
Brain Tumor and Its Segmentation From Brain MRI Sequences 39
Sanjay Saxena, International Institute of Information Technology, India
Puspanjali Mohapatra, International Institute of Information Technology, India
Swati Pattnaik, International Institute of Information Technology, India

Chapter 5
Early Detection of Parkinson's Disease: An Intelligent Diagnostic Approach.................................... 61
Debashree Devi, National Institute of Technology Silchar, India
Saroj K. Biswas, National Institute of Technology Silchar, India
Biswajit Purkayastha, National Institute of Technology Silchar, India

Chapter 6
Soft Computing-Based Early Detection of Parkinson's Disease Using Non-Invasive Method
Based on Speech Analysis 96
Chandrasekar Ravi, National Institute of Technology Puducherry, India

Chapter 7
Assessment of Gait Disorder in Parkinson's Disease 108
Divya Govindaraju, Anna University, India
Gururaj Nagarajan, Birla Institute of Technology and Science, India
Paramasivam Alagumariappan, B.S. Abdur Rahman Crescent Institute of Science and Technology, India

Chapter 8
Tremor Identification Using Machine Learning in Parkinson's Disease 128
Angana Saikia, North-Eastern Hill University Shillong, India
Vinayak Majhi, North-Eastern Hill University Shillong, India
Masaraf Hussain, North-Eastern Indira Gandhi Regional Institute of Health and Medical Sciences, India
Sudip Paul, North-Eastern Hill University Shillong, India
Amitava Datta, The University of Western Australia, Australia

Chapter 9
Epileptic Seizure Detection and Classification Using Machine Learning 152
Rekh Ram Janghel, National Institute of Technology Raipur, India
Yogesh Kumar Rathore, National Institute of Technology Raipur, India
Gautam Tatiparti, National Institute of Technology Raipur, India

Chapter 10
Neurocognitive Mechanisms for Detecting Early Phase of Depressive Disorder: Analysis of Event-Related Potentials in Human Brain 165
Shashikanta Tarai, National Institute of Technology Raipur, India

Chapter 11
Social Media Analytics to Predict Depression Level in the Users... 199
Mohammad Shahid Husain, Ibri College of Applied Sciences, Oman

Chapter 12
Linguistic Markers in Individuals With Symptoms of Depression in Bi-Multilingual Context......... 216
Anbu Savekar, National Institute of Technology Raipur, India
Shashikanta Tarai, National Institute of Technology Raipur, India
Moksha Singh, National Institute of Technology Raipur, India

Chapter 13
Motor Imagery Classification Using EEG Signals for Brain-Computer Interface Applications 241
Subrota Mazumdar, Kalinga Institute of Industrial Technology University, India
Rohit Chaudhary, Kalinga Institute of Industrial Technology University, India
Suruchi Suruchi, Kalinga Institute of Industrial Technology University, India
Suman Mohanty, Kalinga Institute of Industrial Technology University, India
Divya Kumari, Kalinga Institute of Industrial Technology University, India
Aleena Swetapadma, Kalinga Institute of Industrial Technology University, India

Chapter 14
Intelligent Big Data Analytics in Health 252
Ebru Aydindag Bayrak, Istanbul University – Cerrahpaşa, Turkey
Pinar Kirci, Istanbul University – Cerrahpaşa, Turkey

Chapter 15
Medical Image Segmentation: An Advanced Approach 292
Ramgopal Kashyap, Amity University Chhattisgarh, India
Surendra Rahamatkar, Amity University Chhattisgarh, India

Compilation of References 322

About the Contributors 369

Index 375

Detailed Table of Contents

Preface xiv

Chapter 1
Mapping the Intellectual Structure of the Field Neurological Disorders: A Bibliometric Analysis....... 1
S. Ravikumar, North-Eastern Hill University Shillong, India

The chapter utilizes bibliometric tools to explore papers in the field of neurological disorders and to examine the scientific development in the above subject domain. The research data were retrieved from the WOS database, which consists of 16,830 papers on the above phrase, but for the current study was limited to only those articles that have received more than four citations. Using this criterion, the data was narrowed to 10,694 as of 25/6/18. Using bibliometric tools, the author has identified the most productive authors, most productive countries, annual scientific production with an average growth rate of 4.82, and average article citations per year was 44.85. Network analysis was carried out to find co-citation network pattern, and with co-word analysis, found the conceptual structure of a field of neurological disorders.

Chapter 2
Neurofeedback: Retrain the Brain 13
Meena Gupta, North-Eastern Hill University Shillong, India
Dinesh Bhatia, North-Eastern Hill University Shillong, India

Neurofeedback (NF) is a type of brain wave training based on operant learning. NF has been employed in research and clinical settings for the investigation and treatment of a growing number of psychological illnesses. This technique involves detection of electroencephalographic (EEG) information from the surface of the scalp of a subject by separating its frequency decomposition into its component waveform (alpha, beta, theta, gamma, and delta) and making these components visible usually as polygraphic traces on a computer screen. Neurofeedback is being considered as a promising new method for restoring brain function in a large number of mental disorder cases. NF takes into account behavioral, cognitive, and subjective aspects as well as the brain activity of the concerned individual. About 25 years ago, NF was employed for clinical and research purposes in psychological illness. These psychological illnesses include attention deficit disorder, addiction to drug, depression, stress, and eating disorders.

Chapter 3
Neurological Disorders, Rehabilitation, and Associated Technologies: An Overview 26
Sateesh Reddy Avutu, North-Eastern Hill University Shillong, India
Dinesh Bhatia, North-Eastern Hill University Shillong, India

Patients with neurological disorders are increasing globally due to various factors such as change in lifestyle patterns, professional and personal stress, small nuclear families, etc. Neurological rehabilitation is an area focused by the several research and development organizations and scientists from different disciplines to invent new and advanced rehabilitation devices. This chapter starts with the classification of different neurological disorders and their potential causes. The rehabilitation devices available globally for neurological patients with their underlying associated technologies are explained in the chapter. Towards the end of the chapter, the reader can acquire the fundamental knowledge about the different neurological disorders and the mal-functionality associated with the corresponding organs. The utilization of advanced technologies such as artificial intelligence, machine learning, and deep learning by researchers to fabricate neuro rehabilitation devices to improve patients' quality of life (QOL) are discussed in concluding section of the chapter.

Chapter 4
Brain Tumor and Its Segmentation From Brain MRI Sequences 39
Sanjay Saxena, International Institute of Information Technology, India
Puspanjali Mohapatra, International Institute of Information Technology, India
Swati Pattnaik, International Institute of Information Technology, India

Automated segmentation of tumorous region from the brain magnetic resonance image (MRI) is the procedure of extrication anomalous tissues from regular tissues, such as white matter (WM), gray matter (GM), and cerebrospinal fluid (CSF). The process of accurate and efficient segmentation is still exigent because of the diversity of location, size, and shape of the tumorous region. Brain MRI provides metabolic process, psychological process, and descriptive information of the brain. Brain tumor segmentation using MRI is drawing the attention of the researchers due to its non-invasive nature and good soft tissue contrast of MRI sequences. The main motive of this chapter is to provide a broad overview of the methods of brain tumor segmentation based on MRI. This chapter provides the information of the brain tumor, its types, brief introduction of the MRI, and its diverse types, and lastly, this chapter gives the brief overview with benefits and limitations about diverse techniques used for brain tumor segmentation by different researchers and scientists.

Chapter 5
Early Detection of Parkinson's Disease: An Intelligent Diagnostic Approach.................................... 61
Debashree Devi, National Institute of Technology Silchar, India
Saroj K. Biswas, National Institute of Technology Silchar, India
Biswajit Purkayastha, National Institute of Technology Silchar, India

Parkinson's disease (PD) is a neurodegenerative disorder that occurs due to corrosion of the substantia nigra, located in the thalamic region of the human brain, and is responsible for transmission of neural signals throughout the human body by means of a brain chemical, termed as "dopamine." Diagnosis of PD is difficult, as it is often affected by the characteristics of the medical data of the patients, which include presence of various indicators, imbalance cases of patients' data records, similar cases of healthy/ affected persons, etc. Through this chapter, an intelligent diagnostic system is proposed by integrating one-class SVM, extreme learning machine, and data preprocessing technique. The proposed diagnostic model is validated with six existing techniques and four learning models. The experimental results prove the combination of proposed method with ELM learning model to be highly effective in case of early detection of Parkinson's disease, even in presence of underlying data issues.

Chapter 6
Soft Computing-Based Early Detection of Parkinson's Disease Using Non-Invasive Method Based on Speech Analysis 96
Chandrasekar Ravi, National Institute of Technology Puducherry, India

This chapter aims to use the speech signals that are a behavioral bio-marker for Parkinson's disease. The victim's vocabulary is mostly lost, or big gaps are observed when they are talking or the conversation is abruptly stopped. Therefore, speech analysis could help to identify the complications in conversation from the inception of the symptoms of Parkinson's disease in initial phases itself. Speech can be regularly logged in an unobstructed approach and machine learning techniques can be applied and analyzed. Fuzzy logic-based classifier is proposed for learning from the training speech signals and classifying the test speech signals. Brainstorm optimization algorithm is proposed for extracting the fuzzy rules from the speech data, which is used by fuzzy classifier for learning and classification. The performance of the proposed classifier is evaluated using metrics like accuracy, specificity, and sensitivity, and compared with benchmark classifiers like SVM, naïve Bayes, k-means, and decision tree. It is observed that the proposed classifier outperforms the benchmark classifiers.

Chapter 7
Assessment of Gait Disorder in Parkinson's Disease 108
Divya Govindaraju, Anna University, India
Gururaj Nagarajan, Birla Institute of Technology and Science, India
Paramasivam Alagumariappan, B.S. Abdur Rahman Crescent Institute of Science and Technology, India

Neurological disorders are some of the leading chronic disorders that impose a massive burden on low-income and developing countries. The disability resulting from the neurological disorder increases the severity and costs during the primary healthcare and for entire lifetime. Parkinson's disease (PD) is the second most common chronic neurodegenerative disorder which is slowly progressive with decrease in the motor and non-motor function of the nervous system due to cognitive impairment leading to gait abnormality. PD is most common in the age group of 40-65years leading to increase in gait disorders associated with slowing down of the movement, balance instability, rigidness in the muscles, and difficulty in performing everyday tasks. The assessment of gait plays a significant role in maintaining the balance disorders in Parkinson's disease. In patients with PD, the neurons present in substantia nigra region of the brain get injured, and they progressively decline during their lifetime. Therefore, the patients lose their ability to perform movement and also lose their stability. The symptoms of PD can be monitored and controlled by assessing gait parameters based on gait disorder.

Chapter 8
Tremor Identification Using Machine Learning in Parkinson's Disease 128
Angana Saikia, North-Eastern Hill University Shillong, India
Vinayak Majhi, North-Eastern Hill University Shillong, India
Masaraf Hussain, North-Eastern Indira Gandhi Regional Institute of Health and Medical Sciences, India
Sudip Paul, North-Eastern Hill University Shillong, India
Amitava Datta, The University of Western Australia, Australia

Tremor is an involuntary quivering movement or shake. Characteristically occurring at rest, the classic slow, rhythmic tremor of Parkinson's disease (PD) typically starts in one hand, foot, or leg and can eventually affect both sides of the body. The resting tremor of PD can also occur in the jaw, chin, mouth, or tongue. Loss of dopamine leads to the symptoms of Parkinson's disease and may include a tremor. For some people, a tremor might be the first symptom of PD. Various studies have proposed measurable technologies and the analysis of the characteristics of Parkinsonian tremors using different techniques. Various machine-learning algorithms such as a support vector machine (SVM) with three kernels, a discriminant analysis, a random forest, and a kNN algorithm are also used to classify and identify various kinds of tremors. This chapter focuses on an in-depth review on identification and classification of various Parkinsonian tremors using machine learning algorithms.

Chapter 9
Epileptic Seizure Detection and Classification Using Machine Learning 152
Rekh Ram Janghel, National Institute of Technology Raipur, India
Yogesh Kumar Rathore, National Institute of Technology Raipur, India
Gautam Tatiparti, National Institute of Technology Raipur, India

Epilepsy is a brain ailment identified by unpredictable interruptions of normal brain activity. Around 1% of mankind experience epileptic seizures. Around 10% of the United States population experiences at least a single seizure in their life. Epilepsy is distinguished by the tendency of the brain to generate unexpected bursts of unusual electrical activity that disrupts the normal functioning of the brain. As seizures usually occur rarely and are unforeseeable, seizure recognition systems are recommended for seizure detection during long-term electroencephalography (EEG). In this chapter, ANN models, namely, BPA, RNN, CL, PNN, and LVQ, have been implemented. A prominent dataset was employed to assess the proposed method. The proposed method is capable of achieving an accuracy of 97.5%; the high accuracy obtained has confirmed the great success of the method.

Chapter 10
Neurocognitive Mechanisms for Detecting Early Phase of Depressive Disorder: Analysis of Event-Related Potentials in Human Brain 165
Shashikanta Tarai, National Institute of Technology Raipur, India

This chapter discusses neurocognitive mechanisms in terms of latency and amplitudes of EEG signals in depression that are presented in the form of event-related potentials (ERPs). Reviewing the available literature on depression, this chapter classifies early P100, ERN, N100, N170, P200, N200, and late P300 ERP components in frontal, mid-frontal, temporal, and parietal lobes. Using auditory oddball paradigm, most of the studies testing depressive patients have found robust P300 amplitude reduction. Proposing EEG methods and summarizing behavioral, neuroanatomical, and electrophysiological findings, this chapter discusses how the different tasks, paradigms, and stimuli contribute to the cohesiveness of neural signatures and psychobiological markers for identifying the patients with depression. Existing research gaps are directed to conduct ERP studies following go/no-go, flanker interference, and Stroop tasks on global and local attentional stimuli associated with happy and sad emotions to examine anterior cingulate cortex (ACC) dysfunction in depression.

Chapter 11
Social Media Analytics to Predict Depression Level in the Users.. 199
Mohammad Shahid Husain, Ibri College of Applied Sciences, Oman

As people around the world are spending increasing amounts of time online, the question of how online experiences are linked to health and wellbeing is essential. Depression has become a public health concern around the world. Traditional methods for detecting depression rely on self-report techniques, which suffer from inefficient data collection and processing. Research shows that symptoms linked to mental illness are detectable on social media like Twitter, Facebook, and web forums, and automatic methods are more and more able to locate inactivity and other mental disease. The pattern of social media usage can be very helpful to predict the mental state of a user. This chapter also presents how activities on Facebook are associated with the depressive states of users. Based on online logs, we can predict the mental state of users.

Chapter 12
Linguistic Markers in Individuals With Symptoms of Depression in Bi-Multilingual Context......... 216
Anbu Savekar, National Institute of Technology Raipur, India
Shashikanta Tarai, National Institute of Technology Raipur, India
Moksha Singh, National Institute of Technology Raipur, India

Depression has been identified as the most prevalent mental disorder worldwide. Due to the stigma of mental illness, the population remains unidentified, undiagnosed, and untreated. Various studies have been carried out to detect and track depression following symptoms of dichotomous thinking, absolutist thinking, linguistic markers, and linguistic behavior. However, there is little study focused on the linguistic behavior of bilingual and multilingual with anxiety and depression. This chapter aims to identify the bi-multilingual linguistic markers by analyzing the recorded verbal content of depressive discourse resulting from life situations and stressors causing anxiety, depression, and suicidal ideation. Different contextual domains of word usage, content words, function words (pronouns), and negative valance words have been identified as indicators of psychological process affecting cognitive behavior, emotional health, and mental illness. These findings are discussed within the framework of Beck's model of depression to support the linguistic connection to mental illness-depression.

Chapter 13
Motor Imagery Classification Using EEG Signals for Brain-Computer Interface Applications........ 241
Subrota Mazumdar, Kalinga Institute of Industrial Technology University, India
Rohit Chaudhary, Kalinga Institute of Industrial Technology University, India
Suruchi Suruchi, Kalinga Institute of Industrial Technology University, India
Suman Mohanty, Kalinga Institute of Industrial Technology University, India
Divya Kumari, Kalinga Institute of Industrial Technology University, India
Aleena Swetapadma, Kalinga Institute of Industrial Technology University, India

In this chapter, a nearest neighbor (k-NN)-based method for efficient classification of motor imagery using EEG for brain-computer interfacing (BCI) applications has been proposed. Electroencephalogram (EEG) signals are obtained from multiple channels from brain. These EEG signals are taken as input features and given to the k-NN-based classifier to classify motor imagery. More specifically, the chapter gives an outline of the Berlin brain-computer interface that can be operated with minimal subject change. All the design and simulation works are carried out with MATLAB software. k-NN-based classifier is trained with data from continuous signals of EEG channels. After the network is trained, it is tested with various test cases. Performance of the network is checked in terms of percentage accuracy, which is found to be 99.25%. The result suggested that the proposed method is accurate for BCI applications.

Chapter 14
Intelligent Big Data Analytics in Health 252
Ebru Aydindag Bayrak, Istanbul University – Cerrahpaşa, Turkey
Pinar Kirci, Istanbul University – Cerrahpaşa, Turkey

Intelligent big data analytics and machine learning systems have been introduced to explain for the early diagnosis of neurological disorders. A number of scholarly researches about intelligent big data analytics in healthcare and machine learning system used in the healthcare system have been mentioned. The authors have explained the definition of big data, big data samples, and big data analytics. But the main goal is helping researchers or specialists in providing opinion about diagnosing or predicting neurological disorders using intelligent big data analytics and machine learning. Therefore, they focused on the healthcare systems using these innovative ways in particular. The information of platform and tools about big data analytics in healthcare is investigated. Numerous academic studies based on the detection of neurological disorders using both machine learning methods and big data analytics have been reviewed.

Chapter 15
Medical Image Segmentation: An Advanced Approach.. 292
Ramgopal Kashyap, Amity University Chhattisgarh, India
Surendra Rahamatkar, Amity University Chhattisgarh, India

Today, IoT in therapeutic administrations has ended up being more productive in light of the fact that the correspondence among authorities and patients has been improved with versatile applications. These applications are made by the associations with the objective that the pros can screen the patient's prosperity. If any issue has hopped out at the patient, by then the authority approaches the patient and gives the correct treatment. In this proposition, particular focus is given to infant human administrations, in light of the fact that the greatest fear of gatekeepers is that they would lose their infant kids at whatever point. Therefore, in this part, a business contraption has been recognized which screens the consistent information about the infant's heart rate, oxygen levels, resting position. In case anything happens to the tyke, the information will get to the adaptable application, which has been made by an association and is mechanically available by finishing a representation field test for the kid; the information is recorded and examined.

Compilation of References 322

About the Contributors 369

Index... 375

Preface

This book basically focuses on the early detection of various neurological disorders using machine learning techniques. Computer Aided Diagnosis is a rapidly growing dynamic area of research in medical industry. The recent researchers in machine learning promise the improved accuracy of perception and diagnosis of disease. Here the computers are enabled to think by developing intelligence by learning. Machine learning is one element of Artificial Intelligence, whereby a computer is programmed with the ability to self-teach and improve its performance of a specific task. In essence, machine learning is all about analyzing big data, the automatic extraction of information and using it to make predictions, decipher whether the prediction was correct, and if incorrect, learning from that to make a more correct prediction in the future. There are many types of Machine Learning Techniques that are used to classify the data sets. They are Supervised, Unsupervised Semi-Supervised, Reinforcement, Evolutionary learning, and Deep learning algorithms. The chapters included mostly are on various brain disorders like Parkinson's disease, Epilepsy, and Tremor etc. Various diagnostic techniques have been described for the early detection of neurological disorders. Some of the topics included in this book are artificial intelligence, data analysis, and biomedical informatics.

Machine learning is bringing a paradigm shift to healthcare, by increasing availability of healthcare data and rapid progress of analytics techniques. Hence, the disease diagnosis using various machine learning techniques will be a effective tool for fast and early diagnosis of the diseases. As a result of which the disease progression can be reduced. Machine learning algorithms provide enhanced accuracy on detection of various diseases. Machine learning is far less sinister, and it's actually not something of the far-off future. It's here today, and it's shaping and simplifying the way we live, work, travel and communicate. Recently Machine learning techniques have made vast developments across healthcare sectors. We believe that human physicians will not be replaced by machines in the foreseeable future, but machine learning can definitely assist physicians to make better clinical decisions or even replace human judgments in certain functional areas of healthcare. The increasing availability of healthcare data and rapid development of analytic methods has made possible the recent successful applications of machine learning in healthcare. Machine learning offers a principled approach for developing sophisticated, automatic, and objective algorithms for analysis of high-dimensional and multimodal biomedical data. Machine learning can use sophisticated algorithms to 'learn' features from a large volume of healthcare data, and then use the obtained insights to assist clinical practice. It can also be equipped with learning and self-correcting abilities to improve its accuracy based on feedback. A machine learning system can assist physicians by providing up-to-date medical information from journals, textbooks and clinical practices to inform proper patient care. In addition, it can help to reduce diagnostic and therapeutic errors that are inevitable in the human clinical practice. It extracts useful information from a large patient population to assist making real-time inferences for health risk alert and health outcome prediction. Hence we can say that, Machine learning would be most effective tool in today's world for early detection of the diseases. Computers can now analyze data much better than people, only due to Machine Learning. It can be used to identify the patterns and trends in amongst lots of data. This book is designed mainly for clinicians, doctors, neurologists, physiotherapists, neuro-rehabilitation specialists, scholars, academics, and students interested in topics centered on biomedical engineering, bio-electronics, medical electronics, physiology, neurosciences, life sciences, and physics. A person living in a place that is far away from a hospital or do not have sufficient money to cover up the hospital bill or do not have enough time to take off work. In such cases, the disease diagnosis through sophisticated machines would be lifesaving. Scientists had developed numerous artificially intelligent diagnosis algorithms for detecting various diseases like Rheumatoid Arthritis, Cancer, Lung Diseases, Heart Diseases, Diabetic Retinopathy, Hepatitis Disease, Alzheimer's disease, Liver Disease, Dengue Disease and Parkinson Disease. Machine learning technique allows the computers to self-learn on their own without the need for human programming. The implications of machine learning on industries, professions and the workforce are considered miraculous by some and catastrophic by others. Machine learning has the potential to automate a large portion of skilled labor, but the degree to which this affects a workforce depends on the level of difficulty involved in the job. Machine learning at present allows the automation of singular tasks, whereas many jobs involve multiple tasks and even multitasking at level machine learning isn't capable of yet.

There are near about more than 380 neurological disorders are identified with their unique characteristics based on their symptoms. Each disease related to nervous systems can be treated as a neurological disorder. As each of them have many common or different symptoms, which is very difficult to identify without proper guided diagnosis. Here is the significance of our book. In our book we try to identify different types of neurological disorder by using machine learning. Through this book we are trying to demonstrate different types of machine learning technique that are used or can be used in future for the diagnosis of different neurological disorders.

In this book we mainly focus on the different diagnostic technique where machine learning can be applied or being applied like Image processing, Image Segmentations, EEG signal analysis, Gait analysis, and also speech analysis. Each method has its unique potential to identify different symptoms with their features. Where machine learning technique is applied for feature extraction for specific disease like Parkinson's disease, Brain Tumor, Depression etc. Another approach we implemented in this book is the application of Bigdata analysis for identifying neurological disorders. The impact of social media in our life takes very important role. Billions of people are connected through social network apps and sites where each and every one shares their emotions and activity of daily life. This social media is the mirror image of a person's life. This social media analysis can predict the characteristic of each person's which is proved as a good material for the diagnosis of any disease. In our book we contribute a chapter where social network data based depression analysis is being discussed. Biometric analysis is a field generally used in security application through face recognition, fingerprint, or retina-based identification. The advancement of the biometric sensor can also detect different facial expression and emotion, which can be used for identification of depression and other neurological symptoms. Analysis of facial expression through machine learning technique is one of the new dimensions for identifying neurological disorder.

The 1st chapter of this book cover this novel technique which manly focus for finding different types of neurological disorder. In 2nd and 3rd chapter we discussed a different neurological disorder associated with the brain and also the rehabilitation technique for overcome such disorder with applying technological advancement by applying the input as neurological feedback technique. In 4th and 15th chapter we discussed about the different image processing technique which is very helpful for identification of different neurological disorder through MRI, CT scan, PET scan etc. To identify the cause of neurological disorder the general diagnosis method is image-based analysis. Both these chapters contain the segmentation technique of image in which the 4th chapter specifically describes about the image segmentation technique of MRI sequence for identification of brain tumor. Parkinson's disease is one of the neurodegenerative diseases next to the Alzheimer disease millions of people suffer in Parkinson's disease throughout the world. As we know PD cannot be cured fully so the early detection of PD is very much essential for preventive purpose. In this book we contribute few chapters based on identification of the Parkinson's disease in early stages. The 5th chapter describes the different technique of identifying PD in early stages. Parkinson disease can be identified through speech analysis also in 6th chapter we describe the soft computing-based speech analysis method for early detection of Parkinson's disease. Posture and Gait disorder is also an important identification marker in Parkinson's disease. The 7th chapter also describes the gait disorder and its identification technique for the identification of Parkinson's disease. Tremor is one of the common symptoms of Parkinson's disease, in 8th chapter we try to describe the tremor identification using machine learning for the detection of Parkinson's disease. Epileptic Seizure identification and classification using machine learning is a practical approach now a day. The electrical activity of the brain can be identified using EEG technique. The EEG classification using machine learning also proved to be helpful for the identification of neurological disorder. In 13th chapter machine learning for EEG classification for brain computer interfacing is describe where reader can get a detail overview of the brain computing technique using EEG signal. Whereas in 9th chapter the Epileptic Seizure classification is described where the reader will get a brief knowledge about the electrical activity of the brain and in the disturbance of this electrical activity how Epileptic Seizure symptoms can be highlighted gradually. In 10th, 11th and 12th chapter we focused about the most common neuropsychiatric disorder Depression. In this chapters we focused on early symptoms of depression and its identification method through event related potential method, also through the analysis of social network activity analysis and finally through speech analysis. In these three different approaches we discussed about how we can identify depression in the early stage with the hierarchy of depression level. In 14th chapter we describe the big data analysis method for identification of neurological disorder and how intelligent system can be used for processing of Big data in the field of medical diagnosis.

Overall the audience of this book will have a great and big review of the machine learning system and its application in the field of medical science and how the possible different technique can be applied for identification of neurological disorder.

Chapter 1
Mapping the Intellectual Structure of the Field Neurological Disorders:
A Bibliometric Analysis

S. Ravikumar
North-Eastern Hill University Shillong, India

ABSTRACT

The chapter utilizes bibliometric tools to explore papers in the field of neurological disorders and to examine the scientific development in the above subject domain. The research data were retrieved from the WOS database, which consists of 16,830 papers on the above phrase, but for the current study was limited to only those articles that have received more than four citations. Using this criterion, the data was narrowed to 10,694 as of 25/6/18. Using bibliometric tools, the author has identified the most productive authors, most productive countries, annual scientific production with an average growth rate of 4.82, and average article citations per year was 44.85. Network analysis was carried out to find co-citation network pattern, and with co-word analysis, found the conceptual structure of a field of neurological disorders.

INTRODUCTION

Neurological clutters are infections of the mind, spine and the nerves that interface them. There are in excess of 600 maladies of the sensory system, for example, cerebrum tumours, epilepsy, Parkinson's sickness and stroke and in addition less natural ones, for example, front temporal dementia. The investigation of nervous system science and neurosurgery goes back to ancient occasions; however the scholarly trains did not start until the sixteenth century. From an observational science they built up an efficient method for moving toward the sensory system and conceivable mediations in neurological infection. John Fothergill (1712–1780), James Parkinson (1755–1824) and on three writers of early nineteenth-century British neurological texts, namely John Cooke (1756–1838), Charles Bell (1774–1841) and Marshall Hall (1790–1857), are considered prolific contributions to the history of the neurosciences (Clifford. F,

DOI: 10.4018/978-1-5225-8567-1.ch001

1999). The ebb and flow study will distinguish the breakthrough in the improvement of the subject area of "neurological disorder" over the timeframe and connected scientometric strategies into logical writing of this field and we have endeavoured to think about the development of subject over the timeframe and who are the most productive writers in this field and to examine the commitment by different writers and nations to this exploration front.

BIBLIOMETRICS AND ITS UTILIZATION

Bibliometrics is stressed over the examination of research subject to citation counts and precedents. The individual assessments used are in like manner routinely insinuated as bibliometrics, or citation estimations. They can be used to survey the effect of an individual research yield, for instance, a journal article, or a collection of research yields, for instance, all works by an explicit author, research social occasion or institution.

Bibliometrics can be used as an indication of the hugeness and impact of your work or that of a research social event, office or school, and therefore of its motivating force to the more broad research arrange. Bibliometrics are continuously being used to measure and rank research yield both inside institutions and on a national or worldwide measurement. School rankings may consider and they are utilized in the Research Excellence Framework (REF).Bibliometrics can be used as a gadget to recognize research characteristics and light up decisions about future research interests.

Bibliometrics ponder helps to understand research productivity (Counts of papers) in explicit subject space. Impact of the distribution in a region can be evaluated utilizing Citation checks which help us to consider the Indirect acknowledgment/impact (second-age citation tallies) and papers and journals are positioned utilizing normal citation per paper which has bring forth Journal Impact factor and H-Index . Research fronts, Collaboration markers and Trend examination (Time arrangement) can be considers utilizing bibliometrics

LITERATURE REVIEW

Bibliometrics is an arrangement of numerical and factual strategies used to dissect and measure the amount and nature of books, articles and different types of production. There are three sorts of bibliometric pointers: Quantity markers, which measure the efficiency of a specific research, quality markers which estimate the nature of an exploration's yield, and basic pointers, which measure associations between distributions (Durieux, 2010). Inside the wide zone of neurological science, many subject-particular examinations have been completed; one of the vital research fronts is epilepsy which had pulled in noticeable reference (Ibrahim, 2012). Bibliometric study on the literature output on the area of bipolar disorder and schizophrenia research and its funding pattern was assessed. There is a general deficiency of research exercises on bipolar disorder differentiated and schizophrenia (Clement & Singh, 2003). Recovery was under-spoken to in the neurological writing on incapacitating infections. The finding featured that over the different neurologic conditions, the heaviness of Rehab writing was extremely negligible. The outcomes recommend that nervous system science is as yet hesitant to confront the incapacity challenges (Tesio & Gamba, 1995). The examination enthusiasm for uncommon neurological conditions is excessively bigger than that in like manner conditions. Our outcomes bolster an adjustment in the focal point of therapeutic research towards the most well-known conditions that are in charge of the best incapacity, demise, financial hardship, and loss of personal satisfaction. It is perceived that subsidizing for examination into an illness ought to be relative to that ailment's weight on society; in any case, conditions that represent 90% of the worldwide weight of ailment get short of what one-tenth of the world's wellbeing spending plan (Al-Shahi & Will, 2001).

Publishers these days confront the issues of choosing which of the numerous papers they get are of higher quality for distribution in their journals (Hanks, Blinderman, & Cherny, 2005). Article evaluation utilized in companion survey process (Horrobin, 2001). A few quantitative measurements related with logical generation, one such measurement is citation tally. Predictive models can help to conjecture the citation include of paper published a branch of knowledge (Brody, Harnad, & Carr, 2006).

From the writing audit, it's clear that bibliometric thinks about on nervous system science have been taken in different pockets none of the investigations have broken down aggregate distribution in the zone of neurological disorder. The current examination attempts to overcome any issues by the perception the aggregate writing yield which is ordered in the Web of Science database.

METHODOLOGY

The focal point of the examination is constrained to the subject "Neurological disorders". The wellspring of the information exhibited in this investigation is from Web of Science. A hunt was performed on Web of Science Core Collection utilizing the key work "Neurological disorders" inside section/beds. WoS has filed the reports beginning from 1989 to till date. From the above inquiry 16,830 reports on "Neurological disorders" were recovered. The recovered outcome was additionally refined utilizing the most cited paper concept (MCP) (Tas, 2014). Among them, 6,136 (36%) distributions were distinguished that met the previously mentioned criteria; referred to equivalent or in excess of multiple times (Tas, 2014). Bibliometrix programming was utilized to perform different bibliometric examinations (Aria & Cuccurullo, 2016).

DATA ANALYSIS

Unmistakable measurements of the informational collection comprise of 10753 records among with 10634 are articles, 77 from books and monograph, and 42 articles from procedures. These above papers were written by 44623 writers. Out of those 450 reports are of the single-composed article and 44173 are of multi-wrote records. Normal reports per creator are 0.241, creator per article 4.15 and co-creators per record is 5.71 the coordinated effort list is 4.4.

The yearly development of writing was in a positive heading, toward the finish of the period declining pattern is seen, which was a direct result of reference; as our example depended on the most referred to paper. Subsequently the pattern is negative amid the end organize. The yearly level of development rate is 4.82.The most productive year were 2013,2014 and 2015 with a publication count 857, 818 and 804 respectively.

When it comes to author specific analysis Li Y was the most beneficial creator with 46 productions in his record pursued by Zhang Y with 44 distribution and Wang J with 39 distributions.

Figure 1. Annual scientific production

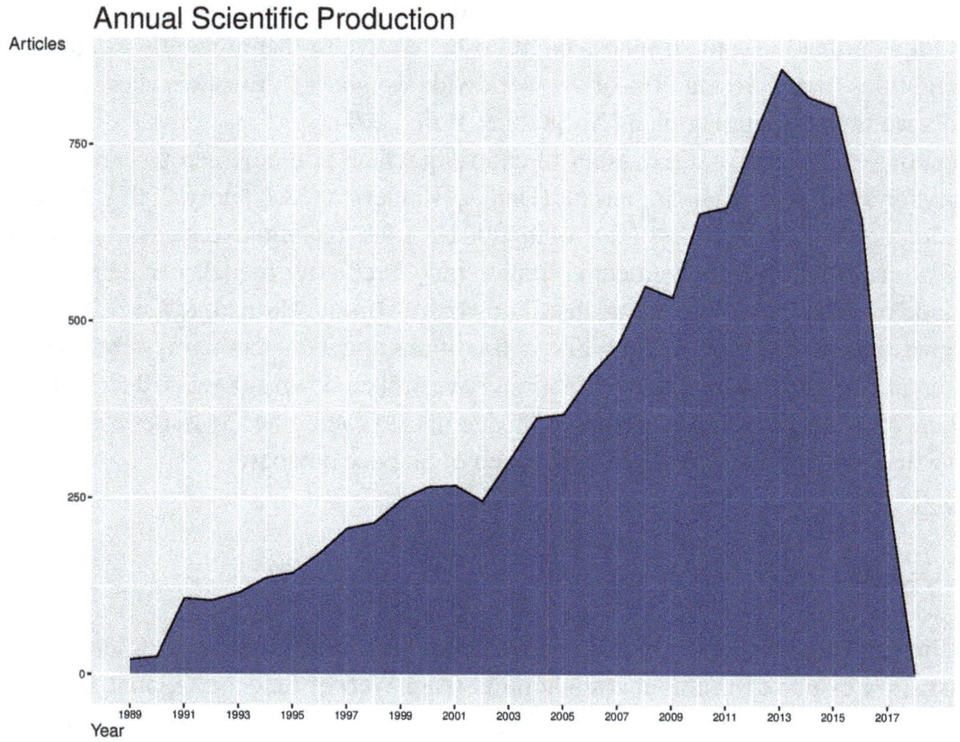

With the end goal to standardize for contrasts in citation conduct among fields, citations can be partially checked proportionately to the length of the reference records in the referring to papers. Mattson MP, finished the table with the fractionalized score of 16.87 pursued by Louis Ed with 10.4 and Farooqui AA with 9.87.

Most referred to paper/creator was Roman GC, 1993 had gotten a sum of 3387 citations with a normal 135.5 citation for each year, alongside him was Goldberger AL, 2000 was referred to multiple times and third creator as Klimesch W, 1999 has pulled in 2637 affirmation, however, Vos T, 2015 has increased more unmistakable quality in a brief timeframe with 1323 citation with a normal rate of 441 every year.

Most Productive Authors

See Table 1 and Figure 2.

Most Cited Authors

See Table 2 and Figure 3.

Most Productive Countries

See Table 3.

Table 1. Top ten productive authors

S.No	Author	Articles	Authors	Articles Fractionalized
1	LI Y	46	MATTSON MP	16.87
2	ZHANG Y	44	LOUIS ED	10.4
3	WANG J	39	FAROOQUI AA	9.87
4	WANG X	39	LIU X	7.38
5	WANG Y	38	LI Y	7.05
6	LOUIS ED	36	DALAKAS MC	6.88
7	LIU X	34	ZHANG Y	6.81
8	MATTSON MP	34	HORROCKS LA	6.3
9	BORLONGAN CV	32	KUMAR A	6.23
10	LI X	31	JANKOVIC J	6.08

Figure 2. Most productive author

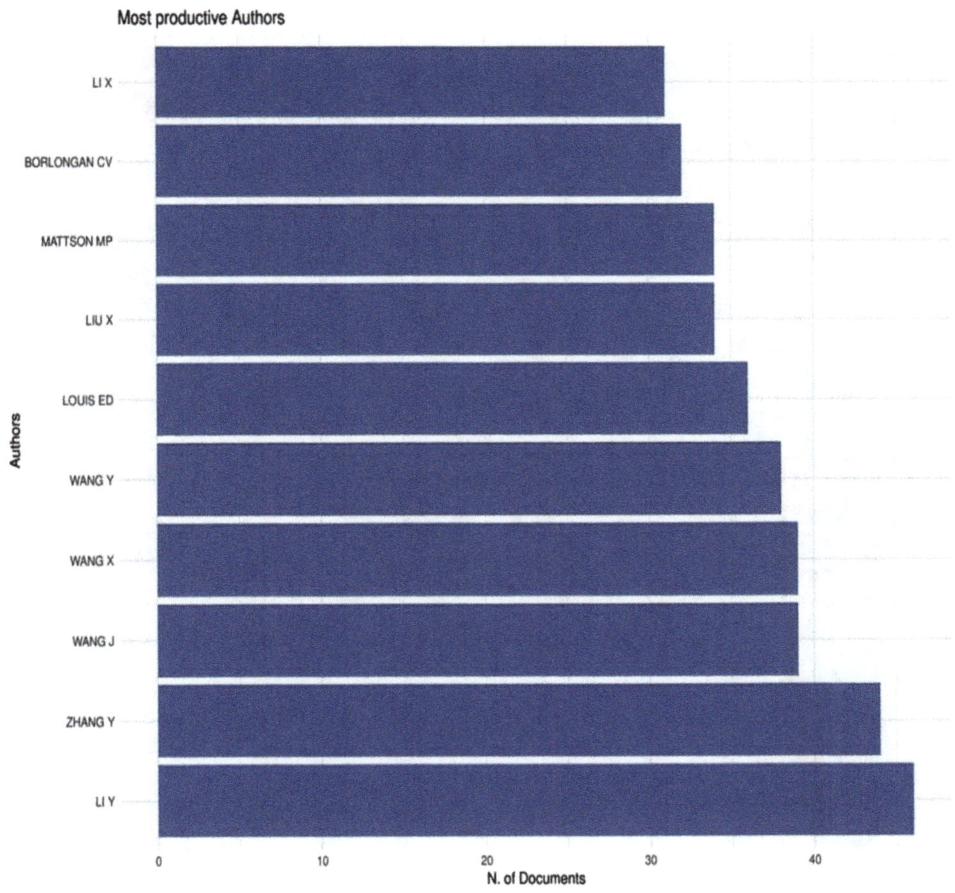

Table 2. Most cited authors

S.No	Name of Author and Source	Tc	Tc per Year
1	ROMAN GC, 1993, NEUROLOGY	3387	135.5
2	GOLDBERGER AL, 2000, CIRCULATION	3366	187
3	KLIMESCH W, 1999, BRAIN RES REV	2637	138.8
4	BEAULIEU C, 2002, NMR BIOMED	2373	148.3
5	HORWITZ J, 1992, PROC NATL ACAD SCI U S A	1496	57.5
6	BARD F, 2000, NAT MED	1474	81.9
7	LITVAN I, 1996, NEUROLOGY	1451	66
8	KRIAUCIONIS S, 2009, SCIENCE	1396	155.1
9	STENMARK H, 2009, NAT REV MOL CELL BIOL	1350	150
10	VOS T, 2015, LANCET	1323	441

Figure 3. Most productive countries and their collaboration pattern

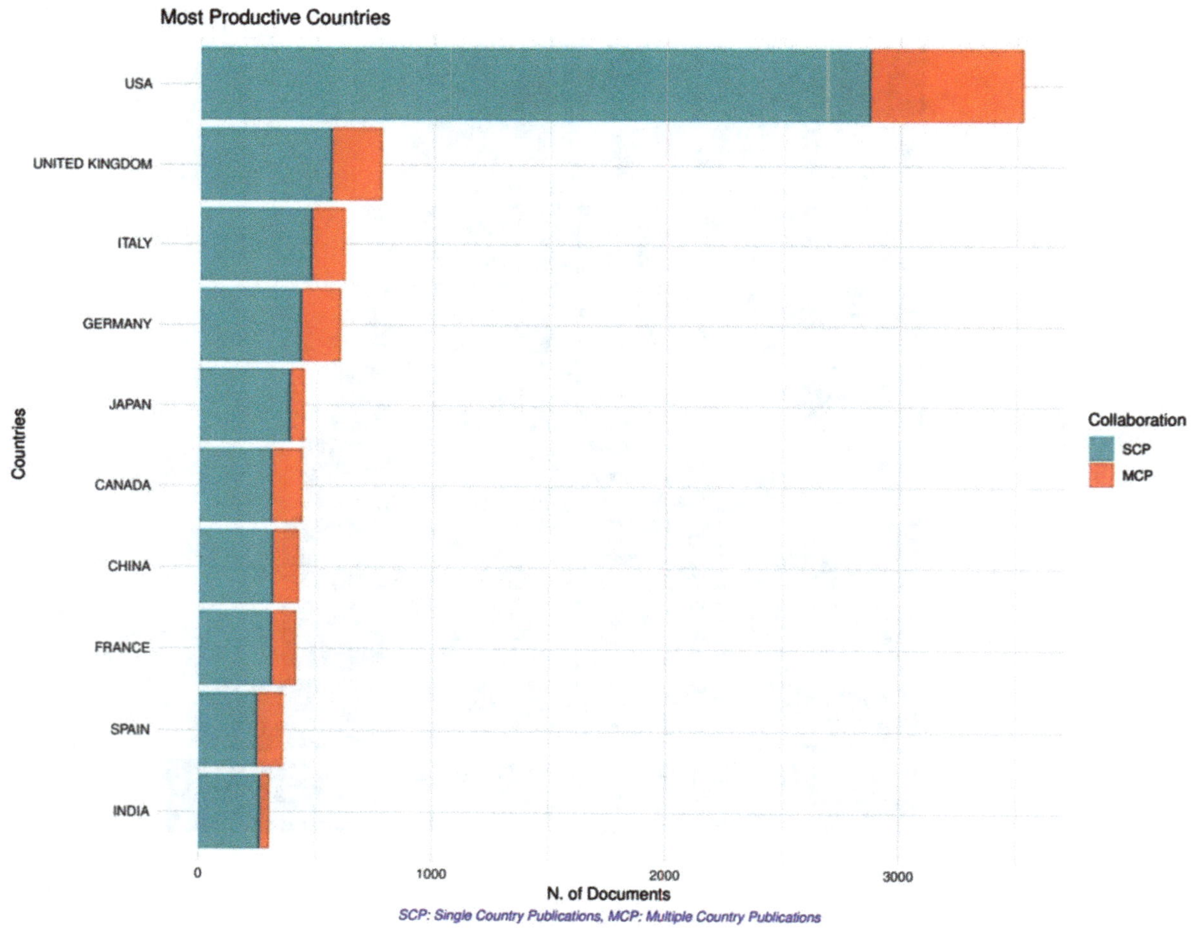

Table 3. Top ten countries productivity, citation

S.No	Country	Articles	Freq	SCP	MCP	MCP_ratio
1	UAS	3525	0.332	2868	657	0.186
2	UK	774	0.0729	560	214	0.276
3	ITALY	617	0.0581	475	142	0.23
4	GERMANY	600	0.0565	432	168	0.28
5	JAPAN	446	0.042	386	60	0.135
6	CANADA	438	0.0412	309	129	0.295
7	CHINA	424	0.0399	314	110	0.247
8	FRANCE	413	0.0389	311	102	0.247
9	SPAIN	359	0.0338	248	111	0.309
10	INDIA	301	0.0283	261	40	0.133

Top Cited Countries

See Table 4.

Most Relevant Sources

See Table 5.

Analysis Based on Country and Type of Source

As indicated by the Clarivate Analytic report, 2017 greater part of the world exceptionally referred to inquire about is from the USA. From the present examination informational index, it was discovered that USA finished the table with 3525 research paper with 2868 papers with single nation distribution

Table 4. Top ten countries based on citation

S.No	Country	Total Citation	Average Article Citation
1	UAS	202835	57.54
2	UK	40118	51.83
3	GERMANY	28525	47.54
4	ITALY	25927	42.02
5	CANADA	23168	52.89
6	JAPAN	15428	34.59
7	FRANCE	15279	37
8	SPAIN	11361	31.65
9	ISRAEL	9240	77
10	NETHERLANDS	8404	43.1

Table 5. Top ten favourite publication source

S.No	Sources	Articles
1	PLOS ONE	210
2	JOURNAL OF NEUROSCIENCE	139
3	STROKE	126
4	JOURNAL OF NEUROCHEMISTRY	114
5	JOURNAL OF THE NEUROLOGICAL SCIENCES	112
6	BRAIN RESEARCH	96
7	NEUROSCIENCE	94
8	PROCEEDINGS OF THE NATIONAL ACADEMY OF SCIENCES OF THE UNITED STATES OF AMERICA	88
9	JOURNAL OF BIOLOGICAL CHEMISTRY	82
10	BRAIN	74

and 657 articles with the multi-nation distribution, second in the line was the UK with 774 reports and pursued by Italy with 617 paper among the best ten gainful nations.

UAS has gotten a sum of 202835 citations with normal article citation with 57.54 rates, second in the table was the UK with 40118 and the third country was Germany with 28525. The citation contrasts between the USA and different countries were extremely huge.

Production source assumes an essential job in conveying the data to its perusers. From information in it was discovered that greater part of the writers working in the territory of “Neurological Disorder” will, in general, distribute their examination result in the journal titled “PLOS ONE” with 210 articles, trailed by “Journal of Neuroscience” with 139 compositions, third in line was “Stroke” with 126 articles. The above table gives us a reasonable image of the most conspicuous source in the region of “Neurosciences”.

Analysis of Keyword Co-Occurrences

Keyword co-occurrence network empowers the per users to envision different subspace which has risen over the timeframe. Four bunches have risen up out of the best 50 keywords dependent on their co-occurrence. The principal bunch had 20 keywords with Alzheimer ailment, Central Nervous system, and Parkinson maladies a noteworthy on-screen character in that group. The second group has 13 factors; the significant performing artists were Brain, articulation, and Protein. The third bunch was a gathering with 9 sub-domains and in that group pretty much every one of the hubs was having measure up to weight in the network. The fourth bunch was gathered with 8 keywords with three unmistakable players like neurological disorder, multiple sclerosis, and disorders. The aggregate size of the network was 28247 with the normal thickness of 0.001 and with a transitivity of 0.061, the average eigenvector centrality was at 0.985 and the normal way length between the hubs was 2.88.

The best three vertices dependent on the degree of centrality was Alzheimer diseases (0.1859) Central sensory system (0.1545) and Parkinson malady (0.1370) and the Hub score f the above best three were 1.000, 0.883 and 0.836 separately.

Figure 4. Keyword co-occurrence

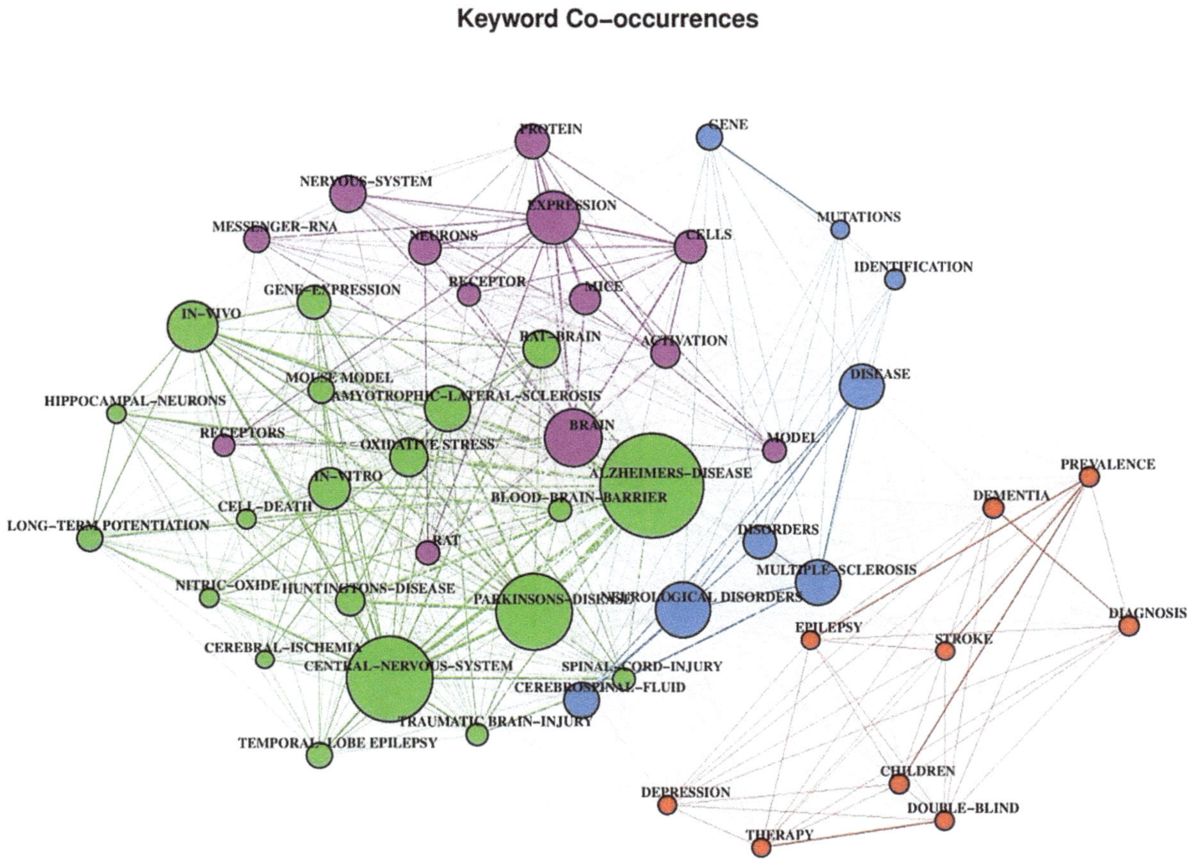

Analysis of Co-Citation Network

Co-citation is a report coupling concept which depends on the recurrence with which two archives are referred to together. The groups of co-referred to papers give another approach to contemplate the claim to fame structure of science.

From our informational collection, we acquired a network chart with 10589 hubs with less thickness estimation of 0.003 between the hubs and with a transitivity of 0.076. Eigenvector centrality of the diagram is 0.975 and the normal way length is 2.55. According to the general positioning, the main three vertices are Neuroscience, Neuro-Chicago, and Neuro Report. Betweenness centrality of best three vertices is 0.1398, 0.1048 and 0.0580.

In this network diagram of the best 30 sources, we got two conspicuous bunches with Neurosciences as the significant performer in group 1 and Neuropharmacology as a noteworthy player in the second bunch.

Analysis of Historical Citation Network

History of science depends on a scholarly model of the logical procedure. The coordinated chart orchestrated on a level plane in sequential request to speak to papers and bolts to speak to the references

Figure 5. Co-citation network graph

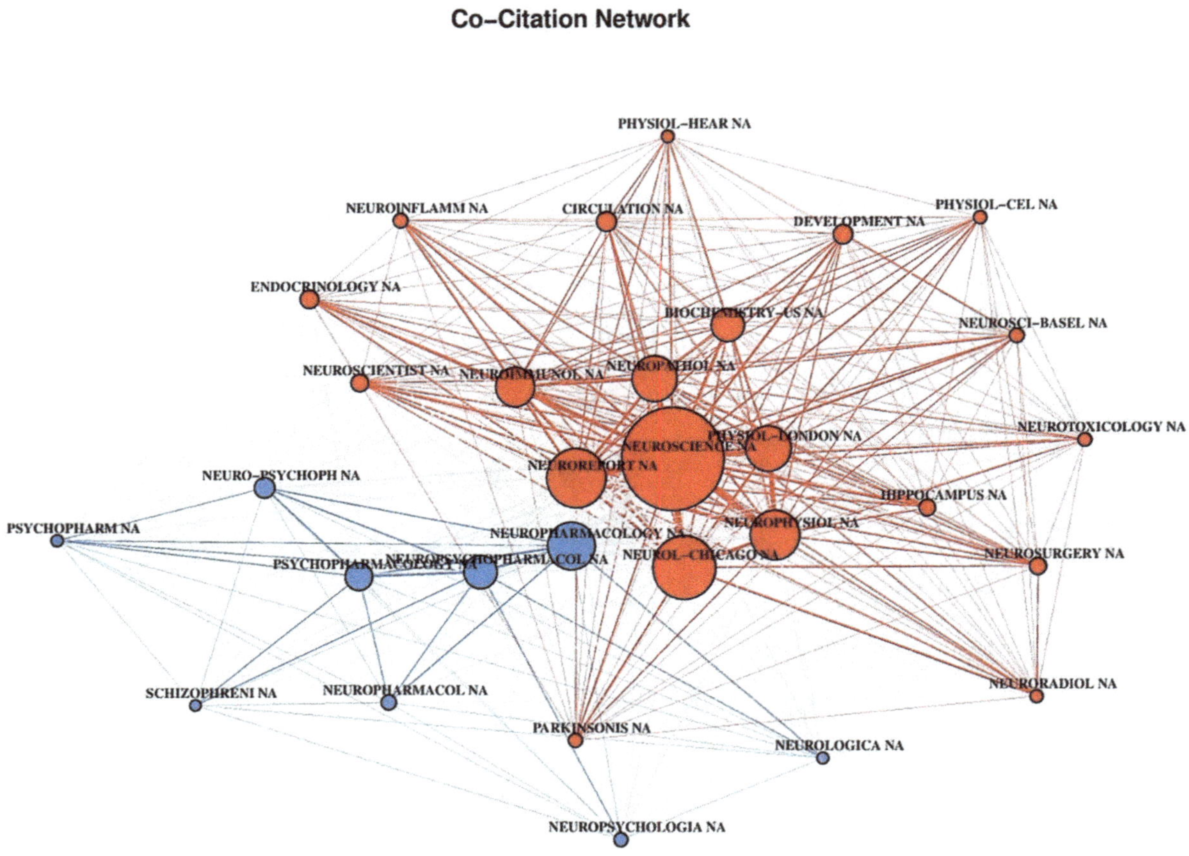

between papers. From the above graph the historical network between Penzes P, 2011 and Farooqui AA 1991 and for legend paper of Hussian MM, 1989. Reference investigation, at that point, is by all accounts a strategy that enormously disentangles the exertion included in building the arrangement of occasions and web of connections that fill in as the beginning stage for the assessments, understandings, and clarifications that are the substance of chronicled investigate.

FINDINGS

From the present investigation is discovered that a decent quantum of research is been done in the subject of neurological science from the informational collection, it was seen a steady increment in distribution in the above research area. The informational index additionally determines that the real offer of production is from a created country and USA finished rundown with more distribution and high citation. From breaking down different research front utilizing catchphrase it was discovered that Alzheimer, Central Nervous system and Parkinson disease has pulled in more research which is reflected from the writing yield. The favoured hotspot for production has been seen as PLOS One. The creator sound chronicled citation organize was seen for the paper distributed by Farooqui AA, 1991.

Figure 6. Historical citation network

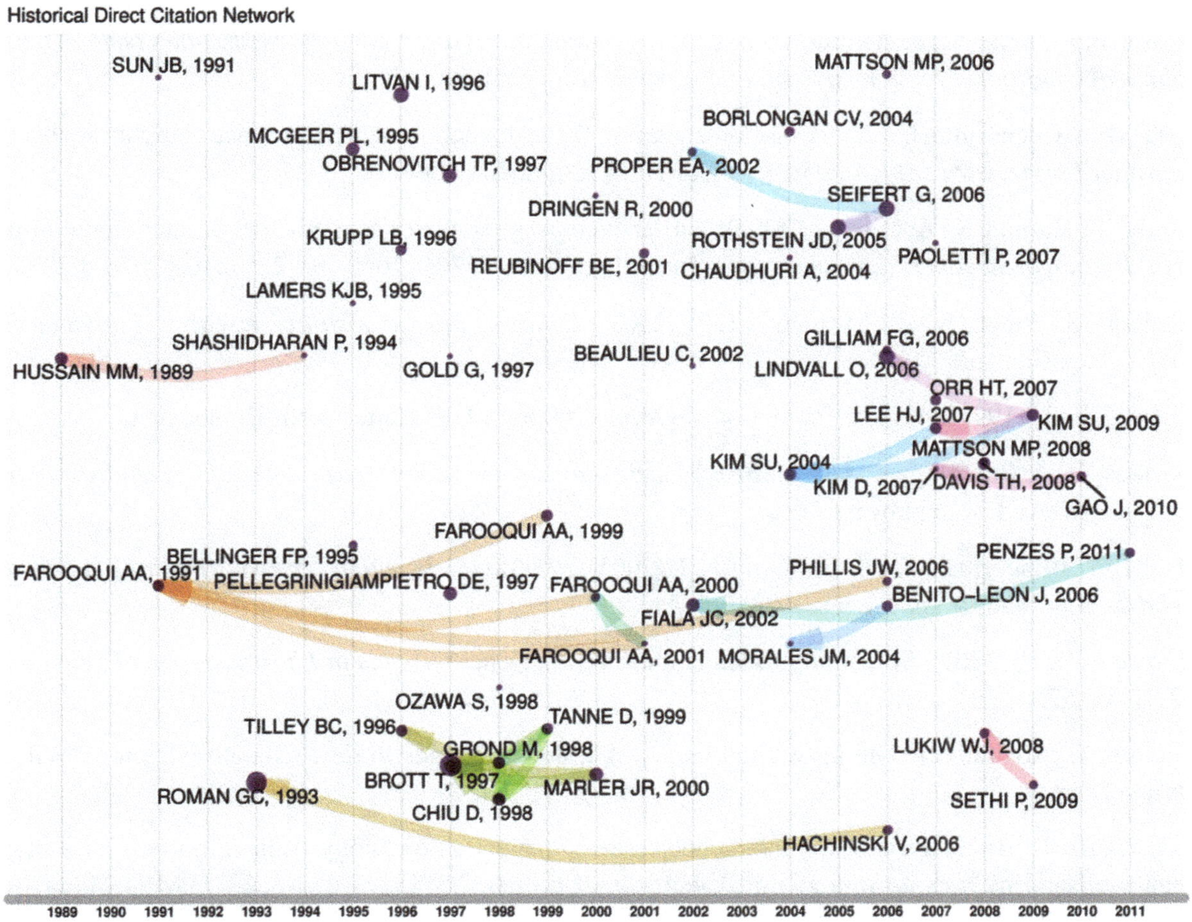

CONCLUSION

The present investigation is a examination of logical writing in the field of the neurological disorder in worldwide shape amid period 1989-2017. The examination has unfurled profitable data on in general research efficiency, the profitability of unmistakable creators, noticeable journals. Discoveries demonstrated an exponential development in research profitability of efficiency from 1989-2017. The most profitable year was from 2013 to 2015. From the informational index, it was seen an unfaltering increment in the original design and diminishing pattern single creator paper. Creators had demonstrated their enthusiasm to distribute in unmistakable journals with spreads the centre subject of neurosciences. Finding additionally hit a considerable increment in the three unmistakable research zones to be specific Alzheimer, Central Nervous system, and Parkinson disease.

REFERENCES

Al-Shahi, R., Will, R., & Journal, C.-B. (2001). *Amount of research interest in rare and common neurological conditions: bibliometric study*. Retrieved from ncbi.nlm.nih.gov

Aria, M., & Cuccurullo, C. (2017). bibliometrix : An R-tool for comprehensive science mapping analysis. *Journal of Informetrics, 11*(4), 959–975. doi:10.1016/j.joi.2017.08.007

Brody, T., Harnad, S., & Carr, L. (2006). Earlier Web usage statistics as predictors of later citation impact. *Journal of the American Society for Information Science, 57*(8), 1060–1072. doi:10.1002/asi.20373

Clement, S., Singh, S., & Psychiatry, T.-T. (2003). *Status of bipolar disorder research: bibliometric study*. Cambridge.org.

Clifford, F. R. (1999). *A Short History of Neurology*. Oxford, UK: Butterworth-Heinemann.

Durieux, V., & Radiology, P. (2010). *Bibliometric indicators: quality measurements of scientific publication*. Retrieved from pubs.rsna.org

Hanks, G., Blinderman, C. D., & Cherny, N. I. (2005). *Peer review in action: The contribution of referees to advancing reliable knowledge*. Academic Press.

Horrobin, D. F. (2001). Something rotten at the core of science? *Trends in Pharmacological Sciences, 22*(2), 51–52.

Ibrahim, G., III. (2012). The most cited works in epilepsy: Trends in the "Citation Classics". Wiley Online Library.

Tas, F. (2014). An analysis of the most-cited research papers on oncology: Which journals have they been published in? *Tumour Biology, 35*(5), 4645–4649. doi:10.100713277-014-1608-7 PMID:24414487

Tesio, L., & Gamba, C. (1995). Rehabilitation: the Cinderella of neurological research? A bibliometric study. Springer.

Chapter 2
Neurofeedback:
Retrain the Brain

Meena Gupta
North-Eastern Hill University Shillong, India

Dinesh Bhatia
North-Eastern Hill University Shillong, India

ABSTRACT

Neurofeedback (NF) is a type of brain wave training based on operant learning. NF has been employed in research and clinical settings for the investigation and treatment of a growing number of psychological illnesses. This technique involves detection of electroencephalographic (EEG) information from the surface of the scalp of a subject by separating its frequency decomposition into its component waveform (alpha, beta, theta, gamma, and delta) and making these components visible usually as polygraphic traces on a computer screen. Neurofeedback is being considered as a promising new method for restoring brain function in a large number of mental disorder cases. NF takes into account behavioral, cognitive, and subjective aspects as well as the brain activity of the concerned individual. About 25 years ago, NF was employed for clinical and research purposes in psychological illness. These psychological illnesses include attention deficit disorder, addiction to drug, depression, stress, and eating disorders.

INTRODUCTION

Neurofeedback (NBF) is a technique of self-regulation in which parameters of electroencephalography (EEG) recorded from subject's present cognitive status represents the subject's brain functioning and any pathological abnormality. NFB is a one of the special application of biofeedback (BFB) for visualizing and training the electrical activity of the human brain. Visualization of EEG helps the brain to learn to better self-regulate brain activity based on operant conditioning. It focuses on optimization of the brain functioning rather than suppressing symptoms which is done in case of medication and drugs (Prinsloo et al., 2017).

DOI: 10.4018/978-1-5225-8567-1.ch002

In other words, NFB is a type of brain wave training, based on operant learning. In this training, our brain determines everything which we feel and do. NFB has been employed in research and clinical settings for the investigation and treatment of a growing number of psychological illnesses. This technique involves detection of EEG information from the surface of the scalp of a subject by employing frequency decomposition technique and separating brain waves into its component waveforms (alpha, beta, theta, gamma, and delta) and making these components visible usually as polygraphic traces on a computer screen. Neurofeedback is being considered as a promising new method for restoring brain function in mental disorders (Escolano, Aguilar, & Minguez, 2011). It takes into account the behavioral, cognitive, and subjective aspects as well as brain activity. For the past 25 years, NF has been employed for clinical and research purpose in psychological illness (Lubar, 1997). These psychological illnesses include attention deficit disorder, addiction to drug, depression, stress and eating disorders. But in recent years NFB studies are gaining much attention to determine human cognitive ability according to several published research studies (Pope & Palsson, 2001). In NFB training many researchers concluded that it revealed its therapeutic effects in the treatment of varieties of neurological and psychological disorders and improves certain cognitive aptitudes. Apart from this NFB training in healthy human users have been reported in many works (Vernon, 2005). NF training principles are based on brain activities, patterns of brain interest and positive or negative stimuli and the stimuli can be any visual or auditory modalities.

LITERATURE REVIEW

In their review article, Grefkes and Fink (2011) suggested that balance within the motor network may be critically disturbed after stroke when the lesion either directly affects any of the brain areas or damages related white matter. A growing body of evidence suggests that abnormal interactions among cortical region remote from the ischemic lesion might also contribute to the motor impairment after stroke. They suggested that pathological intra and inter hemisphere among key motor regions of the brain constitute an important pathophysiological aspect of motor impairment after subcortical stroke. They demonstrated therapeutic interventions such as repetitive transcranial magnetic stimulation, which aims to interfere with abnormal cortical activity that may correct pathological connectivity not only at the stimulation site but also distant brain regions (Grefkes & Fink, 2011).

In their paper, Escolano, Aguilar, and Minguez (2011) have revealed therapeutic effect of Neurofeedback to treat a variety of neurological and psychological disorders and have demonstrated its feasibility to improve certain aptitudes in healthy users. Their aim was to improve working memory performance in healthy users by the enhancement of upper alpha band. In their study EEG assessment in active and passive eyes open state were conducted pre and post neurofeedback training. It showed significance improvement in working memory of the healthy users (Escolano, Aguilar, & Minguez 2011).

In their study, Scharnowski and Weiskopt (2015) used alpha rhythm to conduct brain induced training. It proposed the use of Bluetooth low energy to connect the EEG signals to the smart phone. The result of their experiments indicated that the power of alpha waves demonstrated on the phone had a significant memory increase as a result of the memory of cognition brain training (Scharnowski & Weiskopt, 2015).

In Margaret E. Ayers's (2004) study on cerebral palsy and neurofeedback suggested sensorimotor inhibition can be obtained solely by inhibiting theta activity on the appropriated sensory motor areas utilizing bipolar hookup and analog or all digital real time feedback. Cerebral palsy is considered to be one of the most rewarding neurological challenges in neurofeedback (Ayers, 2004).

Gomez-Pilar and Corralejo (2014) used electroencephalogram (EEG) signal-based brain computer interface systems in order to assist and improve the quality of life of people with disabilities. In this regard they developed Neurofeedback training tool using motor imagery based brain computer interface. This training comprised of imagery motor exercises combined with, memory and logical relation tasks. Results show a significant improvement of three cognitive features after performing the NFT, visual perception, expressive speech and immediate memory. The evidences showed that the performance of a NFT tool based on motor imagery could be a positive activity for slowing down the aging effects (Gomez-Pilar & Corralejo, 2014).

Gonzalez-Ortega, Diaz-Pernas, and Martinez-Zarzuela (2014) used 3D computer vision system for cognitive assessment and rehabilitation. 3D computer vision system easily implemented with a consumer grade computer for left and right-hand tracking and for face and facial feature detection. This 3D system was capable of human limb monitoring and analyzing the psychomotor exercises (Gonzalez-Ortega, Diaz-Pernas, & Martinez-Zarzuela, 2014).

In Lohaugen, Beneventi, and Andersen's (2014) clinical trial study on cerebral palsy patient they implemented computerized working memory training for cognition enhancement. This study shows that training of working memory also induced neurobiological changes such as increased activity in the prefrontal cortex and parietal lobe (Lohaugen, Beneventi, & Andersen, 2014).

NEUROFEEDBACK PROCESS

In neurofeedback process brain signal such as electroencephalography (EEG) are recorded by employing electronics and computers to create a representation of that signal to teach the brain to change. In EEG recording sensors are placed firmly on the scalp of the subject to record the electrical activity of the brain. The process of representation electrical activities is known as feedback and it's generated from the scalp of the brain so called as neurofeedback. In NFB training first EEG is recorded from the subject scale to see the change in EEG after completion of session and EEG is the most used recording which is cheap, portable and cost-effective which need low set up to treat the patients as shown in Figure 1.

SIGNAL PROCESSING

Signal processing is a process from which raw EEG signals are extracted. This signal processing consists of mathematical operations that are implemented either in hardware or in software and its providing suitable measure for extracting EEG data. It is important that signal processing is done in real time. Fourier transformation is the very common transform for signal processing in NF training. In signal processing for NF training mathematical analysis of the EEG is required. In signals processing brain waves frequency measures are given in Table 1.

However, the neurologists and other EEG analysts directly view these waveforms. However, the basic operations yield estimates of important parameters such as the amount of power in a certain frequency band. Signal processing also provides the speed of each EEG signal, the presence or the absence of signals and it also reflexes the quality of connections between brain regions.

Figure 1. Neurofeedback training of cerebral palsy child

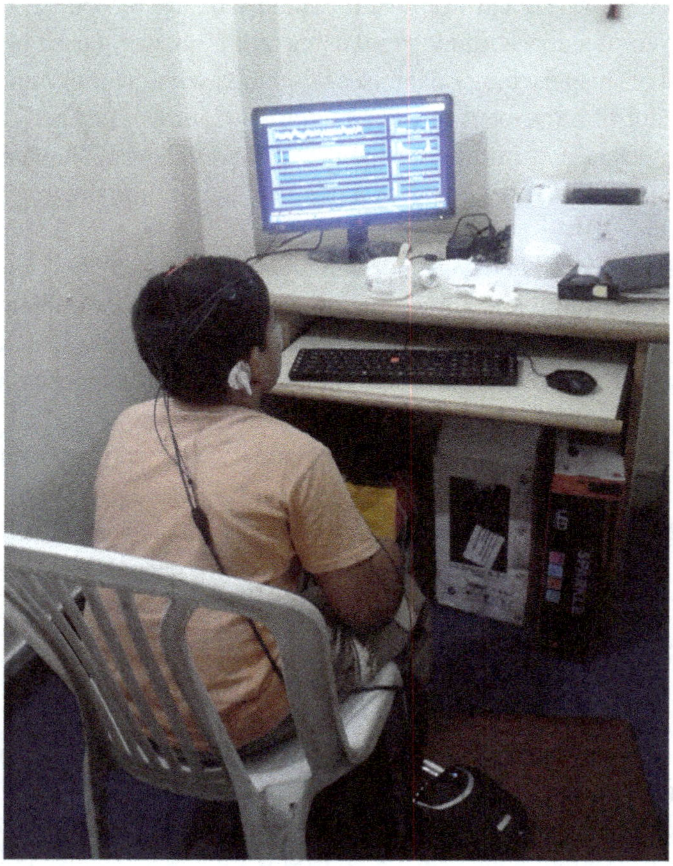

Table 1. Brain waves and their frequencies

Type of Brain Waves	Frequency
Delta	1-3 Hz
Theta	4-7 Hz
Alpha	8-12 Hz
Low Beta	12-15 Hz
Beta	15-20 Hz
High Beta	20-35 Hz
Gamma	35-40 Hz

OPERANT CONDITIONING

Whenever an organism either human or animal provides feedback in the form of reward and consequently learns to perform the desired behavior is known as operant conditioning learning. Operant conditioning is also defined as a type of learning in which strength of the behavior is modified by its consequences such as reward or punishment. The behavior is controlled by an antecedent called as negative reinforcement. There are several learning mechanisms as mentioned in Table 2.

Classical Learning

Classical learning (CL) is also known as Pavlovian or respondent conditioning (Legg, 2018). CL is learning procedure which involves forming an association between two stimuli resulting in a learned response. There are three basic phases of CL process

- **Before Conditioning**: Natural occurrence stimulus that automatically elicits response such as salivation in response of smell of food.
- **During Conditioning**: During conditioning the previously neutral stimulus is repeatedly paired with the unconditioned stimulus.
- **After Conditioning**: Presenting the conditioned stimulus alone will come to evoke a response even without the unconditioned stimulus.
- **Habituation Learning**: It is a form of non-associative learning sometimes also called implicit learning. Non-associative learning is a change in a response to a stimulus that does not involve associating the presented stimulus with another stimulus or event such as a reward or punishment (Thompson & Spencer, 1966). It can be distinguished from other behavioral changes such as sensory adaptation and fatigue. In this form of learning repeated presentation of stimulus will causes decrease in reaction. Some related phenomena to habituation include sensitization and stimulus generalization/discrimination. Sensitization is the opposite process to habituation, i.e. an increase in the elicited behavior from repeated presentation of a stimulus.
- **Self-Efficacy Learning**: It depends on individual belief in their ability to achieve goals or we can say how well one can execute courses of action required to deal with prospective stimulations (Bandura, 1982). It also involves determination and preservation to overcome obstacles that would interfere with utilizing those innate abilities to achieve goals (Bandura, 1977).
- **Generalization learning**: Response to one stimulus will be generalized to another as a function of the distance between the two stimuli is known as generalization learning. In generalized learning humans and animals use their past learning in present situation of learning if the situation is similar and it directly tied to the transfer of knowledge across multiple situations (Walker, Shea, &

Table 2. Neurofeedback learning mechanism

S. No	Neurofeedback Learning Mechanism
1	Classical learning
2	Habituation learning
3	Self-efficacy learning
4	Generalization learning
5	Transference learning
6	Concurrent learning
7	Nonlinear learning

Bauer, 2016). This idea rivals the theory of situated cognition, instead stating that one can apply past knowledge to learning in new situations and environments.

Goals of NFB Training

- Improve self-regulation
- Achieve flexible and appropriate brain states
- Normalize connectivity
- Address functionality, not symptoms
- Provide lasting change

NEUROFEEDBACK MODALITIES

Neurofeedback modalities can be divided into two categories. First, clinicians who employ a symptom-based approach and a treatment approach guided by a pretreatment qualitative electroencephalogram (QEEG). Second clinicians who apply neurofeedback to present complaints without a quantitative analysis are symptom-based practitioners and those who utilize age-normed data in assessment and training are said to be QEEG based (Nasehi & Pourghassem, 2011).

QEEG Metrics

QEEG metric is a computed value derived from the EEG known as metrics. Qualitative analysis is based on the use of a reference database. Other modalities include an analysis of EEG waveforms to design NF protocol. For understanding the pathological or compensatory deviations it's important to understand the functional neuro-anatomy of the brain. QEEG metric helps to evaluate network dynamics through metrics that relate the relationship between pairs of the channel. Other connectivity metrics includes modulation and spectral correlation coefficient that reflects the magnitude between the signals and the correlation between amplitude spectra, respectively.

QEEG BASED NFB ENHANCE/INHIBIT TRAINING

Inhibit or enhance training is the traditional method of NF training. It is based on providing rewards when particular frequency bands are either present in excess and so are inhibited or when they are insufficient and so enhanced according to their inhibit or enhance pattern. This is known as enhance/inhibit NF training. These trainings commonly employ traditional method of NF training such as theta, beta, alpha, low beta or high beta training. Enhanced training is also called up training while inhibit training is known as down training.

Z-Score Training

The training is based on the principle of using statistical z-scores in real time, rather than using raw signal amplitudes or other variables (Cook, O'Hara, Uijtdehaage, Mandelkern, & Leuchter, 1998). In Z score training pre-post treatment qEEG maps are collected before and after Z-score training (Kroemer & Kroemer-Elbert, 2001).

NEUROFEEDBACK MODALITIES: SYMPTOM-BASED APPROACHES

Symptoms based approaches rely on applying the appropriate training protocols to specific problems. These symptoms based approaches were established after several applied differentially determined by client feedback, from different functional locations in the brain area and after huge clinical experiences by various clinicians. The symptom-based approach began with the alpha band training program and followed by sensory motor rhythm (SMR) and alpha/theta training (Nidal & Malik, 2017). This symptom-based approach also utilized in QEEG based treatment in the clinical field.

Alpha Training

Alpha training mostly used for the relaxation, peak performance, anxiety and for reducing the pain. Alpha training is basically used in the posterior region of cortex and most frequently in the parietal region (Hardt & Kamiya, 1978).

SMR Training

Barry Sterman first develops SMR training to reduce the seizures disorders. Joel Lubar after his research utilized this training for ADHD. SMR band training studies 12-15 Hz. This SMR training is often used to improve attention and reduction of restless or motoric stillness.

Alpha-Theta Training

This training is also referred to as deep status work. Eugene Penniston and Paul Kulikowski later applied this alpha-theta training in rehabilitation intervention for alcoholics and in post-traumatic stress disorder (Penniston & Kulkosky, 1991). The goal of the training is to enter a "crossover" state wherein the theta band is greater in amplitude than the alpha band (Penniston & Kulkosky, 1989).

Alpha Asymmetry Training

In mid-1990s Peter Rosenfeld and Elsa and Rufus Baehr first developed Alpha asymmetry training (Rosenfeld, Baehr, Baehr, Gotlib, & Ranganath, 1996). They search very strong relationship between asymmetries in alpha absolute power in the frontal lobes and mood distress. For alpha asymmetry training the targeted area on the montage at F3/F4 and reference to CZ.

PATIENT ASSESSMENT

NFB has been employed for nearly 25 years in research and clinical setting for the years in research and clinical setting for the investigation and treatment of growing number of psychological and neurological disorders (Lubar, 1997). These include attention deficit disorder, addictions, depression, eating disorder and post-traumatic stress disorder. In NFB the techniques involves detecting EEG information from the surface of the scalp of a subject, separating it by frequency decomposition into its component waveforms and make component visible on computer screen. For the assessment of the patient for NFB training clinician generally use various psychological assessment tools, subjective symptom questionnaires, objective question, and qualitative EEG. But pre and post QEEG is more frequently used as a testing purpose. QEEG is a noninvasive, painless assessment process which assesses all areas of the brain and detects area which needs to be trained. Apart from the QEEG, some subjective questionnaires can be utilized for the assessment. In recent years neurofeedback studies have gained much attention among human cognitive researchers.

FUNDAMENTAL OF EEG SIGNAL PROCESSING

The EEG signal contains information about the behavior or nature of some phenomenon. These biological signals processing generally extract useful information contained in the signal. These signals generally extract useful information contained in the signals. The method used to extract this information depends on the nature of the signal and kind of information contained in the signals.

Continuous-Time and Discrete-Time Signals

Many biomedical measurements such as EEG, ECG or arterial blood pressure are inherently defined at all instants of time. The signals resulting from these measurements are called continuous time signals and it is traditional to represent their functions of time in the form and so forth. On the contrary we could sample the values of the continuous time signal at integral multiples of a fundamental time increment called the sampling time and obtain a signal that consists of sequences of samples, each corresponding to one instant of time. This signal is called a discrete time signal.

Classification of Discrete Time Systems

It is classified based on their input and output relationship into the following classes.

Liner Systems

A discrete time system is called linear if it possesses the important property of superposition. if the input consist of the weighted sum of several signals then the output is the weighted sum of the responses of the system.

Time Invariant Systems

The system is time invariant if the behavior and characteristics of the system are fixed over time. If a system is time invariant if a time shift in the input signal results in an identical time shift in the output signal.

Linear Time Invariants System

We call a system that possesses the properties of both linearity and time invariance a linear time interval system. Such a system is amendable to simple mathematical analysis and characterization, which makes it widely used.

Causal Systems and Stable System

If the output at any time depends on values of only the present and past inputs called causal system and in stable system input produces a bounded output. This type of stability is called bounded-input bounded output stability.

Process of NFB Training

During NFB training the subjects is seated in front of a computer for 30 minutes to 45 minutes. Before starting the training non disposable electrodes were place in frontal lobe of the head and reference electrode behind the right ear lobe. On computer screen many games are running. According to the child clinical features the training such as alpha/ beta training, SMR training, and theta –beta training is decided after clinical examination. This training act as a drug free solution for many neurological as well as psychological illnesses.

CLINICAL USE OF EEG IN COGNITIVE DISORDERS

The diagnosis of most of the cognitive disorders is clinically based on EEG. It plays an important role in evaluating, classifying, and following some of these disorders. In many findings regarding the clinical used of quantitative EEG is awaiting validation by independent investigation and for clinical follow-ups.

Encephalopathies and Delirium

Quantitative EEG is described as a tool for evaluating encephalopathies associated to diverse causes including uremic (Jonkman et al., 1992), ischemia (Doyle et al., 2007), hepatic (Popkena, Kropvelda, Oostingb, & Chamuleau, 1983) and methamphetamine abstinence (Kullmann et al., 2001). The diagnosis of the any disease such as delirium is critical and urgent because of life threating medical complication associated with its high morbidity and mortality. qEEG has considerable potential as clinical diagnosis of an organic syndrome. Relative power in the alpha frequency band enables qEEG to distinguish normal from enchalopathic subjects. The non-delirium patient includes the amount of EEG theta activity (Brenner, 1991), relative power in the delta frequency band and the amount of activity in the slow wave bands compared to the alpha band (Jacobson, Leuchter, & Walter, 1993) .

Learning Disorders

In many studies qEEG is complementing the investigation and evaluating of learning disability. In learning disability qEEG discriminant accuracy ranged (Coburn et al., 2006) from 46-98%. The correlation between intelligence and EEG measures can be tasted by EEG power and EEG network properties such as coherence and phase delays and non- linear dynamical models of network complexity. EEG power shows neurophysiological sense and it represents the sum of neurons discharge. It also measures the capacity or performance of cortical information processing.

Attention Disorders

It's a neuropsychological disorder of childhood affecting 3-5% school aged children (Kilmesch, 1999). A literature survey from 1997 to 2008 reveled EEG associated with the terms attention deficit and children with diagnosis of ADHD have high slow-wave power and adolescent children with ADHD have reduce beta power compared with their respective normal children (John, 2002).

DISCUSSION AND CONCLUSION

This chapter has presented a new technology called NFB which helps to improve cognition and retrain the brain in various neurological and psychological disorders. It shows trainability and independence of brain waves such as alpha during the active stage of task. This is shows significance enhancement of working memory. This manuscript also suggests various condition where the research is going on and many researches working to develop new protocol for training the brain. Recently, researchers began to pay attention to training and focused on how to build appropriate neurofeedback based training program at initial several training sessions comparing with normal training.

REFERENCES

Ayers, M. E. (2004). Neurofeedback for cerebral palsy. *Journal of Neurotherapy*, *8*(2), 93–94. doi:10.1300/J184v08n02_07

Bandura, A. (1977). Self-efficacy: Toward a Unifying Theory of Behavioral Change. *Psychological Review*, *84*(2), 191–215. doi:10.1037/0033-295X.84.2.191 PMID:847061

Bandura, A. (1982). Self-efficacy mechanism in human agency. *The American Psychologist*, *37*(2), 122–147. doi:10.1037/0003-066X.37.2.122

Brenner, R. P. (1991). Utility of EEG in Delirium: Past Views and Current Practice. *International Psychogeriatrics*, *3*(2), 211–229. doi:10.1017/S1041610291000686 PMID:1811775

Coburn, K. L., Lauterbach, E. C., Boutros, N. N., Black, K. J., Arciniegas, D. B., & Coffey, C. E. (2006). The Value of Quantitative Electroencephalography in Clinical Psychiatry: A Report by the Committee on Research of the American Neuropsychiatric Association. *The Journal of Neuropsychiatry and Clinical Neurosciences*, *18*(4), 460–500. doi:10.1176/jnp.2006.18.4.460 PMID:17135374

Cook, I. A., O'Hara, R., Uijtdehaage, S. H., Mandelkern, M., & Leuchter, A. F. (1998). Assessing the accuracy of topographic EEG mapping for determining local brain function. *Electroencephalography and Clinical Neurophysiology*, *107*(6), 408–414. doi:10.1016/S0013-4694(98)00092-3 PMID:9922086

Doyle, O. M., Greene, B. R., Murray, D. M., Marnane, L., Lightbody, G., & Boylan, G. B. (2007). The effect of frequency band on quantitative EEG measures in neonates with hypoxic-ischaemic encephalopathy. *Conference Proceedings; ... Annual International Conference of the IEEE Engineering in Medicine and Biology Society. IEEE Engineering in Medicine and Biology Society. Conference*, 717–721. doi:10.1109/IEMBS.2007.4352391 PMID:18002057

Escolano, C., Aguilar, M., & Minguez, J. (2011). EEG-based upper alpha neurofeedback training improves working memory performance. *Proc. 33rd Annual International Conference of the IEEE*, 2327-2330 10.1109/IEMBS.2011.6090651

Escolano, C., Navarro-Gil, M., Garcia-Campayo, J., Congedo, M., De Ridder, D., & Minguez, J. (2014). A controlled study on the cognitive effect of alpha neurofeedback training in patients with major depression disorder. *Frontiers in Behavioral Neuroscience*, *8*, 296. doi:10.3389/fnbeh.2014.00296 PMID:25228864

Ganzalez-Ortega, D., Diaz-Pernas, F. J., & Martinez-Zarzuela, M. (2014). A Kinect-based system for cognition rehabilitation exercise monitoring. *Computer Methods and Programs in Biomedicine*, *113*(2), 620–631. doi:10.1016/j.cmpb.2013.10.014 PMID:24263055

Gomez-Pilar, J., & Corralejo, R. (2014). Assessment of neurofeedback training by means of motor imagery based-BCI for cognitive rehabilitation. *Proc Engineering in Medicine and Biology Society (EMBC), 36th Annual International Conference of the IEEE*, 3630-3633. 10.1109/EMBC.2014.6944409

Grefkes, C., & Fink, G. R. (2011). Reorganization of cerebral network after stroke: New insights from neuroimaging with connectivity approaches. *Brain*, *134*(5), 1264–1276. doi:10.1093/brain/awr033 PMID:21414995

Hardt, J. V., & Kamiya, J. (1978). Anxiety change through electroencephalographic alpha feedback seen only in high anxiety subjects. *Science*, *201*(4350), 79–81. doi:10.1126cience.663641 PMID:663641

Jacobson, S. A., Leuchter, A. F., & Walter, D. O. (1993). Conventional and quantitative EEG in the diagnosis of delirium among the elderly. *Journal of Neurology, Neurosurgery, and Psychiatry*, *56*(2), 153–158. doi:10.1136/jnnp.56.2.153 PMID:8437004

John, E. R. (2002). The Neurophysics of Consciousness. *Brain Research. Brain Research Reviews*, *39*(1), 1–28. doi:10.1016/S0165-0173(02)00142-X PMID:12086706

Jonkman, J., de Weerd, A. W., Portvliet, D. C., Veldhuizen, R. J., van Duijn, H., Rozeman, C. A., & Laman, M. (1992). Neurometrics in cerebral ischemia and uremic encephalopathy. *Brain Topography*, *4*(4), 277–284. doi:10.1007/BF01135565 PMID:1510871

Klimesch, W. (1999). EEG alpha and theta oscillations reflect cognitive and memory performance: A review and analysis. *Brain Research. Brain Research Reviews*, *29*(2-3), 169–195. doi:10.1016/S0165-0173(98)00056-3 PMID:10209231

Kroemer, K., & Kroemer-Elbert, E. (2001). *Ergonomics: How to Design for Ease and Efficiency*. Englewood Cliffs, NJ: Prentice Hall.

Kullmann, F., Hollerbach, S., Lock, G., Holstege, A., Dierks, T., & Scholmerich, J. (2001). Brain electrical activity mapping of EEG for the diagnosis of (sub)clinical hepatic encephalopathy in chronic liver disease. *European Journal of Gastroenterology & Hepatology*, *13*(5), 513–522. doi:10.1097/00042737-200105000-00009 PMID:11396530

Legg, T. J. (2018). Is neurofeedback effective for treating ADHD. *Medical News Today*. Retrieved from https://www.medicalnewstoday.com/articles/315261.php

Lohaugen, G. C., Beneventi, H., & Andersen, G. L. (2014). Do children with cerebral palsy benefit from computerized working memory training – Study protocol for a randomized controlled trail. *BioMed Central*, *15*(269), 2–9.

Lubar, J. F. (1997). Neocortical Dynamics: Implications for Understanding the Role of Neurofeedback and Related Techniques for the Enhancement of Attention. *Applied Psychophysiology and Biofeedback*, *22*(2), 111–126. doi:10.1023/A:1026276228832 PMID:9341967

Lubar, J. F. (1997). Neocortical Dynamics: Implications for Understanding the Role ofNeurofeedback and Related Techniques for the Enhancement of Attention. *Applied Psychophysiology and Biofeedback*, *22*(2), 111–126. doi:10.1023/A:1026276228832 PMID:9341967

Nasehi, S., & Pourghassem, H. (2011). Epileptic seizure onset detection algorithm using dynamic cascade feed-forward neural networks. *2011 International Conference on Intelligent Computation and Bio-Medical Instrumentation (ICBMI)*, 196–199. 10.1109/ICBMI.2011.59

Nidal, K., & Malik, A. S. (2017). *EEG/ERP Analysis method and applications*. Boca Raton, FL: CRC Press.

Penniston, E., & Kulkosky, P. (1991). Alpha-theta brainwave neurofeedback for Vietnam veterans with combat related post-traumatic stress disorder. *Medical Psychotherapy*, *4*, 47–60.

Penniston, E. G., & Kulkosky, P. J. (1989). Alpha-theta brainwave training and betaendorphin levels in alcoholics. *Alcoholism, Clinical and Experimental Research*, *13*(2), 271–279. doi:10.1111/j.1530-0277.1989.tb00325.x PMID:2524976

Pope, A. T., & Palsson, O. S. (2001). *Helping video games "Rewire our minds."* Retrieved from https://ntrs.nasa.gov/archive/nasa/casi.ntrs.nasa.gov/20040086464.pdf

Prinsloo, S., Novy, D., Driver, L., Lyle, R., Ramondetta, L., Eng, C., ... Cohen, L. (2017). Randomized controlled trial of neurofeedback on chemotherapy-induced peripheral neuropathy: A pilot study. *Cancer*, *123*(11), 1989–1997. doi:10.1002/cncr.30649 PMID:28257146

Rosenfeld, J. P., Baehr, E., Baehr, R., Gotlib, I. H., & Ranganath, C. (1996). Ranganath. (1996). Preliminary evidence that daily changes in frontal alpha asymmetry correlate with changes in affect in therapy sessions. *International Journal of Psychophysiology*, *23*(1-2), 137–141. doi:10.1016/0167-8760(96)00037-2 PMID:8880374

Scharnowski, F., & Weiskopt, N. (2015). Cognitive enhancement through real-time fMRI neurofeedback. *Current Opinion in Behavioral Sciences*, *4*(1), 122–127. doi:10.1016/j.cobeha.2015.05.001

Thompson, R., & Spencer, W. (1966). Habituation: A model phenomenon for the study of neuronal substrates of behavior. *Psychological Review*, *73*(1), 16–43. doi:10.1037/h0022681 PMID:5324565

Vernon, D. J. (2005). Can neurofeedback training enhance performance? An evaluation of the evidence with implications for future research. *Applied Psychophysiology and Biofeedback*, *30*(4), 347–364. doi:10.100710484-005-8421-4 PMID:16385423

Walker, J. E., Shea, T. M., & Bauer, A. M. (2016). *Generalization and the Effects of Consequences*. Retrieved from www.education.com

KEY TERMS AND DEFINITIONS

ADHD: Attention deficit hyperactive disorder.
CL: Classical learning.
CZ: Central zone.
NFB: Neurofeedback.
OC: Operant conditioning.
QEEG: Qualitative electroencephalogram.
SMR: Sensory motor rhythm.

Chapter 3
Neurological Disorders, Rehabilitation, and Associated Technologies:
An Overview

Sateesh Reddy Avutu
North-Eastern Hill University Shillong, India

Dinesh Bhatia
North-Eastern Hill University Shillong, India

ABSTRACT

Patients with neurological disorders are increasing globally due to various factors such as change in lifestyle patterns, professional and personal stress, small nuclear families, etc. Neurological rehabilitation is an area focused by the several research and development organizations and scientists from different disciplines to invent new and advanced rehabilitation devices. This chapter starts with the classification of different neurological disorders and their potential causes. The rehabilitation devices available globally for neurological patients with their underlying associated technologies are explained in the chapter. Towards the end of the chapter, the reader can acquire the fundamental knowledge about the different neurological disorders and the mal-functionality associated with the corresponding organs. The utilization of advanced technologies such as artificial intelligence, machine learning, and deep learning by researchers to fabricate neuro rehabilitation devices to improve patients' quality of life (QOL) are discussed in concluding section of the chapter.

INTRODUCTION

In human's, disease or injury due to nervous system is treated as neurological disorder. The malfunction of either central or peripheral nerves system due to biochemical, electrical or structural abnormalities can cause neurological disorders. The neurological disorders are categorized as movement, sensory and mental. Abnormalities in the central nervous system will affect the functionality of brain and spinal-cord.

DOI: 10.4018/978-1-5225-8567-1.ch003

The functionality of hands, legs and other sensory organs are depending on performance of peripheral nervous system. Rehabilitation to neurological patient depends on kind of neurological disorder, age, gender, living atmosphere and life style. Based on situation and purpose the rehabilitation devices are helpful for physiotherapist and nurses to make their task easy and reduces the burden on patient. The rehabilitation device will play the role for neurological patient throughout their life-spam. The advanced technology such as artificial intelligence, machine-learning and deep-learning in the field of computer science and robotics facilitate the bio medical engineer to design multipurpose devices rather than single application oriented devices and size of the devices are tremendously decreased which lead to easy transportation. New physiotherapy techniques are discovered based on the advanced technology. Irrespective of the technology, the purpose of any rehabilitation device is to facilitate the user to do their daily activities by themselves without any risk. However, independent of technology used each device has its own merits and demerits. The objective of this chapter is to provide fundamental knowledge of different neurological disorders and classification. The working principle and associated technology, along with merits and demerits of various rehabilitation devices and therapy techniques are briefly explained. The future scope of the current technology in neuro-rehabilitation engineering is discussed in the concluding section of this chapter.

NEUROLOGICAL DISORDERS AND CLASSIFICATION

Based on the literature survey it can be concluded that humans are suffering from more than 600 types known neurological disorders. According to the Global Burden of Diseases (GBD) Neurological disorders are the leading cause for disability and sometimes lead to death. Feigin et al gave the brief summary on global, regional and national wide burden of neurological disorders for the period from 1996 to 2015 (Headache, dizziness, raised intracranial pressure, unconsciousness, Neurological problems and Neurological disorders). The international classification of functioning, disability and health (ICF) provides the description of health and related states. In order to design best or innovative rehabilitation device/therapy, the designer must possess the basic knowledge of various neurological disorders, causes and effects on performance of the organs. Any neurological disorder can cause impairment in movement, sensory and mental. The classification of the neurological disorder based on the nature of impairment is shown in table 1.

REHABILITATION FOR NEUROLOGICAL DISORDERS

Rehabilitation services provide help to improve the abilities against the impairment of disabled people and not focus on the disease. The impairment may have related to consciousness, cognition, speech, vision, sensory and physical movement. The level of impairment depends on the neurologic function across multiple domains. The various scales such as Glasgow Coma Scale and American Spinal Injury Association Impairment are used to evaluate patient's condition. The patient's ability to perform their routine tasks are measured in terms of daily living activities and functional independence measure. Rehabilitation will be achieved through learning compensatory techniques and adaptation to promote neurological recovery. Over the past two decades' tremendous growth in neuro rehabilitation technologies such as robotic systems, electrical stimulators and wearable sensors to check the actual performance.

Table 1. The classification of neurological disorders based on cause of impairment

Movement Related Neurological Disorders	Sensory Related Neurological Disorders	Mental Related Neurological Disorders
Ataxia Cervical dystonia Chorea Dystonia Functional movement disorder Huntington's disease Multiple system atrophy Myoclonus Parkinson's disease Progressive supranuclear palsy Restless legs syndrome Rett Syndrome Spasticity Tardive dyskinesia Tourette syndrome Tremor Wilson's disease	Autism spectrum disorder (ASD) Blindness and low vision Hearing loss and deafness Sensory processing disorder Sensory hypersensitivity	Anger Anxiety and panic attacks Bipolar disorder Body dysmorphic disorder Borderline personality disorder Depression Dissociative disorders Recreational drugs and alcohol Hypomania and mania Loneliness

Since, the rehabilitation is combination of multiple technical expanses, multi-disciplinary professionals are needed to provide effective and efficient rehabilitation for people with long term neurological problems. The different component related to rehabilitation is shown in figure 1.

ADVANCES IN NUERO REHABILITATION DEVICES AND THERAPY TECHNIQUES

The advances in technology offers more practical applications in both engineering and medical field. It allows the doctor to give better treatment for patient and allows an engineer to design a suitable rehabilitation device. From past two decades, tremendous technological advancement and change has taken place in manufacturing the rehabilitation devices. All kind of neurologic patients are benefited with advanced rehabilitation techniques. The role of rehabilitation for various kind of neurological disorders are explained in the section titled "Rehabilitation For Neurological Disorders." Globally available rehabilitation devices and various therapy techniques along with merits and demerits are elaborated in following sections.

Rehabilitation Devices

Movement disorder due to neurological syndrome results an excess of movement or unnatural movement. In the year 2011, Stanley Fahn explained the classification of movement disorders including parkinsonism, Dystonia, and tremor (Fahn, 2011). Irrespective of the movement disorder classification, the main objective of rehabilitation device, or technique/method is to provide balance in movement, gait and posture. Based on the disorder and requirement, the patient can choose the devices like wheelchair, robotic arms, exoskeletons etc. to fulfil their movement related tasks.

Figure 1. The different components related to rehabilitation
(source: Saans Saksham Rehabilitation and Home Care)

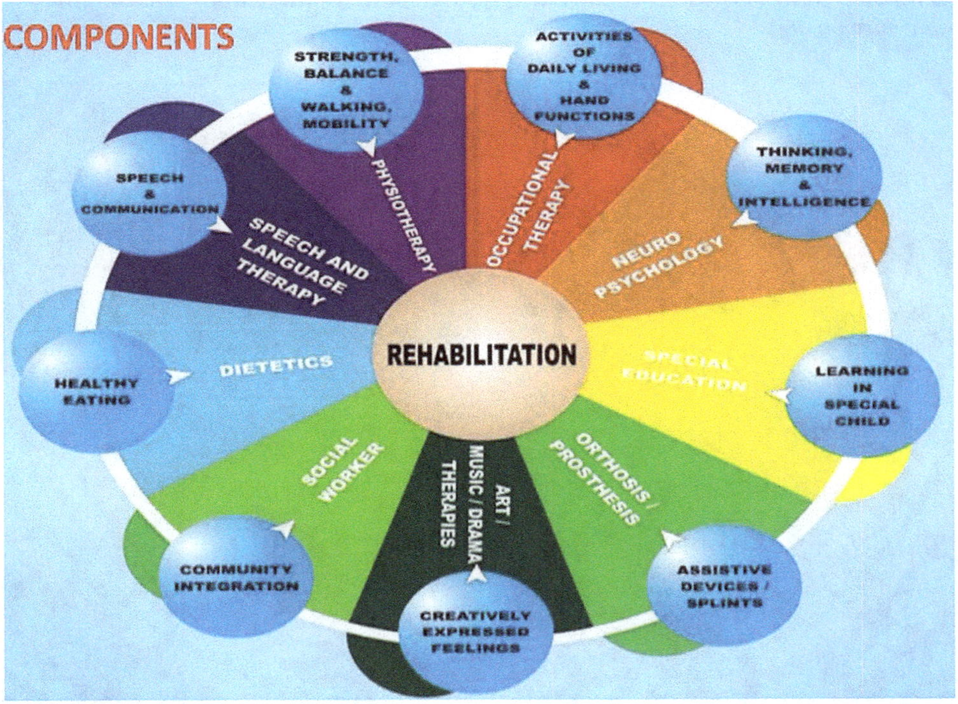

Wheelchair

Wheelchair is an ancient rehabilitation device used to overcome the mobility disorder. The first wheelchair was invented in 1595 and called as invalid's chair. The Bath wheelchair was invented in 19th century. After making so many improvements a wheelchair model was invented with rear push wheels and small front wheels and patented in 1869. The first spoked wheels and motorized wheelchair was invented in 1900 and 1916 respectively. Unfortunately, motorized wheelchairs were not available commercially in 1916. The first folding wheelchair was invented by Harry Jennings, in 1932 which is similar to the traditional manual wheelchair available globally. George Klein, a Canadian scientist put more effort to improve the motorized wheelchair. In 1956, Everest and Jennings started manufacturing electric wheelchair on mass scale. The various wheelchair models from past to present is shown in figure 2.

In 19th century people used wood to make wheelchair frame and parts. In 20th century various materials are used by the manufacturing industry to design a wheelchair without violating the design ethics. The innovation in design of the wheelchair facilitate the user in comfort seating and safety in all- terrains during the ride. But, controlling the wheelchair movement is difficult for neurological disorder patient compared with other patients, these people should depend on either add-on devices or caregivers as per their safety concern. The doctors will prescribe the powered wheelchair to neurological disorder patients in the absence of care givers. Joy stick is common device used to control the wheelchair movement. However, the modern wheelchairs are added with touch panels to control the wheelchair at less physical effort. Operating the touch panel is difficult for people not able to control their finger movements, in such cases external controlling device must be added to wheelchair to help the rider and trained profes-

Figure 2. The various wheelchair design models from past to present [A] Spain wheelchair [B] Steven Farffler wheelchair [C] Bath chair [D] First wheelchair with spokes [E] Basic manual wheelchair [F] Basic powered wheelchair [G] I-bot wheelchair [H] Direct drive hub motor wheelchair
(Source: https://abilitytools.org)

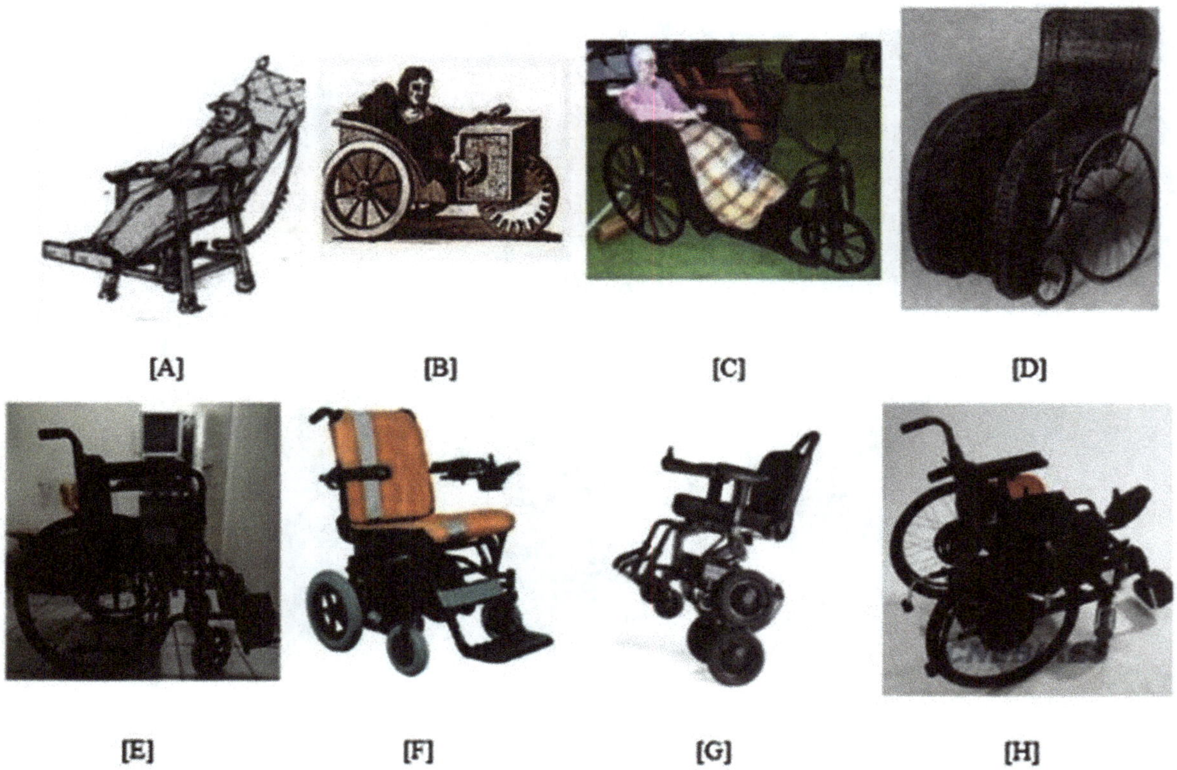

sional is mandatary to demonstrate the device. The performance, accuracy and reliability of the device will decide the safety of the rider. The various smart control methods are:

- Brain computer interface (BCI)
- Voice control method
- Various physiological signals

Brain computer interface (BCI) is a direct neural interface that enables the direct communication pathway between the brain and wheelchair and classified as Active BCI, Reactive BCI and Passive BCI. In Passive BCI, the command signal is from spontaneous brain activity instead of voluntary control. Irrespective of classification, BCI is combination of hardware and software and consists of signal acquisition and processing unit to generate the control signal. The signal processing unit made with algorithms to perform the tasks such as feature extraction and data translation (Hassanien & Azar, 2015). In 2005, Tanaka et al proposed the first BCI controlled wheelchair based on Electroencephalogram (EEG). Bi et al did the survey on EEG based brain controlled robots and explored the various kind of algorithms used (Bi, Fan, & Liu, 2013). In 2017, Ramadan et al explained the various controlled signals, types and classification used for BCI. The various electrodes used for data acquisition, its merits and demerits and challenges associated with current technology which restricts the accuracy of BCI are elaborated (Ramadan & Vasilakos, 2017). The accuracy of the whole BCI system depends on user and their requirements are depending on nature of the disability. Unfortunately, the guidelines have to be followed by the BCI developers are not yet standardized and till fully autonomous BCI controlled wheelchair are not commercialized in global market.

Voice control method is the best remedy to control the wheelchair movement and recommended for wheelchair bounded patients. It is easy to attach a Vo powered wheelchair. The input voice signal can be generated by the wheelchair user or collected from the bio signals. A microphone is used to take the input from the wheelchair rider and electrodes are used to collect the bio signals. Irrespective of input signal the accuracy of the output depends on signal processing algorithms. Separate algorithms are required for voice processing and bio signal processing. The two major disadvantages with voice control are, human voice is not unique and the features of the voice signal is depending on the emotional status of the user.

Hansen et al explained about the problems associated with the speaker recognition (Hansen & Hasan, 2015). Schultz et al (2017) explained the bio signal based speech processing algorithms. Tirumala et al (2017) discussed various speaker recognition algorithms. The development tree for neural-inspired algorithms and hardware architecture is shown in figure 3.

Robotic Arms

The Robotic arm is used as assistive device to fulfil the tasks done by human arm. It may be a complete prosthetic device or augmentation device made with lightweight materials and low power consumption

Figure 3. The development tree of neural-inspired algorithms and hardware architecture
(James et al., 2017)

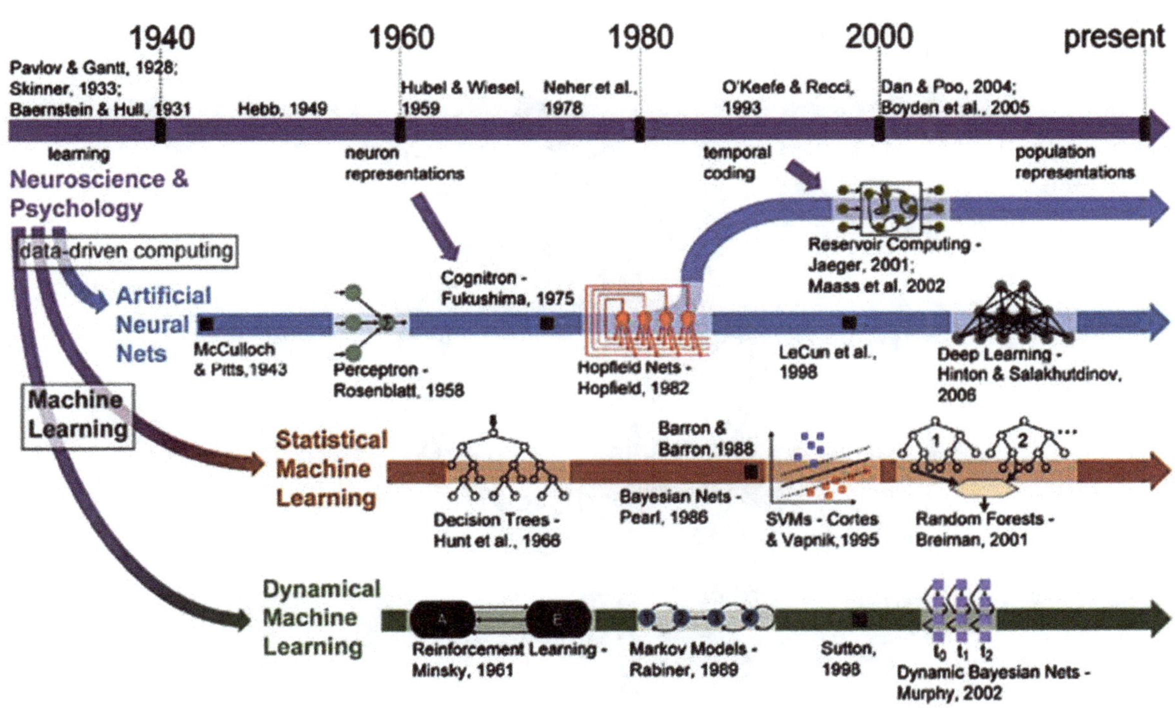

motors. In case of amputee patients, the robotic arm is directly attached to patient hand and movement was controlled by electromyogram (EMG) signals. It can be fixed with support of rigid body for patients with neurological disorders. In case of wheelchair or bed redounded patients it can be used to feed the patient. The accuracy and efficiency of robotic arm movement depends on quality of hardware components and algorithms used. The degree of freedom (DOF) define the number of hand or finger movements in different directions. The people with muscle impairment prefer augmentation device for extra support so that they can do the task easily. Saikia et al (2016) explored the recent advancements and history in prosthetic hand design. In year 2016, the defense advanced research projects Agency (DARPA) released food and drug administration (FDA) approved mind – controlled robotic arm as shown in figure 4. It has an ability to bend, rotate, and twist in 27 different ways like a normal human hand.

Exoskeleton

An external skeleton made with lightweight material and mechatronic devices to support the internal skeleton is treated as exoskeleton and these are classified as full body, upper extremities and lower extremities. The upper extremities are used to support arms and trunk. The lower extremities are used to control the parts below the trunk such as hip, knee and ankle or its combination. Exoskeletons with batteries to run the sensors and actuators is treated as powered exoskeleton otherwise it is treated as passive exoskeletons. The powered exoskeletons are classified as static and dynamic. The passive exo-skeletons are used for weight re-distribution, energy capture, dampening and locking. The exoskeletons based on functional electrical simulation (FES) is treated as hybrid-exoskeletons. The exoskeletons can be controlled by biosignals such as EEG or EMG signals. The Berkeley lower extremity exoskeleton

Figure 4. DARPA'S prosthetic hand
(Source: www.darpa.mil)

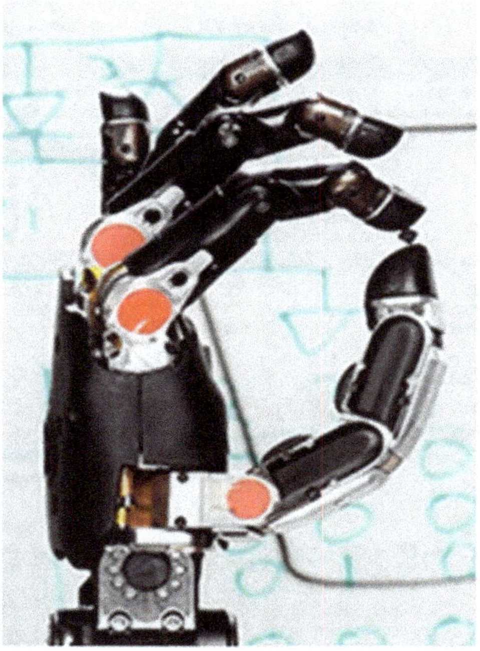

(BLEEX), hybrid assistive limb (HAL), XoR, Body Extender, hydraulic lower extremity exoskeleton (HLEE), Institute for machine and cognition mobility assist exoskeleton (IHMC MAE), MIT Exoskeleton are the few models developed by the research and development organizations. Ansari et al (2015) gave the brief explanation about performance and mathematical modeling for above models.

The full body exoskeletons can change the life style of wheelchair or bedridden patients due to neurological disorders. However, it is mandatory to check the walking style to avoid the damage of another biological system or organs of the patient. The difference in nature of human walking can estimated by using the gait lab. In BLEEX and HAL they used the EMG and pressure sensors to collect the walking data. Machine learning classification and clustering algorithms are required for off line data mining to predict the movement of lower limb. In 2012, Zhao, Zhang, & Guo (2012) explained the application of the machine-learning algorithms and various lower limb movements for motion analysis. Caldas et al (2017) explained the adaptive algorithms used to analyze the gait cycles based on inertial sensor data.

Rehabilitation for Sensory Related Disorders

Sensory receptors are specialized cells to detect specific stimuli occurring in the human body. These cells are classified as interoceptors and Exteroceptors. The mall function in exteroceptors will result in the impairment in the ability to taste, smell, vision, and hearing. The impairment in the sensory organs such as Eyes, Ears, Nose, Tongue and Skin can cause low vision/blindness, partial/complete loss of ability to hear, smell, taste and touch feel respectively. The low vision/blindness is due to chronic visual deficit which is not compensated by ordinary glasses and lens. The advanced devices such as video magnifiers, sonic cane, mini-guide, victor reader stream, haptic shoes and navigation bracelet are mostly expensive and unfamiliar to common people. The modern smart phones available in the global market allows the patients to do multitasking with the help of some add-on applications. The various electronic gadgets available in the global market to serve the visually impaired people are classified as travelling, path oriented and position locator devices and their performance is depending on following aspects.

- Exchange of information between user and sensors in an indoor and outdoor environment will help to avoid the obstacles
- The sensors should work at any condition of light i.e., day and night
- The range of obstacle detection should be more than five meters as safety concern
- An ability to differentiate the static and dynamic objects

Elmanni and Elleithy (2017) elaborated the broad classification visual assistive technologies and brief explanation about the sensor based assistive devices along with working principle and future aspects.

The hearing loss can be categorized as sensorineural and conductive hearing loss or combination of both. The damage in the cochlear/vestibulocochlear nerve can cause sensorineural hearing loss. The impairment of physical and mechanical obstruction to air conduction channel of ears can cause the conductive hearing loss. Hearing machines/aids are used to avoid the problems associated with ears impairment and classified as implanted and non-implanted devices. Implanted devices are fixed in ear and non-implanted devices are placed outside of ear. The broad classification of implantable devices is shown in figure 5.

Figure 5. Classification of implantable sensors for hearing devices
(Brody, Smith, & Ray, 2018).

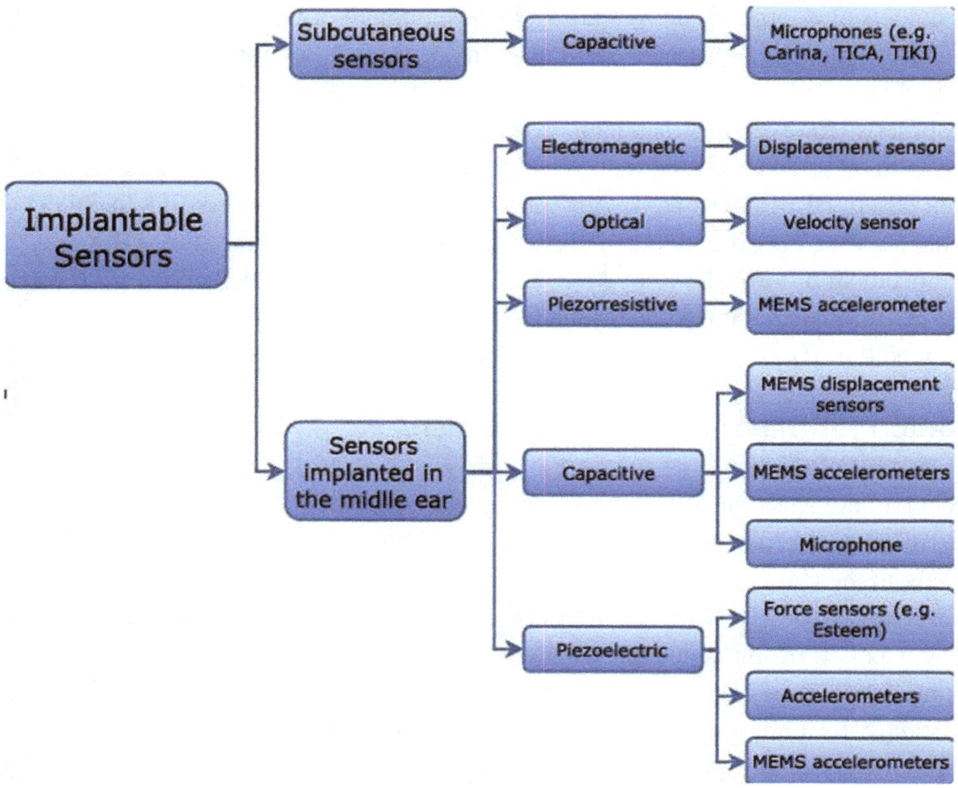

Hearing aid is simple electronic device consisting of microphone, an amplifier and speaker. The power is needed for amplifier to boost up the signal strength and the quality of the device is based on performance of signal processing algorithms. The development in the hardware and software technology leads to reduce the physical size of the hearing aids drastically and current research is ongoing to develop a self-rechargeable implantable hearing device. Calero et al described the technical development of implantable sensors (Brodie, Smith, & Ray, 2018). Brodie, Smith, and Ray (2018) did the survey to explain the impact of hearing aids on quality of life of hearing loss patients (Calero, Paul, Gesing, Alves, & Cordioli, 2018).

The inability to smell and taste is treated as olfactory. It is the common problem occurred in adults aged between 65 to 80 years. There are multiple factors such as olfactory epithelium damage, age-related nasal epithelium atrophy, decrease in nasal mucosal metabolizing enzymes that are responsible for olfactory sensation (Wongrakpanich, Petchlorlian, & Rosenzweig, 2016). Patel (2017) reviewed the various therapy techniques to improve the ability of olfactory patients. Tongue is an organ made with muscles and capable to move without any bone support. The restrictions in the tongue movement results in dysfunction of mastication, deglutition and speech. The rehabilitation to this patient depends on the nature of glossectomy. Therapy techniques are mandatory along with prosthetic tongue.

Rehabilitation for Stroke and Trauma Patients

The sudden death of neurons inside the human brain can be treated as stroke. Ischemic stroke and hemorrhagic stroke are the two common types. The rehabilitation for stroke patients depends on several factors such as nature of stroke, age and living atmosphere and class of evidence. The class of evidences are well explained by American heart association (AHA) and American stroke association (ASA). According to the guide lines given by AHA/ASA (Winstein et al., 2016) large team support is needed for adult stroke rehabilitation. Suarez-Escobar et al briefly explained the technology developments of robotic/mechanical devices for post stroke rehabilitation (Suarez-Escobar & Rendon-Velez, 2018).

Any physical injury which leads to severe wounds, broken bones or internal organ damage can be treated as trauma. The severity of injury is calculated by injury severity score (ISS). The rehabilitation to the trauma patients depends on the severity of the injury or nature of the damaged organ. Long and Koyfman (2018) explained the advances in neuro-trauma management.

ADVANCES IN THERAPY TECHNIQUES

Psychotherapy is kind of treatment used to cure the mental related disorders. According to American psychiatric association (APA) the therapy techniques are classified as cognitive behavioral therapy, interpersonal therapy, psychodynamic therapy and psychoanalysis. Based on the patient's disorder and circumstances the doctor will suggest the suitable therapy technique (American Psychiatric Association, 2011). Evidence based practice (EBP) is the common technique used by many psychotherapists. The drivers of EBP is shown in the figure 6.

Akyuz et al explained about the physical therapy modalities to cure the neuropathic pain (Akyuz & Kenis, 2014). Sullivan, briefly explained the various manual therapy techniques for chronic and low back pain disorders (O'Sullivan, 2005).

Figure 6. The drivers of EBP
(Lennon & Stokes, 2009)

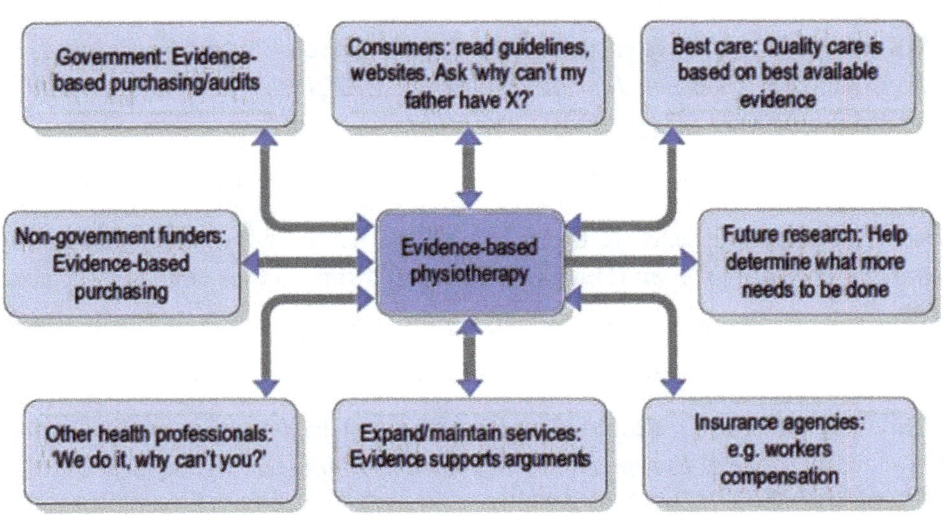

CONCLUSION

We have classified Neurological disorders as Movement, Sensory and Cerebral. Movement disorders are those where the Neurological injury restricts the movement of the patient. Sensory disorders are those where the some or most of the senses (sight, sound, touch, smell) are disturbed and the patient is unable to function normally. Mental disorders are those where the patient has lost the balance of his mind. However, with some technological help such patients can be normal or near normal and carry on their daily activities. The main difficulties in the movement and sensory disorder patients are:

- Movement from one place to another
- Performing daily tasks (such as closing doors, crossing roads, climbing stairs)
- Performing tasks involving effort such as lifting weights.

The principal utilities to help such patients are:

- **Automated Wheelchairs:** These are wheel chairs which are battery operated and can be controlled with available controls (movement, speed, breaks) on the arm rests or foot pedals, as desired by the patient These chairs require no further assistance making the patient fully independent. More advanced versions have additional features such as step climbing and therapeutic abilities.
- **Robotic Arms:** Robotic arms are extensions of human arms. These arms are either controlled via a BCI (Brain Computer Interface) or are attached to the arms themselves and controlled via mouse/keyboard. Typically, these Robotic arms can lift weights, can perform very precise tasks or tasks which require great skill. For example, robotic arms are used by surgeons to perform intricate surgery with great success.
- **Exoskeletons:** Exoskeletons are for those who cannot move their arms or legs. The exoskeleton allows control/movement of robotic arms and legs. Thus, paraplegic patients can use such a system to both move and perform tasks with ease and control.

REFERENCES

Akyuz, G., & Kenis, O. (2014). Physical therapy modalities and rehabilitation techniques in the management of neuropathic pain. *American Journal of Physical Medicine & Rehabilitation*, *93*(3), 253–259. doi:10.1097/PHM.0000000000000037 PMID:24322437

American Psychiatric Association. (2011). Talk facts, Healthy Minds. *Healthy Minds Healthy Lives, 2.*

Ansari, A., Atkeson, C. G., Choset, H., & Travers, M. (2015). *A Survey of Current Exoskeletons and Their Control Architectures and Algorithms* (Draft 4.0). Retrieved from www.cs.cmu.edu/~cga/exo/survey.pdf

Bi, L., Fan, X. A., & Liu, Y. (2013). EEG-based brain-controlled mobile robots: A survey. *IEEE Transactions on Human-Machine Systems*, *43*(2), 161–176. doi:10.1109/TSMCC.2012.2219046

Brodie, A., Smith, B., & Ray, J. (2018). The impact of rehabilitation on quality of life after hearing loss: A systematic review. *European Archives of Oto-Rhino-Laryngology*, *275*(10), 2435–2440. doi:10.100700405-018-5100-7 PMID:30159730

Caldas, R., Mundt, M., Potthast, W., Buarque de Lima Neto, F., & Markert, B. (2017). A systematic review of gait analysis methods based on inertial sensors and adaptive algorithms. *Gait & Posture*, *57*(February), 204–210. doi:10.1016/j.gaitpost.2017.06.019 PMID:28666178

Calero, D., Paul, S., Gesing, A., Alves, F., & Cordioli, J. A. (2018). A technical review and evaluation of implantable sensors for hearing devices. *Biomedical Engineering Online*, *17*(1), 1–26. doi:10.118612938-018-0454-z PMID:29433516

Elmannai, W., & Elleithy, K. (2017). Sensor-based assistive devices for visually-impaired people: Current status, challenges, and future directions. *Sensors (Switzerland)*, *17*(3), 565. doi:10.339017030565 PMID:28287451

Fahn, S. (2011). Classification of movement disorders. *Movement Disorders*, *26*(6), 947–957. doi:10.1002/mds.23759 PMID:21626541

Hansen, J. H. L., & Hasan, T. (2015). Speaker recognition by machines and humans: A tutorial review. *IEEE Signal Processing Magazine*, *32*(6), 74–99. doi:10.1109/MSP.2015.2462851

Hassanien, A.E. & Azar, A.T. (2015). *Brain Computer Interfaces: Current Trends and Applications* (Vol. 143). doi:10.1007/978-3-319-10978-7

Hutcheson, J. A., & Kimberley, M. O. (1999). A pragmatic approach to characterising insect communities in New Zealand: Malaise trapped beetles. *New Zealand Journal of Ecology*, *23*(1), 69–79. doi:10.1016/S1474-4422(17)30299-5

James, C. D., Aimone, J. B., Miner, N. E., Vineyard, C. M., Rothganger, F. H., Carlson, K. D., & Plimpton, S. J. (2017). A historical survey of algorithms and hardware architectures for neural-inspired and neuromorphic computing applications. *Biologically Inspired Cognitive Architectures*, *19*, 49–54. doi:10.1016/j.bica.2016.11.002

Lennon, S., & Stokes, M. (2009). *Pocket book of Neurologcial physciotherapy.* Elsevier Publication.

Long, B., & Koyfman, A. (2018). Secondary Gains: Advances in Neurotrauma Management. *Emergency Medicine Clinics of North America*, *36*(1), 107–133. doi:10.1016/j.emc.2017.08.007 PMID:29132572

O'Sullivan, P. (2005). Diagnosis and classification of chronic low back pain disorders: Maladaptive movement and motor control impairment as underlying mechanism. *Manual Therapy*, *10*(4), 242–255. doi:10.1016/j.math.2005.07.001 PMID:16154380

Patel, Z. M. (2017). The evidence for olfactory training in treating patients with olfactory loss. *Current Opinion in Otolaryngology & Head & Neck Surgery*, *25*(1), 43–46. doi:10.1097/MOO.0000000000000328 PMID:27841770

Ramadan, R. A., & Vasilakos, A. V. (2017). Brain computer interface: control signals review. *Neurocomputing*, *223*, 26–44. doi:10.1016/j.neucom.2016.10.024

Saikia, A., Mazumdar, S., Sahai, N., Paul, S., Bhatia, D., Verma, S., & Rohilla, P. K. (2016). Recent advancements in prosthetic hand technology. *Journal of Medical Engineering & Technology*, *40*(5), 255–264. doi:10.3109/03091902.2016.1167971 PMID:27098838

Schultz, T., Wand, M., Hueber, T., Krusienski, D. J., Herff, C., & Brumberg, J. S. (2017). Biosignal-Based Spoken Communication: A Survey. *IEEE/ACM Transactions on Audio Speech and Language Processing, 25*(12), 2257–2271. doi:10.1109/TASLP.2017.2752365

Suarez-Escobar, M., & Rendon-Velez, E. (2018). An overview of robotic/mechanical devices for post-stroke thumb rehabilitation. *Disability and Rehabilitation. Assistive Technology, 13*(7), 683–703. doi:10.1080/17483107.2018.1425746 PMID:29334274

Tirumala, S. S., Shahamiri, S. R., Garhwal, A. S., & Wang, R. (2017). Speaker identification features extraction methods: A systematic review. *Expert Systems with Applications, 90*, 250–271. doi:10.1016/j.eswa.2017.08.015

Winstein, C. J., Stein, J., Arena, R., Bates, B., Cherney, L. R., Cramer, S. C., … Zorowitz, R. D. (2016). Guidelines for Adult Stroke Rehabilitation and Recovery: A Guideline for Healthcare Professionals from the American Heart Association/American Stroke Association. *Stroke, 47*. doi:10.1161/STR.0000000000000098

Wongrakpanich, S., Petchlorlian, A., & Rosenzweig, A. (2016). Sensorineural Organs Dysfunction and Cognitive Decline: A Review Article. *Aging and Disease, 7*(6), 763. doi:10.14336/AD.2016.0515 PMID:28053826

Zhao, C. Y., Zhang, X. G., & Guo, Q. (2012). The application of machine-learning on lower limb motion analysis in human exoskeleton system. Lecture Notes in Computer Science, 7621, 600–611. doi:10.1007/978-3-642-34103-8_61

Chapter 4
Brain Tumor and Its Segmentation From Brain MRI Sequences

Sanjay Saxena
International Institute of Information Technology, India

Puspanjali Mohapatra
International Institute of Information Technology, India

Swati Pattnaik
International Institute of Information Technology, India

ABSTRACT

Automated segmentation of tumorous region from the brain magnetic resonance image (MRI) is the procedure of extrication anomalous tissues from regular tissues, such as white matter (WM), gray matter (GM), and cerebrospinal fluid (CSF). The process of accurate and efficient segmentation is still exigent because of the diversity of location, size, and shape of the tumorous region. Brain MRI provides metabolic process, psychological process, and descriptive information of the brain. Brain tumor segmentation using MRI is drawing the attention of the researchers due to its non-invasive nature and good soft tissue contrast of MRI sequences. The main motive of this chapter is to provide a broad overview of the methods of brain tumor segmentation based on MRI. This chapter provides the information of the brain tumor, its types, brief introduction of the MRI, and its diverse types, and lastly, this chapter gives the brief overview with benefits and limitations about diverse techniques used for brain tumor segmentation by different researchers and scientists.

DOI: 10.4018/978-1-5225-8567-1.ch004

1. INTRODUCTION

Human brain is the most vital part in human body. It is a complex composition that exhibits neural activity on numerous spatial scales. It is the main and only reason of our each and every emotion, thought, memory and action in the world. If any situation arises of brain getting affected then, whole human body system gets affected. Out of many such scenarios, brain tumor is the worst case scenario. Among all life threatening diseases which are increasing in quick rate, Brain tumor is one of the most serious life threatening disease. It is basically a mass of tissue which is generally formed due to unstructured growth of abnormal cells in brain at any random location. The prevalence of research on human brain imaging focuses on the covered structure of the cerebral cortex gray matter.

A tumor (sometimes it is called lesion or neoplasm) is anomalous tissue that grows by irrepressible division of cells. Standard cell grows in controlled approach as old or damaged cells are replaced by new cells. Taking into consideration about the brain tumor, it can be separated into two types' primary tumor and metastatic or secondary tumor.

A primary brain tumor is an anomalous growth that initiates in the brain and generally does not spread to another part of the body. It may be malignant or benign. The benign tumor grows gradually, is having discrete boundaries, and hardly ever spread. While a malignant tumor grows rapidly and having asymmetrical boundaries. Secondary (metastatic) brain tumor begins as cancer somewhere else in the body and spread to the brain. They form where the cancer cells are conceded in the blood stream of the brain. There are almost 120 different types of brain tumor. Ordinary brain tumor includes glioma, lymphoma, craniopharyngioma, schwannoma, epidermoid, meningioma, pituitary adenoma, medulloplastoma, pinealoma, and many more. This chapter will give the brief introduction of the different types of commonly brain tumor as per WHO (World Health Organization). American Brain Tumour Association (ABTA) presented that in the year 2015, nearly 78,000 new human cases of primary brain tumours have been diagnosed. That includes just about 53,000 nonmalignant and 25,000 primary malignant brain tumours. The growth of brain tumour amongst the people and people expire out of brain tumour are increasing in every year amid the developed countries and that is approximated by National Brain Tumour Foundation (NBTF) (El-Dahshan, Mohsen, Revett & Salem, 2014). Grading for brain tumours is issued by the World Health Organization (WHO) (Louis, Ohgaki, Wiestler, Burger, Jouve & Kleihues, 2007) in which Grade I (pilocytic astrocytoma) are least violent and cultivate gradually and Some Grade II (low-grade astrocytoma) replicate and affect close by tissues. Grade III (anaplastic astrocytoma) are the malignant tumour that replicate cells and impinge on tissues. Grade IV (glioblastoma) are the mainly malignant tumours that usually imitate quickly and affect close by normal brain tissue.

Further, identification of exact brain tumor is also an essential and critical task. One of the most significant ways of diagnosing brain tumor is MRI. It is a non invasive medical test that uses radio frequency waves and magnetic field to give a descriptive view of the soft tissue of the brain. It views the brain 3 dimensionally in slices which can be taken from the side or can be taken from the top as a cross section. A contrast agent may be inserted into the patient's blood stream. MRI is one of the important tools for analyzing brain tumor. There are several types of brain MRI sequences available such as T1-weightetd MRI, T2-weighted MRI, Diffusion weighted MRI, Fluid attenuation Inversion Recovery (FLAIR) MRI, Diffusion Tensor Imaging, Gradient Record MRI, functional MRI. This chapter provides the detailed information of the different kinds of MRI. How they are useful and what are the uses and significance. Though, MRI gives the detailed information of the brain such as structure and shape of the tumor, if it is there. However, it is very difficult task for a medical practitioner for analyzing brain tumor manually from the slices of brain MRI. For this, automated system for brain tumor segmentation is significantly recommended and it plays a very important role for treatment planning.

Till now there are several techniques and methods are developed for brain tumor localization. Broadly brain MRI segmentation can be divided into two categories manual and automated segmentation. Manual segmentation deals with extracting the region manually by an expert. While automated segmentation deals with extracting the region of interest automatically by applying numerous methods such as intensity based methods which deal with the gray levels of the brain MRI slices for example thresholding, edge based segmentation, region growing, region splitting and merging. Atlas based methods it exploits knowledge from previously labeled training images to segment the target image. The atlas contains information about the brain anatomy (e.g., it contains the information about the location of different brain structures) and it is used as a reference (a prior knowledge) for segmenting new images. Surface based methods for example active contouring methods and deformable methods. Hybrid segmentation methods it includes methods based on combining expectation-maximization segmentation, binary mathematical morphology, and active contours models. Few researchers have developed a combined 3D brain MRI segmentation algorithm which iterates between a classification step to identify tissues and an elastic matching step to align a template of normal brain anatomy with the classified tissues. Apart from these some approaches are machine learning based such as ANN (Artificial Neural Network), fuzzy, neuro-fuzzy, deep learning and many more. Now a day's researches have implemented some advance methods for brain MRI segmentation for example Intensity and patch normalization, CNN (Convolution neural network) based classification system is used. CNN based techniques are used to achieve high performance using a new two-way architecture. In Generative-discriminative model technique as advanced method is also implemented for brain MRI segmentation. Some researchers have implemented PSO(Particle Swarm Optimization) and its various forms for example Enhanced Darwinian Particle Swarm Optimization (EDPSO) and Fractional-Order Darwinian Particle Swarm Optimization(FODPSO). Experimental result shows that feature extraction from FODPSO segmented images provides higher performance than the classical PSO and EDPSO. Apart from these there are number of methods used for brain tumor segmentation. This chapter mainly focuses on the three aspects firstly brain tumor and its types, brain MRI image sequencing and its different types and several brain MRI segmentation techniques and its analysis. The structure of the chapter in such a way that section 2 describes about the brain tumor and its types. In section 3, effect of the brain tumours in neurological disorders are explained. Detailed information about the MRI is given in section 4. Section 5 presents the description of different techniques with their pros and cons. Conclusion of the chapter is given in section 6. Finally references are given in section 7.

2. BRAIN TUMORS AND THEIR TYPES

Just like other tumors, a brain tumor is a compilation of cells that increase at a speedy rate. The tumor may cause harm by spreading into hale and hearty portion of the brain and prying with function. It can be malignant or benign. They can build up inside or outside the brain. A benign tumor is noncancerous but not essentially risk-free. It tends to cultivate gradually. Symptoms of the benign tumor may not emerge for a long time. These kinds of tumor are often detected incidentally. For example, it may be revealed when a brain scan is implemented because of a nuisance or after a calamity. A benign tumor generally has discrete borders and is less expected to root damage to neighbouring tissue. Malignant tumors are strictly cancerous. It tends to grow uncompromisingly and extend to neighbouring tissues.

In spite of treatment, they may persist either in the similar place or in different location. If a malignant tumor left untreated it can eventually lead to death. This kind of tumours are among the most hard types of cancer to brawl. Malignant brain tumors are categorized as either primary or secondary. A primary means with in the brain the cancerous cells start. In a metastatic or secondary tumor, the cancerous cells begin somewhere else in the human body. Further, they extend during the brain's bloodstream. This procedure is known as metastasis. About more than 120 diverse types of brain tumors have been identified("Understanding brain tumors", 1999).

There are over 120 different types of brain tumors ("Understanding brain tumors", 1999). List of the most common brain tumors are given below

1. Glioma
2. Craniopharyngioma
3. Epidermoid
4. Lymphoma
5. Meningioma
6. Schwannoma (neuroma)
7. Pituitary adenoma
8. Pinealoma (pineocytoma, pineoblastoma)
9. Medulloblastoma

Among brain tumors, gliomas are the most common and aggressive, leading to a very short life expectancy in their highest grade. Gliomas are the brain tumors with the highest mortality rate and prevalence. These neoplasms can be graded into Low Grade Gliomas (LGG) and High Grade Gliomas (HGG), with the former being less aggressive and infiltrative than the latter (Louis, Ohgaki, Wiestler, Burger, Jouve & Kleihues, 2007), (Bauer, Wiest, Nolte & Reyes, 2013),("Brain tumors: An Introduction", 2016). Following figures shows HGG (High Grade Glioma)

Different types of the Gliomas are given below in figure 2.

Figure 1. High Grade Glioma
Isensee et al. (2018)

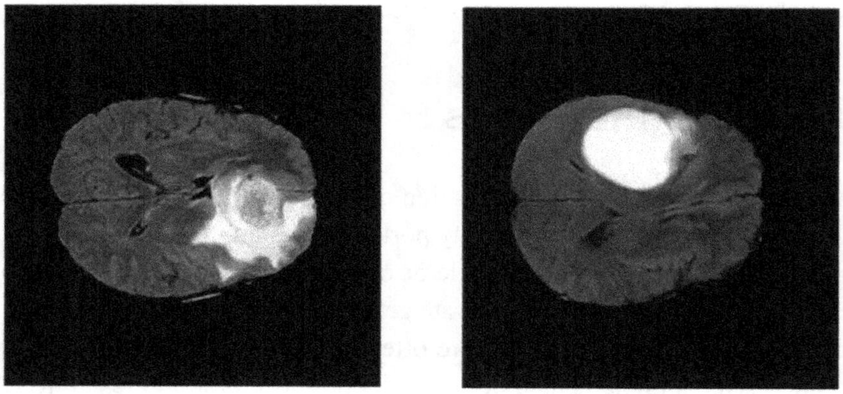

Figure 2. Different Types of Gliomas
("Brain tumors: An Introduction", 2016)

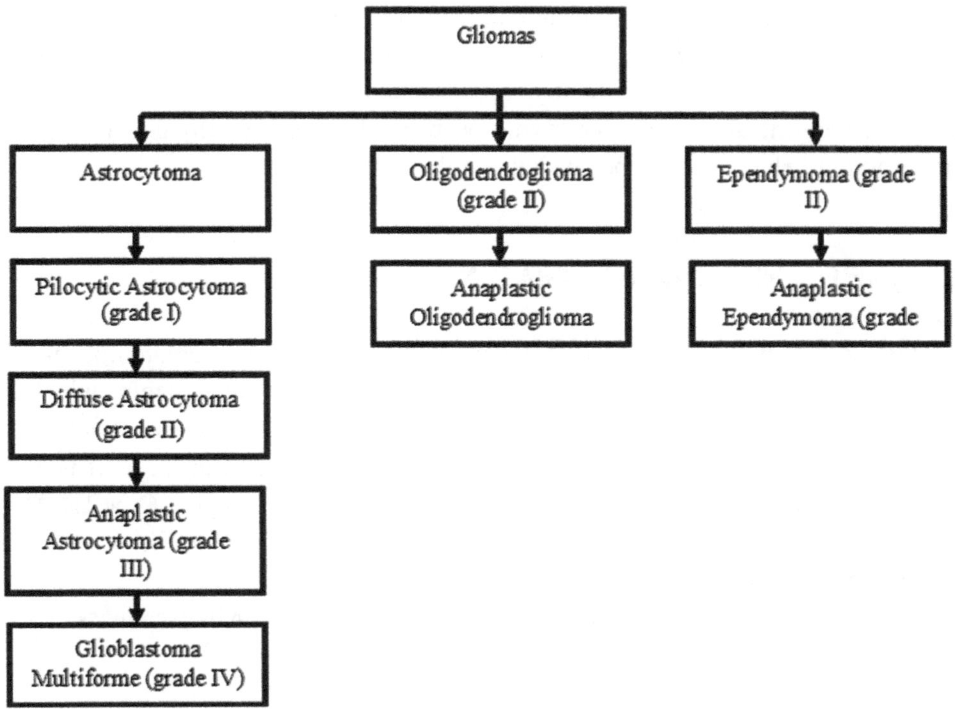

The World Health Organization (WHO) developed a classification and grading system to standardize communication, treatment planning, and predict outcomes for brain tumors. Tumors are classified by their cell type and grade by viewing the cells, usually taken during a biopsy, under a microscope.

1. Cell type. Refers to the cell of origin of the tumor. For example, nerve cells (neurons) and support cells (glial and schwann cells) give rise to tumors. About half of all primary brain tumors grow from glial cells (gliomas). There are many types of gliomas because there are different kinds of glial cells.
2. Grade. Refers to the way tumor cells look under the microscope and is an indication of aggressiveness (e.g., low grade means least aggressive and high grade means most aggressive). Tumors often have a mix of cell grades and can change as they grow. Differentiated and anaplastic are terms used to describe how similar or abnormal the tumor cells appear compared to normal cells.

3. NEUROLOGICAL DISORDER AS A REASON OF BRAIN TUMOR

Patients with prime inherent brain tumours can experience cognitive, neurological, and psychiatric symptoms that significantly disturb everyday lifecycle. As discussed Gliomas (Grade II, III, or IV) are the utmost common main malignant brain tumours, with an occurrence of six per 100,000 presented by World Health Organization. By means of the tumour growths, numerous indications consequential from the sickness often become more noticeable. As both the ailment and its handling have a straight consequence on brain effective, patients usually experience cognitive, nervous, and psychiatric symptoms. Neurobehavioral indications may disturb the patient's aptitude to involve with clinical decision-making and eventually may affect existence. Furthermore, these signs can damagingly distress patients' straight social environment, such as partners, family affiliates, and nearby friends. Neurobehavioral indications are general in brain tumour patients, frequently happen concomitantly, and are problematic to tell apart. For instance, affective illnesses can co-occur with or mirror fatigue, alexithymia, and apathy, however a dissimilar method in behaviour may be needed (Boele, 2015).

4. MRI (MAGNETIC RESONANCE IMAGING)

One of the many medical imaging techniques that are used in radiology to create images of the human being structure and its physiological processes is called Magnetic Resonance Imaging which is developed in the era of 1970s and 1980s, since then MRI has demonstrated to be a extremely adaptable imaging technique and is much acceptable for not having any identify regional effects. MRI is also known as magnetic resonance tomography (MRT), nuclear magnetic resonance imaging (NMRI). MRI Scanners are the devices that are used to produce these images. MRI scanner is a tube-like structure surrounded by a large circular magnet shown in Figure 3.

The patient is placed in a moveable bed and inserted into the tube. MRI scanners use strong radio waves, magnetic fields, and magnetic field gradients.

Figure 3. MRI Scanner
(PET/MRI Scan. (n.d.), 2018)

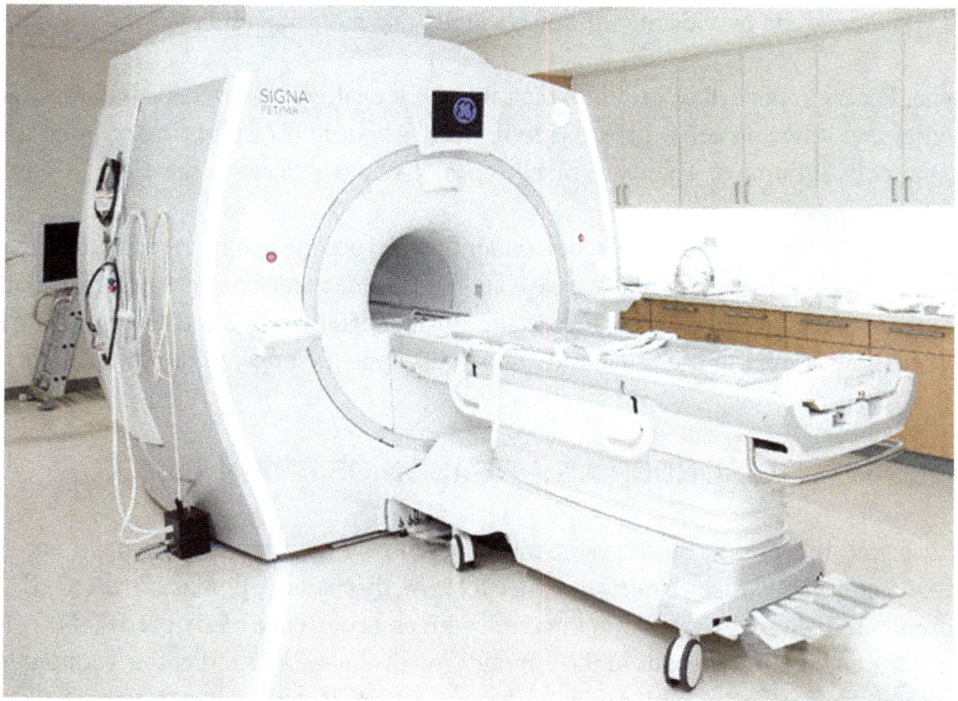

The primary difference between MRI and CT or PET scan is that it does not use X-rays or ionization radiation. Although in recent years the demerits of X-rays have been controlled, MRI is still a better choice than CT. MRI is popularly used in hospitals and clinics for medical diagnosis, staging of diseases and follow up without using introducing radiations to the body, however, it may yield different diagnostic information concerning the CT. Compared to CT scan, MRI takes longer, and the patient is required to enter a narrow, confining tube-like structure (MR Scanner). Furthermore, patients with medical implants or other nonremovable metal implants in the body are unable to undergo an MRI examination successfully.

MRI is the most preferred imaging technique used for investigation in the preoperative staging of rectal and prostate cancer.

Applications of MRI

MRI has a wide range of application in medical imaging, and more than 25,000 medical scanners are estimated to be in use worldwide.

Classifying MRI by functionality:

1. Neuroimaging: In the case of Neurological cancer MRI is predominantly used because it gives better resolution than CT scan. It offers better visualization of the posterior cranial fossa, containing the brainstem and the cerebellum. It provides a contrast between the grey matter and white matter, and this feature of the MRI makes it the best choice for many conditions of the central nervous system including epilepsy, infectious diseases, cerebrovascular disease, dementia, Alzheimer's disease, and demyelinating diseases.
2. Cardiovascular: Cardiac MRI works in combination with other imaging techniques, such as such as cardiac CT, echocardiography, and nuclear medicine and together they provide a complete diagnostic. Its applications include assessment of iron overload, myocardial ischemia and viability, myocarditis, cardiomyopathies, vascular diseases, and congenital heart disease.
3. Musculoskeletal: One of the significant use of MRI is spinal imaging, assessment of joint disease (system includes the knee, shoulder, ankle, wrist, and elbow) and soft tissue tumors.
4. Liver and gastrointestinal: MRI can also detect and characterize lesions of the liver, bile duct, and pancreases. Such an MRI is named Hepatobiliary MRI.
5. Magnetic Resonance Angiography(MRA): It is a non-invasive diagnostic procedure that uses MRI in combination with intravenous (IV) contrast dye to visualize blood vessels. The dye causes blood vessels to appear opaque on the MRI image and enables the physicians in visualizing the concerned blood vessels. It is generally used to access the blood flow in the heart and other soft tissue.
6. Functional MRI (fMRI): While taking the fMRI, the patient is asked to perform physical activities to help the surgeons map the functional areas of the brain. fMRI usually takes place pre-surgery.
7. Magnetic resonance venography(MRV): It uses a combination of a large magnet, radio frequencies, and a computer to produce detailed images of organs inside the body. MRV process is similar to the MRA and also uses magnetic resonance technique in combination with intravenous (IV) contrast dye to visualize the veins. MRV is useful in some cases as it may help to perceive causes of leg pain other than problems of vein.

8. Breast MRI: Patients at high risk of breast cancer are required to undergo breast MRI. It can single out areas of concern earlier with higher accuracy and in ways not possible with other breast imaging techniques. It is a painless procedure in which patients lie flat on their stomach for 45 minutes with their breast in the scanner to produce the internal structure of the breast.

To extract brain tumor and its types MRI plays a very vital role. Reimer, 2010 has presented different types of sequences of the brain given as shown in Table 1 with their specific indications.

5. BRAIN TUMOR SEGMENTATION TECHNIQUES FROM BRAIN MRI SEQUENCES

There are several techniques available for segmentation of brain tumor from brain MRI sequences(Angulakshmi & Priya, 2017). In this section, some of the important techniques are discussed.

Table 1. Different types of MRI sequences

FLAIR	• Common for lesion detection, usually for the white matter • Less sensitive in the posterior fossa • Applied for coronal or axial images • Usually combined with fat saturation to decrease the "glare" of bright subcutaneous fat
FLAIR + Gd	• Detection of leptomeningeal disease
PD/T2	• Proton density (first echo) is used as an alternative to FLAIR and is more sensitive for the detection of posterior fossa lesions • T2-WI (second echo) is the principal sequence for detection of long T2 lesions
DWI/ADC	• Mandatory for all patients with suspicion of stroke or cerebrovascular disease • Evaluation of cystic lesions • Useful during trauma to detect diffuse axonal injury (DAI) and hemorrhagic lesions • Brain tumors to assess cell density
SWI	• A sequence which combines magnitude and phase information • Detection of intracranial calcifications or hemosiderin deposits • Sensitive to the detection of "microbleeds" than gradient echo T2*-WI
T2*	• Gradient echo sequence provides information about hemoglobin breakdown products and calcifications • Sensitivity to susceptibility effects is proportional to TE and field strength
T1±Gd	• Portion of the most habitual brain imaging protocols • Usually applied in sagittal, axial or coronal imaging planes, depending on the indication • Identical imaging plane must be used prior to and subsequent to gadolinium-chelate injection
MP-RAGE, 3D SPGR(±Gd)	• Isotropic 3D T1-W sequence allows reformatting in other imaging planes • Provides the mechanism to differentiate between gray and white matter with high accuracy • Used to detect migration disorders (e.g., gray matter heterotopia, etc.) • Less responsive to enhancement in comparison with SE or TSE T1-W sequences
Fat-sat T2, STIR	• Indicated to notice white matter-lesions in "hard areas," for example in the optic nerve (optic neuritis)
TOF MRA	• Examine intracranial vessels and circle of Willis
Contrast-enhanced MRA	• Follow-up after endovascular aneurysm coiling • Time-resolved angiography (unravelling draining veins and afferent arteries)

Thresholding Method

Thresholding is the one of the simplest segmentation methods. The pixels present in the image are partitioned depending on their values of intensity.

Global thresholding is a kind of thresholding that uses an appropriate threshold T:

$$n(x,y) = \begin{cases} 1, & if\, m(x,y) > T \\ 0, & if\, m(x,y) \le T \end{cases} \quad (1)$$

Variable thresholding is a thresholding in which if T can change over the whole image.

If T depends on the neighborhood of the pixel(x, y) then it is called local thresholding. If T is the function of (x, y) then it is called adaptive thresholding.

Multiple thresholding:

$$n(x,y) = \begin{cases} p, & if\, m(x,y) > T2 \\ q, & if\, T1 < m(x,y) \le T2 \\ r, & if\, m(x,y) \le T1 \end{cases} \quad (2)$$

Choosing the appropriate threshold is one of the important tasks. Following figures represent histogram of the images with different peaks and valleys. That can be helpful in choosing the appropriate threshold(s).

Like in figure 1 T can be the appropriate threshold while in other figure T1 and T2 will be the good one. Few important factors that affect the appropriateness of the histogram for guiding the option of the appropriate threshold are:

1. the separation among peaks
2. the content of noise present in the image
3. the comparative size of background and objects

Figure 4. Histograms of different objects with different thresholds

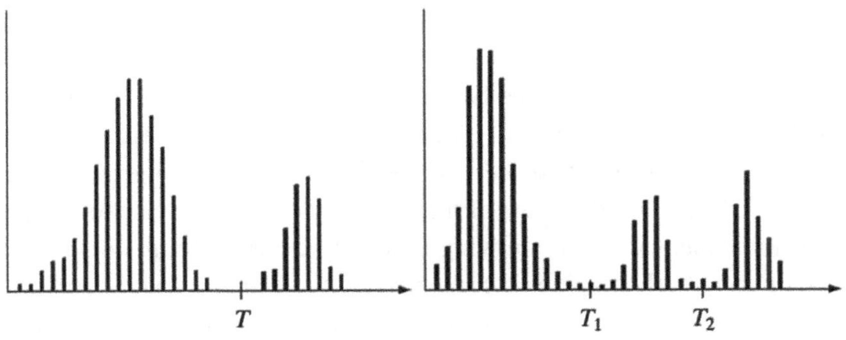

4. the consistency of the illumination
5. the evenness of the reflectance

Saad et al. (2011) has implemented brain lesion segmentation based on thresolding method. The important benefits of implementing this method it works fantastically for standardized image. However, the choice of the optimal threshold is not easy.

Edge-Based Method

Edges are confined changes in the intensity of the image. Edges normally transpire on the boundaries between two distinguished regions. The main features of the particular object can be computed from the edges of an image. Edge detection has a very significant role in image analysis.

There are numerous edge detection techniques available in the existing literatures. Those techniques are Roberts edge detection, Prewitt edge detection, Sobel Edge Detection, Marr-Hildreth edge detection, Kirsch edge detection, Robinson edge detection, LoG edge detection and Canny Edge Detection.

Aslam et al. (2015) have implemented edge based segmentation for brain tumor segmentation. In this literature an image dependent thresholding is implemented, that used with the combination with sobel operator to identify boundaries of the brain lesion. Further, the tumorous region is then localized using algorithm of closed contouring and object separation based segmentation. The outcomes of the developed technique are enhanced as per the traditional method that uses sobel operator. However, there were more depth on the boundary lines of the detected edges.

Mathur et al. (2016) the procedure of edge detection for segmentation is performed using the Fuzzy Inference System. The automatic thresholding is desined using fuzzy rule based on K-means. The disadvantage of this approach is it is too computationally expensive.

Region Growing Method

Region-growing method exploits the imperative fact that pixels that are close together are having analogous gray values. Start with a pixel i.e. called seed pixel and add new pixels. Following is the algorithm of region growing

1. Pick the seed pixel.
2. Ensure the neighboring pixels and insert them to the region if they are alike to the seed.
3. Repeat step 2 for every of the recently added pixels; discontinue if further no more pixels can be added.

Lin et al. (2012) proposed fuzzy knowledge-based seeded region growing for multispectral MR images. By considering the benefits of correlation and spatial information from multispectral images, similarity and fuzzy edges are used for defining first seed in modified seeded region growing method to localise brain tumour from MRI slices. Disadvantage of this method is that seed selection is quite difficult.

Viji et al. (2013) implemented region growing based on texture is. In the developed method, local texture in sequence of neighborhood pixel is computed. In this method texture and intensity threshold for a pixel are taken into account for region growing to localize tumorous region. Execution time is too high that can be considered as the drawback.

Watershed Algorithm

Watershed method is a dominant arithmetical morphological tool for the segmenting the image into its constituents regions. It is more accepted in the areas such as computer vision and biomedical image processing. In geography, means of watershed the ridges that divide regions drained by diverse river systems. Suppose image is viewed as geological landscape, the lines of watershed decide boundaries that divide regions of image. The watershed transform calculates ridgelines and catchment basins that is also known as watershed lines, where catchment basins corresponding to image regions and ridgelines relating to region boundaries. Segmentation by watershed embodies many of the concepts of the three techniques such as threshold based, edge based and region based segmentation.

Pandav et al. (2014) has implemented watershed transform for brain tumor segmentation. The main advantage of their work is that huge number of segmented region in edges is condensed by marker controlled watershed segmentation. However, forefront objects and the locations of background must be marked previously to get superior segmentation result.

Genetic Algorithm

It is the technique used for optimization and is based on the growth of a population of solutions which beneath the action of a few specific optimized rules. A GA manipulates a population of fixed size. This population is formed by chromosomes. Each chromosome represents the coding of a potential solution to the problem to be solved; it is formed by a set of genes belonging to an alphabet (Genetic Algorithms Tutorial, n.d.). At each iteration is formed a new population by applying the different genetic operators: selection, crossover and mutation. GA chooses in selection the most pertinent candidates. Crossover consists in building 2 new chromosomes from 2 old ones referred to as the parents. Mutation realizes the inversion of one or several genes in a chromosome. Following figure shows steps of genetic algorithm GA.

Chandra et al. (2016) used Genetic Algorithm for optimizing the localized results of brain tumour from MRI sequences, through evaluation criteria. In the proposed method, clusters of K -means algorithm is used as starting population. Centers that are clustered are evaluated by a fitness function. The main advantages of this method that it is good in selecting optimal number of region for segmentation. However, selection of fitness function is difficult.

Fuzzy Clustering

Fuzzy c-means (FCM), it is a method of clustering which that permits one piece of data to belong to two or more clusters. It is based on minimization of the following objective function:

$$J_m = \sum_{i=1}^{N}\sum_{j=1}^{C} u_{ij}^m x_i - c_j^2 ; 1 \le m \le \infty \tag{3}$$

where m is any real number greater than 1, u_{ij} is the degree of membership of x_i in the cluster j, x_i is the ith of d-dimensional measured data, c_j is the d-dimension center of the cluster, and ||*|| is any norm expressing the similarity between any measured data and the center.

Figure 5. General steps of genetic algorithm

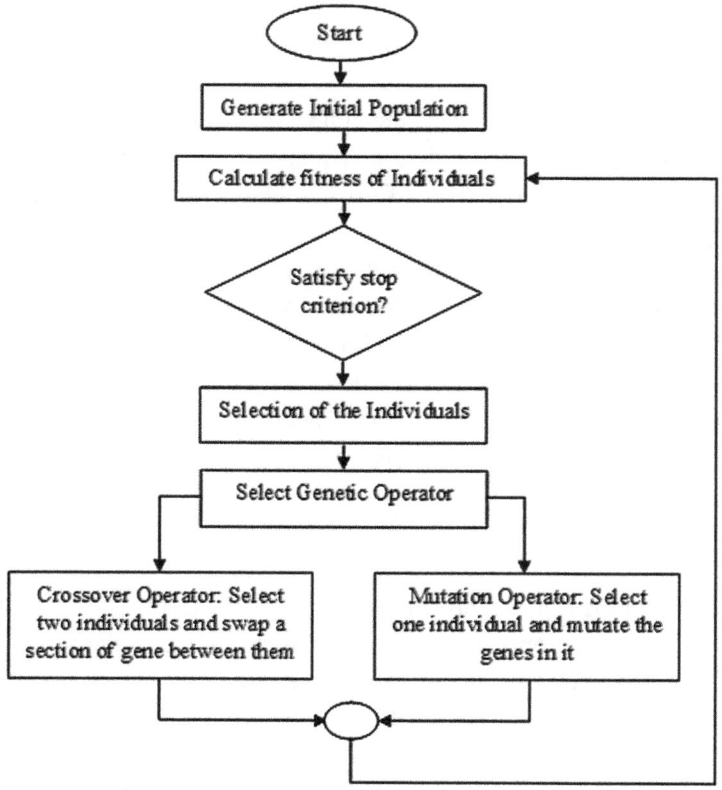

Fuzzy partitioning is carried out through an iterative optimization of the objective function shown above, with the update of membership u_{ij} and the cluster centers c_j by:

$$u_{ij} = \frac{1}{\sum_{k=1}^{C}\left(\frac{x_i - c_j}{x_i - c_k}\right)^{\frac{2}{m-1}}} \tag{4}$$

$$C_j = \frac{\sum_{i=1}^{N} u_{ij}^{m} \cdot x_i}{\sum_{i=1}^{N} u_{ij}^{m}} \tag{5}$$

This iteration will stop when $\max_{ij}\left\{\left|u_{ij}^{(k+1)}\right|u_{ij}^{(k)}\right\} < \epsilon$ where ϵ is a termination criterion between 0 and 1, whereas k are the iteration steps. So many researchers have implemented fuzzy c means clustering method for brain tumor localization.

Aina et al. (2014) author developed a multi-stage system. First stage is brain tumour diagnosis and the second is tumour region extraction. In first stage, different texture features are extracted from the brain MR slices. For classifying tumours ensemble based support vector machine (SVM) classification. In the second stage, brain region extraction, skull removal and brain tumour segmentation are implemented to take out the brain tumour. Drawback of this method is that it requires high computational complexity for combining different methods.

Verma et al. (2016) implemented an enhanced IFCM(Intuitionistic FCM) clustering algorithm, which includes the local spatial gray level information used in IFCM. The splitting method of Discrete Curve Evolution (DCE) methods are used to locate cluster for T1, T2 and PD MR Brain image segmentation. Drawback of this method is that Local spatial information is not incorporated in process of segmentation. Therefore this method is very much sustainable to noisy brain MR Slices.

Ji et al. (2014) developed AS-FLGMM (adaptive scale FLGMM) algorithm for brain MR image segmentation. They implemented a local scale inference method to estimate the variances of the Gaussian mixture model locally. Further, this is combined with Fuzzy C-means for localization. The initialisation of FCM is enhanced by the aforesaid method.

Dubey et al. (2016) implemented rough set based intuitionist fuzzy clustering. The initialisation of cluster centre is implemented using intuitionistic rough set. Membership of the cluster center is rationalized using intuitionistic rough set resemblance measure. The technique used to localize brain tumor an image into the CSF, WM, and GM, which is very useful for the diagnosis of brain diseases. Disadvantages of this approach is Setting the lower and upper estimate value for Roughness assess is hard.

Morphological-Based Method

Morphology is a enormous amount operations of image processing that modifies the images based on structure and shapes. It is well thought-out to be one of the data processing proceedure useful in image processing. It has many applications like noise elimination, texture analysis, boundary extraction and many more. Binary images may enclose innumerable defects. In a few circumstances binary regions constructed by simple thresholding are distorted by some noise and textures. The goal of morphological image processing is to remove all the defects discussed and while maintaining structure of an image. These operations are certain only on the connected ordering values of the pixels, than their numerical values, hence they are specifically focused more on binary images, however it can also be implement in greyscale images.

Morphological techniques probe an image with a template or small shape called as a structuring element(SE). The SE is located at all possible locations in the image and compared with the analogous neighbourhood of pixels. Some operations check whether the element fits within the neighbourhood, while others check whether it hits the neighbourhood. Dilation and Erosion are the basic two operation in image processing. Other algorithms based on dilation and erosion. The erosion of a binary image f by a SE s (denoted by $f \ominus s$) produces a new binary image $g = f \ominus s$ with ones in all locations (x, y) of a SE's source at which that SE s fits the input image f, i.e. $g(x,y) = 1$ is s fits f and 0 otherwise, repeating for all pixel coordinates (x, y). The dilation of an image f by a SE s (denoted by $f \oplus s$) produces a new binary image $g = f \oplus s$ with ones in all locations (x,y) of a structuring element's orogin at which that structuring element s hits the the input image f, i.e. $g(x,y) = 1$ if s hits f and 0 otherwise, repeating for all pixel coordinates (x,y)("Morphological Image Processing "(n.d.)).

Sudharani et al. (2016) has implemented a method to segment tumor in low intensity images. The method consists a number of steps to extract tumour from the MR slices, image enhancement, resampling of image, histogram application, color plane extraction, an advanced morphological operation to segment tumour region. In this method, morphological operations are principally used as the filter to eradicate low-frequency pixels and pixels present in the boundary. Different parameters of the tumour such as area and length are identified effectively for treatment planning and diagnosis of the tumour. The main drawback of this method is that this method uses so many repetitive steps for image segmentation.

K-Means Clustering

K-means clustering is a kind of unsupervised learning, that is used when we have unlabeled data (the data devoid of defined groups or categories). The objective of the K-means is to find groups in the unstructured data, with the numeral of groups presented by the variable *K*. This technique works iteratively to allocate each and every data point to one of *K* groups on the basis of the features that are given. Data points are clustered based on similarity of feature. The outcome of the *K*-means clustering algorithm are given below:

1. The centroids of the *K* clusters, which can be used to label new data
2. Labels for the training data

Rather than defining the groups previous to looking at the data, clustering allows us to analyze and find the groups that are formed organically (Trevino, n.d.).

Nimeesha et al. (2013) have modelled FCM and K-means on T1 contrast axial plane MRI sequences for extraction of brain tumour with the histogram guided initialization of the cluster. K-means is capable to cluster the regions relatively superior than FCM. FCM identifies barely three tissue classes, however K-means identifies all the six classes. Main drawback of this method is that Few WM(white matter) is characterized as edema and vice versa in using K-means.

Atlas Based Segmentation

In this kind of segmentation and atlas is developed that contains the combination of intensity image and the segmented image which is called as atlas labels. In this, the scrupulous case of deforming a brain atlas into a subject's brain is done with the intention of creating a new individualized brain atlas. Which is known as atlas-based segmentation and it relies on the existence of a reference MRI within which structures of interest have been previously segmented (labelled image). Then, a non-rigid registration between the reference and MRI of a subject is done. The resulting transformation encodes a pixel-by-pixel or voxel-by-voxel correspondence between the two MR images that can be applied to the reference labelled image in order to find out the structures of interest of the subject. We can say that once the non rigid registration can be efficiently applied between an atlas and a patient, segmentation becomes an easy task. Some possible applications of atlas-based segmentation include surgical planning, radiation therapy planning, automatic labelling or morphological and morphometrical studies of brain anatomy. Atlas-Based Segmentation of medical images is an image analysis task which involves labelling a desired anatomy or set of anatomy from images generated by medical imaging modalities. The overall goal of atlas-based segmentation is to assist radiologists in the detection and diagnosis of diseases. By extracting the relevant anatomy from medical images and presenting it in an appropriate view, their work-flow can be optimised.

Al-Shaikhli et al. (2014) have used the topological graph previous with information of atlas in a customized multilevel set formulation for multiregional localization of brain tumour MRI slices. Disadvantage of this method is accuracy of the proposed method depends on accurateness of topological graph priors.

Diaz et al. (2015) implemented mesh-free total Lagrangian explicit dynamic (TLED) method to pact model with atlas deformation and utilized the shape of the tumour segmented from multimodal MRI to derive a new tumour growth model. This method is able to handle large deformation without remeshing. The tumour growth models use actual shape of tumour instead of irregular shape and require no seed initialization. The method increased robustness to parameter variations and reduced computational time by means of parallel processing. Drawback of the proposed method is pre-processing of the brain MRI slices need to implemented for better results.

Artificial Neural Network (ANN)

Artificial Neural Network (ANN) is an well-organized computing system whose fundamental theme is rented from the correspondence of biological neural networks. It is also named as "parallel distributed processing systems," or "artificial neural systems," or "connectionist systems." It acquires a huge assortment of units that are interrelated in various patterns to permit messages among the units. These units are also referred to as neurons or nodes. These are simple processors that operate in parallel. Each and every neuron is associated with another neuron through a link. Each connection link is connected with a weight that consist information about the input signal. This is the most practical information for neurons to resolve a fastidious problem as the weight generally inhibits or excites the signal which is being communicated. Each and every neuron has an inner state, that is called a signal of activation. Output signals that are produced after incorporating the activation rule and input signals may be sent to another units (Artificial Intelligence Neural Networks (n.d.).).

Dahab et al. (2012) used modified probabilistic neural network (PNN) with linear vector quantization (LVQ) modeling procedure for classification for particular ROI(Region of Interest). The features set are extracted from each and every ROI to approximate brain tumour, each ROI is assigned a particular weight. These assigned weights are implemented for modelling network based on LVQ.

Mei et al. (2015) proposed a process that showed the impact of SOM (selforganizing map) in brain tumour extraction. In SOM, the training is based on topological map and competitive learning. The output result shows that the dented tissues are detached well from normal tissues. The system is proficient to cluster diverse areas with the tumour.

De et al. (2015) proposed a method to include spatial data and gray value of pixels in process of segmentation using LQV method. An adaptive segmentation algorithm is implemented for search of the segment number (codebook). The LVQ based on codebook learning is done by SOM. The common restraint of SOM is the lack of the accuracy of distance for input vectors and also to obtain the ideal mapping.

Marcov Random Field (MRF)

Segmentation is measured in a general framework, i.e. called image labeling, where the predicament is abridged to assigning particular labels to particular pixels. If we consider probabilistic approach, dependencies of the label are modeled by Markov random fields (MRF). Further, an optimal labeling is dogged by Bayesian estimation, in meticulous highest a posteriori (MAP) estimation. The major benefit of MRF models is that earlier information can be obligatory close by through clique potentials. MRF model incorporates spatial information into process of clustering. This deducts segmentation overlap and noise's effect in the segmentation. This special feature motivates different researchers to exploit MRF in segmentation.

Subbanna et al. (2012) proposed a method that uses the combined space feature to pull out the model using Gabor decomposition, to split tumour and nontumour region which includes edema as well. Further, the Bayesian classification with texture-based feature extraction is implemented to localize tumour and edema. The obtained results were auxiliary polished using MRF segmentation. Drawback of this method is that information of boundary is not captured precisely as process is based only on information of texture.

Subbanna et al. (2014) developed an iterative MRF frame work to include voxel-based MRF, adopted MRF, and regional MRF. The implemented framework was also used to categorize all the sub class of the brain image. The main restriction of MRF is its computational complexity and effective selection of parameters. However, it is frequently used to model properties of texture and intensity in homogeneity.

Deep Learning Method

Deep learning brought a new machine approach since 2006. Sometimes it is called as deep structured learning or hierarchical learning. It is an promising field of machine learning (ML) research. It consists of numerous hidden layers of ANN(artificial neural networks). For the large database, this kind of methodology applies model abstractions and nonlinear transformations. The topical advancements in deep learning architectures within plentiful fields have previously provided noteworthy assistance in the field of artificial intelligence. CNN (Convolutional Neural Network) is the competent way of implementing deep learning methodologies. It is generally unruffled with the layers set which can be gathered by their functionalities.

Shen et al. (2018) have developed a contemporaneous fully Convolutional Networks(CFCN) structure that contains three FCN. Mean filter, Gaussian filter and Median filter have been chosen for preprocessing the novel multimodal MRI sequences. Further, they fused the outcomes from three concurrent networks. At last, a Fully Connected Conditional Random Field (Fully Connected CRF) have been used to complete the post-processing part, by improving the generated model's ability of detecting structures of minuscule. For the future perspective, authors can compel on the modifications about the structure of FCN in order to reduce the errors of segmentation for the particular network. That can produce additional accurate results of segmentation.

In Havaei et al. (2016) authors have presented a fully automatic brain tumor segmentation method based on Deep Neural Networks (DNNs). Developed networks are personalized to high and low-grade glioblastomas. BRATS 2013 data set have been used for training and validation. They have achieved significant speed up and DSC (Dice Similarity Coefficient).

Rao et al. (2018) have also developed deep learning methods for brain tumor segmentation on BRATS 2015 challenges. Their method is to finding tumors in brain MR slices to accomplish a pixel-wise classification. They have used deep depictions for each pixel based on its locality in each modality such as T1, T2, FLAIR for learning and syndicate these to form a multimodal depiction for each pixel. They have accomplished the network with areas around 25000 arbitrarily elected pixels. Further, experimented the pixels so that their tags were in line with the circulation of the labels in the whole dataset.

In Seetha et al. (2018), authors have classified brain tumor using convolutional neural network. Instead of using large filters they have used small kernels. Experimental results demonstrate that the CNN archives rate of 97.5% correctness with low intricacy and associated with the all other state of arts methods. This classification method doesn't require feature extraction steps distinctly. The feature value is occupied from CNN itself. Hence the involvedness and time of computation is low and precision is high.

PSO (Particle Swarm Optimization) Based Method

Particle swarm optimization (PSO) algorithms are basically population-based and nature-inspired metaheuristic algorithms in the beginning. PSO impersonate the bird's social behavior of fishes schooling and flocking. Basically, PSO tries to enhance the solutions according to a quality measure i.e. fitness function form a haphazardly dispersed set of particles i.e. potential solutions.

Vijay et al. (2016) implemented Enhanced Darwinian Particle Swarm Optimization (EDPSO) for automated brain tumor segmentation that overcomes the negative aspect of existing PSO (Particle Swarm Optimization). This pioneering process basically consists of four steps. Pre-processing is the first step. In this film artifacts and superfluous portions of MRI sequences are disconnected using a particular tracking algorithm. The second step consists the procedure of removing the high frequency component and noises using Gaussian filter. In the third step, segmentation is implemented using Darwinian Particle Swarm Optimization. Further on the fourth step classification is implemented, that is done by using Adaptive Neuro Fuzzy Inference System. In the practical image dataset contained 101 brain MRI slices, which includes 87 tumorous brain images while other 14 brain images without tumor. Disadvantage of this approach is that performance is not up to the level of mark. In future several optimization algorithms can be combined in order to progress the system's performance in terms of robustness.

Normalized Cut Method

A normalized cut method is an annexe of using graph partitioning in order to achieve efficient and accurate segmentation. Graph partitioning can be implemented by combining a graph hooked on two disjoint sets of vertices. Basically, the grouping is based on the divergence among the two distinct pieces. Further, the cut measure is the sum of the capacities among the two distinct regions under deliberation. The optimal partitioning of the graph minimizes this cut transversely the whole graph, beneath only the least cut measure

Pezoulas et al. (2017) attempted to grant an application of these practices on brain tumor segmentation from MR Image sequences. More particularly, a novel skull stripping method is developed based on approach of normalized cut and histogram classification method is implemented on skull free MR sequences for more accurate segmentation. However, to achieve more accuracy more data need to be tested.

Hybrid Methods

The hybrid method incorporates the benefits of two or more types of methods used for brain tumour localization and segmentation. These methods are strong, speedy, and precise. The major benefit of hybrid method is that it uses the advantages of numerous diverse processes and produces the enhanced result. The main shortcoming is huge computational costs.

Demirhann and Guler (2011) proposed stationary wavelet transform (SWT) to acquire sub-images that include multi-resolution information. Spatial filtering procedure is then applied to pull out statistical features of different sub images. A multi-dimensional feature vector is created by combining coefficients of SWT and their corresponding statistical features. Further, this feature vector is used as input to the particular SOM. At last, LVQ is applied to refrain the end result. The correctness is extremely less for extracting white matter from brain MRI image which is the major drawback.

El-Sayed et al., (2015) implemented feedback pulse-coupled neural network(PCNN) technique for segmentation, discrete wavelet transform(DWT) for feature extraction, principal component analysis(PCA) for dimensionality reduction and further feed forward back-propagation neural network to classify inputs into abnormal or normal. The proposed process is accurate, hybrid, fast, and robust. In this method training phase takes more time.

Sachdeva et al. (2016) proposed content-based active contour to localize brain tumours. Obtained features are high-dimensional. To reduce those GA is implemented. GA with ANN and GA with SVM are implemented for brain tumour segmentation and classification and the results are compared. GA with SVM gives more benefits in terms of processing speed, and GA with ANN produce better accuracy. Again the problem in this case, is that computational complexity increases due to hybridization.

6. CONCLUSION

In this chapter, brain tumor and its types, brain MRI sequences, its various types with its applications have been discussed. In today's scenario MRI-based brain tumour segmentation techniques are implemented more for the segmentation of brain tumours due to the non-invasive nature of MRI and good soft tissue contrast. Various automated segmentation techniques of brain tumour from brain MRI sequences have been reviewed. Basically, the brief introductions of the implemented methods, their benefits, their precincts, have been discussed to give insight into various implemented methods such as thresholding, watershed, morphological, genetic algorithm, deep learning based and many more. Though, there are several automated methods are available for accurate brain tumor segmentation. However, efficient automated methods are very complicated to use in real time applications by the medical practitioner for treatment planning due to the lacking of the interpretability. In future, enhancement in the numerous class classifications of the brain tumors, tumor volume estimation, and many more will bring more interest of the researchers in this area. The automated brain tumor segmentation unquestionably demonstrate enormous prospective in future.

REFERENCES

Ain, Q., Jaffar, M. A., & Choi, T. (2014). Fuzzy anisotropic diffusion based segmentation and texture based ensemble classification of brain tumor. *Applied Soft Computing*, *21*, 330–340. doi:10.1016/j.asoc.2014.03.019

Al-Shaikhli, S. D., Yang, M. Y., & Rosenhahn, B. (2014). Multi-region labeling and segmentation using a graph topology prior and atlas information in brain images. *Computerized Medical Imaging and Graphics*, *38*(8), 725–734. doi:10.1016/j.compmedimag.2014.06.008 PMID:24998760

Angulakshmi, M., & Priya, G. L. (2017). Automated brain tumour segmentation techniques- A review. *International Journal of Imaging Systems and Technology*, *27*(1), 66–77. doi:10.1002/ima.22211

Artificial Intelligence. (n.d.). *Neural Networks*. Retrieved from https://www.tutorialspoint.com/artificial_intelligence/artificial_intelligence_neural_networks.htm

Aslam, A., Khan, E., & Beg, M. S. (2015). Improved Edge Detection Algorithm for Brain Tumor Segmentation. *Procedia Computer Science*, *58*, 430–437. doi:10.1016/j.procs.2015.08.057

Bauer, S., Wiest, R., Nolte, L., & Reyes, M. (2013). A survey of MRI-based medical image analysis for brain tumor studies. *Physics in Medicine and Biology*, *58*(13), R97–R129. doi:10.1088/0031-9155/58/13/R97 PMID:23743802

Boele, F., Rooney, A., Grant, R., & Klein, M. (2015). Psychiatric symptoms in glioma patients: From diagnosis to management. *Neuropsychiatric Disease and Treatment*, *1413*. doi:10.2147/ndt.s65874 PMID:26089669

Brain tumors: An Introduction. (2016). Retrieved from https://www.mayfieldclinic.com/PDF/PE-TumorIntro.pdf

Chandra, G. R., & Rao, K. R. (2016). Tumor Detection In Brain Using Genetic Algorithm. *Procedia Computer Science*, *79*, 449–457. doi:10.1016/j.procs.2016.03.058

Dahab, Ghoniemy, Gamal, & Selim. (2012). Automated brain tumour detection and identification using image processing and probabilistic neural network techniques. *Int J Image Process Visual Commun.*

De, A., & Guo, C. (2015). An adaptive vector quantization approach for image segmentation based on SOM network. *Neurocomputing*, *149*, 48–58. doi:10.1016/j.neucom.2014.02.069

Diaz, I., & Boulanger, P. (2015). Atlas to patient registration with brain tumor based on a mesh-free method. *2015 37th Annual International Conference of the IEEE Engineering in Medicine and Biology Society (EMBC)*. doi:10.1109/embc.2015.7319004

Dubey, Y. K., Mushrif, M. M., & Mitra, K. (2016). Segmentation of brain MR images using rough set based intuitionistic fuzzy clustering. *Biocybernetics and Biomedical Engineering*, *36*(2), 413–426. doi:10.1016/j.bbe.2016.01.001

El-Dahshan, E. A., Mohsen, H. M., Revett, K., & Salem, A. M. (2014). Computer-aided diagnosis of human brain tumor through MRI: A survey and a new algorithm. *Expert Systems with Applications*, *41*(11), 5526–5545. doi:10.1016/j.eswa.2014.01.021

Havaei, M., Davy, A., Farley, D. W., Biard, A., Courville, A., Bengio, Y., ... Larochelle, H. (2016). Brain tumor segmentation with Deep neural networks. *Medical Image Analysis*, *35*, 18–31. doi:10.1016/j.media.2016.05.004 PMID:27310171

Isensee, F., Kickingereder, P., Wick, W., Bendszus, M., & Maier-Hein, K. H. (2018). Brain Tumor Segmentation and Radiomics Survival Prediction: Contribution to the BRATS 2017 Challenge. Brainlesion: Glioma, Multiple Sclerosis, Stroke and Traumatic Brain Injuries Lecture Notes in Computer Science, 287-297. doi:10.1007/978-3-319-75238-9_25

Ji, Z., Xia, Y., Sun, Q., Chen, Q., & Feng, D. (2014). Adaptive scale fuzzy local Gaussian mixture model for brain MR image segmentation. *Neurocomputing*, *134*, 60–69. doi:10.1016/j.neucom.2012.12.067

Lin, G., Wang, W., Kang, C., & Wang, C. (2012). Multispectral MR images segmentation based on fuzzy knowledge and modified seeded region growing. *Magnetic Resonance Imaging*, *30*(2), 230–246. doi:10.1016/j.mri.2011.09.008 PMID:22133286

Louis, D. N., Ohgaki, H., Wiestler, O. D., Cavenee, W. K., Burger, P. C., Jouvet, A., ... Kleihues, P. (2007). The 2007 WHO Classification of Tumours of the Central Nervous System. *Acta Neuropathologica*, *114*(2), 97–109. doi:10.100700401-007-0243-4 PMID:17618441

Mathur, N., Mathur, S., & Mathur, D. (2016). A Novel Approach to Improve Sobel Edge Detector. *Procedia Computer Science*, *93*, 431–438. doi:10.1016/j.procs.2016.07.230

Mei, P. A., Carneiro, C. D., Fraser, S. J., Min, L. L., & Reis, F. (2015). Analysis of neoplastic lesions in magnetic resonance imaging using self-organizing maps. *Journal of the Neurological Sciences*, *359*(1-2), 78–83. doi:10.1016/j.jns.2015.10.032 PMID:26671090

Morphological Image Processing. (n.d.). Retrieved from https://www.cs.auckland.ac.nz/courses/compsci773s1c/lectures/ImageProcessing-html/topic4.htm

Nimeesha, K.M., & Gowda, R.M. (2013). Brain tumour segmentation using Kmeans and fuzzy c-means clustering algorithm. *Int J Comput Sci Inf Technol Res Excell*, 60–65.

Pandav, S. (2014). Brain tumor extraction using marker controlled watershed segmentation. *Int J Eng Res Technol.*

Pereira, S., Pinto, A., Alves, V., & Silva, C. A. (2016). Brain Tumor Segmentation Using Convolutional Neural Networks in MRI Images. *IEEE Transactions on Medical Imaging*, *35*(5), 1240–1251. doi:10.1109/TMI.2016.2538465 PMID:26960222

PET/MRI Scan. (n.d.). Retrieved from https://stanfordhealthcare.org/medical-tests/p/pet-mri-scan.html

Pezoulas, V. C., Zervakis, M., Pologiorgi, I., Seferlis, S., Tsalikis, G. M., Zarifis, G., & Giakos, G. C. (2017). A tissue classification approach for brain tumor segmentation using MRI. *2017 IEEE International Conference on Imaging Systems and Techniques (IST)*. 10.1109/IST.2017.8261542

Reimer, P. (2010). *Clinical MR imaging: A practical approach.* Heidelberg, Germany: Springer. doi:10.1007/978-3-540-74504-4

Saad, N. M., Abu-Bakar, S. A., Muda, S., & Mokji, M. (2011). Segmentation of brain lesions in diffusion-weighted MRI using thresholding technique. *2011 IEEE International Conference on Signal and Image Processing Applications (ICSIPA)*. 10.1109/ICSIPA.2011.6144092

Sachdeva, J., Kumar, V., Gupta, I., Khandelwal, N., & Ahuja, C. K. (2016). A package-SFERCB-"Segmentation, feature extraction, reduction and classification analysis by both SVM and ANN for brain tumors. *Applied Soft Computing*, *47*, 151–167. doi:10.1016/j.asoc.2016.05.020

Seetha, J., & Raja, S. S. (2018). Brain Tumor Classification Using Convolutional Neural Networks. *Biomedical & Pharmacology Journal*, *11*(3), 1457–1461. doi:10.13005/bpj/1511

Shen, G., Ding, Y., Lan, T., Chen, H., & Qin, Z. (2018). Brain Tumor Segmentation Using Concurrent Fully Convolutional Networks and Conditional Random Fields. *Proceedings of the 3rd International Conference on Multimedia and Image Processing - ICMIP 2018*. 10.1145/3195588.3195590

Subbanna, N., Precup, D., & Arbel, T. (2014). Iterative Multilevel MRF Leveraging Context and Voxel Information for Brain Tumour Segmentation in MRI. *2014 IEEE Conference on Computer Vision and Pattern Recognition*. 10.1109/CVPR.2014.58

Subbanna, N. K., & Arbel, T. (2012). Probabilistic Gabor and Markov random fields, segmentation of brain tumours in MRI volumes. *Proceedings of the MICCAI-BRATS.*

Sudharani, K., Sarma, T., & Prasad, K. S. (2016). Advanced Morphological Technique for Automatic Brain Tumor Detection and Evaluation of Statistical Parameters. *Procedia Technology*, *24*, 1374–1387. doi:10.1016/j.protcy.2016.05.153

Trevino, A. (n.d.). *Introduction to K-means Clustering.* Retrieved from https://www.datascience.com/blog/k-means-clustering

Tutorialspoint.com. (n.d.). *Genetic Algorithms Tutorial.* Retrieved from https://www.tutorialspoint.com/genetic_algorithms/

Understanding Brain Tumors. (1999). Retrieved from https://www.brainandlife.org/siteassets/about-us/about-brain--life/understanding-brain-tumors.pdf

Verma, H., Agrawal, R., & Sharan, A. (2016). An improved intuitionistic fuzzy c-means clustering algorithm incorporating local information for brain image segmentation. *Applied Soft Computing*, *46*, 543–557. doi:10.1016/j.asoc.2015.12.022

Vijay, V., Kavitha, A., & Rebecca, S. R. (2016). Automated Brain Tumor Segmentation and Detection in MRI Using Enhanced Darwinian Particle Swarm Optimization (EDPSO). *Procedia Computer Science*, *92*, 475–480. doi:10.1016/j.procs.2016.07.370

Viji, K. S., & Jayakumari, J. (2013). Modified texture based region growing segmentation of MR brain images. *2013 IEEE Conference On Information And Communication Technologies*. 10.1109/CICT.2013.6558183

Zhao, X., Wu, Y., Song, G., Li, Z., Fan, Y., & Zhang, Y. (2016). Brain Tumor Segmentation Using a Fully Convolutional Neural Network with Conditional Random Fields. Brainlesion: Glioma, Multiple Sclerosis, Stroke and Traumatic Brain Injuries Lecture Notes in Computer Science, 75-87. doi:10.1007/978-3-319-55524-9_8

Chapter 5
Early Detection of Parkinson's Disease:
An Intelligent Diagnostic Approach

Debashree Devi
National Institute of Technology Silchar, India

Saroj K. Biswas
National Institute of Technology Silchar, India

Biswajit Purkayastha
National Institute of Technology Silchar, India

ABSTRACT

Parkinson's disease (PD) is a neurodegenerative disorder that occurs due to corrosion of the substantia nigra, located in the thalamic region of the human brain, and is responsible for transmission of neural signals throughout the human body by means of a brain chemical, termed as "dopamine." Diagnosis of PD is difficult, as it is often affected by the characteristics of the medical data of the patients, which include presence of various indicators, imbalance cases of patients' data records, similar cases of healthy/ affected persons, etc. Through this chapter, an intelligent diagnostic system is proposed by integrating one-class SVM, extreme learning machine, and data preprocessing technique. The proposed diagnostic model is validated with six existing techniques and four learning models. The experimental results prove the combination of proposed method with ELM learning model to be highly effective in case of early detection of Parkinson's disease, even in presence of underlying data issues.

DOI: 10.4018/978-1-5225-8567-1.ch005

INTRODUCTION

Parkinson's Disease (PD) is a progressive, neurodegenerative disorder that basically effects the motor system of a human being which causes physical problems such as shaking, stiffness, and difficulty in walking, balancing and coordinating movements (Parkinson's disease) (Mohamed, 2016). PD is basically central nervous system oriented disease, occurred due to disintegration of a region called "substantia nigra" in the thalamic region of human brain (Figure 1).

This substantia nigra secretes a neurochemical named "dopamine" which is responsible for transmitting of neural signals to the different organs and parts of the human body (Figure 2).

With increase of dopamine loss in the course of time, the PD progresses gradually which ultimately leads to mental disorder such as thinking and behavioral disability, dementia, depression and anxiety, sleep disorder, lack of emotions etc. (Olanrewaju, Sahari, Musa, Hakiem, 2014).The various movement-difficulties experienced by PD-suffered individuals are collectively addressed by the term "Parkinsonism". It has been revealed in a recent survey in 2015 that approximately there are 7-10 million people are suffering from PD in the worldwide. The occurrence of PD is much higher in case of elderly people, typically over the age of 60 years; with a male-to-female ratio of 3:2 (Parkinson's disease) (Mohamed, 2016).

Parkinsonism is defined by "Bradykinesia", a spectrum of movement disorder, commonly known as hypokinesia. Bradykinesia refers to a situation when a person's movement or initiation of voluntary body-movement has slowed down, due to disruption in basal ganglia of human brain, with an increasing reduction of speed and range of repetitive actions (Parkinson's disease). Bradykinesia is considered to be one of the four key symptoms of PD, along with rigidity, tremor, and postural instability (Pahwa and Lyons, 2013).

Figure 1. Location of Substantia nigra in human brain (Parkinson's disease)

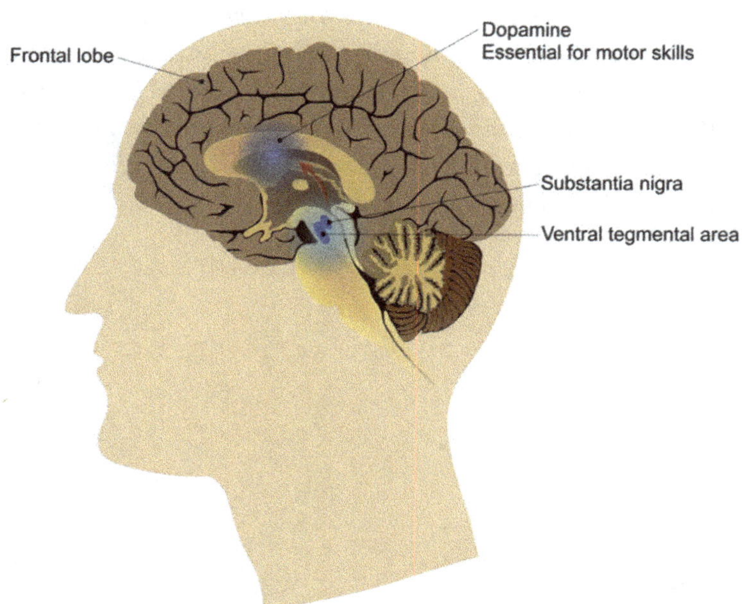

Figure 2. Comparison of neurons of normal and PD-affected persons (Parkinson's disease)

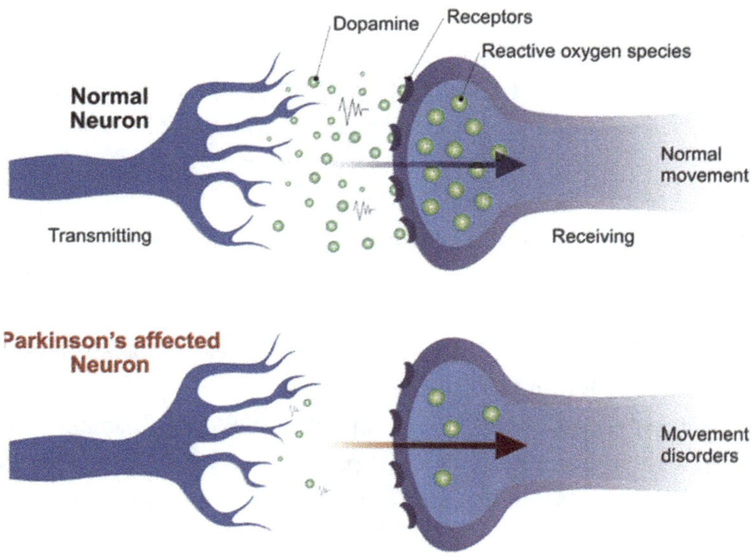

There is no remedy or prevention available for PD. However, PD can be controlled if diagnosed at an early stage. Basically, in clinical diagnosis, PD is diagnosed with the presence of two or three of the four key motor-sign symptoms, namely tremor, rigidity, Bradykinesia and postural disability. The risk factor of PD tends to increase with the age of an individual. Most of the motor-sign symptoms are remained unnoticed as they are similar to the aging-sign of an elderly individual. By early detection of PD, its effect can be minimized on the affected person and proper treatment can be offered. One of the advanced and recent method of early detection of PD is using of biomarkers. Biomarker namely DaTscan, which is approved by FDA, to be used in diagnosis test of PD. The DaTscan (Ioflupane ^{123}I injection, also known as phenyltropane) is a radiopharmaceutical agent which is injected into a patient's veins in a procedure referred to as SPECT imaging (DAT-scanning) (DaTSCAN, 2011). It is used to detect the loss of nerve cells in the striatum region of human brain, specifically the cells that release dopamine. However, the use of DaTscan also carries risk of allergic reaction, especially in case of pregnant women (DaTSCAN, 2011). Hence, there is a demand for development of intelligent data mining techniques which can provide efficient and early detection and diagnosis of PD, without risking the side-effects of treatments. A number of research works have been proposed in recent years based on this idea (Olanrewaju, Sahari, Musa, Hakiem, 2014) (Alemami and Almazaydeh, 2014) (Mohamed, 2016) (Caliskan, Badem, Baştürk, Yüksel, 2017) (Anita and Aruna Priya, 2016).

On application of data mining techniques to clinical diagnosis, they are more often affected by the characteristics of the underlying dataset. Clinical data are characterized by the presence of similar/overlapping cases, data imbalance and data redundancy. The similarities of the symptoms of PD with the other neurodegenerative disorders, such supranuclear palsy and multiple system atrophy (Olanrewaju, Sahari, Musa, Hakiem, 2014) (Ahmed, Santosh, Kumar, Christlet, 2009); make it difficult to precisely diagnose PD. Moreover, most of the clinical datasets have imbalanced data, which infer a scenario where cases of a specific category are found to be very high as compared to the other category. This is commonly termed as the "data imbalance" where data associated to the cases have skewed distribution which leads to produce results biased towards the majority case, when standard learning models are employed. Another issue is data redundancy, which is a common erroneous feature available in case of clinical data, as the medical history of a specific person can be recorded multiple times for diagnosis purpose. All these factors bring forward the requirement of developing an intelligent diagnostic system which can facilitate efficient and early detection of PD, from a set of clinical data even in presence issues such as overlapping cases, data imbalance, and data redundancy. The objectives of this chapter are listed as below:

1. **Detection of Overlapping Cases**: For detection of overlapping cases, one-class SVM model is employed to extract the outliers. The outliers are defined as the case instances which are not belonging to the range of novel instances, within a definite case. One-class SVM, is commonly known as ϑ -SVM (Vlasveld, 2013) defines the parameter, ϑ which denotes the percentage of similar/overlapping cases within a definite case.
2. **Cleaning Up of Overlapping Cases:** The concept of Tomek-link (Tomek, 1976) pair is refined to obtain the set of Abnormal Tomek- link (ATL) pairs whose significance is rare for classification purpose. The overlapping cases belong to ATL are selected for elimination. Following this, sparse neighborhood of majority overlapping cases is determined with higher misclassification probability. Cleaning up of overlapping zone is achieved by joint application of ATL and sparse neighborhood.
3. **Undersampling of the Majority Instances**: Basic Tomek-link pair (Tomek, 1976) concept, defined as Normal Tomek link (NTL) is used to detect the boundary majority instances contributing noise. The factor of data redundancy and intra-cluster significance is then incorporated with NTL to obtain a set of noisy, redundant and least significant majority instance cases. Redundancy among the instances is determined as the similarity among them while intra-cluster significance is defined as the respective distances of the majority instances to the centroid of the majority class. The detected instance cases are subjected to elimination.
4. **An Effective Data-Preprocessing Framework:** A new data processing framework is defined by incorporating the concepts of ATL, sparse neighborhood, NTL, redundancy and intra-cluster significance to compress the overlapping zone while balancing the data imbalance. The improvement of the classifier performance in the proposed scheme is evaluated with respect to Feed Forward Neural Network (FFNN), Support Vector Machine (SVM), Extreme Learning Machine (ELM), and Naive Bayes classifiers. A comparative analysis with seven state-of-the-art techniques is also carried out in this chapter.

BACKGROUND

The early detection of PD is very much crucial from adequate diagnosis point of view. The diagnosis of PD fails to detect the disease, before the patient has a significant loss of dopamine (Olanrewaju, Sahari, Musa, Hakiem, 2014). The movement-disability symptoms carry similarity with other neurological disorders, which create ambiguity during diagnosis. On discussing the PD, individuals with PD tend to lose the nerve endings that produce norepinephrine, the prime chemical messenger of the sympathetic nervous system, which controls many automatic functions of the body, such as heart rate and blood pressure (Pahwa and Lyons, 2013).The brain cells of patients affected with PD, contain Lewy bodies, which are unusual clumps of the protein alpha-synuclein. Scientists are in a mission to understand the normal and abnormal functions of alpha-synuclein and its relationship to genetic mutations that impact PD and Lewy body dementia (Pahwa and Lyons, 2013).

Although, in general the occurrence of PD in an individual appears to be hereditary, and a few can be traced to specific genetic mutations, in most of the cases the disease occurs randomly and does not seem to run in families. Many researchers have revealed the fact that PD is resultant of a combination of genetic factors and environmental factors such as exposure to toxins.

To discuss the various symptoms of PD, they can be listed down as below: (Pahwa and Lyons, 2013) (Parkinson's disease)

Basic motor-sign symptoms:

- Tremor (trembling) in hands, arms, legs, jaw, or head.
- Stiffness of the limbs and legs
- Bradykinesia: Slowness of movement
- Postural disability i.e. impaired balance and coordination

Additional symptoms include:

- Depression
- Dementia
- Emotional breakdown or lack of emotions
- Difficulty swallowing, chewing, and speaking
- Urinary problems or constipation
- skin problems
- Sleep disruptions.
- Blood pressure variation.
- Smell dysfunction
- Fatigue.
- Sexual dysfunction.

Early symptoms of Parkinson's disease are subtle and occur gradually. For example, affected people may feel mild tremors or have difficulty getting out of a chair. It is also noticed that they speak too softly or that their handwriting is slow and looks cramped or small. Parkinsonian gait (Pahwa and Lyons, 2013) is a common body deformity gained by PD- patients that involves a tendency to lean forward, associated with small quick steps as if hurrying forward, and reduced swinging of the arms. They also may have trouble on initiating or continuing body movement.

On discussing the risk factors of PD, these include the followings (Pahwa and Lyons, 2013):

- **Age**: Age carries a big risk factor in case of PD-affected people. Generally people with age>60 or more, easily develop this disease. About 5-10% of people have "early-onset" PD, which begins before the age of 50.
- **Heredity**: Having a close relative with Parkinson's disease increases the chances of developing the disease.
- **Sex:** Men are more likely to develop Parkinson's disease than women.

- **Exposure to Toxins**: Ongoing exposure to herbicides and pesticides may slightly increase the risk of Parkinson's disease.

Treatment of Parkinson's Disease

There is no standard treatment or remedy available for Parkinson's disease. There are some medicines, surgical treatments, and other therapies which can reduce the effect of PD.

Medicines prescribed for Parkinson's disease include:

- Drugs those increase the level of dopamine in the brain.
- Drugs those affect other brain chemicals in the body.
- Drugs those help to control motor-sign symptoms.

Alternative mode of treatments involves:

- **Deep Brain Stimulation:** For people with severe PD who has stopped responding to medications, deep brain stimulation, or **DBS,** may be an appropriate mode of treatment. DBS is a surgical procedure that surgically implants electrodes into part of the brain and connects them to a small electrical device implanted in the chest. The device and electrodes painlessly stimulate the brain in a way that helps stop many of the movement-disability of PD, such as tremor, slowness of movement, and rigidity.
- **Therapies**: A number of therapies are available which can be used for treatment of PD. These include physical, occupational, and speech therapies, which help with gait and voice disorders, tremors and rigidity, and decline in mental functions. Other supportive therapies include a healthy diet and exercises to strengthen muscles and improve balance.

DIAGNOSIS OF PARKINSON'S DISEASE

The early signs of PD are often misconceptualized as signs of aging. As a result, treatments are not sought at the early stage. The available treatments of PD are likely to be more effective when it's started in its early stage. Moreover, a number of neurological disorders have symptoms similar to those of PD. So, there are higher chances of misdiagnosis. The medical conditions with similar features to PD are listed below (Pahwa and Lyons, 2013):

- Drug-induced Parkinsonism
- Head trauma
- Encephalitis
- Stroke
- Lewy body dementia
- Corticobasal degeneration
- Multiple system atrophy
- Progressive supranuclear palsy

Since the diseases have similar features as PD but require different treatments, it is important to make an exact diagnosis as soon as possible. There are currently no blood or laboratory tests are available to diagnose non-genetic cases of PD. Diagnosis is done based on a person's medical history and a neurological examination. This way of clinical diagnosis can also be erroneous due to the presence of various indicators, similar cases of patients, data imbalance, and redundant data. In presence of data imbalance, there is a higher chance misdiagnosing a patient as the healthy one, if the cases of affected individuals create the minority class. In such scenario, it is very important to diagnose PD accurately since if a patient is misdiagnosed as healthy, his condition might worsen over the time.

Due to all these factors, a number of researchers have adopted data mining tools and techniques for precise diagnosis of PD. Some of the research works are discussed below:

- M. S. Islam *et al.* (Islam, Parvez, Deng, Goswami, 2014) conducted a comparative analysis for effective detection on Parkinson's disease using Random tree (RT), SVM and Feed forward Back Propagation Neural Network (FBPNN).
- A. Sharma and Ram Nivas (Sharma and Giri, 2014) evaluated the performance of the model build using Artificial Neural Networks (ANN), K-Nearest Neighbor (KNN), and SVM with radial basis function.
- A. H. Hadjahamadi and T. J. Askari (Hadjahamadi and Askari, 2012) compared various classification methods (Bayesian Network, C5.1, SVM, ANN) for diagnosis of PD. They indicated that the role of computing of the variable (feature) is an important issue in many applied problems complementing variable selection by interpretation issues.
- Y. Alemami and L. Almazaydeh (Alemami and Almazaydeh, 2014) developed and validated classification algorithms based on Naïve Bayes and KNN; their results show that the automated classification algorithm, Naïve Bayes, and KNN obtained a high degree of accuracy around 93.3%.
- Olanrewaju *et al.* (Olanrewaju, Sahari, Musa, Hakiem, 2014) proposed a model in early detection and diagnosis of PD by using the Multi-Layer Feedforward Neural Network (MLFNN) with Back-propagation (BP) algorithm. The output of the network is classified into healthy or PD by using K-Means Clustering algorithm.
- Caliskan *et al.* (Caliskan, Badem, Baştürk, Yüksel, 2017) proposed a deep neural network model using stacked autoencoder and softmax classifier for diagnosis of PD.
- G. S. Mohamed (Mohamed, 2016) discussed the effect of attribute selection and discretization of PD dataset over the diagnosis of PD.
- Anita *et al.* (Anita, S. and Aruna Priya. P, 2016) have developed an ANN model for prediction of Gamma-Amino Butyric Acid (GABA) concentration level for PD and Healthy Group (HG).
- Finberg *et al.* (Finberg *et al.*, 2013) has proposed an advanced technique of PD detection, by detecting of volatile molecules in exhaled breath (sensor array), and thus chances of person having PD or not.
- Chatterjee, Saxena, Vyas, and Mehra (Chatterjee, Saxena, Vyas, Mehra, 2018) have proposed cepstral feature based real-time program for detection of neurological health of a person, based on analysis of the utterance of "aah" by a person. Then, SVM classifier is used to identify the odds of PD based on various audio samples of both healthy as well as affected people.
- De Souza et al. (De Souza, Almeida, Rebouças Filho, 2017) proposed a similarity extraction approach by using structural similarity, mean squared error and peak signal-to-noise ratio measures, to evaluate the variations obtained in exam template and the handwritten trace generated by the

PD patient. Each of these variations was used together with the Naive Bayes, OPF, and SVM classifiers.

- Schindlbeck and Eidelberg (Schindlbeck and Eidelberg, 2018) have proposed PD-related functional network imaging which can capture the whole brain and the responses of the patients are recorded.
- Parisi et al. (Parisi, RaviChandran, Manaog, 2018) has proposed a Multi-Layer Perceptron based feature selection technique in integration Lagrangian Support Vector Machine for classification of people, affected with PD.
- Hariharana, Polat, and Sindhu (Hariharana, Polat, Sindhu, 2014) have proposed a hybrid intelligent system by combining feature pre-processing, feature reduction/selection and classification tasks. For feature pre-processing, Model-based clustering (Gaussian mixture model) is used. Feature selection is done by using principal component analysis (PCA), linear discriminant analysis (LDA), sequential for-ward selection (SFS) and sequential backward selection (SBS). For classification task, Least-Square Support Vector Machine (LS-SVM), Probabilistic Neural Network (PNN) and General Regression Neural Network (GRNN) are employed.
- Nilashi *et al.* (Nilashi, Ibrahim, Ahmadi, Shahmoradi, Farahmand, 2018) defined the concept of Unified Parkinson's Disease Rating Scale (UPDRS) in detection of PD, and have proposed incremental SVM based prediction system for prediction of Total- UPDRS and Motor- UPDRS.
- Chen *et al.* (Chen, Huang, Yu, Xu, Sun, Wang, Wang, 2013) have proposed Principal Component Analysis (PCA) based feature selection method for selecting the features, which are then classified by using non-linear classifier to detect the patients with PD.
- Picillo *et al.* (Picillo, Moccia, Spina, Barone, Pellecchia, 2015) have performed a comparison analysis of different biomarkers (clinical, biochemical or imaging), to retrieve the best combination of biomarkers for detection of PD in its different stages.

DIAGONOSIS OF PARKINSON'S DISEASE

Issues

The treatment of PD is generally done based on medical history of the patient and the neurological analysis. Hence, the collected medical data carries a vital role in the developing an efficient diagnostic system. Data collected for clinical diagnosis are used to be incomplete, imbalanced, and redundant, due to lack of effective data collection techniques. Moreover, the available real-life medical data are usually random data, collected from random sources. Profiling and offering treatment of a patient based on these data would carry a higher risk. Data pre-processing techniques allow mending the raw data to minimize incompleteness, imbalance and redundancy of data.

SOLUTIONS AND RECOMMENDATIONS

As a solution to the issues experienced during diagnosis of PD, the authors of this chapter have come with a concept of intelligent diagnostic system. An intelligent diagnostic system offers to deliver an efficient and rapid early detection of PD, with an aim of reduced misdiagnosis rate, even in the presence of similar/overlapping cases of patients (overlapping cases) and data imbalance. An effective data pre-processing technique is a mandatory stage for treatment of overlapping cases, data imbalance, and data redundancy. ELM classification model is considered for detection of PD, in a test individual. The motivation of an intelligent diagnostic system is to offer rapid and efficient early detection of PD, in patients in presence of different adversities.

Proposed Methodology for Intelligent Diagnosis System

The proposed methodology can be categorized into two stages, namely a) *data preprocessing stage* and b) *learning stage*. The data preprocessing stage involves mining the initial training data before learning. It involves two sub-stages, namely 1) *detection of class overlapping cases*, and 2) *cleaning up of the overlapping cases and undersampling of imbalanced data.*

The initial case set is fed to one-class SVM model to detect the overlapping cases. The cases detected as outliers are extracted to generate the overlapping zone. In the next stage, cleaning up of the most insignificant overlapping cases is performed by detecting *Abnormal Tomek-Link pairs (ATL)*. The *ATL* pair concept is introduced for efficient detection of similar cases out of healthy and affected patients. Following to this, the issue of data imbalance has been treated in terms of redundancy and intra-cluster significance among the patients' cases. The refined case set is then fed to the learning stage for diagnosis/ classification of the PD (affected/ healthy). Extreme Learning Machine (ELM) learner is used for diagnosis of the disease, against a set of test cases, and then, the performance of the method is evaluated. The pictorial representation of the proposed methodology is presented in figure 3.

For comprehensive understanding of the proposed system, the following notations are considered. Table 1 represents corresponding description of each notation.

Data Pre-Processing Stage

This stage involves preprocessing the initial case set with aspects of class overlapping and data imbalance. One-class SVM is implemented for detection of overlapping cases. The presence of data imbalance is then treated with consent of overlapping cases in order to achieve a refined case set with balanced class distribution and a compressed overlapping zone. Figure 4 presents the block diagram of the various sub-stages in step-by-step manner. The sub-stages are discussed in details as below:

Figure 3. Framework of the proposed scheme

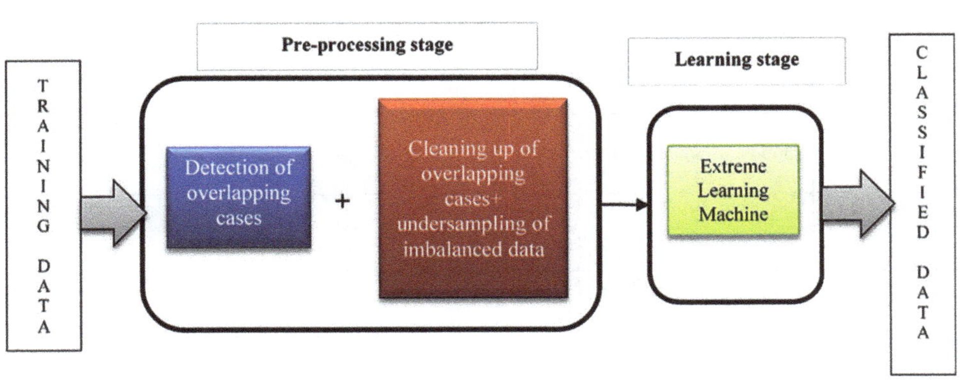

Table 1. Notations and descriptions

Notations	Descriptions
$S_{n\times l}$	An imbalanced training dataset, with *n*- number of total instances and $l - number$ of total features
$\vec{x}_a$	$= \left(x_{a1}, x_{a2}, \cdots\cdots x_{al}\right)$; input vector of ath - instance of $S_{n\times l}$, with a total of *l*-features
y_b	$= \left(y_1, y_2, \cdots\cdots y_c\right)$ = set of designated class labels for instances in $S_{n\times l}$ with a total of *c*-classes
S_{min}	Set of minority class instances, where $S_{min} : \left\{x_i \mid i = 1,2,\ldots.,p\right\}$, where p is the total minority-class instances
S_{maj}	Set of majority class instances, where $S_{maj} : \left\{x_m \mid m = 1,2,\ldots,q\right\}$, where q is the total majority-class instances
NN_{maj}	Nearest neighbor from majority class
TL	Set of Tomek-link pairs
reg_{ovr}	Overlapping region
ovr_reg_{min}	Overlapping region of minority class
ovr_reg_{maj}	Overlapping region of majority class
nov_reg_{min}	Set of novel minority instances
nov_reg_{maj}	Set of novel majority instances
$NN_{hits}\left(x_m\right)$	K-NN hits of x_m where $class\left(x_m\right) = class\left(NN\right)$
$NN_{miss}\left(x_m\right)$	K-NN misses of x_m, where $class\left(x_m\right) \neq class\left(NN\right)$
sp_{NN}	Set of instances with sparse neighborhood
$d\left(x_a, x_b\right)$	Euclidean distance between instances x_a and x_b
d_{intra_cen}	Intra-centroid distance of x_m
cen_{maj}	Centroid of majority set, S_{maj}

Figure 4. Step-by-step block diagram of the working of data pre-processing stage

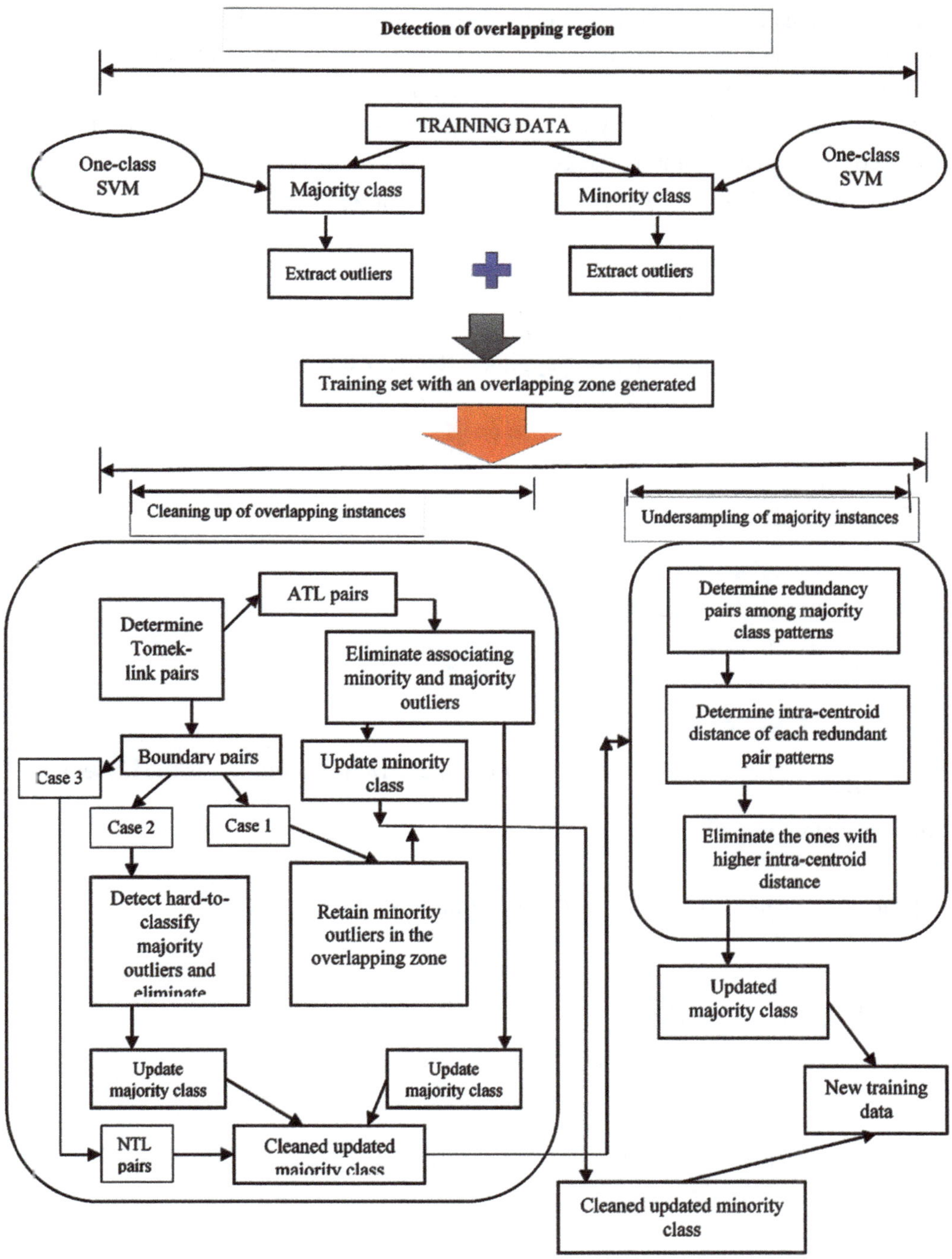

Detection of Overlapping Region

One-class SVM defines a domain-based novelty detection, by setting a boundary to extract the transformed case instances with maximum margin in the feature space. The case instances not falling in the proximity of the maximum margin are termed as "outliers". In the proposed methodology, the one-class SVM model is applied to both minority and majority case sets to obtain the set of outliers from each case. These set of outliers are combined together to generate the overlapping zone, reg_{ovr} for the entire training data. Formal depiction of this stage is presented below:

Input: $S_{\min}$, S_{maj}

Step 1: Apply one-class SVM to $S_{\min}$ and S_{maj}.

Step 2: Extract the outliers to obtain the overlapping instances from S_{maj} and store in the set, ovr_reg_{maj} as:

$$ovr_{regmaj} = \left\{x_m' \mid f\left(x_m'\right) < 0; x_m' \in S_{maj}\right\} \tag{1}$$

$$nov\_reg_{maj} = \left\{x_m' \mid f\left(x_m'\right) > 0; x_m' \in S_{maj}\right\} \tag{2}$$

where $f\left(x_m'\right) = \sum_{m=1}^{q} \alpha_m K\left(x_m', x\right) - \rho$; for $K\left(x_m', x\right)$ is the kernel function, ρ is the offset and α_m is the center of majority class region.

Step 3: Repeat step (1) and (2) for $S_{\min}$ and the resultant is

$$ovr\_reg_{\min} = \left\{x_i' \mid f\left(x_i'\right) < 0; x_i' \in S_{\min}\right\} \tag{3}$$

$$nov\_reg_{\min} = \left\{x_i' \mid f\left(x_i'\right) > 0; x_i' \in S_{\min}\right\} \tag{4}$$

where $f\left(x_i'\right) = \sum_{i=1}^{p} \alpha_i K\left(x_i', x\right) - \rho$; for $K\left(x_i', x\right)$ is the kernel function, ρ is the offset and α_i is the center of minority class region.

Step 4: Generate overlapping zone for entire training data as:

$$reg_{ovr} = ovr\_reg_{\min} + ovr\_reg_{maj} \tag{5}$$

Output: ovr_reg_{maj}, ovr_reg_{min}, reg_{ovr}.

The process of overlapping region detection is summarized in Algorithm 1.

Cleaning Up of the Overlapping Instances and Undersampling of Negative Instance

This stage involves to eliminate the trivial overlapping instances from both minority and majority case sets, in order to reduce the overlapping zone, reg_{ovr}. To accomplish the objective, the concept of Tomek-link pair is refined to retrieve Abnormal Tomek-link pair (*ATL*). The concept of Tomek-link pair basically addressed the boundary instances which promote noise along the decision boundary. However, the presence of significant borderline instances is also important to accurately define the decision boundary.

Algorithm 1.

Input: $S_{\min}$, S_{maj}	
1	$ovr\_reg_{min} \leftarrow one\_class\_SVM\left(S_{min}\right)$
2	$ovr\_reg_{maj} \leftarrow one\_class\_SVM\left(S_{maj}\right)$
3	$reg_{ovr} = ovr\_reg_{min} + ovr\_reg_{maj}$
one_class_SVM	
4	For $m = 1.....q$, q is the total number of instances in S_{maj}
	a) $f\left(x_m'\right) = \sum_{m=1}^{q} \alpha_m K\left(x_m', x\right) - \rho$ b) If $f\left(x_m'\right) < 0$ c) $x_m' \leftarrow outlier$ d) Else e) $x_m' \leftarrow novel$ f) $ovr\_reg_{maj} = \left\{x_m' \mid x_m' \; is outlier \; ; x_m' \in S_{maj}\right\}$
5	For $i = 1.....p$, p is the total number of instances in S_{min}, repeat steps 4(a)-4(f).
Output: ovr_reg_{maj}, $ovr\_reg_{\min}$, reg_{ovr}	

In case of class overlapping, overlapping cases often occurred near the decision boundary. Random elimination of boundary instances in such cases can drift apart the decision boundary between minority and majority cases which in turn can degrade the learning process. Hence, in the proposed model, an effective way of pre-processing is defined which facilitates to eliminate only the trivial boundary cases as well as insignificant redundant majority cases without distorting the decision boundary while balancing data distribution. The behavior of instances near the decision boundary in presence of class overlapping has been deeply explored in the present study and based on the study; some inferences have been made as follows:

Tomek-Link Pairs

Tomek-link pairs, formed by instances lying in the overlapping zone may not always endorse boundary instances. But, there is a higher chance of these instances promoting noise; as it's difficult to draw a crisp decision boundary along these instances, in presence of overlapping cases. Hence, the concept of *ATL* pair is defined. The instances forming *ATL* pairs are promoting maximum noise as a slight deviation in feature values will lead to misclassify them. Hence, both minority and majority cases of *ATL* pairs are selected for elimination.

Input: S_{min}, S_{maj}, ovr_reg_{maj}, ovr_reg_{min}, reg_{ovr}, K1= K-NN of minority instance, K2= K-NN of majority patter, K3= K-NN of overlapped majority instance, set K1=1, K2=5, K3=1.

Step 1: For $\forall\ x_i \in S_{min}$, determine its K1-NN from $S_{n \times l}$, for K1=1, by using Euclidean distance.

Step 2: for $\forall\ x_i \in S_{min}$, determine NN_{maj}, i.e. nearest neighbor belonging to S_{maj}; and create the set TL as:

$$TL = \left\{ \left(x_i, x_m \right) \mid x_m = NN_{maj}\left(x_i \right); x_i \in S_{\min}, x_m \in S_{maj} \right\} \tag{6}$$

Step 3: Extract the Abnormal Tomek- link, ATL pairs as:

$$ATL = \left\{ \left(x_c, x_d \right) \mid x_c, x_d \in TL; x_c \in ovr\_reg_{\min}, x_d \in ovr\_reg_{maj} \right\} \tag{7}$$

Step 4: For $\forall\ \left(x_c, x_d \right) \in ATL$, eliminate x_c and x_d from ovr_reg_{min} and ovr_reg_{maj} respectively, and update ovr_reg_{maj}, ovr_reg_{min}, reg_{ovr}.

$$ovr\_reg_{maj}' = ovr\_reg_{maj} - \left\{ x_d \right\}; x_d \in ATL \tag{8}$$

$$ovr\_reg_{min}' = ovr\_reg_{min} - \left\{ x_c \right\}; x_c \in ATL \tag{9}$$

$$reg_{ovr}' = ovr_{regmaj}' + ovr_{regmin}' \tag{10}$$

Step 5: Update S_{min} and S_{maj} as

$$S'_{min} = S_{min} - \{x_d\}; x_d \in ATL \tag{11}$$

$$S'_{maj} = S_{maj} - \{x_d\}; x_d \in ATL \tag{12}$$

Step 6: Update TL to TL' as

$$TL' = \{(x_c', x_d') \mid x_c', x_d' \notin ATL; x_c' \in S'_{\min}, x_d' \in S'_{maj}\} \tag{13}$$

The Instances in TL'

The instances in TL' are considered as potential boundary cases and crucial in defining a distinctive decision boundary. Based on the existence of the associating instances either in overlapping zone or non-overlapping zone; three different scenarios are investigated:

Scenario 1: If the minority case associating instance resides in the overlapping zone while majority case associated instance lies in the non-overlapping zone; the minority instances are retained in the training case set. Elimination of such minority case instances can incline the decision boundary more towards the majority case which will lead to degrade the classification rate of minority cases.

Step 7: *Scenario 1:*

For $\forall(x_c', x_d') \in TL'$; if $x_c' \in ovr\_reg'_{min}$ and $x_d' \notin ovr\_reg'_{maj}$; then retain x_c' in S'_{min}.

Scenario 2: If the majority associating instance resides in the overlapping region with minority being in the non-overlapping region; the concept of sparse neighborhood is employed to detect the hard-to-classify outlier majority case instances. Sparse neighborhood is defined as K-NN estimation of a case instance where most of its neighbors have different class labels. For an outlier with sparser neighborhood, it will carry maximum chances of misclassification and hence is selected for elimination.

Step 8: *Scenario 2:*

For $\forall(x_c', x_d') \in TL'$; if $x_d' \in ovr\_reg'_{maj}$ and $x_c' \notin ovr\_reg'_{min}$; x_d' is extracted and stored in the set, ovr_{out_maj} as

$$ovr_{out\_maj} = \{x_d^{ovr} \mid x_d^{ovr} \leftarrow x_d', x_d' \in TL', x_d' \in ovr\_reg'_{maj}\} \tag{14}$$

Step 9: For ovr_{out_maj}, detection of sparse-neighborhood is performed with the following sub-steps:

a. For $\forall x_d^{ovr} \in ovr_{out\_maj}$, determine K2-NN from reg_{ovr}' for K2=5.

b. Determine $NN_{hits}(x_d^{ovr})$.

c. Determine $NN_{miss}(x_d^{ovr})$.

d. For $\forall x_d^{ovr}$, compare $NN_{hits}(x_d^{ovr})$ and $NN_{miss}(x_d^{ovr})$.

e. If $NN_{miss}(x_d^{ovr}) > NN_{hits}(x_d^{ovr})$; extract x_d^{ovr} and store in a set sp_{NN} as

$$sp_{NN} = \left\{x_d^{ovr} \mid NN_{miss}\left(x_d^{ovr}\right) > NN_{hits}\left(x_d^{ovr}\right)\right\} \tag{15}$$

f. Otherwise, retain x_d^{ovr} in ovr_{out_maj}.

g. Update ovr_{out_maj} as

$$ovr'_{out_{maj}} = ovr_{out_{maj}} - sp_{NN} \tag{16}$$

h. Update TL' as

$$TL'' = TL' - sp_{NN} \tag{17}$$

i. Update ovr_reg_{maj}' as

$$ovr_{regmaj}'' = ovr_{regmaj}' - sp_{NN} \tag{18}$$

j. Update S'_{maj} *as*

$$S_{maj}'' = S'_{maj} - sp_{NN} \tag{19}$$

Scenario 3: If both the associating case instances reside outside the overlapping region; they are assumed to be the *Normal Tomek-link* (*NTL*) pairs. The majority instances forming *NTL* pairs are subjected to redundancy check. The most redundant instances with least significance are selected for elimination, out of each redundant pair. The significance of an instance is determined through intra-cluster significance.

Step 10: *Scenario 3:*

For $\forall\left(x_c', x_d'\right) \in TL'$; if $x_c', x_d' \notin reg_{ovr}$; extract x_c', x_d' and store in a set, NTL as

$$NTL = \left\{\left(x_c'', x_d''\right) \mid x_c'' \leftarrow x_c', x_d'' \leftarrow x_c', x_c'', x_d'' \notin reg_{ovr}'; x_c'' \in S'_{\min}, x_d'' \in S'_{maj}\right\} \tag{20}$$

Step 11: *Redundancy check*:

For $\forall x_d" \in NTL$, determine its redundant pair, x_e from $S_{maj}"$, by using K3-NN rule and Euclidean distance, for K3=1 and create a set $REDN$ as:

$$REDN = \left\{ \left(x_d", x_e\right) \mid x_d" \in NTL, S_{maj}; x_e \in S_{maj}; d\left(x_d", x_e\right) is\ minimum \right\} \tag{21}$$

Step 12: *Check intra-cluster significance:*

Determine the centroid of S_{maj}' as

$$cen_{maj}\left(x_1, x_2, \ldots\ldots\ldots, x_l\right) = \frac{1}{q'} \left\{ \sum_{d''=1}^{q'} \left(x_{d1}", x_{d2}", \ldots\ldots\ldots, x_{dl}"\right) \right\} \tag{22}$$

where q' is total number of instances in S_{maj}'.

Step 13: For $\forall x_d"$, determine $d_{intra\_cen}\left(x_d"\right)$ as

$$d_{intra\_cen}\left(x_d'\right) = \frac{1}{q'} \left[\sum_{d''=1}^{q'} \left\{ \left(x_{d1}" - cen_{maj}\left(x_1\right)\right)^2 + \left(x_{d2}" - cen_{maj}\left(x_2\right)\right)^2 + \ldots\ldots\ldots + \left(x_{dl}" - cen_{maj}\left(x_l\right)\right)^2 \right\} \right] \tag{23}$$

Step 14: *Detection of least significant redundant instance:*

For each $\left(x_d", x_e\right)$ pair, if $d_{intra\_cen}\left(x_d"\right) > d_{intra\_cen}\left(x_e\right)$; then $x_d"$ is supposed to be less significant and is selected for elimination. Update $S_{maj}"$ as:

$$S_{maj}^{new} = S_{maj}" - \left\{x_d"\right\} \tag{24}$$

Step 15: Obtain the new training set S_{new}. as:

$$S_{new} = S_{maj}^{new} + S_{min}' \tag{25}$$

Output: S_{new}, reg_{ovr}'

All those inferences furnish to develop an effective data pre-processing technique to solve issues of both of data imbalance and overlapping cases. The refined case set S_{new} then fed to the learning stage for training. A summarized algorithm for the above stage is presented below in algorithm 2:

Learning Stage

In the learning stage, the refined case set, S_{new} is trained with ELM classifier which is then validated against a set of test cases, to detect whether a person is affected or healthy. ELM is an advanced Feed Forward Neural Network (FFNN) model which can work without hidden layer parameter tuning (Huang, Zhu, Siew, 2006) (Huang, Zhu, Siew, 2004). ELM is considered to have more generalization capability, and requires less learning time, than the standard Back Propagation Neural Network (BPNN). That is why, ELM has been considered for detection of PD in the learning stage. A brief illustration on working of ELM learning model is presented below:

For a training set, $S_{n\times l} = \left\{\left(x_i, t_i\right) \mid i = 1, 2, \ldots\ldots n\right\}$, with x_i is the training data vector, t_i is the target of each sample, and L denoting the number of hidden nodes, the output function for L-hidden nodes is given by (Tang, Deng, 2016):

$$f_L\left(x\right) = \sum_{i=1}^{L} \beta_i h_i\left(x\right) \tag{26}$$

where β_i is the output weight of $i-th$ hidden node, and $h_i\left(x\right) = G\left(a_i, b_i, x\right)$ is the output function of $i-th$. hidden node.

The hidden-layer output matrix, H of ELM is given by:

$$H = \begin{bmatrix} h\left(x_1\right) \\ \vdots \\ h\left(x_N\right) \end{bmatrix} = \begin{bmatrix} G\left(a_1, b_1, x_1\right) & \cdots & G\left(a_L, b_L, x_1\right) \\ \vdots & \vdots & \vdots \\ G\left(a_1, b_1, x_n\right) & \cdots & G\left(a_L, b_l, x_N\right) \end{bmatrix} \tag{27}$$

where $h\left(x\right) = \left[G\left(h_i\left(x\right), \ldots\ldots. h_L\left(x\right)\right)\right]$ defines the hidden-layer output mapping.

From the view of learning, ELM provides to achieve the smallest training error as well as the minimum output weight during training. The objective function of ELM theory can be given as:

$$\text{Minimize: } \beta_p^{\sigma_1} + CH\beta - T_q^{\sigma_2} \tag{28}$$

Where $\sigma_1 > 0, \sigma_2 > 0, p, q = 0, \frac{1}{2}, 1, 2, \ldots + \infty$, and T is training data target matrix, denoted as

Algorithm 2.

Input: $S_{\min}$, S_{maj}, ovr_reg_{maj}, $ovr\_reg_{\min}$, reg_{ovr}, K1= K-NN of minority instance, K2= K-NN of majority patter, K3= K-NN of overlapping majority instance, set K1=1, K2=5, K3=1.	
1	For $\forall x_i \in S_{min}$,determine $TL = \left\{ \left(x_i, x_m \right) \mid x_m = NN_{maj}\left(x_i \right); x_i \in S_{\min}, x_m \in S_{maj} \right\}$
2	Extract *ATL*, $ATL = \left\{ \left(x_c, x_d \right) \mid x_c, x_d \in TL; x_c \in ovr\_reg_{\min}, x_d \in ovr\_reg_{maj} \right\}$
3	Update ovr_reg_{maj}, ovr_reg_{min}, S_{maj}, S_{min}, reg_{ovr}, TL by using steps 4-6. Retrieve updated $ovr\_reg_{maj}{}'$, $ovr\_reg_{min}{}'$, $reg_{ovr}{}'$, $S_{maj}{}'$, $S_{min}{}'$, TL'
4	For $\forall \left(x_c{}', x_d{}' \right) \in TL'$, a) If case 1 has occurred, retain $x_c{}'$ in $S_{min}{}'$. b) If case 2 has occurred, estimate sparse neighborhood, sp_{NN} of $x_d{}'$ by using steps 8(a) - 8(f). c) Update $S_{maj}{}'$, $reg_{ovr}{}'$, TL' by using steps 8(g)- 8(j). Retrieve $S_{maj}{}''$, $reg_{ovr}{}''$, TL''. d) If case 3 has occurred, determine NTL, $NTL = \left\{ \left(x_c{}'', x_d{}'' \right) \mid x_c'' \leftarrow x_c', x_d'' \leftarrow x_c', x_c{}'', x_d{}'' \notin reg_{ovr}{}'; x_c'' \in S'_{min}, x_d{}'' \in S'_{maj} \right\}$ e) Determine $REDN$, $REDN = \left\{ \left(x_d'', x_e \right) \mid x_d'' \in NTL, S_{maj}; x_e \in S_{maj}; d\left(x_d'', x_e \right) is\, minimum \right\}$ f) Determine $d_{intra\_cen}\left(x_d'' \right)$ by using steps 12-13. g) For each $\left(x_d'', x_e \right)$, if $d_{intra\_cen}\left(x_d'' \right) > d_{intra\_cen}\left(x_e \right)$ h) Eliminate x_d'' i) Else j) Eliminate x_e k) Retrieve S_{maj}^{new} as $S_{maj}^{new} = S_{maj}{}'' - \left\{ x_d'' \right\}$
5	Retrieve refined case set, $S_{new} = S_{maj}^{new} + S_{min}{}'$
Output: S_{new}, $reg_{ovr}{}'$	

$$T = \begin{bmatrix} t_1 \\ \vdots \\ t_N \end{bmatrix} \tag{29}$$

The ELM learning algorithm has the following steps:

1. For $L-$ hidden nodes, randomly assign the input weights, a_i and the biases, b_i as the hidden-node parameters.
2. Calculate the matrix, H
3. Calculate the output-weight vector, β as:

$$\beta = H^{\dagger}T \tag{30}$$

With $T = \left[t_1, \ldots\ldots, t_N\right]^T$; $H^{\dagger}$ is the Moore-Penrose generalized inverse of the matrix, H.

$H^{\dagger}$ can be calculated as $H^{\dagger} = \left(H^T H\right)^{-1} H^T$; providing $H^T H$ is non-singular; or $H^{\dagger} = H^T\left(H^T H\right)^{-1}$; providing HH^T is non-singular

According to ridge regression theory, a positive value $\left(\frac{1}{\lambda}\right)$ is suggested to be add to the diagonal of HH^T or $H^T H$; which facilitates the resultant to be equivalent to ELM optimization solution with $\sigma_1 = \sigma_2 = p = q = 2$.

Hence, the optimal output weight and output function can be given as shown in Table 2.

Experimentations, Results, and Discussions

A number of experimentations are performed to evaluate the proficiency of the proposed methodology in detection of PD, while in comparison with state-of-the-art techniques and standard learning systems. Publicly available dataset for Parkinson Disease are considered for the experimentation purpose. The performance of the proposed intelligent diagnostic system has been evaluated in terms of average accuracy, confusion matrix and ROC curve.

Table 2. Output weight and output function formulation of ELM

Optimal Output Weight	Optimal Output Function
$\beta = H^T\left(\frac{1}{\lambda} + HH^T\right)^{-1} T$	$f(x) = h(x)\beta = h(x)H^T\left(\frac{1}{\lambda} + HH^T\right)^{-1} T$
$\beta = \left(\frac{1}{\lambda} + HH^T\right)^{-1} H^T T$	$f(x) = h(x)\beta = h(x)\left(\frac{1}{\lambda} + HH^T\right)^{-1} H^T T$

Dataset Description

Parkinson Dataset [source: UCI machine learning repository] (UCI Machine Learning Repository) (Mohamed, 2016)

The Parkinson dataset was created by Max Little of the University of Oxford, in collaboration with the National Centre for Voice and Speech, Denver, Colorado, who recorded the speech signals. The dataset is composed of a range of biomedical voice measurements from 31 people, 23 of which effected with PD. The motive of the dataset is to classify healthy people from the affected ones, with two classes, 0 (zero) denoting the healthy individuals while 1 (one) denotes the affected individual with PD. The attributes (columns) denotes a particular voice measure while each row denotes an individual, with a total of 195 individuals. The details of the attributes are given in Table 3.

Table 3. Attribute information of Parkinson dataset

Sl. No	Attributes	Information
1	name	ASCII subject name and recording number
2	MDVP:Fo(Hz)	Average vocal fundamental frequency
3	MDVP:Fhi(Hz)	Maximum vocal fundamental frequency
4	MDVP:Flo(Hz)	Minimum vocal fundamental frequency
5	MDVP:Jitter(%)	Several measures of variation in fundamental frequency
6	MDVP:Jitter(Abs)	
7	MDVP:RAP	
8	MDVP:PPQ	
9	Jitter:DDP	
10	MDVP:Shimmer	Several measures of variation in amplitude
11	MDVP:Shimmer(dB)	
12	Shimmer:APQ3	
13	Shimmer:APQ5	
14	MDVP:APQ	
15	Shimmer:DDA	
16	NHR	Two measures of ratio of noise to tonal components in the voice
17	HNR	
18	RPDE	Two nonlinear dynamical complexity measures
19	Spread1	
20	Spread2	
21	PPE	Pitch Period Entropy
22	D2	Recurrence Period Density Analysis
23	DFA	Signal fractal scaling exponent
	status	Health status of the subject (one) - Parkinson's, (zero) - healthy

It is obvious from the data description that the dataset comprises of two classes, namely healthy and affected individuals. Hence, from the perspective of data imbalance, measure of imbalanced cases is determined by Imbalance Ratio (IR), which is defined as follows:

$$IR = \frac{no.of\, majority\, patterns}{no.of\, minority\, patterns} \quad (31)$$

The data imbalance (IR) in the dataset is obtained as **3.06** which can be considered as a case of moderately low data imbalance.

For clear depiction of various nomenclatures used in this paper, their respective notations are presented in Table 4.

Comparison With State-of-the-Art Data Pre-Processing Methods

As a part of the comparison analysis, the proposed methodology has been compared with six state-of-the-art techniques, proposed in (Yang & Gao, 2013). The performance of the proposed methodology has been evaluated in terms efficiency of the defined data pre-processing stage which offers treatment of overlapping cases, data imbalance, and data redundancy. The following data pre-processing methods are considered for comparison analysis:

- **Neighborhood Cleaning Rule (NCL):** The NCL methods works on the principle of Edited Nearest Neighbor (ENN) (More, 2016). ENN can be defined as an undersampling approach which eliminates majority instances on the context of K-Nearest Neighbors of different class.

Table 4. Notations of nomenclatures

Model/Classifier	Technical Term/ Nomenclature	Notation
Classifier	Feed Forward Neural network	FFNN
	Support Vector Machine	SVM
	Naïve Bayes	NB
	Extreme Learning Machine	ELM
Model	Neighborhood Cleaning Rule	NCL
	Neighborhood Cleaning Rule+ Borderline Noise Factor	NCL+BNF
	One Sided Selection+ Tomek-link	OSS+TL
	One Sided Selection+ Borderline Noise Factor	OSS+BNF
	SMOTE+ Tomek-link	SMOTE+TL
	SMOTE+ Borderline Noise Factor	SMOTE+BNF
	Proposed model with FFNN classifier	Proposed+ FFNN
	Proposed model with SVM classifier	Proposed +SVM
	Proposed model with Naïve Bayes classifier	Proposed +NB
	Proposed model with ELM classifier	Proposed+ELM

- **NCL+BNF:** Borderline Noise Factor (BNF) defines the degree of remoteness of a borderline instance, based on its neighborhood. In (Yang & Gao, 2013), the concept of BNF is defined as an outlier detection approach to clean up the overlapping cases. In NCL+BNF method, undersampling of majority instances is performed by NCL technique, followed by BNF technique to detect and clean-up the outliers.
- **OSS+TL:** In OSS+TL, One-sided-selection (OSS) (Kubat & Matwin, 1997) technique is used to eliminate significant majority instances, followed by removal of noisy cases by Tomek-link pair detection. Cleaning up of outliers is achieved through noise (noisy instances) removal. The approach of OSS+TL is deployed in this chapter is same as in defined in (Yang & Gao, 2013).
- **OSS+BNF:** A hybrid of OSS and BNF is employed which provides to undersample the majority instances by using OSS method while outlier detection and elimination are achieved by using BNF. The mechanism of OSS+BNF is employed from (Yang & Gao, 2013).
- **SMOTE+TL:** Synthetic Minority Oversampling Technique (SMOTE) (Chawla *et al.,* 2002) facilitates to generate synthetic minority instances, and to rebalance the data space. SMOTE is integrated by Tomek-link (TL) method for treating the overlapping of classes. The SMOTE+TL approach discussed in (Yang & Gao, 2013) is deployed in this chapter.
- **SMOTE+BNF:** SMOTE is employed to reduce the imbalance ratio, while BNF is implemented to detect and clean-up the overlapping instances. The mechanism of SMOTE+BNF considered in this chapter is same as defined in (Yang & Gao, 2013).

Parameter Settings

The various parameter settings for comparison analyses with the considered state-of-the art methods are discussed below:

1. *Threshold, t1*: The parameter, *t1* in BNF has defined a threshold for detecting overlapping instances, based on its estimated BNF-value. By experimenting, the best range of *t1*-values has been attained as [2.35-2.55], and the one yielding highest performance is considered for further experimentation. The K-NN estimation in BNF technique is performed for K=5.
2. For SMOTE algorithm, the K-NN estimation is performed for K=5.
3. For the proposed method, the K-NN estimation for detection of hard-to-classify outlier majority cases. is done for K=5. Typically, the value of K is considered to be an odd number, so as to detect maximum number of possible cases for hard-to-classify outlier majority instances, occurred in the overlapping zone.

Results and Discussions

The proposed method and the state-of-the-art techniques are validated with the Parkinson dataset, with ELM used as the learning model. Prior to testing, the data space is normalized by using Min-Max Normalization in the range [0, 1]. By performing 10-fold cross validation, the proposed model is validated with 10 independent training and testing sets of cases. The treatments of overlapping and imbalanced cases have been implemented with respect to each 10-fold. The average of 10-fold is considered as the concluding performance marker. Figures 5 presents the graphical representations of the average accuracies obtained for the proposed method and the considered state-of-the-art methods. By analyzing the experimental results, it is observed that the proposed method has outperformed the considered state-of-the-art methods in most of the cases.

Figure 5. Average accuracy graph of comparison analysis with state-of-the-art data pre-processing methods for ELM classifier

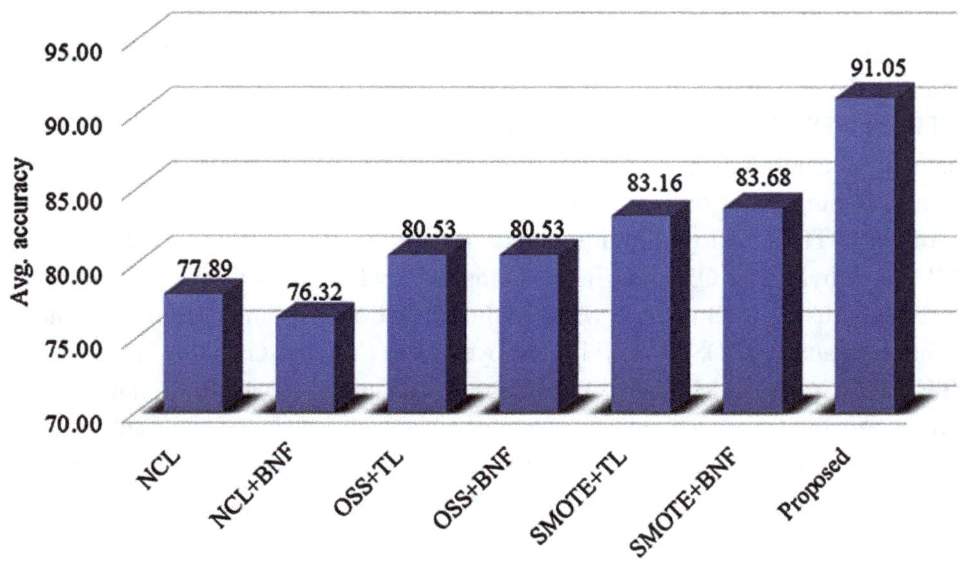

It is observed from Figure 5 that the proposed data pre-processing method has outperformed the considered state-of-the-art data pre-processing techniques for effective detection of PD (accuracy: 91.05%). Analysis of the experimental scenario, the following conclusions can be drawn:

1. The proposed data pre-processing method performs well in case of datasets with low or moderately low IR. In such scenario, undersampling of majority instances is a good choice as it requires elimination of only less significant cases to achieve a balanced data distribution. The considered Parkinson dataset has a moderate IR of IR=3.06 which establishes this inference.
2. The proposed data pre-processing method is successful in minimizing the misdiagnosis rate in detection of PD, even in presence of similar/ overlapping cases of patients. The defined Abnormal Tomek Link (*ATL*) pair offers to eliminate the overlapping cases. *ATL* furnishes to eliminate the Tomek-link paired instances, with both the associating instance cases residing in overlapping zone, but not necessarily along the decision boundary; thus are completely insignificant from classification point of view.
3. The proposed method is effective in treating issues of data imbalance and data redundancy. In the proposed method, an adaptive undersampling strategy is employed which provides elimination of hard-to-classify majority cases followed by elimination of Normal Tomek-link (*NTL*) pairs with the aspects of redundancy and intra-cluster significance. It results the proposed model to perform well than the state-of-the art sampling techniques such as NCL, OSS and SMOTE. Detection of the hard-to-classify outlier majority cases provides to eliminate the instances with higher probabilities of misclassification from the overlapping zone. Moreover, it furnishes to reduce the size of the majority cases as well the size of the overlapping zone; thus treat the both the overlapping and imbalance cases and issues concurrently.

Comparison With State-of-the-Art Learning Models

As part of the comparison analysis, the proposed method of intelligent diagnostic system is evaluated with state-of-the-art learning models. The analytical results provide to yield the best paring of the proposed data pre-processing method, with considered four state-of-the-art learning models, which are as follows:

- Extreme Learning Machine (ELM) (Huang, Zhu, Siew, 2006) (Huang, Zhu, Siew, 2004)
- Feed Forward Neural Network (FFNN). (Siddiquee, Mazumder, Kamruzzaman, 2010)
- Support Vector Machine (SVM). (Fradkin & Muchnik, 2000)
- Naïve Bayes (NB). (Murphy,2006)

The classifiers considered are state-of-the-art in the domain of machine learning, used in many past and recent studies (Li *et al.*, 2010) (Das *et al.*, 2013) (Krawczyk *et al.*, 2016) (Nguyen *et al.*, 2010). The proposed intelligent diagnostic system model provides a data pre-processing method which furnished to alter the prior probability of the classes during data pre-processing. Hence, for learning, a set of both of probabilistic (Naïve Bayes) and non-probabilistic (FFNN, SVM, ELM) classifiers is considered which can validate the proposed model in both the scenarios.

Parameter Settings

1. Non-single hidden layered neural network has the fault of local minima. Hence, neural network model with single hidden layer is chosen, and the optimal network structure is determined by varying the number of neurons in the hidden layer. The number of neurons in the hidden layer for FFNN learner is varied in between (k+1) to 2k where k depicts number of inputs in the input layer. In the present study, "k" implies to number of attributes of the considered Parkinson dataset. With this consideration, the optimal architecture is obtained as 23-37-1, which is in the form of (input layer node- hidden layer node-output layer node). The parameter values which yield minimum training errors are selected.
2. Table 5 presents a statistics of different parameters used in SVM and Naive Bayes classification models. The optimal parameter settings are achieved through adjusting the learning models with varying parameter values and the parameter values which produce the highest average accuracy are taken for further experimentation.

Table 5. Parameter settings for SVM and naïve bayes classifiers

Classifier	Parameter Name	Value of the Parameter Considered
SVM	Kernel function	Gaussian Radial Basis function
	Method	Least squares (LS)
	Scaling factor(rbf_sigma)	1-10
Naïve Bayes	Distribution	Kernel, mvmn
	Prior	Empirical, Uniform

Results and Discussions

The objective of proposed intelligent diagnostic system is to effective early detection of PD. The proposed data pre-processing method offers to mend the case set against adversities of overlapping cases, data imbalance and data redundancy. The task of detecting PD involves some efficient learning mechanism with fast learning and more generalization capability. All these factors require defining a best learning platform. The proposed method is validated in terms of four learning models, to find out the best one, for a given experimental or clinical scenario. The result obtained is presented figure 6.

As shown in Figure 6, the experimental results obtained have manifest the efficiency of ELM learning model as compared to rest state-of-the-art learning models in early detection PD. As discussed earlier, the working principle of ELM offers to learn without hidden layer parameter tuning which is a prime step in FFNN learning model. Both ELM and FFNN learning models performed significantly well in PD detection (FFNN: 87.37%, ELM: 91.05%), while a low performance is achieved in case of Naïve Bayes classifier (accuracy: 77.89%). It is due to the fact of altering of the prior probabilities of the minority and majority cases due to the proposed data pre-processing technique. The performance of SVM classifier is found to be fairly good with the proposed data pre-processing method (accuracy: 84.74%). By analyzing the results, it can be concluded that the proposed method can efficiently detect PD, while employed in a non-probabilistic learning platform.

Performance Analysis

A series of performance analyses tests is performed to evaluate the efficiency of the proposed method as well as the state-of-the art data pre-processing methods. Two well-known performance measures are considered, which are presented below:

Figure 6. Average accuracy graph of the proposed method with respect to four learning models

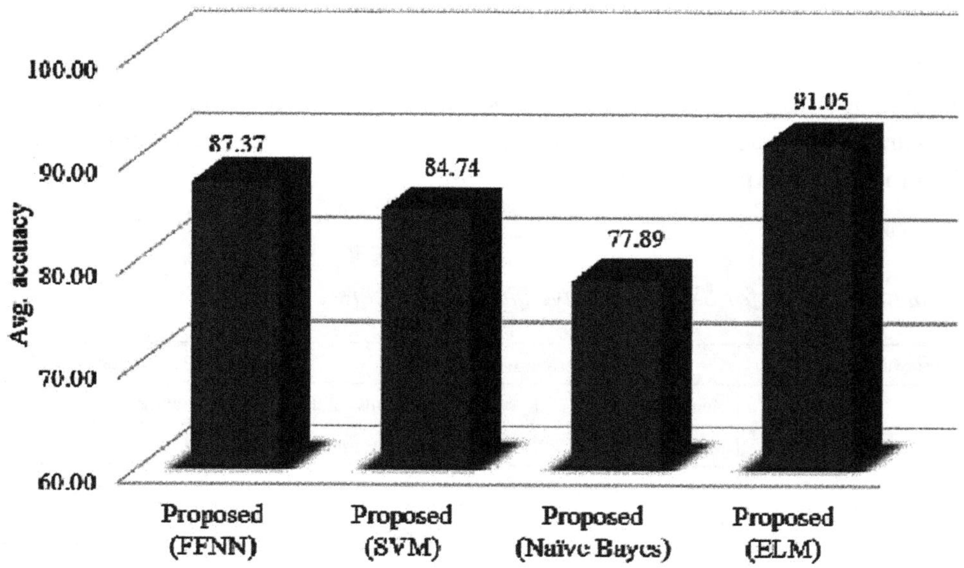

Confusion Matrix

The confusion matrix contains information about actual and predicted classifications done by a classifier. Performance of such classifier is commonly evaluated using the data in the matrix. The confusion matrix for a binary class classifier is presented in table 6 (Sokolova, 2009).

Based on the values of confusion matrix, a number of performance measures can be defined, some of which are considered in this chapter are presented in table 7 (Sokolova, 2009).

Receiver Operating Characteristics (ROC) Curve

ROC curve is a graphical plot that depicts the performance of a binary classifier with respect to its varying discrimination threshold. The ROC curve is formed by plotting False Positive Rate (FPR) along the x-axis and True Positive Rate (TPR) along the y-axis. The convergence of a ROC curve towards top-left corner of the ROC-space defines its proficiency. In table 4, the abbreviations of the legends, used in the ROC graphs are listed down.

Table 6. Confusion matrix for binary classifier

Data Class		Classified	
		Positive	**Negative**
Actual	**Positive**	TP	FN
	Negative	FP	TN

Table 7. Performance measures formulation from confusion matrix

Measure	Formulae
Precision	$\frac{TP}{TP+FP}$
Recall	$\frac{TP}{TP+FN}$
Specificity	$\frac{TN}{TN+FP}$
F-measure	$\frac{2 * precision * recall}{precision + recall}$
MCC	$\frac{TP \times TN - FP \times FN}{\sqrt{(TP+FP)(TP+FN)(TN+FP)(TN+FN)}}$
AUC	$\frac{1}{2} \times \left(\frac{TP}{TP+FN} + \frac{TN}{TN+FP} \right)$

Performance Analysis With State-of-the-Art Data Pre-Processing Techniques

The performance analysis of the proposed method by using confusion matrix in comparison with the considered state-of-the-art data pre-processing techniques is presented table 8.

Through the analysis, it has been observed that the proposed method of data pre-processing has outperformed the considered state-of-the-art methods, for all performance measures considered. In case of the proposed method, higher precision and recall values are achieved for most of the cases than the considered state-of-the-art methods. Achievement of higher precision and recall values is a resultant of higher TP-values which infers increasing of minority case (detection of healthy individuals, in context of this chapter) classification rate. This in turn infers the reducing of misdiagnosis rate of healthy individuals as the affected ones, which is one of the objectives of this chapter. Moving over to F-measure, higher F-measure and specificity values are achieved for the proposed scheme as compared to the state-of–the-art techniques, which infers improving the minority case classification rate without hindering the classification rate of majority cases (i.e., detection of individuals with PD). The MCC values obtained lies in the range [0, +1] which infers accurate predictability of the proposed scheme. The AUC-value obtained for the proposed scheme is of higher range, i.e. (0.9833) than the state-of-the-art methods [0.70-0.85]. This establishes the efficiency of proposed scheme as compared to the considered methods, in terms of all test cases.

Figure 7 has presented the ROC curve based performance analysis assessment of the proposed method with the considered data pre-processing techniques. From the Figure 7, it can be seen that the ROC curve obtained for the proposed model is superior with an AUC of 0.9833, as compared to the rest of the techniques.

Performance Analysis With State-of-the-Art Data Learning Models

Table 9 has presented the performance analysis statistics of the proposed method in comparison with the state-of-the-art learning models.

The obtained performance analysis in table 9 has proven the pairing of proposed method with ELM to be most effective in early detection PD. The performance of the proposed method has been evaluated with four different learning platforms. As discussed earlier, the performance is elevated while working with a non-probabilistic classifier, with all the considered performance measures yielding higher values.

Table 8. Assessment of confusion matrix performance measures for data pre-processing techniques for ELM classifier

Methods	Precision	Recall	Specificity	F-Measure	MCC	AUC
Classifier: Feed Forward Neural Network						
NCL(ELM)	66.8333	82.9167	94.3736	70.5018	0.6424	0.8386
NCL+BNF(ELM)	48.1667	61.25	86.4962	51.6017	0.3837	0.719
OSS+TL(ELM)	61.8571	87.5	96.1635	67.1111	0.6255	0.8509
OSS+BNF(ELM)	60.4048	64.1667	89.5694	59.1313	0.5008	0.7545
SMOTE+TL (ELM)	72.3333	66.25	89.3957	65.9145	0.5913	0.787
SMOTE+BNF(ELM)	65.6667	68.75	89.9296	63.1612	0.5441	0.7896
Proposed(ELM)	98.75	97.5	99.375	97.9048	0.9734	0.9833

Figure 7. ROC graph plot of proposed method with data pre-processing techniques for ELM classifier

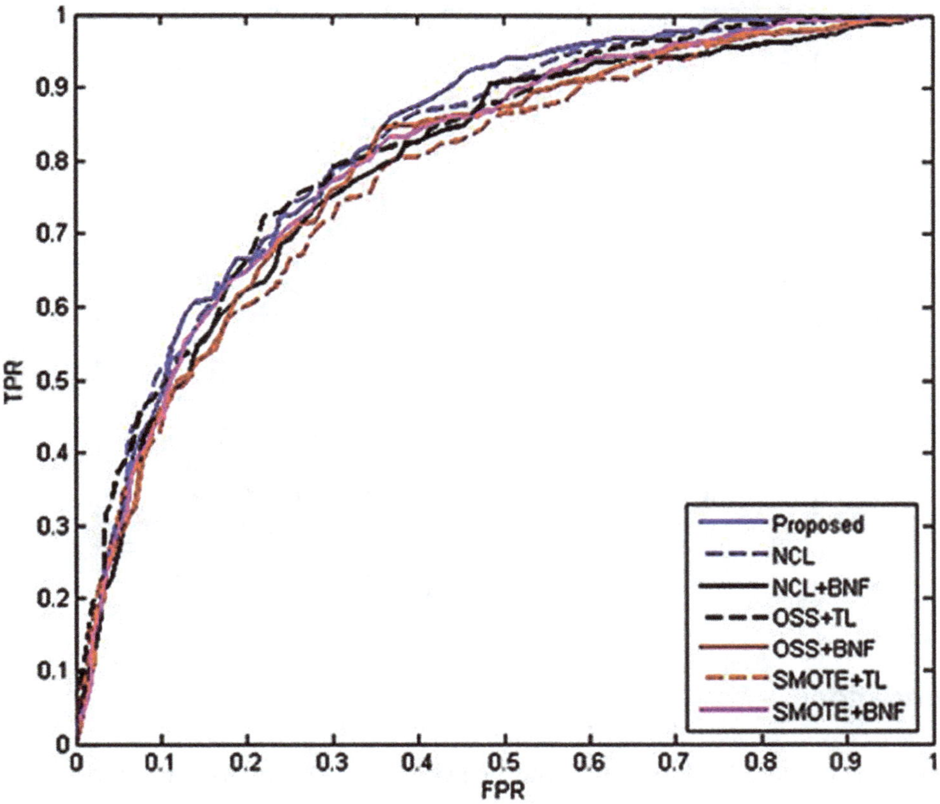

Table 9. Assessment of confusion matrix performance measures for various learning models

Methods	Precision	Recall	Specificity	F-Measure	MCC	AUC
Proposed+FFNN	85.881	75.8333	91.3613	77.5326	0.7321	0.8724
Proposed+Naïve Bayes	50.0303	76.25	90.889	58.3857	0.4575	0.7743
Proposed+SVM	60.5635	80.4167	92.9391	67.6212	0.5858	0.8302
Proposed+ELM	98.75	97.5	99.375	97.9048	0.9734	0.9833

In case of probabilistic classifier (Naïve Bayes), a relatively lower precision and recall values are achieved, which implies increasing of misdiagnosis rate of healthy individuals as the affected ones. Hence, it can be concluded that pairing of the proposed method with probabilistic classifier is not recommended for effective detection of PD.

Figure 8 has presented the ROC curve assessment of the proposed method with the considered learning models. It has been observed that from figure 8, that the combination of proposed method+ELM has outperformed the rest three pairings with learning models. The ROC plot for proposed method+ELM pairing has converged with an AUC-value of 0.9833, which infers its superiority over the rest. From the ROC-curve analysis, the pairing of the proposed method+ELM has the highest recommendation as the intelligent diagnostic system for detection PD.

Figure 8. ROC graph plot of proposed method with standard learning models

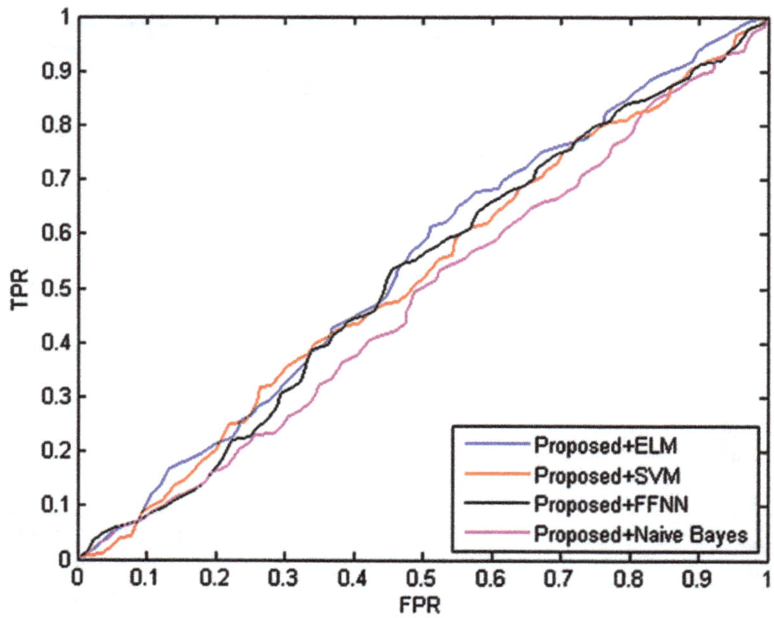

Recommendations

The intention of the proposed intelligent diagnostic system of PD is to offer adequate detection of PD, without compromising any life-value of the individuals. The detection of PD in an affected individual is as much crucial as to detect an individual without PD; as both the situations can be miserable on its opposite side. The proposed diagnostic system involves an advanced data pre-processing technique which offers to mine the case set, to solve the issues of similar/overlapping cases, data imbalance and data redundancy. The manual diagnosis system of PD is often subjective to the various underlying issues of clinical data. Based on the experimental results and performance analysis assessments, the proposed diagnostic system has been proven to be effective against the considered underlying issues of clinical data/ case sets. Hence, the proposed intelligent diagnostic system can be readily recommended for effective and early detection of PD.

FUTURE RESEARCH DIRECTIONS

As direction to future works, a few scopes are listed down below:

- The proposed intelligent diagnostic system can be extended in amalgamation with image processing techniques, to define visual-based diagnostic system.
- The proposed algorithm has not been validated against real-time clinical data, which requires advanced data mining tools, for data pre-processing. In extension of the proposed algorithm, it can be combined with feature extraction/ feature section techniques to extract the important clinical features for learning.

- The treatment of data imbalance and data redundancy can also be investigated through classifier-level solutions or ensemble learning techniques.

CONCLUSION

In this chapter, an intelligent diagnostic system for early detection of Parkinson's disease is proposed. Early detection of PD is much needed as most of the initial symptoms of PD often get unnoticed. By the time, it get diagnosed the loss of dopamine has progressed to a higher level, and PD become incurable. In modern medical science, biomarkers like DaTSCAN are available, which provides to assess the dopamine transporter in the brain through SPECT imaging. However, not many biomarkers are approved as they might hazardous to patient health and the surrounding environment. Clinical diagnosis of PD is effected by the underlying characteristics of patients' data, which come up with issues such similar/ overlapping cases of patients, data imbalance and data redundancy. Statistical techniques which can take up the raw clinical data to mine and then extract the hidden useful information for detection of PD are much of demand.

Through this chapter, the issues occurred during detection of PD in case of clinical diagnosis are discussed in details. An advanced data pre-processing method is proposed to which facilitates to detect the similar cases of patients so that misdiagnosis rate can be minimized. The concept of Tomek-link pair is redefined with respect to the proximity of its associating instance cases, in the overlapping or non-overlapping zone, to yield two sub-concepts, namely Abnormal Tomek-link (*ATL*) and Normal Tomek-link (*NTL*) pairs. Cleaning up of overlapping cases is achieved by *ATL* and sparse neighborhood estimation of majority outliers. *NTL* pairs are integrated with redundancy check and intra-cluster significance to obtain the most redundant and least significant noisy majority cases. The proposed method is validated with four standard learning models, so as to obtain the best paring of data pre-processing and learning method. ELM learning model is found to be most effective for learning during detection of PD. Based on the experimental results; the proposed method with ELM classifier is proven to be effective in early detection of PD. Through the proposed method, the authors have analyzed its effectiveness in various experimental scenarios, against all possible adversities. Both the experimental results and performance analysis assessments have manifested its proficiency in detection of PD, even in presence of similar/ overlapping cases, data imbalance and data redundancy.

With available past medical history records, the proposed diagnostic system can be readily used for detection of healthy/ affected individuals. There is no hardware cost associated while designing the proposed diagnostic system; hence it also feasible to be applied in low-budget maintained medical institutions or clinical diagnostic centers.

ACKNOWLEDGMENT

This research work has not received any kind of specific grant from any funding agency in the public, commercial, or not-for-profit sectors. The authors would like to thank the Department of Computer Science and Engineering of National Institute of Technology, Silchar for its generous support with advanced laboratory facility to carry out the experiments for the present study.

REFERENCES

Ahmed, S. S., Santosh, W., Kumar, S., & Christlet, H. T. (2009). Metabolic profiling of Parkinson's disease: Evidence of biomarker from gene expression analysis and rapid neural network detection. *Journal of Biomedical Science, 16*(63). PMID:19594911

Aich, S., Younga, K., Hui, K. L., Al-Absi, A. A., & Sain, M. (2018). A Nonlinear Decision Tree based Classification Approach to Predict the Parkinson's disease using Different Feature Sets of Voice Data. *International Conference on Advanced Communications Technology (ICACT)*, 638-642.

Alemami, Y., & Almazaydeh, L. (2014). Detecting of Parkinson Disease through Voice Signal Features. *The Journal of American Science*, 10.

Anita, S., & Aruna Priya, P. (2016). Early Prediction of Parkinson's Disease using Artificial Neural Network. *Indian Journal of Science and Technology, 9*(36), 1–7. doi:10.17485/ijst/2016/v9i36/98401

Bhande, S., & Raut, R. (2013). Parkinson Diagnosis using Neural Network: A Survey. *International Journal of Innovative Research in Science. Engineering and Technology, 2*(9), 4843–4846.

Caliskan, A., Badem, H., Baştürk, A., & Yüksel, M. E. (2017). Diagnosis of the Parkinson Disease by Using Deep Neural Network Classifier. *IU-JEEE, 17*(2), 3311–3318.

Chatterjee, J., Saxena, A., Vyas, G., & Mehra, A. (2017). An Efficient Real-Time Approach for Detection of Parkinson's Disease. In Intelligent Systems Design and Applications. ISDA 2017. Advances in Intelligent Systems and Computing. Springer.

Chawla, N. V., Bowyer, K. W., Hall, L. O., & Kegelmeyer, W. P. (2002). SMOTE: Synthetic minority over-sampling technique. *Journal of Artificial Intelligence Research, 16*, 321–357. doi:10.1613/jair.953

Chen, H.-L., Huang, C.-C., Yu, X.-G., Xu, X., Sun, X., Wang, G., & Wang, S.-J. (2013). An efficient diagnosis system for detection of Parkinson's disease using fuzzy k-nearest neighbor approach. *Expert Systems with Applications, 40*(1), 263–271. doi:10.1016/j.eswa.2012.07.014

Das, B., Krishnan, N. C., & Cook, D. J. (2013). Handling Class Overlap and Imbalance to Detect Prompt Situations in Smart Homes. *IEEE 13th Int. Conf. on Data Mining Workshops*, 266-273.

DaTSCAN. (2011). *European Medicines Society*. EMEA/H/C/000266.

De Souza, J. W. M., Almeida, J. S., & Rebouças Filho, P. P. (2017). A New Approach for the Diagnosis of Parkinson's Disease Using a Similarity Feature Extractor. In Intelligent Systems Design and Applications. ISDA 2017. Advances in Intelligent Systems and Computing. Springer.

Finberg, J. P. M., Schwartz, M., Jeries, R., Badarny, S., Nakhleh, M. K., Abu Daoud, E., ... Haick, H. (2018). Sensor Array for Detection of Early Stage Parkinson's Disease before Medication. *ACS Chemical Neuroscience, 9*(11), 2548–2553. doi:10.1021/acschemneuro.8b00245 PMID:29989795

Fradkin, D., & Muchnik, I. (2000). *Support Vector Machines for Classification*. DIMACS Series in Discrete Mathematics and Theoretical Computer Science.

Hadjahamadi, A. H., & Askari, T. J. (2012). A Detection Support System for Parkinson's Disease Diagnosis Using Classification and Regression Tree. *Journal of Mathematics and Computer Science*, *4*(02), 257–263. doi:10.22436/jmcs.04.02.15

Hariharana, M., Polat, K., & Sindhu, R. (2014). A new hybrid intelligent system for accurate detection of Parkinson's disease. *Computer Methods and Programs in Biomedicine*, *113*(3), 904–913. doi:10.1016/j.cmpb.2014.01.004 PMID:24485390

Huang, G.-B., Zhu, Q.-Y., & Siew, C.-K. (2004). Extreme Learning Machine: A New Learning Scheme of Feedforward Neural Networks. *Proc. Of IEEE Int. Joint Conf. on Neural Network*, *2*, 985-990.

Huang, G.-B., Zhu, Q.-Y., & Siew, C.-K. (2006). Extreme learning machine: Theory and applications. *Neurocomputing*, *70*(1-3), 489–501. doi:10.1016/j.neucom.2005.12.126

Islam, M. S., Parvez, I., Deng, H., & Goswami, P. (2014) Performance Comparison of Heterogeneous Classifiers for Detection of Parkinson's Disease Using Voice Disorder (Dysphonia). *3rd International Conference on Informatics, Electronics & Vision*. 10.1109/ICIEV.2014.6850849

Krawczyk, B., Galar, M., Jelen, L., & Herrera, F. (2016). Evolutionary undersampling boosting for imbalanced classification of breast cancer malignancy. *Applied Soft Computing*, *38*, 714–726. doi:10.1016/j.asoc.2015.08.060

Kubat, M., & Matwin, S. (1997). Addressing the curse of imbalanced training sets: one-sided selection. *Proc. Fourteenth International Conference on Machine Learning*, 179-186.

Li, D.-C., Liu, C.-W., & Hu, S. C. (2010). A learning method for the class imbalance problem with medical data sets. *Computers in Biology and Medicine*, *40*(5), 509–518. doi:10.1016/j.compbiomed.2010.03.005 PMID:20347072

Mohamed, G. S. (2016). Parkinson's Disease Diagnosis: Detecting the Effect of Attributes Selection and Discretization of Parkinson's Disease Dataset on the Performance of Classifier Algorithms. *Open Access Library Journal*, *3*, 1–11.

More, A. (2016). *Survey of resampling techniques for improving classification performance in unbalanced datasets*. Cornel University Library.

Murphy, K. P. (2006). *Naive Bayes classifiers, Technical Report.* Available: http://www.cs.ubc.ca/murphyk/ Teaching/CS 340 - Fall 06 /reading/NB.pdf

Nguyen, T.-N., Lars, G., & Zeno, S-T. (2010). Cost-Sensitive Learning Methods for Imbalanced Data. *Int. Joint Conference on Neural Networks*.

Nilashi, M., Ibrahim, O., Ahmadi, H., Shahmoradi, L., & Farahmand, M. (2018). A hybrid intelligent system for the prediction of Parkinson's Disease progression using machine learning techniques. *Biocybernetics and Biomedical Engineering*, *38*(1), 1–15. doi:10.1016/j.bbe.2017.09.002

Olanrewaju, R. F., Sahari, N. S., Musa, A. A., & Hakiem, N. (2014). Application of Neural Networks in Early Detection and Diagnosis of Parkinson's Disease. *Proc. of Int. Conf. on Cyber and IT service Mang. (CITSM)*, 78-82.

Pahwa, R. (Ed.). (2013). *Handbook of Parkinson's Disease*. London: CRC Press. doi:10.3109/9781841849096

Parisi, L., RaviChandran, N., & Manaog, M. L. (2018). Feature-driven machine learning to improve early diagnosis of Parkinson's disease. *Expert Systems with Applications*, *110*, 182–190. doi:10.1016/j.eswa.2018.06.003

Picillo, M., Moccia, M., Spina, E., Barone, P., & Pellecchia, M. T. (2015). Biomarkers of Parkinson's disease: Recent insights, current challenges, and future prospects. *Journal of Parkinsonism and Restless Legs Syndrome*, *6*, 1–13.

Schindlbeck, K. A., & Eidelberg, D. (2018). Network imaging biomarkers: Insights and clinical applications in Parkinson's disease. *Lancet Neurology*, *17*(7), 629–640. doi:10.1016/S1474-4422(18)30169-8 PMID:29914708

Sharma, A., & Giri, R. N. (2014). Automatic Recognition of Parkinson Disease via Artificial Neural Network and Support Vector Machine. *IJITEE*, *4*, 35–41.

Siddiquee, A. B., Mazumder, M., Hoque, E., & Kamruzzaman, S. M. (2010). *A Constructive Algorithm for Feedforward Neural Networks for Medical Diagnostic Reasoning*. Academic Press.

Sokolova, M., & Lapalme, G. (2009). A systematic analysis of performance measures for classification tasks. *Information Processing & Management*, *45*(4), 427–437. doi:10.1016/j.ipm.2009.03.002

Tang, J. X., Deng, C., & Huang, G.-B. (2016). Extreme Learning Machine for Multilayer Perceptron. *IEEE Transactions on Neural Networks and Learning Systems*, *24*(4), 809–821. doi:10.1109/TNNLS.2015.2424995 PMID:25966483

Tomek, I. (1976). Two modifications of CNN. *IEEE Transactions on Systems, Man, and Cybernetics*, 769–772.

Vlasveld, R. (2013). *Introduction to One-class Support Vector Machines*. Retrieved from http://rvlasveld.github.io/blog/2013/07/12/introduction-to-one-class-support-vector-machines/

Yang, Z., & Gao, D. (2013). Classification for Imbalanced and Overlapping Classes Using Outlier Detection and Sampling Techniques. *Applied Mathematics & Information Sciences*, *7*(1), 375–381. doi:10.12785/amis/071L50

ADDITIONAL READING

Ahmed, S. S. S. J., Santosh, W., Kumar, S., & Christlet, T. H. T. (2010). Neural network algorithm for the early detection of Parkinson's disease from blood plasma by FTIR micro-spectroscopy. *Vibrational Spectroscopy*, *53*(2), 181–188. doi:10.1016/j.vibspec.2010.01.019

Gharehchopogh, F. S., Mohammadi, P. (2013). A case Study of Parkinson's disease Diagnosis using Artificial Neural Networks. *International Journal of Computer Applications (0975 – 8887)* 73(19), 1-7.

Gil, A. D., & Johnson, M. B. (2009). Diagnosing Parkinson by Using Artificial Neural Networks And Support Vector Machines. *Global Journal of Computer Science and Technology*, *9*(4), 63–71.

Pan, S., Iplikci, S., Warwick, K., & Aziz, T. Z. (2012). Parkinson's Disease tremor classification – A comparison between Support Vector Machines and neural networks. *Expert Systems with Applications*, *39*(12), 10764–10771. doi:10.1016/j.eswa.2012.02.189

KEY TERMS AND DEFINITIONS

Bradykinesia: Bradykinesia is a symptom of human motor-system that describes slow/difficulty moving of body parts (limbs/legs). It is one of the basic symptoms of Parkinsonism.

Central Nervous System: The central nervous system consists of the brain and spinal cord of the human body and is responsible for incorporating and coordinating activities among all the parts of human body.

Data Imbalance: Data imbalance defines a classification problem where the distribution of data is not even and leads to yield biased results with higher misclassification rate of the minority class data.

Dopamine: Dopamine is defined as a neurotransmitter, which is responsible for transmitting neural signals from the brain to the various body parts and organs.

Extreme Learning Machine: Extreme learning machine is a form of regularized feed-forward neural network without the need of hidden-layer parameter tuning. ELM is popular due to its high regularization ability and low execution time.

One-Class SVM: One-class SVM is a classification model which provides to detect the novel instances, within a region of definite range. It is also known as $\vartheta -$ SVM, as its performance is influenced by the parameter, ϑ.

Overlapping Cases: The cases which have equal probability of belonging to the proximity of two regions are termed as overlapping cases. It is very difficult to distinguish the exact class of these cases.

Tomek-Link: Tomek-link defines the concept boundary pairs in a data distribution. When two instances, *a* and *b* are nearest of each-other, with *class* $(a) \neq$ *class* (b); then the pair *(a,b)* is termed as Tomek-link pair. These pairs are noise-promoting in the data distribution.

Chapter 6
Soft Computing-Based Early Detection of Parkinson's Disease Using Non-Invasive Method Based on Speech Analysis

Chandrasekar Ravi
National Institute of Technology Puducherry, India

ABSTRACT

This chapter aims to use the speech signals that are a behavioral bio-marker for Parkinson's disease. The victim's vocabulary is mostly lost, or big gaps are observed when they are talking or the conversation is abruptly stopped. Therefore, speech analysis could help to identify the complications in conversation from the inception of the symptoms of Parkinson's disease in initial phases itself. Speech can be regularly logged in an unobstructed approach and machine learning techniques can be applied and analyzed. Fuzzy logic-based classifier is proposed for learning from the training speech signals and classifying the test speech signals. Brainstorm optimization algorithm is proposed for extracting the fuzzy rules from the speech data, which is used by fuzzy classifier for learning and classification. The performance of the proposed classifier is evaluated using metrics like accuracy, specificity, and sensitivity, and compared with benchmark classifiers like SVM, naïve Bayes, k-means, and decision tree. It is observed that the proposed classifier outperforms the benchmark classifiers.

DOI: 10.4018/978-1-5225-8567-1.ch006

INTRODUCTION

Parkinson's disease is caused by deteriorating condition of the central nervous system which primarily disturbs the motor function. The symptoms gradually start to appear as time progresses. Common symptoms in the beginning stage of Parkinson are reduced cognition, gait abnormality, decreased body movement, tightness of muscles or oscillating movement of some parts of the body. The brain starts getting affected as the disease starts progressing through advanced stage (Carroll et al., 2016). Mental disorder is yet another common behaviors exhibited by the Parkinson patients. The factor which influences the Parkinson disorder is quite mystery but it is assumed that both genes as well as the environment contributes to the development of the disorder (Lorraine and Anthony, 2015). There is high possibility for the family members to be affected by this disorder. People smoking tobacco and taking hot beverages might have reduced risk while those who suffer from injury in head or having exposure to pest control chemicals have high possibility of getting this disorder.

Periodic automated non-invasive early Parkinson's disease detection method could recover the life of the patients and avert higher treatment costs. This chapter aims to use the speech signals which is a behavioral bio-marker for Parkinson's disease. Although, Parkinson's disease detection could be performed based on psychological, cognitive and physiological bio-markers, speech and conversation will start getting affected from the initial stage onwards. The victim's vocabulary is mostly lost or big gaps are observed when they are talking or the conversation is abruptly stopped. Therefore, speech analysis could help to identify the complications in conversation from the inception of the symptoms of Parkinson's disease in initial phases itself. Speech can be regularly logged in an unobstructed approach and Machine Learning techniques can be applied and analyzed. The Parkinson's dataset from UCI repository is used for Parkinson's disease detection.

Fuzzy Logic based classifier is proposed for learning from the training speech signals and classifying the test speech signals. Brainstorm optimization algorithm is proposed for extracting the fuzzy rules from the speech dataset, which is used by fuzzy classifier for learning and classification. The performance of the proposed classifier is evaluated using metrics like accuracy, specificity and sensitivity and compared with benchmark classifiers like SVM, Naïve Bayes, k-Means and Decision Tree. It is observed that the proposed classifier outperforms the benchmark classifiers. Parkinson Disorder affects the communication of the patient (Smith & Caplan, 2018). This will lead to loss of control on speech and linguistic. The impairment of cognition and motor in open for more research opportunities. Even though several people are affected by this disorder, the symptoms exhibited are varying from one person to another. Diagnosing the disorder in the preliminary stage is vital for accurate remedy because it could extend the life span of the victim (Gupta et al., 2018). Even though several methods are existing for early diagnosis of the disorder, they are inefficient. It is highly necessary to diagnose the disease in early stage because, as the severity of the disorder progresses, it leads to other disabilities related to walking or even standing because the muscles get so rigid in the legs. Thus, analyzing the speech signals would be an effective means to diagnose the disorder in its preliminary stage. Recently, with the advent of sophistications in Artificial Intelligence techniques, automating the learning and analysis of speech signals would be on high expectations.

Amongst the learning mechanisms used by the Machine Learning algorithms, rule-based learning is gaining popularity amongst researchers. Especially in the recent years, biologically inspired optimization algorithms are frequently used for learning purpose. Swarm Intelligence based optimization algorithms like Particle Swarm Optimization, Ant Colony Optimization, Artificial Bee Colony, Bat optimization and so on are based on the swarm intelligence of simple agents like birds, ants, bees, bats and so on. But the brain storm optimization algorithm is based on the brain storming behavior of human beings. Since humans are superior to these small agents and that the cognitive behavior of humans are unique, Brain Storm Optimization algorithm is expected to perform better learning of rules for the Fuzzy System.

Fuzzy Logic classifiers have proven to be effective classifiers due to their ability to handle uncertainty and the much easier to understand Fuzzy rules. Thus, the biologically inspired learning algorithm coupled with Soft Computing technique like Fuzzy Logic classifier would be an ideal option to explore for analyzing the speech signals for detecting the Parkinson disorder.

LITERATURE REVIEW

Table 1 summarizes the related literature review of technique using Fuzzy classifier or Biological Inspired optimization algorithm for detecting Parkinson disorder. (Zhai et al., 2018) extended the Decision Tree to Rough Fuzzy Decision Tree from which Fuzzy rules for classification were derived and applied for Parkinson diagnosis based on voice biomarker. (Gupta et al., 2018) optimized the Cuttlefish algorithm and used it for feature selection from speech dataset from UCI repository. These features were then classified using knn and Decision Tree classifiers. Again, (Gupta et al., 2018) optimized the Crow Search Algorithm and applied to handwriting dataset and extracted the features which were then classified using Decision Tree, K-Nearest Neighbor and Random Forest models. (Ornelas-Vences et al., 2017) used the gait biomarker to measure the turning score using a Fuzzy Inference System. (Shrivastava et al., 2017) used the Modified Cuckoo Search Algorithm, Particle Swarm Optimization, Binary Bat algorithm and Genetic Algorithm to extract features from gait biomarkers. Neural Network was applied on the extracted features for Parkinson diagnosis. (Nilashi et al., 2016) used Principal Component Analysis on speech dataset for dimensionality reduction and applied Support Vector Regression and Adaptive Neuro-Fuzzy Inference System for Parkinson diagnosis. (Abiyev & Abizade, 2016) used Neural Network for feature extraction from voice dataset and clustered them using Fuzzy Inference System. (Chakraborty et al., 2016) used Fuzzy Inference System to diagnose Parkinson using voice dataset. (Liu et al., 2014) integrated Fuzzy Inference System to a tablet game for Parkinson diagnosis. (Chen et al., 2013) applied the Fuzzy based Neural Network on UCI voice data for Parkinson diagnosis. (Zuo et al., 2013) applied the Particle Swarm Optimization algorithm for feature selection on UCI voice data and used Fuzzy based Neural Network for Parkinson diagnosis.

From the literature review, it is evident that the utilization of Fuzzy Inference System or bio inspired optimization techniques have proven to improve the accuracy of classification. Hence a Fuzzy Logic based classifier in combination with a biologically inspired optimization algorithm is proposed in this chapter. Mamdani Fuzzy Inference System is used for classification. The rules and membership functions for the fuzzy inference system are designed using the Brain Storm Optimization, Shi (2011), algorithm which is a biological inspired optimization algorithm. Fuzzy Logic based classifier has the advantage of having interpretable rules and dealing with uncertainty. Brain Storm Optimization (BSO) algorithm is used because it has the advantage of searching based on human idea generation activity called as Brainstorming. Brainstorming is an activity where a group of people work together to propose the solution to a problem. Since the solution is a result of multiple ideas generated from human brain, it is believed to be more efficient. Moreover, when compared to other Swarm Intelligence algorithms like Ant Colony Optimization, Particle Swarm Optimization, Cuckoo Search and so on, Brain Storm Optimization algorithm is assumed to be superior. This is because, Ant Colony Optimization, Particle Swarm Optimization and Cuckoo Search algorithms are based on the group activity done by ants, birds and cuckoo respectively whereas Brain Storm Optimization is based on the brain storming activity of humans. Since, humans are considered to be superior in the hierarchy of the ecosystem, the Brain Storm Optimization is expected to perform superior to other optimization algorithm. On the other hand, the fuzzy inference system can perform well only if the rules and membership functions are robustly designed for it. Hence, the Brain Storm optimization algorithm can be used to search for an optimal combination of membership function and rules that can increase the accuracy of classification of the Fuzzy Inference System.

The Brain Storm Optimization algorithm can help to design a robust rule base with rules having optimal length, size, precision and class variance and a robust membership function having optimal membership function type, count and parameters. Thus the combination of Fuzzy Inference System with biologically inspired algorithm, like Brain Storm Optimization algorithm, which has individually proven to be suitable for Parkinson detection in literature, can be expected to yield high accuracy and efficiency.

Table 1. Literature review summary

Reference	Machine Learning Technique	Advantages
(Zhai et al., 2018)	Rough Set, Fuzzy Set, Decision Tree	Speed of learning is fast
(Gupta et al., 2018)	Crow Search Algorithm, Decision Tree, Random Forest, k-Nearest Neighbor	Reduced features, computational time, accuracy
(Gupta et al., 2018)	Cuttlefish Algorithm, Decision Tree, K-Nearest Neighbor	Optimal features, increased accuracy
(Ornelas-Vences et al., 2017)	Fuzzy Inference System	Scalable, interpretable knowledge
(Shrivastava et al., 2017)	Binary Bat Algorithm, Neural Network	Increased accuracy
(Nilashi et al., 2016)	Principal Component Analysis, Expectation Maximization, Adaptive Neuro-Fuzzy Inference System and Support Vector Regression	Improved accuracy
(Abiyev & Abizade, 2016)	Fuzzy clustering and Gradient Descent Learning algorithms	Improved accuracy
(Chakraborty et al., 2016)	Fuzzy C-Means Clustering, Fuzzy Inference System	Improved accuracy and efficiency
(Liu et al., 2014)	Fuzzy Logic	Better risk prediction
(Chen et al., 2013)	Fuzzy Logic, k-Nearest Neighbor	Improved accuracy, sensitivity, specificity
(Zuo et al., 2013)	Particle Swarm Optimization, Fuzzy k-Nearest Neighbor	Improved accuracy, sensitivity, specificity
(Polat, 2012)	Fuzzy c-Means Clustering, K-Nearest Neighbor	Improved accuracy

PROPOSED METHODOLOGY

The proposed methodology consists of two phases namely the training phase and test phase as shown in Figure 1. In the training phase, the training data is given to the Brain Storm Optimization algorithm. The Brain Storm Optimization algorithm searches for the optimal combination of rules and membership combination that suits the characteristics of the training data and that will yield the best accuracy of classification. Optimal rule base implies the rule base that has the optimal number of rules, with optimal number of attributes, with optimal matching of rules with the training dataset and optimally proportional number of rules for each target class. Optimal membership function implies the optimal membership function types that suits each attribute, optimal number of membership function for each attributes and the optimal parameter values for each membership function of the attributes. This is the output of the training phase. This learned model is applied to the test phase. In the test phase, the fuzzy inference system uses this optimal rule base and optimal membership functions to classify the test data. The fuzzy inference system consists of the fuzzyfier, defuzzyfier, rule base and the inference engine. The fuzzifier and the defuzzifier uses the membership functions derived in the training phase. The rule base derived in the training phase is used as the rule base for the fuzzy inference system.

The Brain Storm Optimization algorithm is tailored, as shown below, for the proposed methodology. The initial population in the Brain Storm Optimization algorithm is called as an idea. The initial ideas in the proposed format along with the configuration inputs and the fitness function tailored for the proposed methodology is given as input to the Brain Storm Optimization algorithm. The initial ideas are clustered and the idea having the highest fitness value in the cluster is made as the center of cluster. Then using some predefined probabilities, some weak ideas are chosen and they are replaced with new ideas. This process is repeated until the optimal idea is generated or until the termination criteria is satisfied.

```
Inputs : Parkinson Training dataset
Output : Optimal rule base and membership function for Fuzzy System
Procedure:
Begin
      Initialize the initial ideas in the proposed format
      Cluster the ideas
      Repeat
            Evaluate fitness of ideas using the proposed fitness function for
            rule base and membership function design
            Generate new ideas
            Replace bad ideas with good ones
      Until termination criteria
      Return the optimal idea
End
```

The initial idea, shown in Figure 2, is formatted as per the requirement suitable for the proposed methodology. The idea is a vector consisting of two parts. The first part represents the rules and second part represents the membership function. The first part consists of 1+(n*r) elements, where 'r' indicates the number of rules and 'n' indicates the number of attributes in the dataset. The 'n' elements of each rule consists of the membership index of the corresponding variable. If a variable is not included in the

Figure 1. Proposed Methodology

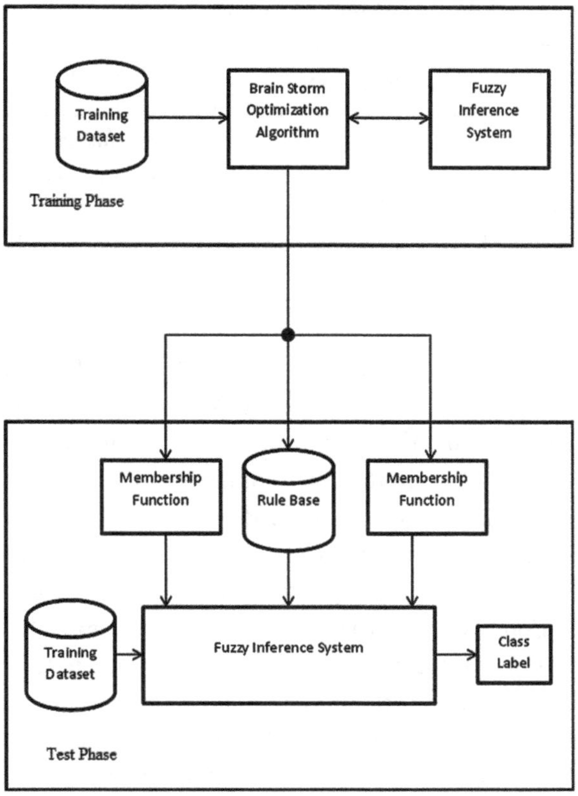

rule, then the corresponding element in the vector is represented by -1. The first element indicates the number of rules. Second to [1+(n*r)] contains all 'n' attributes of all 'r' rules. The 'n' attributes or each rule consists of the (n-1) attributes and the class attribute. The value of the elements from second to [1+(n*r)] contains the membership index of the corresponding variable. The index of the membership function indicates the linguistic term associated with the corresponding variable. This index can range from 1 to #MF which determines the number of membership function for each variable. A sample rule is given in the below figure. It says 1,2,2 which means that there are three variables in the dataset, including the class variable. If the first variable is LOW and second variable is HIGH then the class variable is HIGH. This is the meaning if 1,2,2. If a particular variable need not be included in the rule then it can be mentioned by -1. Say for example, 1,-1,1 indicates that, if first variable is LOW then class variable is LOW invariable of the second attribute. The second half of the idea vector represents the membership function design. It consists of 14*n elements. Out of the 14 elements, first element represents the type of membership function. There are several types of membership functions like triangular membership function, trapezoidal membership function, sigmoidal membership function, Gaussian membership function, Gaussian bell membership function, and so on. These membership functions take atmost four parameters. Upto there membership functions are allowed for each attribute. Hence, we need twelve elements to represent the four parameters of all three membership functions. In addition to these twelve elements, there are the first to elements which indicates the membership function type and the number of membership function. Hence there are totally fourteen elements for each attribute. Second element

Figure 2. Idea format

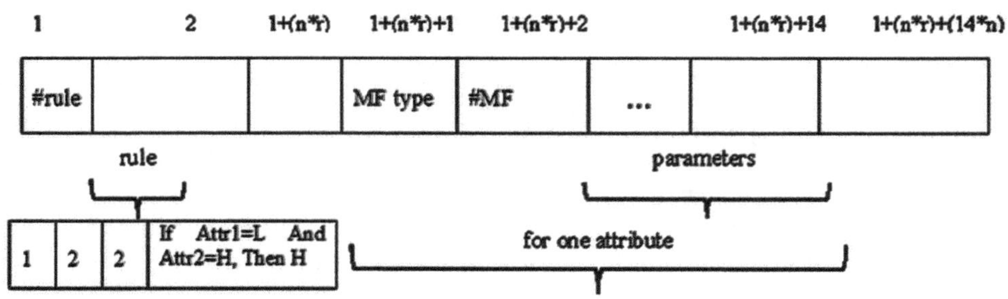

represents the number of membership function and the remaining 12 elements represents the parameters for a maximum of 3 membership functions. Hence for each of the 'n' attributes, there will be (14*n) elements. Thus, in the second part, [1+(n*r)]+1 to [1+(n*r)]+14 holds the membership function information of a single attribute. Thus for 'n' attributes the total number of elements will be [1+(n*r)]+(14*n).

Equation (1) shows the formulation of fitness function for the rule base generated using Brain Storm Optimization algorithm based on the proposed methodology. The fitness function is based on the length of the rule and the correlation of the rule with the dataset. Since rules with lesser length are preferred, the fitness value is inversely proportional to the length of the rule. Since the rules matching the characteristics of data is preferred, fitness of the rule is directly proportional to the preciseness of the rule. The average of two parts are taken to normalize the fitness value in the range of 0 to 1. In the below equation, 'n' indicates the number of attributes, 'r' indicates the number of rules, 'L' indicates the total length of the rules, 'm' indicates the number of instances in the dataset and 'M' indicates the total number of attributes in the rule that matches the dataset. 'L' the total length of the rules is the sum of number of significant attributes in each rule. The denominator in the first half indicates the total number of attributes in all the rule which are both significant as well as insignificant. Hence it is represented by the product of 'n' the number of attributes and 'r' the number of rules. Thus the ration of 'L' and (n*r) will give the significance of the number of attributes in each rule. But since this has to be minimized to have efficient rule base, it is subtracted from 1. 'M' indicates the sum of number of records that each rule matches the dataset. The denominator in the second half indicates the product of number of records and the number of rules in the dataset. Thus the ration of numerator and denominator gives the significance of degree of matching of each rule with the dataset. This ratio has to be maximum to achieve better rules. The average of both the ratios yields the optimal fitness function for the membership function.

$$\mathbf{F} = 0.5 * \left[\left(1 - \frac{\mathbf{L}}{\mathbf{n} * \mathbf{r}} \right) + \left(\frac{\mathbf{M}}{\mathbf{r} * \mathbf{m}} \right) \right] \tag{1}$$

DATASET

The Parkinson's dataset. Little et al. (2007), from UCI repository is used for Parkinson's disease detection. It consists of a collection of voice measurements of thirty-one people, out of which twenty-three were suffering with Parkinson's disease. There are around six recordings per patient totaling about 195 voice recording. The primary objective of this data is to differentiate healthy people from those with Parkinson's disease, according to status attribute which is set as 1 for Parkinson's disease and 0 otherwise. The proposed methodology is compared with benchmark Machine Learning algorithms like Support Vector Machine, Naïve Bayes, k-Means and Decision Tree. Accuracy, Specificity and Sensitivity are used as the comparison metrics.

Results

Equations (2), (3) and (4) shows the formulae for accuracy, specificity and sensitivity. Accuracy is the ratio of number of correctly diagnosed patients to the total number of patients who have undergone the diagnosis. In other words, it is the ratio of sum of true positive and true negative to the sum of true positives, true negatives, false positives and false negatives. Specificity, also called as the true negative rate, is defined as the ratio of true negative to the sum of true negatives and false positives. Sensitivity, also called as the true positive rate, is defined as the ratio of true positive to the sum of true positives and false negatives. Here, True positive is defined as the number of disorder patients diagnosed as disorder patients. False positive is defined as the number of normal patients wrongly diagnosed as disorder patients. True negative is defined as the number of normal patients diagnosed as normal patients. False negative is defined as the number of disorder patients wrongly diagnosed as normal patients.

$$\mathbf{Accuracy} = \frac{\mathbf{TP} + \mathbf{TN}}{\mathbf{TP} + \mathbf{TN} + \mathbf{FP} + \mathbf{FN}} \tag{2}$$

$$\mathbf{Specificity} = \frac{\mathbf{TN}}{\mathbf{TN} + \mathbf{FP}} \tag{3}$$

$$\mathbf{Sensitivity} = \frac{\mathbf{TP}}{\mathbf{TP} + \mathbf{FN}} \tag{4}$$

DISCUSSION

Table 2 compares the performance of the algorithms with the metrics and the same has been plotted in Figure 3, Figure 4 and Figure 5. It is evident from the graphs that the proposed Fuzzy Inference System with the Brain Storm Optimization algorithm outperforms Parkinson disorder detection implemented using benchmark algorithms like Support Vector Machine, Naïve Bayes, k-Means and Decision Tree.

From Table 2, it is observed that, the accuracy of Naïve Bayes classifier, Support Vector Machines classifier, k-Means classifier, Decision Tree classifier and the proposed Soft Computing based classi-

Table 2. Performance Comparison

Machine Learning Technique	Accuracy (%)	Specificity (%)	Sensitivity (%)
NB	70	65	71
SVM	84	75	70
k-Means	78	75	80
Decision Tree	81	65	80
Proposed Methodology	86	81	85

Figure 3. Accuracy Comparison

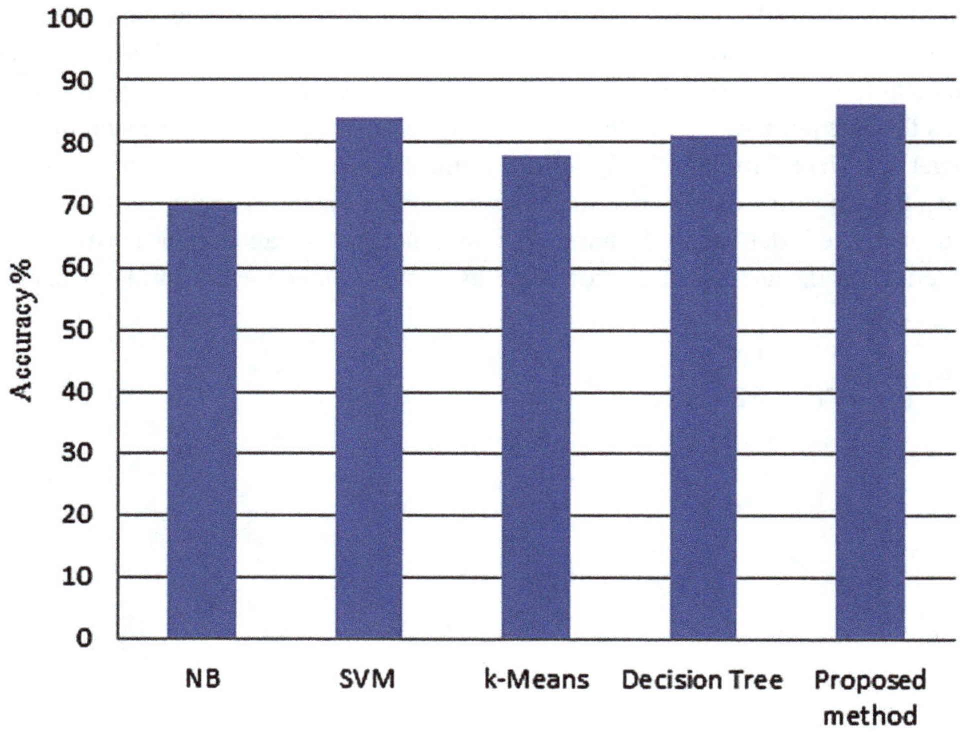

fier are 70%, 84%, 78%, 81% and 86% respectively. Similarly, the specificity of Naïve Bayes classifier, Support Vector Machines classifier, k-Means classifier, Decision Tree classifier and the proposed Soft Computing based classifier are 65%, 75%, 75%, 65% and 81% respectively. Similarly, the sensitivity of Naïve Bayes classifier, Support Vector Machines classifier, k-Means classifier, Decision Tree classifier and the proposed Soft Computing based classifier are 71%, 70%, 80%, 80% and 85% respectively. Hence, it is evident that the proposed Fuzzy Inference System with the Brain Storm Optimization algorithm outperforms Parkinson disorder detection implemented using benchmark algorithms like Support Vector Machine, Naïve Bayes, k-Means and Decision Tree.

Figure 4. Specificity Comparison

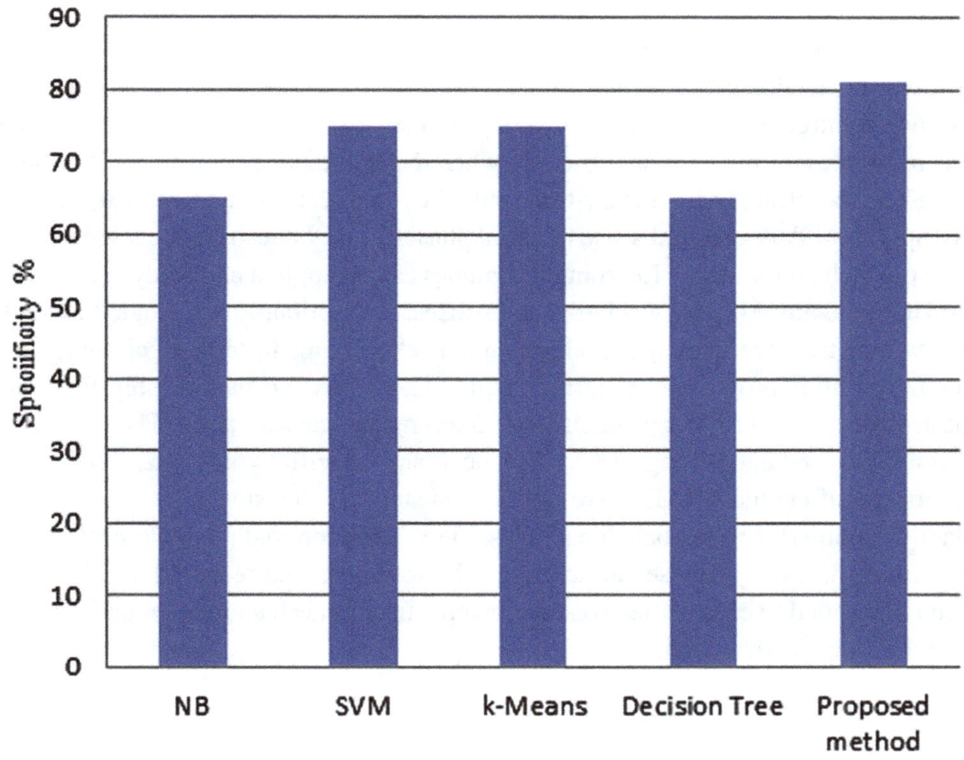

Figure 5. Sensitivity Comparison

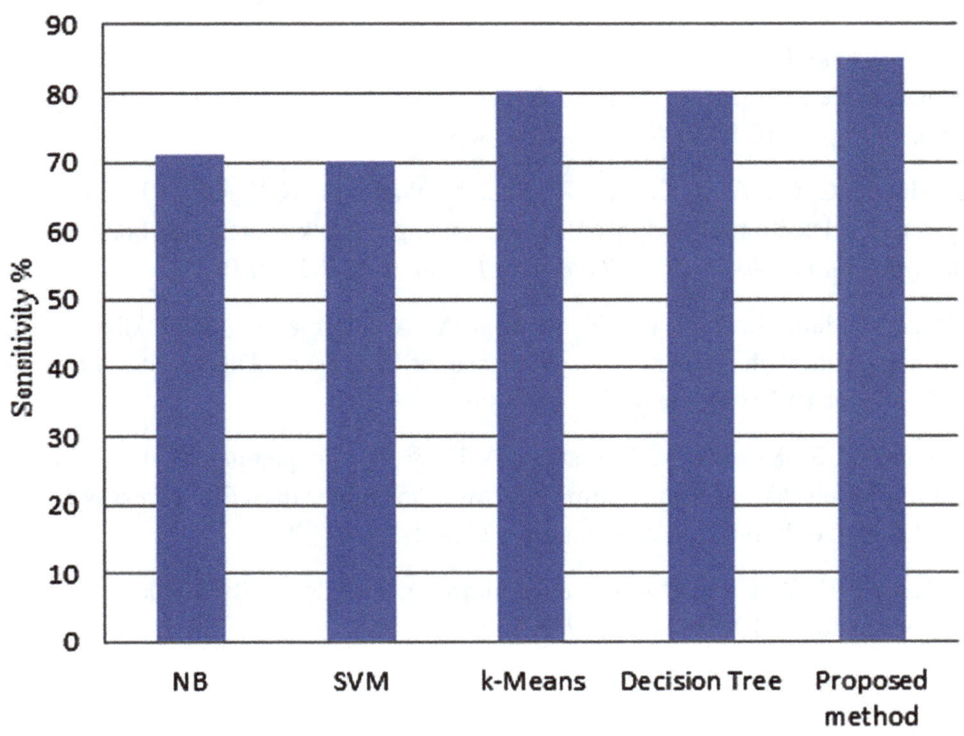

CONCLUSION AND FUTURE SCOPE

This chapter uses the speech signals which is a behavioral bio-marker for Parkinson's disease. Although, Parkinson's disease detection could be performed based on psychological, cognitive and physiological bio-markers, speech and conversation will start getting affected from the initial stage onwards. The victim's vocabulary is mostly lost or big gaps are observed when they are talking or the conversation is abruptly stopped. Therefore, speech analysis will help to identify the complications in conversation from the inception of the symptoms of Parkinson's disease in initial phases itself. Speech can be regularly logged in an unobstructed approach and Machine Learning techniques can be applied and analyzed. The Parkinson's dataset from UCI repository is used for Parkinson's disease detection. Fuzzy Logic based classifier is proposed for learning from the training speech signals and classifying the test speech signals. Brainstorm optimization algorithm is proposed for extracting the fuzzy rules and membership function from the speech dataset, which is used by fuzzy classifier for learning and classification. The performance of the proposed classifier is evaluated using metrics like accuracy, specificity and sensitivity and compared with benchmark classifiers like SVM, Naïve Bayes, k-Means and Decision Tree. It is observed that the proposed classifier outperforms the benchmark classifiers. The proposed methodology can be extended from voice intensity data to speech semantics data. The speech can be recorded and feature extraction algorithms can be applied to extract the semantic features from speech and the proposed method can be applied on it for Parkinson detection.

REFERENCES

Abiyev, R. H., & Abizade, S. (2016). Diagnosing Parkinson's Diseases Using Fuzzy Neural System. *Computational and Mathematical Methods in Medicine, 2016*, 1–9. doi:10.1155/2016/1267919 PMID:26881009

Chakraborty, A., Chakraborty, A., & Mukherjee, B. (2016). Detection of Parkinson's Disease Using Fuzzy Inference System. In *Proceedings of Intelligent Systems Technologies and Applications* (pp. 79–90). Cham: Springer. doi:10.1007/978-3-319-23036-8_7

Chen, H. L., Huang, C. C., Yu, X. G., Xu, X., Sun, X., Wang, G., & Wang, S. J. (2013). An efficient diagnosis system for detection of Parkinson's disease using fuzzy k-nearest neighbor approach. *Expert Systems with Applications*, *40*(1), 263–271. doi:10.1016/j.eswa.2012.07.014

Gupta, D., Julka, A., Jain, S., Aggarwal, T., Khanna, A., Arunkumar, N., & de Albuquerque, V. H. C. (2018). Optimized Cuttlefish Algorithm for Diagnosis of Parkinson's Disease. *Cognitive Systems Research*, *52*, 36–48. doi:10.1016/j.cogsys.2018.06.006

Gupta, D., Sundaram, S., Khanna, A., Hassanien, A. E., & de Albuquerque, V. H. C. (2018). Improved diagnosis of Parkinson's disease using optimized crow search algorithm. *Computers & Electrical Engineering*, *68*, 412–424. doi:10.1016/j.compeleceng.2018.04.014

Lisak, R. P., Truong, D. D., Carroll, W. M., & Bhidayasiri, R. (Eds.). (2016). *International Neurology*. John Wiley & Sons. doi:10.1002/9781118777329

Little, M. A., McSharry, P. E., Roberts, S. J., Costello, D. A., & Moroz, I. M. (2007). Exploiting nonlinear recurrence and fractal scaling properties for voice disorder detection. *Biomedical Engineering Online*, *6*(1), 23. doi:10.1186/1475-925X-6-23 PMID:17594480

Liu, S., Shen, Z., McKeown, M. J., Leung, C., & Miao, C. (2014, July). A fuzzy logic based parkinson's disease risk predictor. In *Proceedings of IEEE International Conference on Fuzzy Systems* (pp. 1624-1631). IEEE. 10.1109/FUZZ-IEEE.2014.6891613

Lorraine, V. K., & Anthony, E. L. (2015). Parkinson's disease. *Lancet*, *386*(9996), 896–912. doi:10.1016/S0140-6736(14)61393-3 PMID:25904081

Nilashi, M., Ibrahim, O., & Ahani, A. (2016). Accuracy improvement for predicting Parkinson's disease progression. *Scientific Reports*, *6*(1), 34181. doi:10.1038rep34181 PMID:27686748

Ornelas-Vences, C., Sanchez-Fernandez, L. P., Sanchez-Perez, L. A., Garza-Rodriguez, A., & Villegas-Bastida, A. (2017). Fuzzy inference model evaluating turn for Parkinson's disease patients. *Computers in Biology and Medicine*, *89*, 379–388. doi:10.1016/j.compbiomed.2017.08.026 PMID:28866303

Polat, K. (2012). Classification of Parkinson's disease using feature weighting method on the basis of fuzzy C-means clustering. *International Journal of Systems Science*, *43*(4), 597–609. doi:10.1080/00207721.2011.581395

Shi, Y. (2011). Brain storm optimization algorithm. In *Proceedings of International Conference in Swarm Intelligence* (pp. 303-309). Springer.

Shrivastava, P., Shukla, A., Vepakomma, P., Bhansali, N., & Verma, K. (2017). A survey of nature-inspired algorithms for feature selection to identify Parkinson's disease. *Computer Methods and Programs in Biomedicine*, *139*, 171–179. doi:10.1016/j.cmpb.2016.07.029 PMID:28187888

Smith, K. M., & Caplan, D. N. (2018). Communication impairment in Parkinson's disease: Impact of motor and cognitive symptoms on speech and language. *Brain and Language*, *185*, 38–46. doi:10.1016/j.bandl.2018.08.002 PMID:30092448

Zhai, J., Wang, X., Zhang, S., & Hou, S. (2018). Tolerance rough fuzzy decision tree. *Information Sciences*, *465*, 425–438. doi:10.1016/j.ins.2018.07.006

Zuo, W. L., Wang, Z. Y., Liu, T., & Chen, H. L. (2013). Effective detection of Parkinson's disease using an adaptive fuzzy k-nearest neighbor approach. *Biomedical Signal Processing and Control*, *8*(4), 364–373. doi:10.1016/j.bspc.2013.02.006

Chapter 7
Assessment of Gait Disorder in Parkinson's Disease

Divya Govindaraju
Anna University, India

Gururaj Nagarajan
Birla Institute of Technology and Science, India

Paramasivam Alagumariappan
B.S. Abdur Rahman Crescent Institute of Science and Technology, India

ABSTRACT

Neurological disorders are some of the leading chronic disorders that impose a massive burden on low-income and developing countries. The disability resulting from the neurological disorder increases the severity and costs during the primary healthcare and for entire lifetime. Parkinson's disease (PD) is the second most common chronic neurodegenerative disorder which is slowly progressive with decrease in the motor and non-motor function of the nervous system due to cognitive impairment leading to gait abnormality. PD is most common in the age group of 40-65years leading to increase in gait disorders associated with slowing down of the movement, balance instability, rigidness in the muscles, and difficulty in performing everyday tasks. The assessment of gait plays a significant role in maintaining the balance disorders in Parkinson's disease. In patients with PD, the neurons present in substantia nigra region of the brain get injured, and they progressively decline during their lifetime. Therefore, the patients lose their ability to perform movement and also lose their stability. The symptoms of PD can be monitored and controlled by assessing gait parameters based on gait disorder.

DOI: 10.4018/978-1-5225-8567-1.ch007

INTRODUCTION

Neurodegenerative disorder primarily affects the neurons present in the human brain leading to the loss or death of the neurons. Aging is one of the greatest risk factor of neurodegenerative disorder. The WHO (World Health Organization) has estimated that the neurological disorder affected more than one billion people worldwide leading to disability and suffering. Gait and balance disorders usually occurs in all major neurological diseases. Parkinson's Disease is the second most progressive neurological disorder which affects the elderly and its prevalence is predicted to increase with respect to the growth of the elderly population. Dr. James Parkinson, a surgeon and physician gave an essay describing the Shaking Palsy which is familiar in the western world. The birthday of Dr. James Parkinson has been chosen as the "World Parkinson's Day" and red tulip flower has been selected as its symbol. The clinical features of the PD combine four major parts of the human body namely changes in the motor function, changes in the cognitive function of the brain, changes in the behaviour and symptoms leading to failure in autonomic nervous systems. Every portion of the brain plays a different and critical role in the human body. The PD develops because there is a loss in the cells present in the basal ganglia portion of the brain. The basal ganglia control the basic human activity like walking and other movements. The abnormality in this portion results in irregulated movements of the human. Normally there are certain specific cells present in the basal ganglia which are responsible for the production of dopamine. The dopamine is one of the neurotransmitters produced in the brain which releases a chemical to communicate with different parts of the brain. Therefore, the progression of PD over many years makes these brain cells to die and there will be reduction in the dopamine level of the brain leading to more complication like resting tremor, bradykinesia, rigidity in the body and balance disorders. The symptom related to PD are unilateral which means one side of the body is more affected than the other side. The disease later progresses to the bilateral findings. Tremor usually occurs during the beginning of the PD and limited to one side of the arm or leg for many years. Bradykinesia which is described as the peculiar and most disabling characteristic of PD leads to slow or absent of movement. Rigidity is the resistance to the movement of the individual. Balance disorder is one the major problem in PD patients leading to frequent falling and postural abnormalities. There are also several minor motor and non-motor functions associated with PD patients namely speech impairment, cognitive impairment and psychological disorder. There are variety of medications available to treat the symptom of PD. At the initial stage the individual has already developed disability and therefore pharmacological treatment is required. The second stage is the development of complications and the third stage is the dopamine deficiency treated using dopamine agonists. Gait Rehabilitation are recommended for PD patients who have speech and mobility problems. The economic cost for the PD patients is high and PD reduces the quality of life of the individual and caregivers. The current research focus on building animal models based on gene therapy and stem cell transplantation.

BACKGROUND

Parkinson's disease (PD) is a neurodegenerative disease which mainly affects the human motor system (Rodriguez-Martin, Sama, Perez-Lopez, Catala, Moreno Arostegui & Cabestany, 2017). PD has many symptoms in which the freezing of Gait (FoG) is one among them. In recent years, the classification systems with several classifiers such as Linear Discriminate Analysis, K-nearest neighbour, K-means, Random forest, Naïve Baiyes, Support Vector Machine (SVM), Artificial Neural Network (ANN) etc.

are utilized as an automated decision support tools for the early detection of diseases of human body. Eventhough, the Naive Bayes classifier is one of the oldest classifier, it is very simple to implement and needs fewer amounts of training data. This simple and efficient classifier is adopted by several researchers on biomedical and other fields for classification (Sarkar, Goswami, Agarwal & Aktar 2014; Wolfson, Bandyopadhyay, Elidrisi, Vazquez-Benitez, Musgrove, Adomavicius, Johnson & O-Connor 2014;Ahmed, Shahjaman, Rana, Mollah & Haque 2017).

Principal Component Analysis (PCA) is a dimensionality reduction technique which is used in various fields such data analytics, bio-signal, image processing etc. where the original dimensionality is too large to process (Chen, Lin, Liao, Lai, Pei, Kuo, Lin, Chang, Chen, Lo & Chen, 2011; Kim, Shin, Shin & Lee, 2009; Hsieh, Lin, Te, Lo, Wu, Chung, Chang, Lin, Lo & Hu, 2017). In bio-signal or image processing, the PCA is used to improve the accuracy of the classifiers. Kikkert et al. (2017) have utilized PCA and extracted 11 gait variables to determine the gait properties. Also, the authors have developed a model using Partial Least Squares-Discriminant Analysis for the assessment of fall risk in geriatric patients. Matsushima et al. (2017) have analysed the characteristics of ataxic gait which is recorded with the help of triaxial accelerometer. Further, the authors have adopted PCA and extracted four principal components in the control subjects and two principal components in the abnormal patients.

Zhao et al. (2013) have designed an ECG identification system using ensemble empirical mode decomposition. Further, the authors have used PCA to reduce the dimensionality of feature space and the K-nearest neighbors (KNN) classifier is utilized as the classification tool.

Feng at al. (2013) have proposed a Naive Bayes based method for the prediction of phage virion proteins. Further, the authors have concluded that the proposed method has a classification accuracy of 79.15% which is superior than other state-of-art classifiers. Sambo et al. (2012) have proposed a Bag of Naive Bayes (BoNB) classification algorithm for the analysis of genome-wide SNP data. Further, the authors have concluded that the proposed BoNB classifier has good classification accuracy which can be used as both classifier and genetic biomarker.

Miranda et al. (2016) have discussed about the detection of risk levels of cardiovascular disease for adults using naive bayes classifier. Further, the authors have assessed three different classifier's performance such as accuracy, sensitivity and specificity. Also, the authors have concluded that the proposed model has the prediction rate of 80%.

SVM is based on statistical learning theory which is highly suitable for semi-structured or unstructured data such as text or images. Also, the SVM with appropriate kernel function can solve any type of complex problems. The various kernel functions are Linear, Quadratic, sigmoid, Gaussian, radial kernel etc (Saberioon, Cisar, Labbe, Soucek, Pelissier&Kerneis, 2018; McDermott, O'Halloran, Porter & Santorelli, 2018). Due to the technological advancements, the SVM classifiers with different kernels are used in wide fields such as image processing, optical text recognition, bio-signal classification etc. McDermott et al. (2018) have discussed about the detection of brain haemorrhages using Electrical Impedance Tomography (EIT) measurement frames and Linear SVM classifiers. Also, the authors have demonstrated that the performance parameter such as sensitivity and specificity of Linear SVM classifier is 90%.

Wu and Xu (2016) have proposed a method in which the block sparse Bayesian learning (BSBL) algorithm is presented to reconstruct an acceleration data. Further, the authors have validated the feasibility of the proposed method for gait telemonitoring application with three different gait classification models such as support vector machine (SVM), multilayer perception (MLP) and KStar.

Nukala et al. (2016) have developed a Wireless Wearable Gait Sensor for the classification of patients with balance disorders and normal subjects. Further, the authors have extracted the features from gait signals which is acquired using gyroscopes and accelerometers and have adopted four different classifiers such as SVM, binary decision trees (BDT), k-nearest neighbours (KNN) and back propagation artificial neural network (BP-ANN) for the classification process. Also, the authors have reported that the SVM has overall classification accuracy of 98%.

Saberioon et al. (2018) have adopted four different classification methods such as Random forest (RF), Support Vector Machine, Logistic regression and KNN to evaluate fish diets. Further, the authors have concluded that the SVM with radial based kernel has highest classification rate of 82% and it is superior to other adopted classifiers.

Wu and Wu (2015) have proposed a novel method for assessment of gait symmetry using advanced statistical learning algorithm. Further, the authors have recorded gait signals from 60 participants using a strain gauge force platform. Also, the authors have designed an advanced statistical learning algorithm such as SVM for binary classification and are utilized to quantitatively evaluate gait symmetry. The authors have reported that the proposed algorithm using SVM can be used as a tool for early identification of the elderly gait asymmetry in the clinical diagnosis.

Simila et al. (2017) have proposed a novel method to detect early stage of shortfalls in balance from gait. Further, the authors have collected gait acceleration data using waist-mounted accelerometer. Also, the authors have concluded that the gait features can be considered for the assessment and prediction of early signs of balance shortfalls. Zhou et al. (2018) have discussed about the impacts of hemodialysis process on gait and balance beyond aging and diabetes condition.

Raknim and Lan (2016) have proposed a Pedestrian dead reckoning based method for continuous assessment of patient's gait signals using smartphone. Also, the authors have concluded that the binary classification-based support vector machine is more significant on classifying walking patterns of a PD patient with overall accuracy of 94%. Thiede et al. (2016) have quantified gait and balance using wearable sensors. Further, the authors have assessed the group differences in frailty using analysis of variance whereas the authors have determined the independent connections within gait and balance using logistic regression models.

Backstrom et al. (2018) have examined mortality and associated risk factors in a community-based population with incident parkinsonism and Parkinson disease. Maqbool et al. (2016) have discussed about the real-time rule based gait event detection for lower limb amputees using shank mounted inertial measurement unit. Further, the authors have stated that the proposed system is highly capable of detecting temporal gait events with detection accuracy of 99.78%. Lee et al. (2014) have analysed the videos which is taken from patients having Parkinson disease. Further, the authors have classified the parameters associated to posture and gait into three classes namely standing, gait and associated symptoms. Also, the authors have concluded that the visual inspection of gait and posture gives reliable information for the diagnosis of Parkinson disease.

Laske et al. (2014) have discussed various diagnostic tools for early detection of Alzheimer's disease. Pistacchi et al. (2017) have investigated an abnormal gait pattern in early Parkinson disease patients. Further, authors have stated that there are some distinguishing characteristics of gait namely ambulation disorders are present in early Parkinson disease patients and they suggested it can be mitigated by proper rehabilitation process.

METHODOLOGY

Assessment of Gait in Healthy Individuals

The neurological condition in which a person slowly develops difficulty in controlling the activities related to movement is termed as movement disorder or gait disorder (Levine, Richards & Whittle, 2012). The ability of the body to maintain stability related to gait and posture with respect to the centre of gravity is defined as balanced gait (Baker, 2018). The analysis of gait can be carried out in two ways namely standard laboratory-based gait analysis or new upcoming methods like wearable and non-invasive measurement methods. The standard laboratory-based measurement is a golden standard for performing gait analysis using EMG(Electromyography) sensor attached to the body motion of the patient or by using optical measurement system and force sensor (Chen, Wang, Liou & Shaw, 2013).The results produced by this method are accurate but only for shorter distance. The wearable and non-invasive measurements use portable digital based equipment which are light, small and less expensive compared to standard method. This type of measurements is used for long term monitoring of patients.

Walking is a most complicated task involving various changes in the gait patterns which is performed by precisely controlling the limb and posture movements. In the brain, cerebral cortex receives input from the visual part, vestibular and proprioceptive part of the brain stream, basal ganglia, cerebellum and integrates it with the neurons which carry signals from muscle stretch receptors. The gait cycle is often assessed during two phases namely swing phase and strike phase. Further, the complexity of walking phase increases the risk of losing stability among elderly people due to age and motor function disorder. Depending upon this, the assessment of gait can be classified into four main stages of the gait cycle (Smulders, Dale, Carlson-Kuhta, Nutt & Horak, 2016). They are

1. First Stage: Walking straight on a flat surface
2. Second Stage: Initiation of gait movement
3. Third Stage: Ability to walk during turning and other rotations
4. Fourth Stage: Adaptability of gait to walk on irregular surface

First Stage: Walking Straight on a Flat Surface

In first stage the motor behaviour is performed automatically in healthy subjects because this stage requires only minimal attention and less cognitive part while walking straight (Hawkes, Del Tredici & Braak, 2010). The stability of gait is determined by calculating the variability in the stride length from step phase to stride phase. This stage does not require much attention because the sensorimotor striatum provides an automatic control to the brain and the operation is performed.

Second Stage: Initiation of Gait Movement

In the second stage, the attentional control gives instruction to the motor cortex because it involves shifting of the posture and balance. The initiation of gait is a goal generated movement which involves more strain to the cortical part. The length of each step and the duration and amplitude are studied during this stage.

Third Stage: Ability to Walk During Turning and Other Rotations

The third stage requires more cognitive control of the attentional and automatic control of the brain for performing the turning action which in turn requires both change in the posture and balance. The turning phase involves uneven rotation of the foot and the upper body. The number of steps taken for rotation, gait speed postural stability with respect to the centre of mass and co-ordination of the feet-head are studied to quantify the turning phase.

Fourth Stage: Adaptability of Gait to Walk on Irregular Surface

The fourth stage is mostly dependent on the cognitive control for adaptability of the gait over obstacles. The obstacles involve walking on an irregular surface, uneven terrain and crowded areas. The output measures of gait adaptability are studied by measuring the success rate in obstacle avoidance, distance measured between the obstacle and the foot and the stability while crossing the obstacle (Xu, Hunt, Foreman, Zhao & Merryweather, 2018).

The recent advances in analysing gait disorder includes portable wireless monitoring of the patient's data, data gathering with the help of intelligent systems by the patient and also wireless sensor monitoring. The portable wireless technology will be the future of gait assessment since it reduces the time complexity and easy for measurement. Further, the force-plate sensors can be fixed into the footwear for measurement which also helps in long-term monitoring of gait irrespective of the stages of the patient. Quantitative measurement makes more accurate measurement of duration, gait speed, stability in gait and gait rhythmicity. Therefore, the advantages of wireless and non-invasive monitoring provide a way to integrate huge number of data depending on the task performed by the individual compared to laboratory based measurement.

Assessment of Gait Disorder in Parkinson's Disease

Parkinson disease is mainly characterised by disability in the motor functions leading to different stages of bradykinesia, cogwheel rigidity, parkinsonian tremor and gait abnormality. The pathology of PD is loss in the energy level of dopamine neurons. Since PD is a chronic and highly progressive disease it has both the motor and non-motor symptoms (Mouradian, 2001). Motor automaticity is associated with the changes in the motor and non-motor function of the PD patients. The PD patients lose the automatic skills or new motor skills due to the impaired function of the sensorimotor striatum. The motor automaticity is usually evaluated during the dual-task paradigm where the secondary action requires equal level of attention as that of the first action (Wu, Hallett & Chan, 2015). When the patients perform dual task in parallel, the attentional resources are limited and divided. An automatic action of this task is accompanied by increased efficiency, minimal attentional demands and little resources to perform the task. The first action includes tasks like getting up from the bed in the morning, eating breakfast, holding a fork/spoon all these requires minimal cognitive action whereas the secondary action requires little attention to the motor function like counting numbers task which requires more cognitive action compared with the first action. The first motor task is said to be automatic if it is performed correctly without any sort of interference. If the performance of any one task lags during the dual task paradigm then the motor action is not performed automatically.

In healthy patients if the motor skills are automatic then (1) the neural functioning of the patient becomes more efficient (2) There will be no need for attentional network (3) The interference will be resisted during the automatic task (4) The support for sensorimotor striatum is critical. If the motor skills are not automatically performed whereas in case of PD patients, they tend to perform all the daily behaviours slower with smaller amplitude than healthy patients. Therefore, the PD patient have difficulty in performing automatic task like arm swing, modulation in speech, facial expression, blinking even during the early stage of the disease. The gait disorder is an early symptom of people with PD and it increases with age leading to disability.If the motor skills are not automatic in PD patients then (1) the movement of the neural coding is less efficient (2) there is a failure in shifting the automated motor skills to the sensorimotor striatum (3) the automatic mode is not stable and it can be disturbed within the striatum (4)mostly they rely on the attention control to execute the movements which are automatically performed by the healthy patients.

First Stage of PD Patients

Bradykinesia, the first stage of symptom in the analysis of PD subjects where they experience smaller steps than usual, and the imbalance associated with it making the people double the time to perform any specific action. The shorter steps at this stage reflects the difficulty in controlling the Centre of Mass (CoM) of the body. The bradykinesia in the upper part of the body results in reduced movement of the arm and reduction in the velocity and range of motion. Further, the changes are also observed during the postural instability which will results in increased risk of falling in PD subjects. Also, there will be at least 50% loss in the level of dopamine(neuron) present in the substantia nigra where these symptoms lead to the starting of PD. Cell loss in this region causes low level of dopamine neurons.

Second Stage of PD Patients

Anticipatory Postural Adjustments (APA) or Akinesia, the second stage of the symptom shows difficulty in APA during the initiation of the gait cycle. The first step length is short, and the movement is also performed slowly by repetitive movements in PD subjects compared to healthy subjects. Depression defined as the premotor symptom plays a major role in the PD patients. The severity of the disease is correlated with the decreased functional connectivity and reduced function of the basal ganglia. Therefore, the automatic control of the PD patient becomes disable and there is no action performed by the sensorimotor to initiate the movement and therefore the attentional control performs the action leading to more time and less force.

Third Stage of PD Patients

Sequential movement, the third stage of the symptom shows difficulty in the co-ordination of eyes and head movement. The turning can be performed only when both cognitive and neural functions of the body work in co-ordination with each other. Therefore, this task of turning and rotating which requires the action of eyes, legs and head simultaneously can only be performed by additional turning and jerky rotational steps sometimes leading to imbalance and increases the risk of instability. The obstacle hit experienced by the PD patients will be more when compared to the healthy patients.The impaired and decreased function of the basal ganglia followed by reduction in the level of dopamine reduces the movement in PD patients. The PD patients performs simple repetitive task with high timing variability compared to the healthy patients.

Fourth Stage of PD Patients

Gait Adaptability, the fourth stage where the patient with PD experience higher number of hit and they are less stable compared with healthy subjects. Sometimes they also experience a breakdown in their motor planning part which makes their situation even worse. The placement of foot relative to that of the obstacle is also smaller and therefore there are more chances of collision. During this stage, the pathology of the disease is widespread, and it is difficult to predict the correlation in the clinical data. A small portion of the PD patients develop changes in the behaviour mainly due to the dopaminergic therapy.

Freezing of Gait

Freezing of gait (FoG), the last stage of PD eventually develops to majority of patient where they have a feeling that their feet are attached to the ground. FoG usually occurs during the dual task paradigm where multiple attention is needed to perform a task like talking or using a device while walking. Therefore, the FoG patients perform these tasks very slowly compared with the PD patients and FoG patients have a shorter stride length and step length. Further, the defective motor functioning in PD patients are also a reason for contributing to FoG. Initiation of gait is usually performed internally in healthy patients. In FoG patients the connectivity of the basal ganglia cortex motor functioning loop is disrupted, and they have difficulty in performing the gait cycle. During the turning phase, FoG patients takes more time to perform the action than PD patients. These patients face a severe cortical damage at the last stage. The damage further results in the impaired taste pathway. Also, the loss of dopaminergic neuron induces a difficulty in executing automatic action in FoG patients. Typically, in this phase the patient is unable to move from a position leading to the advanced stage of the disease.

Comparison of Gait Disorder Between Healthy and PD Patient

Figure 1 shows the assessment of gait in both healthy and PD patients by collecting input from the force sensors that where placed on both the foot of the patient. The old age patients above 60years where considered for assessment. PCA is used for extracting highly correlated features from raw input data obtained from the force sensors. After feature extraction, classification of the healthy and PD patients is performed based on two classifiers namely Naive Bayes (NB) and Linear Support Vector Machine (LSVM). Further, the evaluation of the classifier performance parameters is calculated by considering the accuracy, sensitivity, specificity, positive predictive value and negative predictive value of both the classifiers.

DATA ACQUISITION AND ANALYSIS

In this study, the gait rhythm dataset (Hausdorff, Lertratanakul, Cudkowicz, Peterson, Kaliton & Goldberger, 2000) from the Physiobank was utilized for analysis of gait in PD patients (Zeng, Liu, Wang, Ma & Zhang, 2016). This is one of the large extensively used physiological data for public research

Figure 1. Flowchart for assessment of gait order using classification algorithms

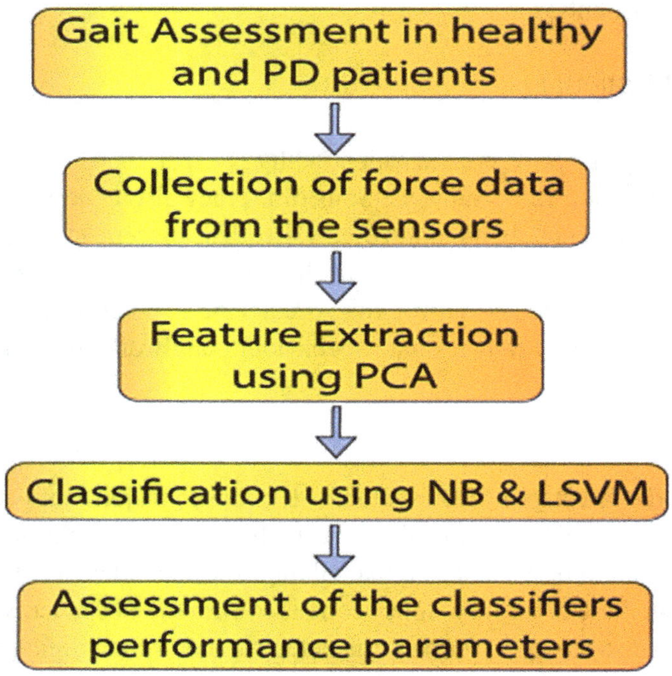

purposes founded by Harvard- MIT institutes. This dataset contains both healthy and PD patient in the age of 66.3 years with 63%men. In the experiment, the patient is required to walk continuously in a flat level ground for a period of two minutes. Under each foot there were 8 sensors that measure the force (in newtons) as a function of time. The output from the sensors are digitized and recorded at 100 samples per second. The stride time (initial contact of one foot to the time taken for the subsequent contact from the same foot), swing time (time taken when one foot is in air with respect to the stride time) and also the centre of pressure can be calculated as a function of time. The stride to stride measurement output can also be calculated from the force sensors. This database also provides information about the severity of the disease and dual task while walking on the flat surface and treadmill. Further, the feature extraction is carried out by transforming the input data obtained from the Physiobank into a set of features which may represent the input data in a well-defined form for performing further analysis of the gait rhythm.

Principal Component Analysis (PCA)

PCA is extensively used in large number of applications in healthcare and industry due to its simplicity and extracting meaningful information from a complex dataset. PCA is easy to understand since it simplifies the confusing dataset to lower dimension (De Maesschalck, Estienne, Verdu-Andres, Candolfi, Centner, Despagne, Jouan-Rimbaud, Walczak, Massart, De Jong & De Noord, 1999). The principle of PCA is to transform the maximum possible number of correlated variables into smaller variables known as principal components. The dimensionality of the PCA is reduced with the help of vector transformation. The reduced dataset makes the interpretation much more clear and easier. The algorithm steps for PCA are as follows:

Step 1: Identify a set of orthogonal coordinate axis from the input data. The new axis obtained is called as first principal component of the data.
Step 2: The interpretation of the first principal component is represented in the form of score plot to identify the correlation in the data.
Step 3: Identify the second principal component axis which is orthogonal to the first principal component and the best direction to approximate the input data.
Step 4: The interpretation of the second principal component is represented in the same above score plot and the loading plot gives the eigen vector values.
Step 5: Covariance is used to measure the correlation between the two variables in the data.

Using these steps, the feature extraction using PCA is carried out for the gait rhythm database. PCA is used for many applications in neuroscience, quantitative analysis of risk management and multivariate calibration in spectroscopy. Next step is the classification of gait rhythm of patients with PD using machine learning algorithms.

Naive Bayes (NB)

The NB classifier is a probabilistic classification method based on the Bayes theorem. Each features of the NB classifier provide independent assumptions. The principle of NB classifier assumes that the particular feature present or absence in a class is unrelated to the presence or absence of the other feature in the same class (Leung, 2007).The Bayesian classifier are based on statistical classifiers which can predict the probability of the data from the given dataset. The algorithm steps involved in NB classifier are as follows:

Step 1: Consider an n-dimensional vector space with a set of training samples, measured values and their class labels.
Step 2: Now given a sample X the classifier will predict the class of X based on the highest probability.
Step 3: In order to reduce the computation steps an assumption is made in the naive classifier by making the value of the attribute independent to one another.
Step 4: The probabilities can be easily calculated with the help of the training data.
Step 5: In case the value of the attribute is categorical, the number of samples in the training data is divided by the number of samples of the original data
Step 6: In case the value of the attribute is continuous, then the values are calculated based on the gaussian distribution with respect to mean and standard deviation.

Some common application of NB classifier is useful in the field of multi-class prediction, real-time prediction, text classification, sentimental analysis and also in automatic medical diagnosis.

Linear Support Vector Machine (LSVM)

SVM is a non-probabilistic linear binary classifier developed from the statistical learning theory and have been applied in numerous numbers of application from time series to biomedical data processing. The principle of SVM are defined by a subset of feature vectors which are known as support vectors. SVM is based on a set of supervised algorithms which is used for prediction, classification and regression based on optimization theory to increase the prediction accuracy and avoid over fitting of the data. The special feature of SVM are (1) the generalization of the matrix is made high by maximizing the margin (2) the non-linear functions are learned efficiently using kernel function. The steps followed in the SVM algorithm are:

The initial form of the LSVM classifier a linear binary classifier where the output obtained from the learned function may be either positive or negative (Yu & Kim, 2012). A multiclass problem can also be computed by means of LSVM by combining multiple binary classifiers together. The main steps are maximization of the margin data and kernel function.

Step 1: Each data point is represented by means of a n dimensional vector. The data points are divided into two categories in case of binary classifier.
Step 2: Linear classifier is used to correctly classify the data in the two-dimensional space with respect to the hyperplane.
Step 3: The LSVM finds the hyperplane with larger margin and maximum separation between the classes.
Step 4: The margin obtained shows the shortest distance separating the hyperplane to the data point nearer to both the categories
Step 5: Similarly, to do mapping of the feature set of the input of the non-linear classification problem kernel function is used.

SVM are used for solving huge number of real-world problems in hand-written characters, classification of images in different fields and also in text and hypertext categorization.

RESULTS AND DISCUSSION

In this chapter, two main events are considered for the recording of force data namely normal walk and Treadmill walk. Also, the individuals of two different groups such as normal or control subjects and PD patients are considered for this study. The force data from both the control subjects and PD patients during normal walk and Treadmill walk are recorded for analysis.

Figure 2 (a) and (b) shows the Total force recorded from control subject during normal walk under the right and left foot, respectively. Further, the total force is given in newtons with respect to time. Figure 3 (a) and (b) shows the Total force recorded from PD patients during normal walk under the right and left foot, respectively. It is seen that there is no significant difference by visually observing the force data's recorded from control subject and PD patient during normal walk.

Figure 4 (a) and (b) shows the Total force recorded from control subject during Treadmill walk under the right and left foot, respectively. Further, the total force is given in newtons with respect to time. Figure 5 (a) and (b) shows the Total force recorded from PD patients during Treadmill walk under the right and left foot, respectively.

In this chapter, the Principal component analyses feature extraction technique is utilized to extract the features from recorded force data. Further, these extracted features are utilized by LSVM and Naïve Bayes classifiers for the classification of normal and PD force data. The standard performance parameters of two different classifiers such as LSVM and Naïve Bayes were obtained using the following equations:

Figure 2. Total force recorded from control subject during normal walk under the (a) right foot (b) left foot

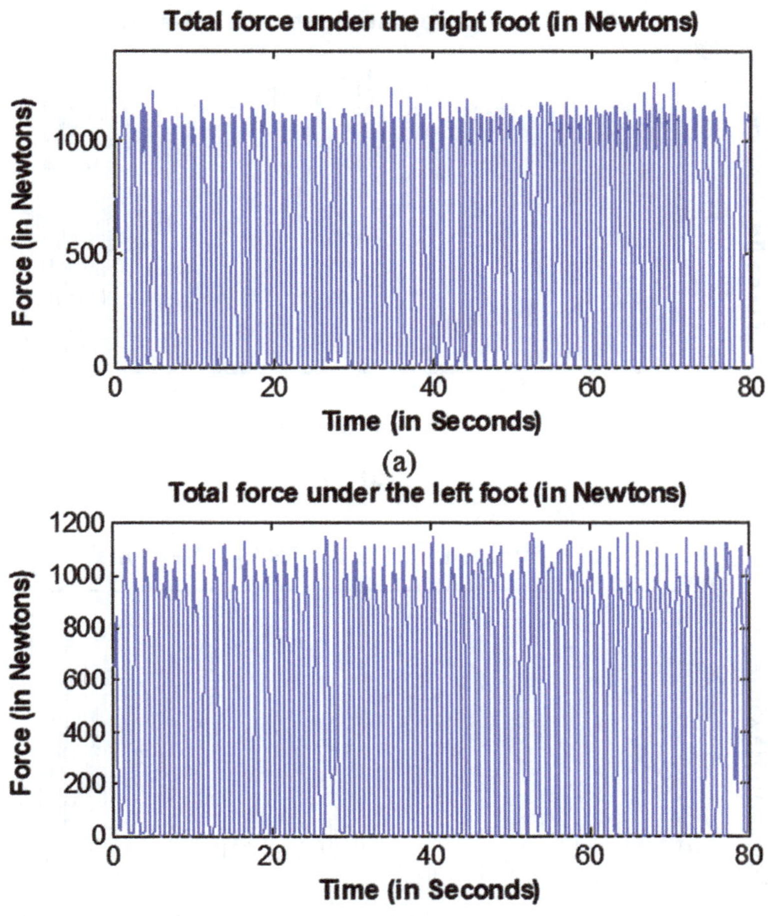

(b)

$$Accuracy = (TP + TN) / (TP + FP + TN + FN) \quad (1)$$

$$Sensitivity = TP / (TP + FN) \quad (2)$$

$$Specificity = TN / (TN + FP) \quad (3)$$

$$Positive\ predictive\ value = TP / (TP + FP) \quad (4)$$

Figure 3. Total force recorded from PD patient during normal walk under the (a) right foot (b) left foot

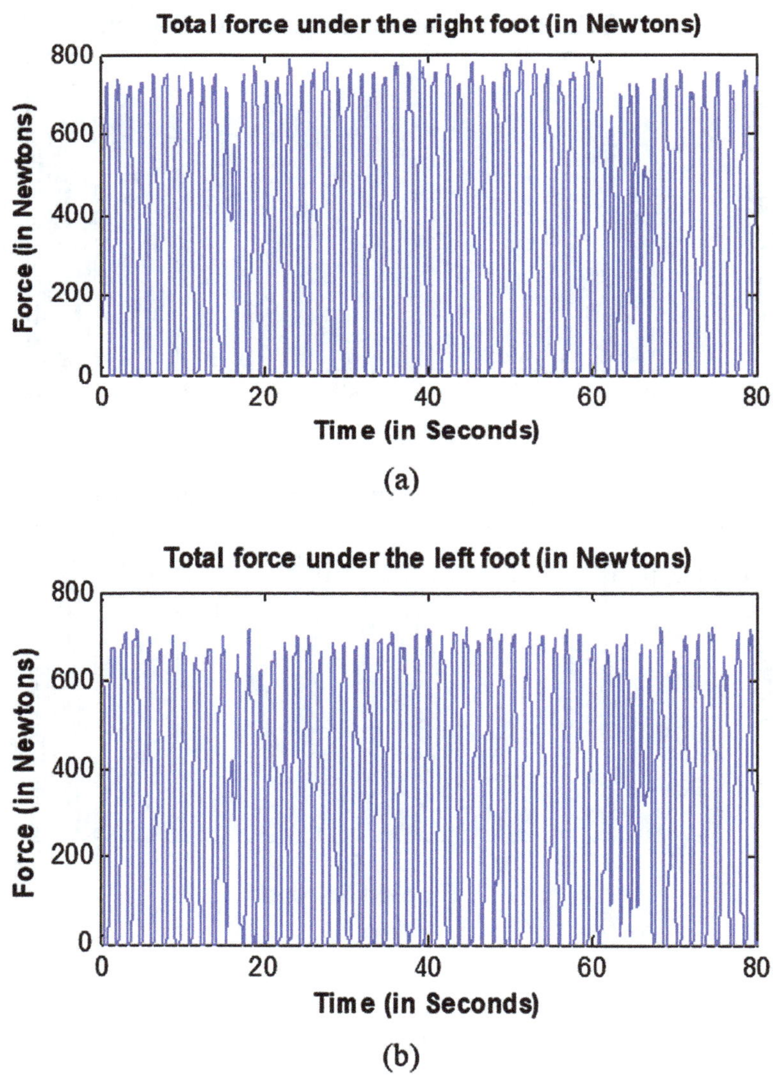

$$Negative\ predictive\ value = TN\ /\ (TN + FN) \tag{5}$$

Figure 6 (a) and (b) show the five different performance parameters such as accuracy, sensitivity, specificity, Positive Predicted Value (PPV) and Negative Predicted Value (NPV) for LSVM and Naïve Bayes classifiers during normal walking event, respectively. Usually, from the output of the classifiers the parameters such as true positive (TP), true negative (TN), false positive (FP) and false negative (FN) are used to assess the standard performance parameters. Further, it is seen that the accuracy of LSVM classifier is 91% and the accuracy of the Naïve Bayes classifier is 73%. It is observed that the Positive Predictive Value of Naïve Bayes is 55% and the Negative Predicted Value is 91. It is seen that the performance of LSVM classifier is good when compared to Naïve Bayes classifier during normal walking. Table 1 presents the performance parameters of LSVM and Naïve Bayes classifiers during normal walking.

Figure 4. Total force recorded from control subject during Treadmill walk under the (a) right foot (b) left foot

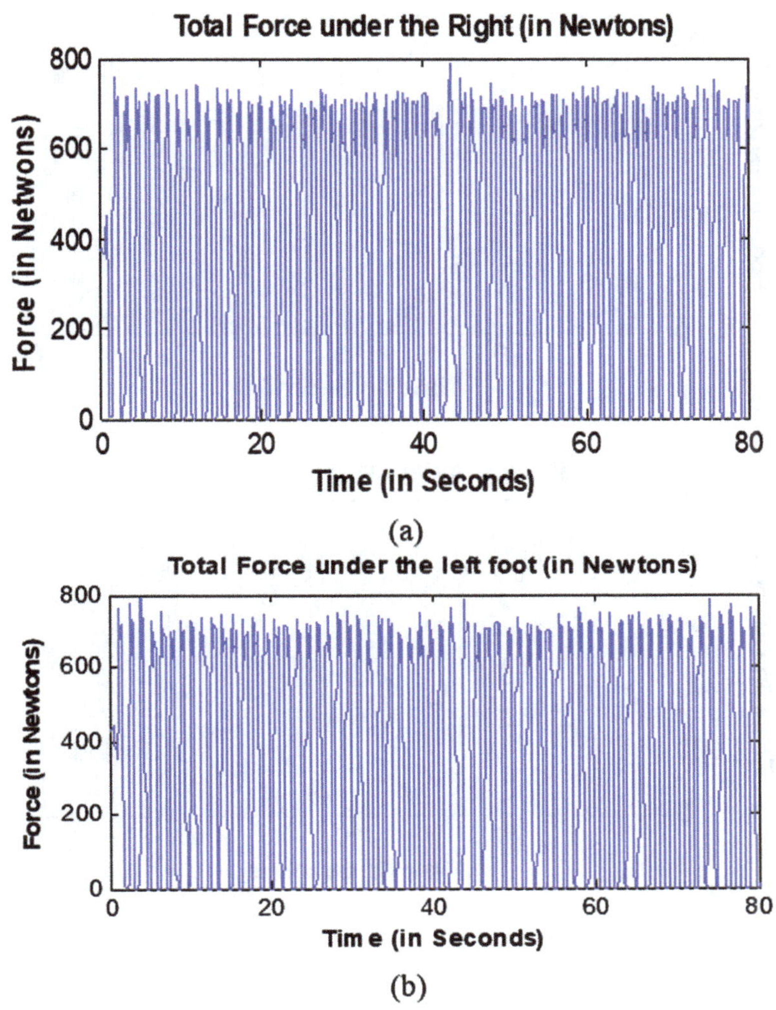

Figure 7 (a) and (b) show the performance parameters such as accuracy, sensitivity, specificity, PPV and NPV for LSVM and Naïve Bayes classifiers during Treadmill walking event, respectively. It is seen that the accuracy of the LSVM classifier is 86% and the accuracy of the Naïve Bayes classifier is 77%. Further, the sensitivity and specificity of LSVM classifier is 83% and 90% respectively. Also, it is inferred that the performance of LSVM classifier is superior to the performance of Naïve Bayes classifier. Table 2 presents the performance parameters of LSVM and Naïve Bayes classifiers during Treadmill walking.

CONCLUSION

The assessment of gait should be performed as a basic initial examination and follow-up for future treatment in every PD patient. The effective treatment of gait reduces the need for medication and further helps

Figure 5. Total force recorded from PD patient during Treadmill walk under the (a) right foot (b) left foot

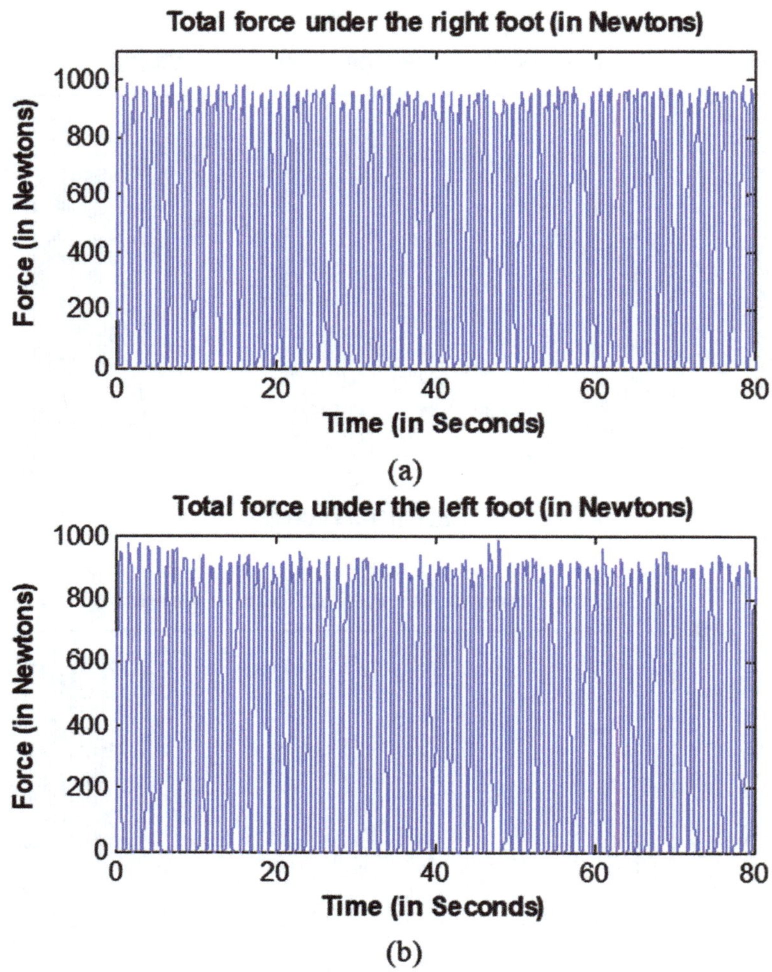

Figure 6. Performance parameters of (a) LSVM and (b) Naïve Bayes classifier during normal walking event

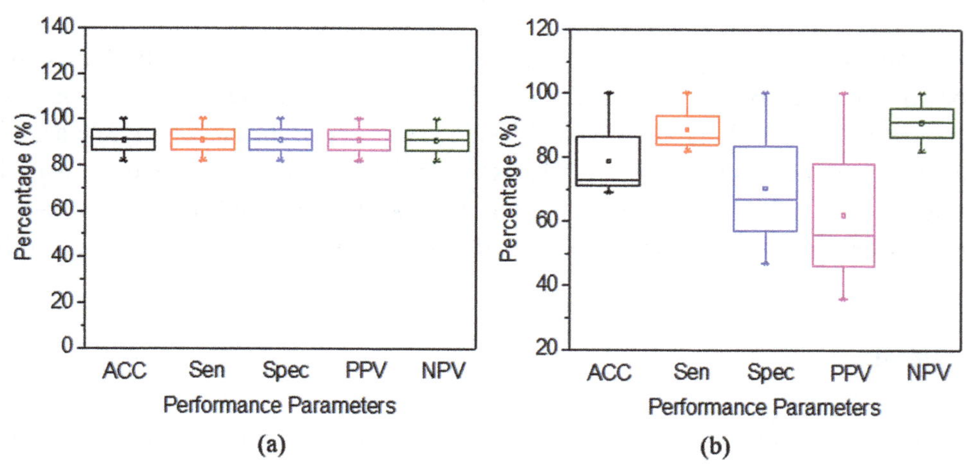

Table 1. Performance parameters of LSVM and Naïve Bayes classifiers during normal walking

Performance Parameters	Normal Walk	
	LSVM classifier (%)	Naïve Bayes classifier (%)
Accuracy	91	73
Sensitivity	91	86
Specificity	91	67
PPV	91	55
NPV	91	91

Figure 7. Performance parameters of (a) LSVM and (b) Naïve Bayes classifier during Treadmill walking event

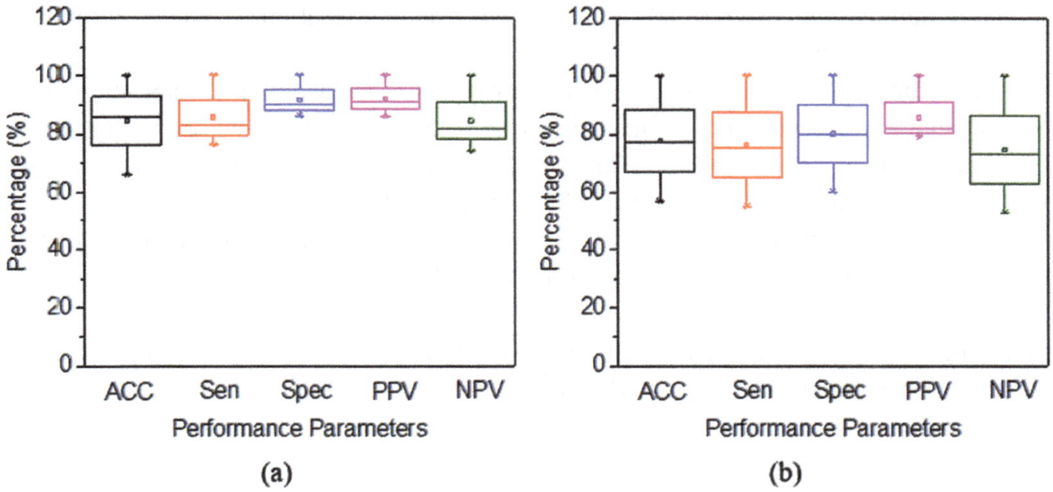

Table 2. Performance parameters of LSVM and Naïve Bayes classifiers during treadmill walking

Performance Parameters	Treadmill Walk	
	LSVM classifier (%)	Naïve Bayes classifier (%)
Accuracy	86	77
Sensitivity	83	75
Specificity	90	80
PPV	91	82
NPV	82	73

in improving the quality of life of PD patients. Further, the symptoms corresponding to the clinical test, neuro-imaging, molecular genetic data and laboratory data should be considered for future diagnosis of the PD patients during the different stages of the disease. Walking test which requires dual task reflect more challenges in the study of PD patients. The patients with PD find it difficult to perform the basic day to day activities and face lot of obstacles. Therefore, the gait rehabilitation can be carried out by increasing the level of dopamine which becomes more effective method for controlling the gait-based disorders in PD patients.

FUTURE WORK

For future analysis,

- The motor automaticity can be analysed by focusing on the attentional control, automatic control and motor cortex networks.
- The reason for bradykinesia can be further investigated by focusing on the non-motor symptoms such as facial movement deficits, micrographia and sleep disorder associated with PD.
- The advances in analysing the gait technology helps in improving the facility by designing intelligent gait system using wearables and wireless data transfer.
- In-vivo and in-vitro studies for diagnostic biomarkers helps in reducing the morbidity and mortality of PD patients (Sharma, Moon, Khoali, Haidous, Chabenne, Ojo, Jelebinkov, Kurdi & Ebadi, 2013).
- Finally, the research on gait rehabilitation can be performed for future diagnosis and long-term assistance of the patients suffering with PD.

REFERENCES

Ahmed, M., Shahjaman, M., Rana, M., Mollah, M., & Haque, N. (2017). Robustification of Naïve Bayes Classifier and Its Application for Microarray Gene Expression Data Analysis. *BioMed Research International*. PMID:28848763

Baker, J. M. (2018). Gait Disorders. *The American Journal of Medicine*, *131*(6), 602–607. doi:10.1016/j.amjmed.2017.11.051 PMID:29288631

Chen, P. H., Wang, R. L., Liou, D. J., & Shaw, J. S. (2013). Gait disorders in Parkinson's disease: Assessment and management. *International Journal of Gerontology*, *7*(4), 189–193. doi:10.1016/j.ijge.2013.03.005

Chen, S. W., Lin, S. H., Liao, L. D., Lai, H. Y., Pei, Y. C., Kuo, T. S., ... Chen, S. Y. (2011). Quantification and recognition of parkinsonian gait from monocular video imaging using kernel-based principal component analysis. *Biomedical Engineering Online*, *10*(1), 99. doi:10.1186/1475-925X-10-99 PMID:22074315

De Maesschalck, R., Estienne, F., Verdú-Andrés, J., Candolfi, A., Centner, V., Despagne, F., ... De Noord, O. E. (1999). The development of calibration models for spectroscopic data using principal component regression. *Internet Journal of Chemistry*, *2*(19), 1.

Feng, P. M., Ding, H., Chen, W., & Lin, H. (2013). Naive Bayes classifier with feature selection to identify phage virion proteins. *Computational and Mathematical Methods in Medicine*. PMID:23762187

Hausdorff, J. M., Lertratanakul, A., Cudkowicz, M. E., Peterson, A. L., Kaliton, D., & Goldberger, A. L. (2000). Gait Dynamics in Neuro-Degenerative Disease Data Base [Data set]. physionet.org. doi:10.13026/C27G6C

Hawkes, C. H., Del Tredici, K., & Braak, H. (2010). A timeline for Parkinson's disease. *Parkinsonism & Related Disorders*, *16*(2), 79–84. doi:10.1016/j.parkreldis.2009.08.007 PMID:19846332

Hsieh, W. H., Lin, C. Y., Te, A. L. D., Lo, M. T., Wu, C. I., Chung, F. P., ... Hu, Y. F. (2017). A novel noninvasive surface ECG analysis using interlead QRS dispersion in arrhythmogenic right ventricular cardiomyopathy. *PLoS One*, *12*(8), e0182364. doi:10.1371/journal.pone.0182364 PMID:28771538

Kikkert, L. H., De Groot, M. H., van Campen, J. P., Beijnen, J. H., Hortobágyi, T., Vuillerme, N., & Lamoth, C. C. (2017). Gait dynamics to optimize fall risk assessment in geriatric patients admitted to an outpatient diagnostic clinic. *PLoS One*, *12*(6), e0178615. doi:10.1371/journal.pone.0178615 PMID:28575126

Kim, J., Shin, H. S., Shin, K., & Lee, M. (2009). Robust algorithm for arrhythmia classification in ECG using extreme learning machine. *Biomedical Engineering Online*, *8*(1), 31. doi:10.1186/1475-925X-8-31 PMID:19863819

Leung, K. M. (2007). *Naive Bayesian classifier.* Polytechnic University Department of Computer Science/Finance and Risk Engineering.

Levine, D., Richards, J., & Whittle, M. W. (2012). *Whittle's Gait Analysis-E-Book.* Elsevier Health Sciences.

Matsushima, A., Yoshida, K., Genno, H., & Ikeda, S. I. (2017). Principal component analysis for ataxic gait using a triaxial accelerometer. *Journal of Neuroengineering and Rehabilitation*, *14*(1), 37. doi:10.118612984-017-0249-7 PMID:28464831

McDermott, B., O'Halloran, M., Porter, E., & Santorelli, A. (2018). Brain haemorrhage detection using a SVM classifier with electrical impedance tomography measurement frames. *PLoS One*, *13*(7), e0200469. doi:10.1371/journal.pone.0200469 PMID:30001401

Miranda, E., Irwansyah, E., Amelga, A. Y., Maribondang, M. M., & Salim, M. (2016). Detection of cardiovascular disease risk's level for adults using naive Bayes classifier. *Healthcare Informatics Research*, *22*(3), 196–205. doi:10.4258/hir.2016.22.3.196 PMID:27525161

Mouradian, M. M. (Ed.). (2001). *Parkinson's Disease: Methods and Protocols* (Vol. 62). Springer Science & Business Media. doi:10.1385/1592591426

Nukala, B. T., Nakano, T., Rodriguez, A., Tsay, J., Lopez, J., Nguyen, T. Q., ... Lie, D. Y. (2016). Real-time classification of patients with balance disorders vs. normal subjects using a low-cost small wireless wearable gait sensor. *Biosensors*, *6*(4), 58. doi:10.3390/bios6040058 PMID:27916817

Rodrıguez-Martın, D., Sama, A., Pérez-López, C., Catala, A., Moreno Arostegui, J. M., Cabestany, J., ... Rodríguez-Molinero, A. (2017). Home detection of freezing of gait using support vector machines through a single waist-worn triaxial accelerometer. *PLoS One*, *12*(2), e0171764. doi:10.1371/journal.pone.0171764 PMID:28199357

Saberioon, M., Císař, P., Labbé, L., Souček, P., Pelissier, P., & Kerneis, T. (2018). Comparative Performance Analysis of Support Vector Machine, Random Forest, Logistic Regression and k-Nearest Neighbours in Rainbow Trout (Oncorhynchus Mykiss) Classification Using Image-Based Features. *Sensors (Basel)*, *18*(4), 1027. doi:10.339018041027 PMID:29596375

Sambo, F., Trifoglio, E., Di Camillo, B., Toffolo, G. M., & Cobelli, C. (2012). Bag of Naïve Bayes: Biomarker selection and classification from genome-wide SNP data. *BMC Bioinformatics*, *13*(14Suppl 14), S2. doi:10.1186/1471-2105-13-S14-S2 PMID:23095127

Sarkar, S. D., Goswami, S., Agarwal, A., & Aktar, J. (2014). A novel feature selection technique for text classification using Naive Bayes. *International Scholarly Research Notices.*

Sharma, S., Moon, C. S., Khogali, A., Haidous, A., Chabenne, A., Ojo, C., ... Ebadi, M. (2013). Biomarkers in Parkinson's disease (recent update). *Neurochemistry International*, *63*(3), 201–229. doi:10.1016/j.neuint.2013.06.005 PMID:23791710

Smulders, K., Dale, M. L., Carlson-Kuhta, P., Nutt, J. G., & Horak, F. B. (2016). Pharmacological treatment in Parkinson's disease: Effects on gait. *Parkinsonism & Related Disorders*, *31*, 3–13. doi:10.1016/j.parkreldis.2016.07.006 PMID:27461783

Wolfson, J., Bandyopadhyay, S., Elidrisi, M., Vazquez-Benitez, G., Musgrove, D., Adomavicius, G., . . . O'Connor, P. (2014). *A Naive Bayes machine learning approach to risk prediction using censored, time-to-event data.* arXiv preprint arXiv:1404.2124

Wu, J., & Wu, B. (2015). The novel quantitative technique for assessment of gait symmetry using advanced statistical learning algorithm. *BioMed Research International*. PMID:25705672

Wu, J., & Xu, H. (2016). An advanced scheme of compressed sensing of acceleration data for telemonintoring of human gait. *Biomedical Engineering Online*, *15*(1), 27. doi:10.118612938-016-0142-9 PMID:26946302

Wu, T., Hallett, M., & Chan, P. (2015). Motor automaticity in Parkinson's disease. *Neurobiology of Disease*, *82*, 226–234. doi:10.1016/j.nbd.2015.06.014 PMID:26102020

Xu, H., Hunt, M., Foreman, K. B., Zhao, J., & Merryweather, A. (2018). Gait alterations on irregular surface in people with Parkinson's disease. *Clinical Biomechanics (Bristol, Avon)*, *57*, 93–98. doi:10.1016/j.clinbiomech.2018.06.013 PMID:29966960

Yu, H., & Kim, S. (2012). SVM tutorial—classification, regression and ranking. In *Handbook of Natural computing* (pp. 479–506). Berlin: Springer. doi:10.1007/978-3-540-92910-9_15

Zeng, W., Liu, F., Wang, Q., Wang, Y., Ma, L., & Zhang, Y. (2016). Parkinson's disease classification using gait analysis via deterministic learning. *Neuroscience Letters*, *633*, 268–278. doi:10.1016/j.neulet.2016.09.043 PMID:27693437

Zhao, Z., Yang, L., Chen, D., & Luo, Y. (2013). A human ECG identification system based on ensemble empirical mode decomposition. *Sensors (Basel)*, *13*(5), 6832–6864. doi:10.3390130506832 PMID:23698274

Chapter 8
Tremor Identification Using Machine Learning in Parkinson's Disease

Angana Saikia
North-Eastern Hill University Shillong, India

Vinayak Majhi
North-Eastern Hill University Shillong, India

Masaraf Hussain
North-Eastern Indira Gandhi Regional Institute of Health and Medical Sciences, India

Sudip Paul
North-Eastern Hill University Shillong, India

Amitava Datta
The University of Western Australia, Australia

ABSTRACT

Tremor is an involuntary quivering movement or shake. Characteristically occurring at rest, the classic slow, rhythmic tremor of Parkinson's disease (PD) typically starts in one hand, foot, or leg and can eventually affect both sides of the body. The resting tremor of PD can also occur in the jaw, chin, mouth, or tongue. Loss of dopamine leads to the symptoms of Parkinson's disease and may include a tremor. For some people, a tremor might be the first symptom of PD. Various studies have proposed measurable technologies and the analysis of the characteristics of Parkinsonian tremors using different techniques. Various machine-learning algorithms such as a support vector machine (SVM) with three kernels, a discriminant analysis, a random forest, and a kNN algorithm are also used to classify and identify various kinds of tremors. This chapter focuses on an in-depth review on identification and classification of various Parkinsonian tremors using machine learning algorithms.

DOI: 10.4018/978-1-5225-8567-1.ch008

INTRODUCTION

Tremor and Its Classifications

An involuntary action which is rhythmic is known as tremor which is caused by either alternating or synchronous contractions of antagonistic muscles. It is movement of muscle contraction and relaxation involving twitching movements of one or more body parts. It affects the hands, arms, eyes, face, head, vocal folds, trunk, and legs. Tremor is the most common of all movement disorders, which occurs in most normal individuals in the form of physiologic tremor (Hallett, 1991).

Tremor is most commonly classified by clinical features, cause or origin. Figure 1 shows the various types of tremors.

- **Cerebellar Tremor (Intention Tremor):** It is a slow, broad tremor of the extremities that occurs at the end of any kind of body movement, such as trying to press a button or touching a finger to the tip of one's nose. It is mostly caused by lesions in or damage to the cerebellum resulting from stroke, tumor, or disease such as multiple sclerosis or any degenerative disorder. It can also result from chronic alcoholism or overuse of some medicines. The tremor is often most prominent when the affected person is active or is maintaining a particular posture. Cerebellar tremor may be accompanied by other manifestations of ataxia, including speech problems, rapid, involuntary rolling of the eyes, gait problems (Elble, 2017).
- **Dystonic Tremor:** It occurs in individuals of all ages who are affected by dystonia. Dystonia is a movement disorder in which sustained involuntary muscle contractions cause twisting and repetitive motions followed by painful and abnormal postures. Dystonic tremor may affect any muscle in the body and is seen most often when the patient is in a certain position or moves a certain way. It occurs irregularly and often can be relieved by complete rest. Touching the affected body part or muscle may reduce tremor severity (Elble, 2017).
- **Essential Tremor**: It is of the most common type of tremor. Although the tremor may be mild and non-progressive in some people, but it is slowly progressive, starting on one side of the body and gradually affecting both sides. The hands are most often affected body part. Other parts like the head, voice, tongue, legs, and trunk may also be involved in some cases. Mild gait disturbance is also a symptom in essential tremor. Tremor frequency may decrease as the person ages, but the severity may increase, affecting the person's ability to perform certain tasks or activities of daily

Figure 1. Types of tremor

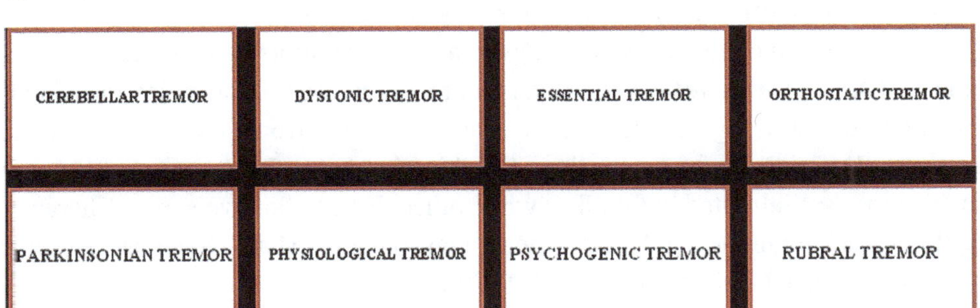

living. Heightened emotion, stress, fever, physical exhaustion, or low blood sugar increases their severity. Onset is most common after age 40, although symptoms can appear at any age (Elble, 2017).

- **Orthostatic Tremor:** It is characterized by fast rhythmic muscle contractions that occur in the legs and trunk immediately after standing. Cramps are felt in the thighs and legs and the patient may shake uncontrollably when asked to stand in one spot. The high frequency of the tremor often makes the tremor look like rippling of leg muscles while standing. Orthostatic tremor may also occur in patients who have essential tremor, and there might be an overlap between these categories of tremor(Elble, 2017).
- **Parkinsonian Tremor:** It is caused by damage within the brain that controls the body movement. This resting tremor is often a precursor to Parkinson's disease but can also be seen in other movement disorders. The tremor, which is classically seen as a "pill-rolling" action of the hands that may also affect the chin, lips, legs, and trunk. This kind of tremor increases by stress or emotion. Onset is generally after age 60. Movement starts in one limb or on one side of the body and usually progresses to include the other side of the body(Marjama-Lyons & Koller, 2000).
- **Physiological Tremor**: It occurs in every normal individual and has no clinical significance. It is rarely visible and may be increased by strong emotion, physical exhaustion, hypoglycemia, hyperthyroidism, heavy metal poisoning, stimulants, alcohol withdrawal or fever. It can be seen in all voluntary muscle groups and can be detected by extending the arms and placing a piece of paper on top of the hands (Elble, 2017).
- **Psychogenic Tremor**: It can occur at rest or during postural or kinetic movement. The characteristics of this kind of tremor may vary but generally include sudden onset and remission, increased incidence with stress. Many patients with psychogenic or another psychiatric disease(Elble, 2017).
- **Rubral Tremor:** It is characterized by slow tremor which is present at rest, at posture and with intention. This tremor is associated with conditions which affect the red nucleus in the midbrain (Elble, 2017).

Figure 2 shows a person having tremor on his hand and leg.

Biological Significance of Tremor

Tremor is associated with disorders in those parts of the brain that control muscles throughout the body or in particular areas, such as the hands or legs. Neurological disorders or conditions that can produce tremor include multiple sclerosis, stroke, traumatic brain injury, chronic kidney disease and a number of neurodegenerative diseases that damage or destroy parts of the brainstem or the cerebellum. Parkinson's disease being the one most often associated with tremor (Louis, 2014).

Other causes of tremor include the use of drugs or alcohol. Tremors can also be seen in infants with sphenylketonuria (PKU), overactive thyroid or liver failure. Tremors can be an indication of hypoglycemia, along with palpitations, sweating and anxiety. It can also be caused from lack of sleep, lack of vitamins, or increased stress. Deficiencies of magnesium and thiamine have also been known to cause tremor. Some forms of tremor are inherited in families, while others have no known cause. Characteristics may include a rhythmic shaking in the hands, arms, head, legs, or trunk; shaky voice; and problems holding things such as a fork or pen (Stein & Oĝuztöreli, 1976).

Figure 2. Tremor on hand and leg

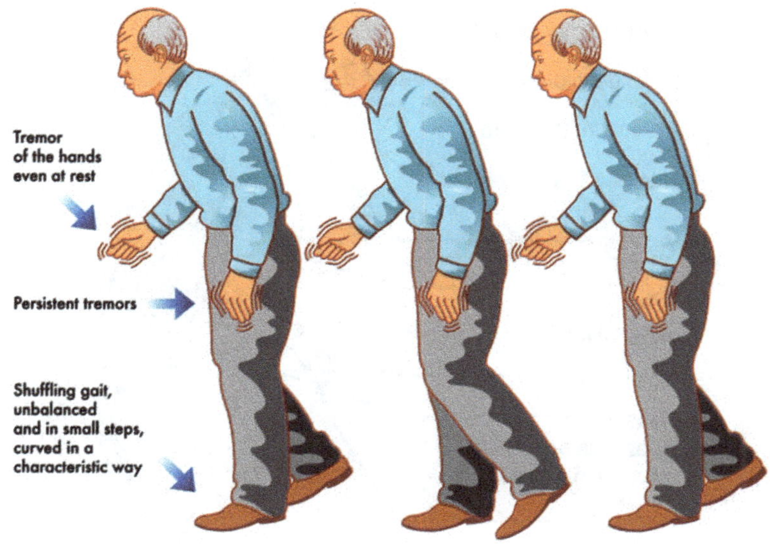

Tremor may occur at any age but is most common in middle-age and older persons. It may be occasional, temporary, or occur intermittently which affects men and women equally.

Tremors Can Result From

- Alcoholism, excessive alcohol consumption, or alcohol withdrawal can kill certain nerve cells, resulting in a tremor known as asterixis. Conversely, small amounts of alcohol may help to decrease familial and essential tremor, but the mechanism behind it is unknown.
- Tremor in peripheral neuropathy may occur when the nerves that supply the body's muscles are traumatized by injury, disease, abnormality in the central nervous system, or as the result of systemic illnesses. Peripheral neuropathy can affect the whole body or certain areas, such as the hands, and may be progressive. Resulting sensory loss may be seen as a tremor or ataxia of the affected limbs and problems with gait and balance.
- Clinical characteristics may be similar to those seen in patients with essential tremor.
- Tobacco withdrawal symptoms also include tremor.

PARKINSON'S DISEASE (PD) AND ITS SYMPTOMS

PD and Its Causes

Parkinson's disease (PD) is a neurodegenerative disorder that affects people over 60 years of age in industrialized countries. It is a progressive disorder that causes motor dysfunctions: involuntary and oscillatory movements (tremor), slowness of movements (bradykinesia), increased muscle tone (rigidity) and postural instability. A common type of Parkinsonian tremors is rest tremor but also postural,

Figure 3. Person suffering from PD (Ejlerskov, 2015)

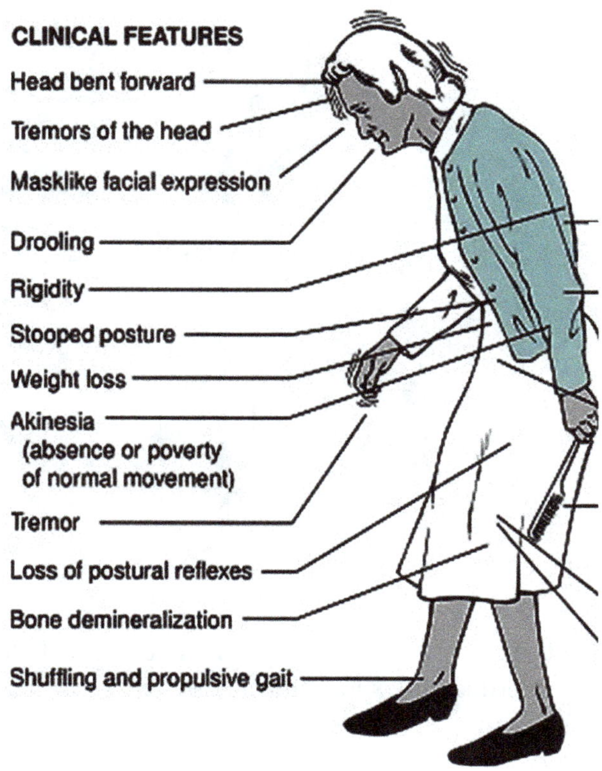

kinetic and intention tremors have been reported. According to current diagnostic criteria, patients can be considered to have PD when they have two of the four symptoms of PD (tremor, bradykinesia, rigidity and postural instability). Although these dysfunctions can be assessed by electromyography, it is still used rarely in the clinical evaluation of PD (Checkoway & Nelson, 1999).

Parkinson's disease occurs when nerve cells, or neurons, in the brain die or become impaired. Although many brain areas are affected, the most common symptoms result from the loss of neurons in an area near the base of the brain called the substantia nigra. Normally, the neurons in this area produce an important brain chemical known as dopamine. Dopamine is a chemical messenger responsible for transmitting signals between the substantia nigra and the next "relay station" of the brain, the corpus striatum, to produce smooth, purposeful movement. Loss of dopamine results in abnormal nerve firing patterns within the brain that cause impaired movement (Bunting-Perry, 2006).

Genetic Factors

Scientists have identified several genetic mutations associated with PD, including the alpha synuclein gene, and many more genes have been tentatively linked to the disorder. Studying the genes responsible for inherited cases of PD can help researchers understand both inherited and sporadic cases. The same genes and proteins that are altered in inherited cases may also be altered in sporadic cases by environmental toxins or other factors. Researchers also hope that discovering genes will help identify new ways of treating PD (Surathi, Jhunjhunwala, Yadav, & Pal, 2016).

Figure 4. Dopamine levels (Medications, 2016)

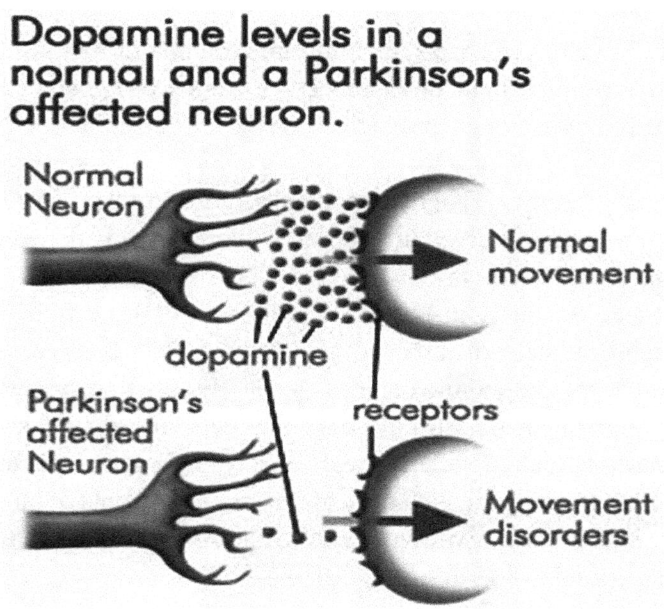

Environmental Factors

Exposure to certain toxins has caused PD symptoms in rare circumstances (such as exposure to MPTP, an illicit drug, or in miners exposed to the metal manganese). Other still unidentified environmental factors may also cause PD in genetically susceptible individuals (Surathi et al., 2016).

Symptoms of PD

Motor Symptoms

- **Bradykinesia:** Bradykinesia means "slow movement." A defining feature of Parkinson's, bradykinesia also describes a general reduction of spontaneous movement, which can give the appearance of abnormal stillness and a decrease in facial expressivity. Bradykinesia causes difficulty with repetitive movements, such as finger tapping (Chapuis, Ouchchane, Metz, Gerbaud, & Durif, 2005).
- **Rigidity:** Rigidity causes stiffness and inflexibility of the limbs, neck and trunk. Muscles normally stretch when they move, and then relax when they are at rest (Chapuis et al., 2005).
- **Tremor:** Tremor, or shaking, often in a hand, arm, or leg, occurs when you're awake and sitting or standing still (resting tremor), and it gets better when you move that body part (Chapuis et al., 2005). Tremor is often the first symptom that people with Parkinson's disease or their family members notice.
- **Postural Instability:** One of the most important signs of Parkinson's is postural instability, a tendency to be unstable when standing upright (Chapuis et al., 2005).

Non-Motor Symptoms

- **Neuropsychiatric:** Neuropsychiatric symptoms are common in Parkinson's disease, even at the earliest stages, and have important consequences for quality of life and daily functioning, are associated with increased care burden and increased risk for nursing home admission (Factor et al., 2003).
- **ICDs**: Impulse control disorders (ICDs), specifically those related to excessive gambling, eating, sex and shopping, have been observed in a subset of people with Parkinson's disease (PD) (Factor et al., 2003).
- **Sleep Disorder**: Sleep disorders in Parkinson's disease (PD) are frequent and have numerous etiologies. Both nighttime sleep disturbances and daytime sleepiness can occur (Wilcox, 2010).
- **Autonomic Dysfunction**: Autonomic nervous system dysfunction symptoms in PD include sexual dysfunction, swallowing and gastrointestinal disorders, bowel and bladder abnormalities, and derangements of cardiovascular regulation, particularly, orthostatic hypotension (Wilcox, 2010).
- **Sensory**: Nineteen of 50 Parkinson patients had sensory complaints of numbness, coldness, burning, or pain. There was no objective sensory loss, and sensory symptoms did not correlate with specific motor or autonomic signs (Wilcox, 2010).

LITERATURE REVIEW

The literature review is shown in Table 1.

PROBLEM DEFINITION AND A WAY TOWARDS SOLUTION

Identification of tremor using an automated or computing system is a bit of difficult process. The following problems are the basic and common nature of identifying the tremor.

The Non-Linear Nature of Each Case

Each human body has the unique nature of itself by which we can differentiate the each and every person even classifying a small sector like retina or fingerprint of whole body. This unique nature also has been seen in the symptoms level for each person. Each tremor level associated with Parkinson's disease is unique in nature for each person. This is the non linear nature of the problem while identifying tremor and this type of problem leads us to find the solution in Non-deterministic algorithm.

Common Symptoms Hazards

In some particular survey it was found that tremor is a common symptom for near about 14 different neurological disorders both in acute and chronic types. Not only tremors but also there are 22 different symptoms including tremor are common in these 14 types of individual neuronal disorder like Parkinson's disease, Huntington disease, Alzheimer's disease, PANDAS etc. So classification of the tremor for identifying PD is also very difficult in this aspect (Chen, Garcia, Huang, & Constantini, 2014).

Table 1.

AUTHOR	YEAR	CONTRIBUTION
Enas Abdulhay. et al	2018	They proposed a machine learning algorithm to diagnose PD using the gait analysis. Various gait features were extracted using the peak detection and pulse duration. An average accuracy of 92.7% was achieved for the diagnosis of PD from gait analysis (Abdulhay, Arunkumar, Narasimhan, Vellaiappan, & Venkatraman, 2018).
Taigo Italo Pedrosa. et al,	2018	Proposed two predictive models using a supervised machine learning approach. These model classify the Parkinson disease's rest tremor between high or low frequencies, showing the intensity of Parkinson's motor symptom. They applied leave-one-out cross-validation methods to classify the level of the PD tremor and reached a classification accuracy of 92.8% (Pedrosa, Vasconcelos, Medeiros, & Silva, 2018).
Hyoseon Jeon. et al	2017	They worked to maximize the scientific validity of automatic tremor-severity classification using machine learning algorithms to score Parkinsonian tremor severity in the same manner as the unified Parkinson's disease rating scale (UPDRS) used to rate scores in real clinical practice. The optimal feature configuration was decided using the wrapper feature selection algorithm or principal component analysis, and decision tree, support vector machine, discriminant analysis, and *k*-nearest neighbor algorithms are considered to develop an automatic scoring system for UPDRS prediction. The highest accuracies are 92.3%, 86.2%, 92.1%, and 89.2% for resting, resting with mental stress, postural, and intention tremors, respectively (Jeon et al., 2017).
Bjoern M. Eskofier. et al	2016	They focused on the detection of bradykinesia in PD. For this, they compared standard machine learning pipelines with deep learning based on convolutional neural networks. Results showed that deep learning outperformed other state-of-the-art machine learning algorithms by at least 4.6% in terms of classification rate(Eskofier et al., 2016).
Andrea Cherubini. et al	2014	Distinguished patients who had tremor-dominant Parkinson's disease (tPD) from those who had essential tremor with rest tremor (rET). They combined voxel-based morphometry-derived gray matter and white matter volumes and diffusion tensor imaging-derived mean diffusivity and fractional anisotropy in a support vector machine (SVM) to evaluate 15 patients with rET and 15 patients with tPD. SVM classification of individual patients showed that no single predictor was able to fully discriminate patients with tPD from those with rET. By contrast, when all predictors were combined in a multi-modal algorithm, SVM distinguished patients with rET from those with tPD with an accuracy of 100% (Cherubini et al., 2014).
S.Gokul. et al	2013	Proposed the application of a Fully Complex-Valued Radial Basis Function network (FC-RBF), Meta-Cognitive Fully Complex-Valued Radial Basis Function network (Mc-FCRBF) and Extreme Learning Machine (ELM) for the prediction of Parkinson's disease. With the help of Unified Parkinson's Disease Rating Scale (UPDRS), the severity of the Parkinson's disease is predicted and for untreated patients, the UPDRS scale spans the range (0-176). The result indicated that the Mc-FCRBF network has good prediction accuracy than ELM and FC-RBF network (Gokul, Sivachitra, & Vijayachitra, 2013).
N.D. Darnall. et al	2012	Compared the accuracy of various data analysis techniques to quantify tremor severity (TS) in a clinical context, with the aim of improving the reliability of tremor evaluation in patients with Parkinson¢s disease (PD) or essential tremor (ET). The machine learning method matched the clinical rating with 82% accuracy, the digital pen with 78% accuracy, and RMS with 42% accuracy. They also obtained the best accuracy of 82% using the decision tree machine learning approach with gyroscope data measured with the Shimmer (Darnall et al., 2012).
Lingmei Ai et al	2011	They worked on a novel approach using singular value decomposition (SVD) to extract the features of intrinsic mode functions (IMFs) and support vector machine (SVM) is proposed to distinguish between them. Due to the accuracy, sensitivity, and specificify could arrive at 98%, 97.5% and 98.33% respectively, thus, practical guiding significance for diagnosing tremor types in clinic is provided (Ai, Wang, & Yao, 2011) .

Identification of Tremor Type

As we discussed earlier that the there are different types of tremor can be present within a person that may not lead the patient to the Parkinson's disease. This type of problem is very difficult to analyze using deterministic algorithms. May be a person can has several types of tremor for different types of disease including Parkinsonian Tremor. So identify and classify tremor type is very much essential in this scenario.

Complexity of the Problems

Complexity analysis is very much crucial factor to find the solution of a particular problem. In computer technology each type of problem can be classified into two broad categories like Time and Space complexity. But in case of solving nondeterministic types of problems; which are very difficult to solve in polynomial time, we need special technique to come in the domain in Polynomial time range or we can say NP-Complete class. Above mention three points lead us to the problem that is nondeterministic type and cannot be solved in polynomial time using conventional algorithm.

Concerning about the above discussion this Nondeterministic polynomial time complexity problem (NP Problem) can be solved using the help of *Machine Learning*; an intelligent domain of computer science belongs to area of Artificial Intelligence. Using Machine learning we can solve the NP Problem within polynomial time and make the NP-Hard problem to NP-Complete Problems.

MACHINE LEARNING SYSTEM

Machine learning can be termed as a subset of artificial intelligence (AI). The aim of machine learning commonly is to figure out the structure of data and fit that into models which can be accepted and utilized by people (Koza, Bennett, Andre, & Keane, 1996; Robert, 2014).

Machine learning is a sector within computer science, but it differs from traditional computational methods. Commonly algorithms are sets of accurately programmed instructions used by computers to calculate or solve problem. Machine learning algorithms rather allow for computers to train on data inputs. Also statistical analysis is used in order to output values that fall within a specific range. As a result, machine learning accelerates computers in building models from sample data in order to automate decision-making processes based on data inputs (Robert, 2014).

Machine learning tasks are typically classified into different categories:

- **Supervised machine learning algorithms** can apply what has been trained in the past to new data using labelled examples to predict future events. Ranging from the analysis of a known training dataset, the learning algorithmic program produces an inferred operates to create predictions regarding the output values. The system is ready to supply targets for any new input after adequate training. The learning algorithm can even compare its output with the proper, supposed output and notice errors in order to change the model consequently(Kotsiantis, Zaharakis, & Pintelas, 2007; Lloyd, Mohseni, & Rebentrost, 2013). The majority of practical machine learning uses supervised learning. Supervised learning is where you have input variables (x) and an output variable (Y) and you use an algorithm to learn the mapping function from the input to the output.

$$Y = f(X) \tag{1}$$

The goal is to approximate the mapping function so well that when you have new input data (x) that you can predict the output variables (Y) for that data. It is called supervised learning because the process of an algorithm learning from the training dataset can be thought of as a teacher supervising the learning process. We know the correct answers; the algorithm iteratively makes predictions on the training data and is corrected by the teacher. Learning stops when the algorithm achieves an acceptable level of performance.

- Supervised learning problems can be further grouped into regression and classification problems.
- Classification: A classification problem is when the output variable is a category, such as "red" or "blue" or "disease" and "no disease".
- Regression: A regression problem is when the output variable is a real value, such as "dollars" or "weight".
- Some common types of problems built on top of classification and regression include recommendation and time series prediction respectively. Some popular examples of supervised machine learning algorithms are:
- Linear regression for regression problems.
- Random forest for classification and regression problems.
- Support vector machines for classification problems.
- Unsupervised machine learning algorithms are used when the information applied to train is neither classified nor categorised. Unsupervised learning studies how systems will infer a performance to explain a hidden structure from unlabeled data. The system doesn't work out the proper output, but it explores the data and may draw inferences from datasets to explain hidden structures from unlabeled data(Lloyd et al., 2013). Unsupervised learning is where you only have input data (X) and no corresponding output variables.

The goal for unsupervised learning is to model the underlying structure or distribution in the data in order to learn more about the data. These are called unsupervised learning because unlike supervised learning above there is no correct answers and there is no teacher. Algorithms are left to their own devises to discover and present the interesting structure in the data.

Unsupervised learning problems can be further grouped into clustering and association problems.

- **Clustering**: A clustering problem is where you want to discover the inherent groupings in the data, such as grouping customers by purchasing behavior.
- **Association**: An association rule learning problem is where you want to discover rules that describe large portions of your data, such as people that buy X also tend to buy Y.
- Some popular examples of unsupervised learning algorithms are:
- k-means for clustering problems.
- Apriori algorithm for association rule learning problems.
- **Semi-supervised machine learning algorithms** come somewhere in between supervised and unsupervised learning, as they use each labelled and unlabeled data for training – usually a small quantity of labelled data and huge quantity of unlabeled data. The systems that use this technique are able to noticeably improve learning accuracy. Usually, semi-supervised learning is chosen

once the acquired labelled data needs competent and relevant resources so as to train it or learn from it. Otherwise, getting unlabeled data usually doesn't need additional resources(Chapelle, Scholkopf, & Zien, 2009). Problems where you have a large amount of input data (X) and only some of the data is labeled (Y) are called semi-supervised learning problems. These problems sit in between both supervised and unsupervised learning. A good example is a photo archive where only some of the images are labeled, (e.g. dog, cat, person) and the majority are unlabeled.

- Many real-world machine learning problems fall into this area. This is because it can be expensive or time-consuming to label data as it may require access to domain experts. Whereas unlabeled data is cheap and easy to collect and store. We can use unsupervised learning techniques to discover and learn the structure in the input variables. It is also use supervised learning techniques to make best guess predictions for the unlabeled data, feed that data back into the supervised learning algorithm as training data and use the model to make predictions on new unseen data.
- Reinforcement machine learning algorithms is a learning method that interacts with its environment through producing actions and discovers problems or rewards. Trial and error search and delayed reward are the most relevant features of reinforcement learning. This method permits machines and software agents to automatically determine the ideal behaviour within a specific context in order to maximize its performance. Simple reward feedback is required for the agent to learn which action is best; this is known as the reinforcement signal (Mnih et al., 2016).

Figure 5. Classification of Machine Learning ("Machine Learning Algorithm - Backbone of emerging technologies")

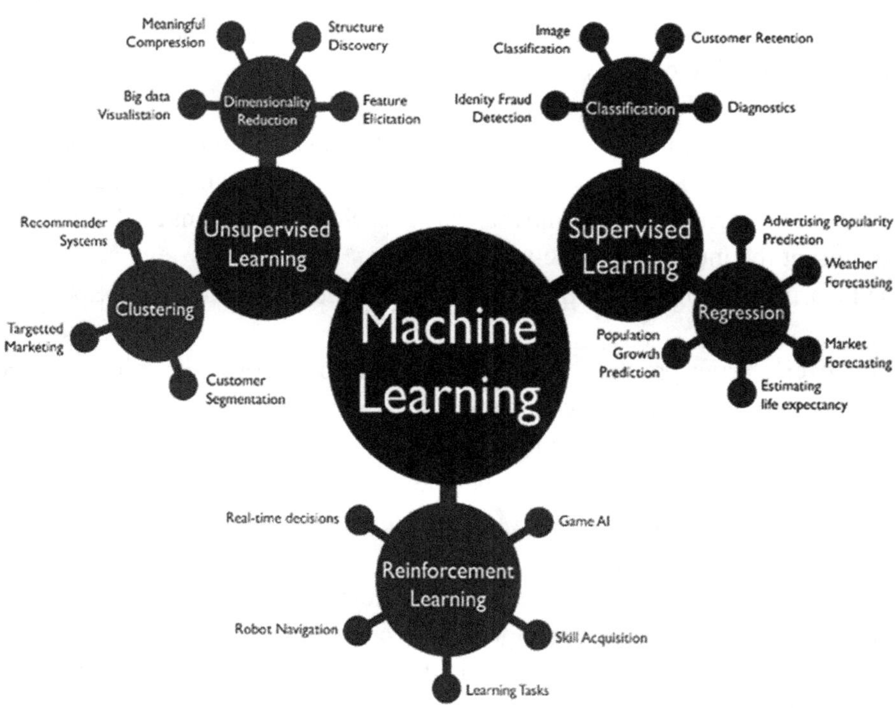

Machine learning allows analysis of huge quantities of data. Whereas it usually delivers quicker, a lot of accurate results in order to spot profitable opportunities or dangerous risks, it may also need extra time and resources to train it properly. Combining machine learning with AI and cognitive technologies will create it even more effective in processing large volumes of information (Robert, 2014).

CLUSTERING

Clustering is a Machine Learning approach that associates the grouping of data points. Given a set of data points, we can use a clustering algorithm to classify each data point into a specific group. In theory, data points that are in the same group should have similar properties and/or features, while data points in different groups should have highly dissimilar properties and/or features. Clustering is a process of unsupervised learning and is a regular process for statistical data analysis used in many fields (Hartigan & Wong, 1979).

Clustering is the task of dividing the population or data points into a number of groups such that data points in the same groups are more similar to other data points in the same group than those in other groups. In simple words, the aim is to segregate groups with similar traits and assign them into clusters.

Figure 6. Different types of Machine Learning Algorithms ("Machine Learning Algorithms Mindmap," 2015)

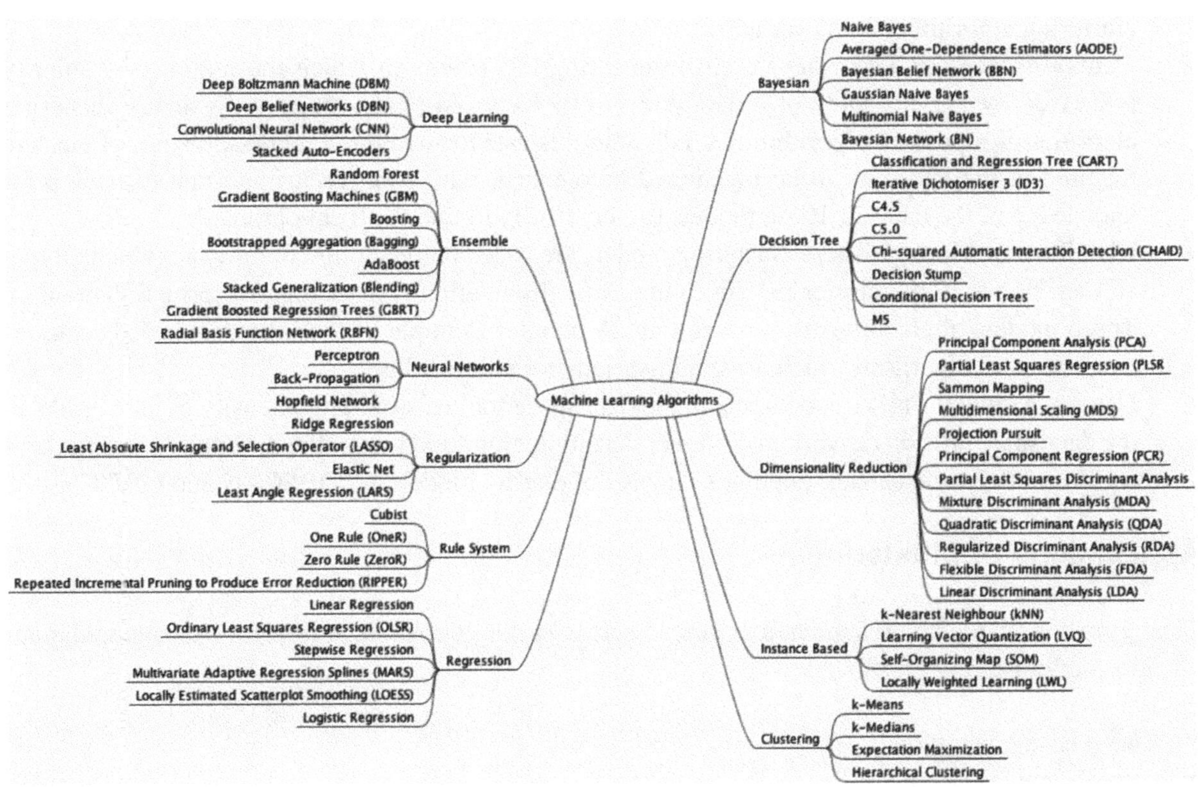

Types of Clustering

Broadly speaking, clustering can be divided into two subgroups:

- **Hard Clustering:** In hard clustering, each data point either belongs to a cluster completely or not. For example, in the above example each customer is put into one group out of the 10 groups.
- **Soft Clustering**: In soft clustering, instead of putting each data point into a separate cluster, a probability or likelihood of that data point to be in those clusters is assigned. For example, from the above scenario each costumer is assigned a probability to be in either of 10 clusters of the retail store.

Types of Clustering Algorithms

There are more than 100 clustering algorithms known. But few of the algorithms are used popularly. They are:

- **Connectivity Models:** As the name suggests, these models are based on the notion that the data points closer in data space exhibit more similarity to each other than the data points lying farther away. These models can follow two approaches. In the first approach, they start with classifying all data points into separate clusters & then aggregating them as the distance decreases. In the second approach, all data points are classified as a single cluster and then partitioned as the distance increases. Also, the choice of distance function is subjective. These models are very easy to interpret but lacks scalability for handling big datasets. Examples of these models are hierarchical clustering algorithm and its variants.
- **Centroid Models:** These are iterative clustering algorithms in which the notion of similarity is derived by the closeness of a data point to the centroid of the clusters. K-Means clustering algorithm is a popular algorithm that falls into this category. In these models, the no. of clusters required at the end have to be mentioned beforehand, which makes it important to have prior knowledge of the dataset. These models run iteratively to find the local optima.
- **Distribution Models:** These clustering models are based on the notion of how probable is it that all data points in the cluster belong to the same distribution (For example: Normal, Gaussian). These models often suffer from overfitting. A popular example of these models is Expectation-maximization algorithm which uses multivariate normal distributions.
- **Density Models:** These models search the data space for areas of varied density of data points in the data space. It isolates various different density regions and assign the data points within these regions in the same cluster. Popular examples of density models are DBSCAN and OPTICS.

Applications of Clustering

Clustering has a large no. of applications spread across various domains. Some of the most popular applications of clustering are:

- Market segmentation
- Social network analysis

- Search result grouping
- Medical imaging
- Image segmentation
- Anomaly detection
- Recommendation engines

K-Means Clustering

K-Means is probably the most well know clustering algorithm. It's taught in a lot of introductory data science and machine learning classes. It's easy to understand and implement in code! Check out the graphic below for an illustration (Kanungo et al., 2002).

1. To begin, we first select a number of groups to use and randomly start their respective centre points. To figure out the number of classes to use, it's good to take a quick look at the data and try to identify any distinct groupings. The centre points are vectors of the same length as each data point vector and are the "X's" in the graphic above.
2. Each data point is allocated by computing the distance between that point and each group centre, and then classifying the point to be in the group whose centre is closest to it.
3. Based on these classified points, we recomputed the group centre by taking the mean of all the vectors in the group.
4. Repeat these steps for a set number of iterations or until the group centres don't change much between iterations. It can also opt to randomly initialize the group centres a few times, and then select the run that looks like it provided the best results.

K-Means has the advantage that it's quite fast, as all we're really doing is computing the distances between points and group centres; clustering has a linear complexity $O(n)$.

On the other hand, K-Means has also disadvantages. It is need to be selected how many groups/classes there are. This isn't always trivial and ideally with a clustering algorithm. K-means also starts with a random choice of cluster centres and therefore it may provide different clustering results on different runs of the algorithm. Thus, the results may not be repeatable and lack consistency.

K-Medians is another clustering algorithm related to K-Means, except rather than re-computing the group centre points using the mean we use the median vector of the group. This technique is lesser sensitive to outliers (because of using the Median) however is much slower for larger datasets as sorting is needed on every iteration when computing the Median vector(Hartigan & Wong, 1979; Kanungo et al., 2002; Likas, Vlassis, & Verbeek, 2003).

Mean-Shift Clustering

Mean shift clustering is a sliding-window-based algorithm that attempts to find compressed areas of data points. It is a centroid-based algorithm meaning that the goal is to locate the centre points of each class, which works by updating candidates for centre points to be the mean of the points within the sliding-window. These candidate windows are then filtered in a post-processing stage to eliminate near-duplicates, forming the final set of centre points and their corresponding groups.

1. To explain mean-shift we will consider a set of points in two-dimensional space like the above illustration. A circular sliding window cantered at a point C (randomly selected) and having radius r as the kernel. Mean shift is a hill climbing algorithm which involves shifting this kernel iteratively to a higher density region on each step until convergence.
2. At every iteration the sliding window is shifted towards regions of higher density by shifting the centre point to the mean of the points within the window. The density within the sliding window is proportional to the number of points inside it. Naturally, by shifting to the mean of the points in the window it will gradually move towards areas of higher point density.
3. We continue shifting the sliding window according to the mean until there is no direction at which a shift can accommodate more points inside the kernel. Check out the graphic above; we keep moving the circle until we no longer are increasing the density (i.e number of points in the window).
4. This process of steps 1 to 3 is done with many sliding windows until all points lie within a window. When multiple sliding windows overlap the window containing the most points is preserved. The data points are then clustered according to the sliding window in which they reside.

In contrast to K-means clustering there is no need to select the number of clusters as mean-shift automatically discovers this. That's a massive advantage. The fact that the cluster centers converge towards the points of maximum density is also quite desirable as it is quite intuitive to understand and fits well in a naturally data-driven sense. The drawback is that the selection of the window size/radius "r" can be non-trivial(Cheng, 1995; Comaniciu & Meer, 1999, 2002).

Density-Based Spatial Clustering of Applications With Noise (DBSCAN)

DBSCAN is a density based clustered algorithm similar to mean-shift, but with a couple of notable advantages.

1. DBSCAN begins with an arbitrary starting data point that has not been visited. The neighbourhood of this point is extracted using a distance epsilon ε (All points which are within the ε distance are neighbourhood points).
2. If there are a sufficient number of points (according to midpoints) within this neighbourhood then the clustering process starts and the current data point becomes the first point in the new cluster. Otherwise, the point will be labelled as noise (later this noisy point might become the part of the cluster). In both cases that point is marked as "visited".
3. For this first point in the new cluster, the points within its ε distance neighbourhood also become part of the same cluster. This procedure of making all points in the ε neighbourhood belong to the same cluster is then repeated for all of the new points that have been just added to the cluster group.
4. This process of steps 2 and 3 is repeated until all points in the cluster are determined i.e all points within the ε neighbourhood of the cluster have been visited and labelled.
5. Once we're done with the current cluster, a new unvisited point is retrieved and processed, leading to the discovery of a further cluster or noise. This process repeats until all points are marked as visited. Since at the end of this all points have been visited, each point well has been marked as either belonging to a cluster or being noise.

DBSCAN poses large advantages over other clustering algorithms. Firstly, it does not require a pre-set number of clusters at all. It also identifies outliers as noises unlike mean-shift which simply throws them into a cluster even if the data point is very different. Additionally, it is able to find arbitrarily sized and arbitrarily shaped clusters quite well.

The main drawback of is that it doesn't perform as well as others when the clusters are of varying density. This is because the setting of the distance threshold ε and midpoints for identifying the neighbourhood points will vary from cluster to cluster when the density varies. This drawback also occurs with very high-dimensional data since again the distance threshold ε becomes challenging to estimate(Tran, Drab, & Daszykowski, 2013; Wang, Wu, Tang, & Hor, 2015).

Expectation–Maximization (EM) Clustering Using Gaussian Mixture Models (GMM)

One of the major drawbacks of K-Means is its naive use of the mean value for the cluster centre. We can see why this isn't the best way of doing things by looking at the image below. On the left hand side it looks quite obvious to the human eye that there are two circular clusters with different radius' centred at the same mean. K-Means can't handle this because the mean values of the clusters are a very close together. K-Means also fails in cases where the clusters are not circular, again as a result of using the mean as cluster centre. Gaussian Mixture Models (GMMs) give us more flexibility than K-Means. With GMMs we assume that the data points are Gaussian distributed; this is a less restrictive assumption than saying they are circular by using the mean. That way, we have two parameters to describe the shape of the clusters: the mean and the standard deviation! Taking an example in two dimensions, this means that the clusters can take any kind of elliptical shape (since we have standard deviation in both the x and y directions). Thus, each Gaussian distribution is assigned to a single cluster. In order to find the parameters of the Gaussian for each cluster (e.g the mean and standard deviation) we will use an optimization algorithm called Expectation–Maximization (EM). Take a look at the graphic below as an illustration of the Gaussians being fitted to the clusters. Then we can proceed on to the process of Expectation–Maximization clustering using GMMs.

1. We begin by selecting the number of clusters (like K-Means does) and randomly initializing the Gaussian distribution parameters for each cluster. One can try to provide a good guesstimate for the initial parameters by taking a quick look at the data too. Though note, as can be seen in the graphic above, this isn't 100% necessary as the Gaussians start our as very poor but are quickly optimized.
2. Given these Gaussian distributions for each cluster, compute the probability that each data point belongs to a particular cluster. The closer a point is to the Gaussian's centre, the more likely it belongs to that cluster. This should make intuitive sense since with a Gaussian distribution we are assuming that most of the data lies closer to the centre of the cluster.
3. Based on these probabilities, we compute a new set of parameters for the Gaussian distributions such that we maximize the probabilities of data points within the clusters. We compute these new parameters using a weighted sum of the data point positions, where the weights are the probabilities of the data point belonging in that particular cluster. To explain this in a visual manner we can take a look at the graphic above, in particular the yellow cluster as an example. The distribution starts off randomly on the first iteration, but we can see that most of the yellow points are to the right

of that distribution. When we compute a sum weighted by the probabilities, even though there are some points near the centre, most of them are on the right. Thus naturally the distribution's mean is shifted closer to those set of points. We can also see that most of the points are "top-right to bottom-left". Therefore the standard deviation changes to create an ellipse that is more fitted to these points, in order to maximize the sum weighted by the probabilities.

4. Steps 2 and 3 are repeated iteratively until convergence, where the distributions don't change much from iteration to iteration.

There are really 2 key advantages to using GMMs. Firstly GMMs are a lot more flexible in terms of cluster covariance than K-Means; due to the standard deviation parameter, the clusters can take on any ellipse shape, rather than being restricted to circles. K-Means is actually a special case of GMM in which each cluster's covariance along all dimensions approaches 0. Secondly, since GMMs use probabilities, they can have multiple clusters per data point. So if a data point is in the middle of two overlapping clusters, we can simply define its class by saying it belongs X-percent to class 1 and Y-percent to class 2 i.e. GMMs support mixed membership (Reynolds & Rose, 1995; Singh, Pal, & Jabr, 2010).

Agglomerative Hierarchical Clustering

Hierarchical clustering algorithms actually fall into 2 categories: top-down or bottom-up. Bottom-up algorithms treat each data point as a single cluster at the outset and then successively merge (or agglomerate) pairs of clusters until all clusters have been merged into a single cluster that contains all data points. Bottom-up hierarchical clustering is therefore called hierarchical agglomerative clustering or HAC. This hierarchy of clusters is represented as a tree (or dendrogram). The root of the tree is the unique cluster that gathers all the samples, the leaves being the clusters with only one sample(Steinbach, Karypis, & Kumar, 2000).

1. We begin by treating each data point as a single cluster i.e if there are X data points in our dataset then we have X clusters. We then select a distance metric that measures the distance between two clusters. As an example we will use *average linkage* which defines the distance between two clusters to be the average distance between data points in the first cluster and data points in the second cluster.
2. On each iteration we combine two clusters into one. The two clusters to be combined are selected as those with the smallest average linkage i.e. according to our selected distance metric, these two clusters have the smallest distance between each other and therefore are the most similar and should be combined.
3. Step 2 is repeated until we reach the root of the tree i.e we only have one cluster which contains all data points. In this way we can select how many clusters we want in the end, simply by choosing when to stop combining the clusters i.e when we stop building the tree!

Hierarchical clustering does not require us to specify the number of clusters and we can even select which number of clusters looks best since we are building a tree. Additionally, the algorithm is not sensitive to the choice of distance metric; all of them tend to work equally well whereas with other clustering algorithms, the choice of distance metric is critical. A particularly good use case of hierarchical clustering methods is when the underlying data has a hierarchical structure and we want to recover the hierarchy;

other clustering algorithms can't do this. These advantages of hierarchical clustering come at the cost of lower efficiency, as it has a time complexity of $O(n^3)$, unlike the linear complexity of K-Means and GMM (Davidson & Ravi, 2005; Steinbach et al., 2000).

APPLICATION OF MACHINE LEARNING IN TREMOR MEASUREMENT

Random Forest, Decision Tree, Nearest Neighbor (NN), Bayes, Multilayer Perceptron (MLP), and Support Vector Machine (SVM) are six classifiers which used in measuring tremor. In a decision tree classifier, entropy is measured as:

$$Entropy\left(S\right) = -p_{+} log_{2} p_{+} - p_{-} log_{2} p_{-} \tag{2}$$

where S is the set of data points, " p_{+} " is the number of data points that belong to the positive class and " p_{-} " is the number of data points that belong to the negative class. The information gain for each attribute is described by the equation:

$$Gain\left(S, A\right) = Entropy\left(S\right) - \sum_{v \in Values\left(A\right)} \frac{S_V}{S} Entropy\left(S_V\right) \tag{3}$$

where Values(A) is the set of all possible values for feature A. Gain(S,A) measures how well a given feature separates the training examples according to their target classification. A tree is grown from independent random vectors using a training set, resulting in a classifier. After a large number of trees is generated, random forest outputs the class that is the mode of the class's output by individual trees. NN calculates instances using Euclidean distance and correspond to points in an n-dimensional space. The algorithm assigns a class label to a data point that represents the most common value among the k training examples nearest to the data point. We used the IBK scheme from Weka with parameter n=1 in our experiment. SVM maximizes the margin between the training examples and the class boundary. SVM generates a hyperplane which provides a class label for each data point described by a set of feature values. Artificial Neural Networks (ANNs) are computational models mimicking a neuronal organizational structure. ANNs are built from an interconnected set of sample units, which takes a number of real-valued inputs and produces a single real-valued output. Using back propagation, ANN minimizes the squared error between the network output and target values. We applied this technique by using Weka's MLP algorithm to classify TS. Naive Bayes Classifier is a probabilistic classifier which assumes the presence of a particular feature of a class is independent of other features. It learns a classification label by mapping features with Bayes' theorem:

$$argmax_{t_i \in T} P(t_i \mid F) = \frac{P(F \mid t_i) P\left(t_i\right)}{P\left(F\right)} \tag{4}$$

where T represents the tremor class label and F represents the features values. P(t_i) is estimated by counting the frequency with which each target value t_i occurs in the training data. P(F) is calculated from the frequency of feature values. Based on the simplifying assumption that feature values are independent given the target values, the probability of observing the features is the product of the probabilities for the individual features.

SIGNIFICANCE OF TREMOR THROUGH ELECTROMYOGRAPHY

Electromyography works usually with surface electrodes, but sometimes needles or fine electrodes can be used. EMG can give the accurate measurement of frequency rhythm city and also the magnitude. It is best to use at least 2 channels and to record EMG together from an antagonist pair so that there will be additional information's.(Milanov, 2001).

Surface electromyography provides essential info on the neurophysiological characteristics of tremor. The tremor frequency, amplitude, burst period and burst pattern are evaluated by surface electromyography examination. On the conception of those parameters, numerous forms of tremor can be recognized. All tremors can be subdivided into two major groups as per the pattern of muscle activation, either synchronous or alternating in the antagonistic muscles. The tremor amplitude is variable and isn't specific for various kinds of tremor and therefore its diagnostic value is restricted whereas tremor frequency more constant parameter. The tremors could be subdivided into low frequency (below 4Hz), middle frequency (4-9 Hz) and high frequency (above 9 Hz) tremors. Spectral analysis of EMG activity of a tremor that shows distinct peaks has sometimes been assumed to point the presence of motor units firing at totally different frequencies. Actually, the peaks could reflect fluctuations in the variety of motor units recruited and interference in the timing of their burst activity.

Figure 7 shows the diagram indicating central nervous system influences on a Limb. There may be a peripheral reflex loop, a central reflex loop and a central oscillator. The central oscillator is characterized by relative isolation from sensory input.

CASE STUDY

Some of the case studies undergone in different hospitals in Assam and Meghalaya for tremor in PD are shown in Table 2.

It has been seen from the case study that tremor is very must common in PD and it starts from the early stage. Mostly it is resting tremor with different symptoms. Various machine learning techniques can be used to classify the symptoms with the kind of tremor. The techniques mentioned in this chapter are used for this classification which is reliable, user friendly and fast technique.

CONCLUSION

Tremors are the results of variety of mechanisms like peripheral and central loops and central oscillators. Tremors may derive from mechanical oscillations, mechanical reflex oscillations, normal central

Figure 7. Diagram indicating central nervous system

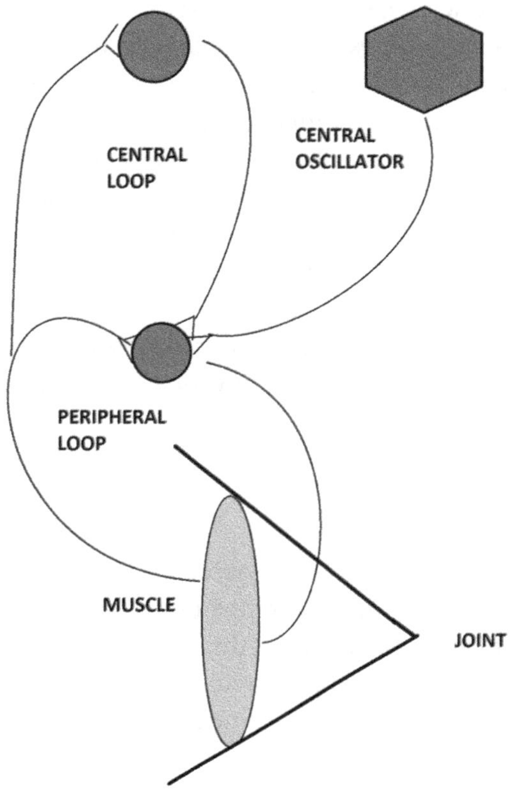

Table 2. Case studies on PD tremor

Patient no	Age	Gender (M:male F:female)	Initial Symptoms	Family History (Immediate Relatives)
1	55	M	Left foot resting tremor.	Mother with PD
2	60	M	Right thumb resting tremor.	Father with tremor
3	62	F	Left hand resting tremor.	None
4	65	F	Right hand resting tremor	Brother with tremor
5	59	M	Right foot resting tremor	Mother and sister with PD
6	70	M	Left hand resting tremor	Mother with tremor
7	73	F	Right thumb resting tremor	None
8	69	M	Left foot resting tremor	None
9	58	M	Right foot resting tremor	Mother with PD and brother with tremor
10	52	M	Left hand resting tremor.	None
11	56	F	Right hand resting tremor	None
12	51	F	Right thumb resting tremor	None
13	77	M	Left foot resting tremor	None
14	73	M	Right foot resting tremor	Father with tremor
15	66	M	Left hand resting tremor	Father with tremor

oscillators and pathologic central oscillators. Methods of studying tremor include accelerometry and electromyography (EMG). Identification of exact location, type and cause of tremor is very much necessary for the detection of various diseases. The physiology of tremor is incompletely known and the definitive identification of a central oscillator for any tremor has not yet been established. Disease like Parkinson's diseases main symptoms starts with early tremor in the fingers and gradually increases in hands and legs followed by tremor in the mouth. Hence its identification is very much essential. Tremor can be identified using various techniques. Nowadays Machine learning is one of the major tools for the tremor identification. Classification of various kinds of tremor can be done by using various machine learning techniques. These techniques are very much accurate and also less time consuming. Hence, this chapter gives a brief review of various kinds of tremor and its classification with respect to Parkinson's disease. Further, this will help the clinicians and researchers to study various kinds of machine learning techniques associated with identification of tremor in various neurological disorders.

ACKNOWLEDGMENT

We would like to acknowledge the Department of Neurology of North Eastern Indira Gandhi Regional Institute of Medical and Health Science, Shillong for their immense help and support. Also our sincerely gratitude to colleagues, faculty members and staffs of the Department of Biomedical Engineering, North-Eastern Hill University, Shillong for providing the required Instrument and laboratory space and also equally grateful to the staffs of School of Computer Science and Software Engineering for software support for providing software support. The corresponding of this paper is thankful to Ministry of Science & Technology, Department of Biotechnology, Government of India for providing the financial support as Biotechnology Overseas Associateship for NE region.

REFERENCES

Abdulhay, E., Arunkumar, N., Narasimhan, K., Vellaiappan, E., & Venkatraman, V. (2018). Gait and tremor investigation using machine learning techniques for the diagnosis of Parkinson disease. *Future Generation Computer Systems*, *83*, 366–373. doi:10.1016/j.future.2018.02.009

Ai, L., Wang, J., & Yao, R. (2011). Classification of parkinsonian and essential tremor using empirical mode decomposition and support vector machine. *Digital Signal Processing*, *21*(4), 543–550. doi:10.1016/j.dsp.2011.01.010

Bunting-Perry, L. K. (2006). Palliative care in Parkinson's disease: Implications for neuroscience nursing. *The Journal of Neuroscience Nursing*, *38*(2), 106. doi:10.1097/01376517-200604000-00006 PMID:16681291

Chapelle, O., Scholkopf, B., & Zien, A. (2009). Semi-supervised learning. IEEE Transactions on Neural Networks, 20(3), 542-542.

Chapuis, S., Ouchchane, L., Metz, O., Gerbaud, L., & Durif, F. (2005). Impact of the motor complications of Parkinson's disease on the quality of life. *Movement Disorders: Official Journal of the Movement Disorder Society, 20*(2), 224-230.

Checkoway, H., & Nelson, L. M. (1999). Epidemiologic approaches to the study of Parkinson's disease etiology. *Epidemiology (Cambridge, Mass.), 10*(3), 327–336. doi:10.1097/00001648-199905000-00023 PMID:10230846

Chen, Y., Garcia, G., Huang, W., & Constantini, S. (2014). The involvement of secondary neuronal damage in the development of neuropsychiatric disorders following brain insults. *Frontiers in Neurology, 5*, 22. doi:10.3389/fneur.2014.00022 PMID:24653712

Cheng, Y. (1995). Mean shift, mode seeking, and clustering. *IEEE Transactions on Pattern Analysis and Machine Intelligence, 17*(8), 790–799. doi:10.1109/34.400568

Cherubini, A., Nisticó, R., Novellino, F., Salsone, M., Nigro, S., Donzuso, G., & Quattrone, A. (2014). Magnetic resonance support vector machine discriminates essential tremor with rest tremor from tremor-dominant Parkinson disease. *Movement Disorders, 29*(9), 1216–1219. doi:10.1002/mds.25869 PMID:24729430

Comaniciu, D., & Meer, P. (1999). Mean shift analysis and applications. *Paper presented at the Computer Vision, 1999. The Proceedings of the Seventh IEEE International Conference on.* 10.1109/ICCV.1999.790416

Comaniciu, D., & Meer, P. (2002). Mean shift: A robust approach toward feature space analysis. *IEEE Transactions on Pattern Analysis and Machine Intelligence, 24*(5), 603–619. doi:10.1109/34.1000236

Darnall, N., Donovan, C., Aktar, S., Tseng, H., Barthelmess, P., Cohen, P., & Lin, D. (2012). Application of machine learning and numerical analysis to classify tremor in patients affected with essential tremor or Parkinson's disease. *Gerontechnology (Valkenswaard), 10*(4), 208–219. doi:10.4017/gt.2012.10.4.002.00

Davidson, I., & Ravi, S. (2005). *Agglomerative hierarchical clustering with constraints: Theoretical and empirical results.* Paper presented at the European Conference on Principles of Data Mining and Knowledge Discovery. 10.1007/11564126_11

Ejlerskov, P. (2015). *Immune gene prevents Parkinson's disease and dementia.* Retrieved from http://www.health.am/psy/more/prevents-parkinsons-disease-and-dementia/

Elble, R. J. (2017). *Tremor. In Neuro-Geriatrics* (pp. 311–326). Springer. doi:10.1007/978-3-319-56484-5_20

Eskofier, B. M., Lee, S. I., Daneault, J.-F., Golabchi, F. N., Ferreira-Carvalho, G., Vergara-Diaz, G., . . . Kautz, T. (2016). *Recent machine learning advancements in sensor-based mobility analysis: deep learning for Parkinson's disease assessment.* Paper presented at the Engineering in Medicine and Biology Society (EMBC), 2016 IEEE 38th Annual International Conference of the. 10.1109/EMBC.2016.7590787

Factor, S., Feustel, P., Friedman, J., Comella, C., Goetz, C., Kurlan, R., ... Group, P. S. (2003). Longitudinal outcome of Parkinson's disease patients with psychosis. *Neurology, 60*(11), 1756–1761. doi:10.1212/01.WNL.0000068010.82167.CF PMID:12796526

Fleuriephysio. (2017). *10 Signs of Parkinson's Disease.* Retrieved from http://fleurieuphysiotherapy.com.au/10-signs-parkinsons-disease/

Gokul, S., Sivachitra, M., & Vijayachitra, S. (2013). *Parkinson's disease prediction using machine learning approaches.* Paper presented at the Advanced Computing (ICoAC), 2013 Fifth International Conference on. 10.1109/ICoAC.2013.6921958

Hallett, M. (1991). Classification and treatment of tremor. *Journal of the American Medical Association, 266*(8), 1115–1117. doi:10.1001/jama.1991.03470080085035 PMID:1650852

Hartigan, J. A., & Wong, M. A. (1979). Algorithm AS 136: A k-means clustering algorithm. *Journal of the Royal Statistical Society. Series C, Applied Statistics, 28*(1), 100–108.

Jeon, H., Lee, W., Park, H., Lee, H. J., Kim, S. K., Kim, H. B., ... Park, K. S. (2017). High-accuracy automatic classification of Parkinsonian tremor severity using machine learning method. *Physiological Measurement, 38*(11), 1980–1999. doi:10.1088/1361-6579/aa8e1f PMID:28933707

Kanungo, T., Mount, D. M., Netanyahu, N. S., Piatko, C. D., Silverman, R., & Wu, A. Y. (2002). An efficient k-means clustering algorithm: Analysis and implementation. *IEEE Transactions on Pattern Analysis and Machine Intelligence, 24*(7), 881–892. doi:10.1109/TPAMI.2002.1017616

Kotsiantis, S. B., Zaharakis, I., & Pintelas, P. (2007). Supervised machine learning: A review of classification techniques. *Emerging Artificial Intelligence Applications in Computer Engineering, 160*, 3-24.

Koza, J. R., Bennett, F. H., Andre, D., & Keane, M. A. (1996). Automated Design of Both the Topology and Sizing of Analog Electrical Circuits Using Genetic Programming. In J. S. Gero & F. Sudweeks (Eds.), *Artificial Intelligence in Design '96* (pp. 151–170). Dordrecht: Springer Netherlands. doi:10.1007/978-94-009-0279-4_9

Likas, A., Vlassis, N., & Verbeek, J. J. (2003). The global k-means clustering algorithm. *Pattern Recognition, 36*(2), 451–461. doi:10.1016/S0031-3203(02)00060-2

Lloyd, S., Mohseni, M., & Rebentrost, P. (2013). *Quantum algorithms for supervised and unsupervised machine learning.* arXiv preprint arXiv:1307.0411

Louis, E. D. (2014). Re-thinking the biology of essential tremor: from models to morphology. *Parkinsonism & Related Disorders, 20*, S88-S93. Retrieved from https://www.techleer.com/articles/203-machine-learning-algorithm-backbone-of-emerging-technologies/ files/74/203-machine-learning-algorithm-backbone-of-emerging-technologies.html

Machine Learning Algorithms Mindmap. (2015). Retrieved from https://jixta.wordpress.com/2015/07/17/machine-learning-algorithms-mindmap/

Marjama-Lyons, J., & Koller, W. (2000). Tremor-predominant Parkinson's disease. *Drugs & Aging, 16*(4), 273–278. doi:10.2165/00002512-200016040-00003 PMID:10874522

Medications, P. (2016). *Causes of Parkinson's Disease.* Retrieved from https://www.atrainceu.com/course-module-short-view/1874200-080_antiparkinson-strategies-module-03

Milanov, I. (2001). Electromyographic differentiation of tremors. *Clinical Neurophysiology, 112*(9), 1626–1632. doi:10.1016/S1388-2457(01)00629-0 PMID:11514245

Mnih, V., Badia, A. P., Mirza, M., Graves, A., Lillicrap, T., Harley, T., . . . Kavukcuoglu, K. (2016). *Asynchronous methods for deep reinforcement learning.* Paper presented at the International conference on machine learning.

Pedrosa, T. Í., Vasconcelos, F. F., Medeiros, L., & Silva, L. D. (2018). Machine Learning Application to Quantify the Tremor Level for Parkinson's Disease Patients. *Procedia Computer Science*, *138*, 215–220. doi:10.1016/j.procs.2018.10.031

Reynolds, D. A., & Rose, R. C. (1995). Robust text-independent speaker identification using Gaussian mixture speaker models. *IEEE Transactions on Speech and Audio Processing*, *3*(1), 72–83. doi:10.1109/89.365379

Robert, C. (2014). Machine Learning, a Probabilistic Perspective. *Chance*, *27*(2), 62–63. doi:10.1080/09332480.2014.914768

Singh, R., Pal, B. C., & Jabr, R. A. (2010). Statistical representation of distribution system loads using Gaussian mixture model. *IEEE Transactions on Power Systems*, *25*(1), 29–37. doi:10.1109/TPWRS.2009.2030271

Stein, R., & Oĝuztöreli, M. (1976). Tremor and other oscillations in neuromuscular systems. *Biological Cybernetics*, *22*(3), 147–157. doi:10.1007/BF00365525 PMID:1276248

Steinbach, M., Karypis, G., & Kumar, V. (2000). *A comparison of document clustering techniques.* Paper presented at the KDD workshop on text mining.

Surathi, P., Jhunjhunwala, K., Yadav, R., & Pal, P. K. (2016). Research in Parkinson's disease in India: A review. *Annals of Indian Academy of Neurology*, *19*(1), 9. doi:10.4103/0972-2327.167713 PMID:27011622

Tran, T. N., Drab, K., & Daszykowski, M. (2013). Revised DBSCAN algorithm to cluster data with dense adjacent clusters. *Chemometrics and Intelligent Laboratory Systems*, *120*, 92–96. doi:10.1016/j.chemolab.2012.11.006

Wang, W.-T., Wu, Y.-L., Tang, C.-Y., & Hor, M.-K. (2015). *Adaptive density-based spatial clustering of applications with noise (DBSCAN) according to data.* Paper presented at the Machine Learning and Cybernetics (ICMLC), 2015 International Conference on.

Wilcox, S. K. (2010). Extending palliative care to patients with Parkinson's disease. *British Journal of Hospital Medicine, 71*(1), 26-30.

Chapter 9
Epileptic Seizure Detection and Classification Using Machine Learning

Rekh Ram Janghel
National Institute of Technology Raipur, India

Yogesh Kumar Rathore
National Institute of Technology Raipur, India

Gautam Tatiparti
National Institute of Technology Raipur, India

ABSTRACT

Epilepsy is a brain ailment identified by unpredictable interruptions of normal brain activity. Around 1% of mankind experience epileptic seizures. Around 10% of the United States population experiences at least a single seizure in their life. Epilepsy is distinguished by the tendency of the brain to generate unexpected bursts of unusual electrical activity that disrupts the normal functioning of the brain. As seizures usually occur rarely and are unforeseeable, seizure recognition systems are recommended for seizure detection during long-term electroencephalography (EEG). In this chapter, ANN models, namely, BPA, RNN, CL, PNN, and LVQ, have been implemented. A prominent dataset was employed to assess the proposed method. The proposed method is capable of achieving an accuracy of 97.5%; the high accuracy obtained has confirmed the great success of the method.

INTRODUCTION

As per International League Against Epilepsy (ILAE) and the International Bureau for Epilepsy (IBE), Epilepsy is a neurological disorder distinguished by repeated unprovoked convulsions which are a consequence of irregular electrical activity in the brain (Guo et al., 2012). According to a study by WHO, Approximately 50 million people suffer from epilepsy universally (Cook, 2013). Approximately 2.4 million new cases of epilepsy are reported every year globally (Acharya et al., 2013). Epilepsy could be of two

DOI: 10.4018/978-1-5225-8567-1.ch009

major types depending upon the area of the brain tissue that is involved, which are, generalized seizures and, partial seizures, generalized seizures roughly involves nearly the whole brain, partial convulsions develop in a particular section of the brain and is restricted to this area (Ling Guo et.al., 2010). Potential risk of mortality makes early diagnosis and treatment of epilepsy a critical task. Electroencephalography (EEG) is a famous electrophysiological technique used to comprehend the complicated activity of the brain (Gandhi et al., 2010). The EEG directly gauges and registers the electrical activity of the brain. Spontaneous EEG signals are classified into several rhythms based on their frequencies, which are δ band(0:3 - 4Hz); ɵ band (4 - 8Hz); α band (8 - 13Hz); β band (13 - 30Hz) (Zhou & Gotman, 2004). An EEG is especially useful at times when the brain is at risk by providing a sensitive indication of cerebral functioning. Such intervals are usually of long time spans, hence an extended EEG recording is needed Early studies have shown evidence of this abnormal activity to be a convenient aid in detection of epilepsy and cerebral tumors. Nowadays EEG signals are used to get information relevant to the diagnosis, prognosis, and treatment of these abnormal conditions. EEG is registered using electrodes placed on the scalp and have small amplitudes of the degree of 20 μV (Selvan & Srinivasan, 1999) The electrodes are placed as per the 10-20 international system which has been shown. Usually EEGs contain massive amounts of information and detection of traces of epilepsy requires a visual inspection of the total span of the EEG by a specialist which is a cumbersome task (Rivero et al., 2009). Hence, developing automated epileptic seizure detection system is noteworthy for assessing EEGs. Studies on automated seizure detection systems started in the 1970s and multiple techniques have been proposed for addressing the problem. Artificial Neural Networks (ANNs) are the most common classifiers that have been used for discriminating the EEGs as per the literature review. Artificial Neural Networks (ANNs) are information processing systems that were inspired by biological nervous system of humans. Artificial Neural Networks are highly parallel and interconnected and consist of simpler non-linear processing elements (Guo et al., 2010). Artificial Neural Networks were chosen as a classifier for the current work as it is capable of performing computations with high accuracy when executed on customized hardware. In this chapter, a unique epileptic seizure recognition system has been discussed.

The method is employs five different Artificial Neural Network (ANN) models, namely, Back Propagation Algorithm (BPA), Competitive Learning (CL), Linear Vector Quantization (LVQ), Probabilistic Neural Networks (PNN), and, Recurrent Neural Networks (RNN). A database consisting of 500 EEG segments is employed. High accuracies acquired designate the outstanding classification accomplishment of the suggested technique in contrast to other approaches.

METHODS AND MATERIALS

Steps involved in methodology and their flow of control is shown in figure 2.

Database Description

The dataset employed in the current work has been described by Andrzejak et al. (2001). The total dataset includes five subsets (designated as Z, O, N, F and S) each subset consisting of 100 single-channel EEG fragments, each fragment being of 23.6s, and were sampled at 173:6Hz. All fragments were chosen from continuous multi-channel EEG recordings after visual inspection for artifacts such as, muscle activity or eye movements. Sets Z, O contain fragments that have been obtained from surface EEG recordings

Figure 1. Standardized electrode placement scheme (Polat et al., 2007)

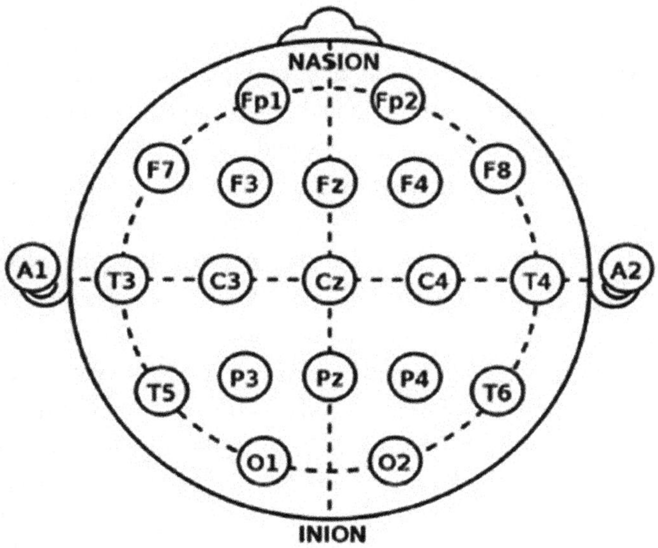

Figure 2. Flowchart of methodology

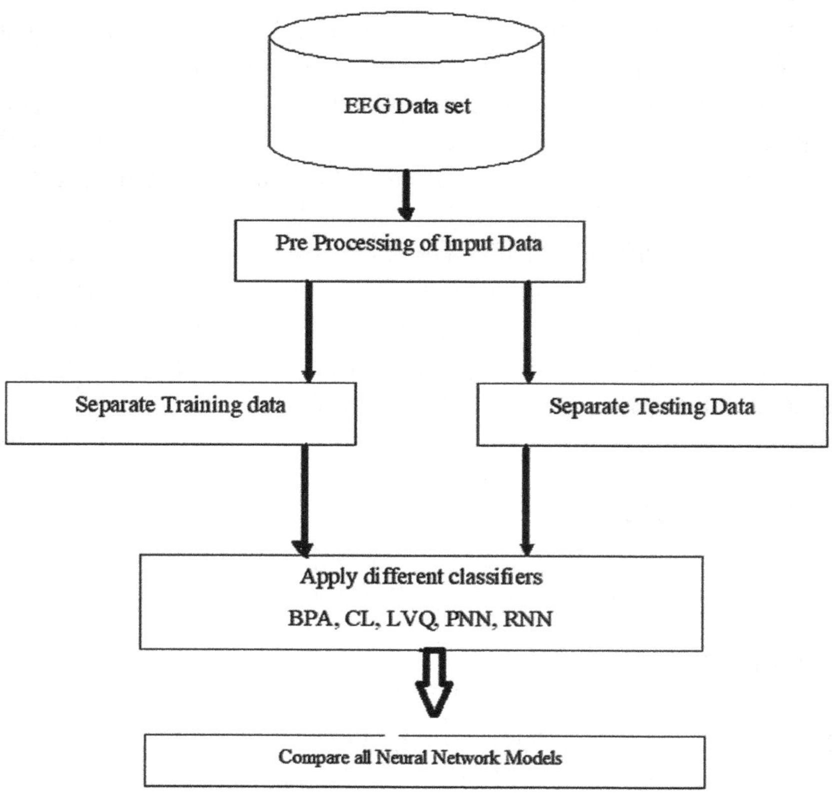

conducted on five healthy subjects. Subjects were in an awaken condition and eyes open (Z) and eyes closed (O) respectively (Srinivasan et al., 2005). Sets N, F and S emerged from an EEG repository of presurgical diagnosis. Fragments in Set F have been registered from the epileptogenic zone, and fragments in set N from the hippocampal formation of the opposite hemisphere of the brain. To do so, Sets N and F encompassed only activity measured during seizure free spans, set S contained only seizure activity. Entire EEG data was recorded using the same 128-channel amplifier system, using an average common reference (Venema et al., 2006). The spectral bandwidth of the data is the same as that of the acquisition system, which ranges from 0.5 Hz to 85 Hz. Representative EEG fragments have been shown below (Polat et al., 2007).

Feature Extraction

The proposed system relies on three features namely, Mean, Standard Deviation, and, Average Power

Figure 3. Raw EEG specimens belonging to the five subsets (Z, F, N, O, and S)

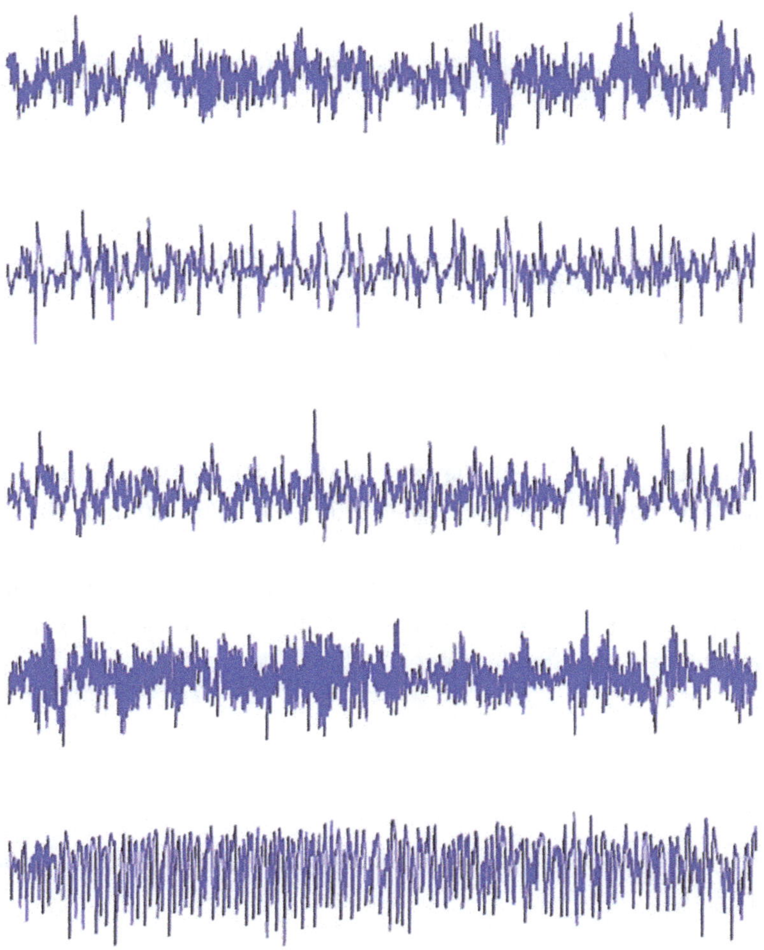

1. **Mean:** Mean of a signal is computed as the summation of all the samples divided by the total samples in the signal, it indicates the average value of the signal over the entire duration.

$$\mu = \sum_{t=0}^{N-1} Xi \tag{1}$$

where μ is mean, N is number of inputs and Xi is value of inputs

2. **Standard Deviation:** Standard Deviation represents the variability or dispersion of a signal about its mean value. Dispersion is measured as a difference between the actual values and the average value. Larger the dispersion around the mean, the higher the dispersion value.

$$\sigma 2 = \frac{1}{N-1} \sum_{t=0}^{N-1} (xi - \mu) \tag{2}$$

where, xi is input and μ is mean of different xi inputs, N shows number of inputs.

3. **Average Power:** The average power denotes the average amount of work done or energy transferred per unit time. The average power of a signal is defined by,

$$p\left(k\right) = \frac{1}{N} \sum_{k=0}^{N} (Xk * Xk) \tag{3}$$

Xk is inputs and N is number of inputs.

Back Propagation Algorithm (BPA)

Back Propagation Algorithm is one among the extensively used algorithms for training Feed Forward Networks the reason being is how efficient they are, however, back propagation is not free of issues, the algorithm doesn't produce required outcomes. In addition to this, the optimum hidden units to be used are not know in advance and are meant to be determined by trial and error (Hinton, 1992). The algorithm has been described in mathematical terms below j is a unit in the output layer and unit i is a unit in the previous layer. A unit in the output layer determines the activity in a two-step manner, Initially, the total weighted input x_j is computed using the formula

$$Xj = \sum_{i} (Yi * Wij) \tag{4}$$

where, Y_i is the activity level of the ith unit in the previous layer and W_{ij} is the weight of the connection between the ith and j^{th} unit.

$$Yi = \frac{1}{1 + e^{-xj}} \quad (5)$$

After the activities of all the output units have been computed, the network calculates the error E, as per (6)

$$E = \frac{1}{2}\sum_{j}\left(Yj - dj\right)^{2} \quad (6)$$

where, Y_j is the activity level of the j_{th} unit in the top layer and dj is the desired output of the j_{th} unit.

Competitive Learning (CL)

Competitive Learning, also known as unsupervised learning, comprises of a network learning that responds correctly on its own without the involvement of any external agent i.e. actual output When an input is presented to the perceptron multiple association neurons get activated which in turn activate some response neurons (Janghel et al., 2012). Competitive Learning systems are typically feed forward multilayer neural network where neurons compete for activation which is induced by randomly sampled pattern vectors, the continuous distribution of the random pattern vectors x is denoted by an unknown probability density function (Janghel et al., 2010). The network is initialized by a random number of neurons. It is better to estimate the number of neurons based on the current understanding of the problem. Usually, the number of output neurons is chosen to be greater than the possible clusters as the redundant neurons can be eliminated. The dimensionality of the input vector is computed based upon the problem (Zarkogianni et al., 2017).

If a neuron wins the competition, its weight vector gets updated. The updated weight is computed as per the following update rule:

$$w_j(n + 1) = w_j(n) + ή(n)(x - w_j(n)) \quad (7)$$

where, ή is the learning rate, and w_j is the weight of the winning neuron j.

Learning Vector Quantization (LVQ)

The fundamental steps in the learning process of an LVQ are:

- **Initialization:** The codebook vectors are placed at random positions in the input space.
- **Training sample:** A training sample p of the training set P is chosen and presented.
- **Winner:** The closest cookbook vector wins, i.e. the one with Learning Process takes place according to the rule

$$\Delta Ci = \eta\left(t\right).h\left(p, Ci\right).(p - Ci) \quad (8)$$

$$Ci\left(t+1\right)=Ci\left(t\right)+\Delta Ci \tag{9}$$

1. ή (t) is time-dependent learning rate which allows us to differentiate between large learning steps and fine tuning.
2. (p - C_i) is the direction towards which the codebook vector ids moved
3. Function h(p,Ci) is the core of the rule, which implements a distinction of cases.
   a. **Assignment Is Correct:** The winning vector is a codebook vector of the class that includes p. In this case, the function provides positive values and the codebook vector moves towards p.
   b. **Assignment Is Wrong:** The winning vector does not represent the class that includes p. Therefore it moves away from p.

The codebook vectors can be understood as neurons which have fixed positions within the input space and it is possible that often one neuron could fire, and inhibit all the other neurons (Janghel et al., 2012; Kriesel, 2005).

Probabilistic Neural Networks (PNN)

Probabilistic Neural Networks were proposed by Specht in the year 1990 (Specht, 1990). A single PNN possess the capability of handling multiclass problem. This is against the one-against-the rest or one-per-class approach taken by some classifiers like SVM, which decompose a multiclass problem into dichotomies and each chotomizer separates a single class from all others (Acharya, 2013). Architecture of PNN has been shown in figure. It consists of multiple processing units or neurons which are inter-connected and organized into successive layers. The input layer does not perform any computation and distributes the input to the neurons in the pattern layer on receiving the pattern x from the input layer, the neuron x_{ij} of pattern layer computes its output by summarizing and averaging all the neurons that belong to the same class (Kala et al., 2011).

$$Pi\left(x\right)=\frac{1}{\left(2\pi\right)^{d/2}*\sigma^{d}}*\frac{1}{N}\sum_{j=1}^{Ni}\exp[-\frac{\left(x-xij\right)^{T}*\left(x-xij\right)}{2\sigma^{2}}] \tag{10}$$

$$\varnothing ij\left(x\right)=\frac{1}{\left(2\pi\right)^{d/2}*\sigma^{d}}*\exp\left[-\frac{\left(x-xij\right)^{T}*\left(x-xij\right)}{2\sigma^{2}}\right] \tag{11}$$

where, d denotes the dimension of the pattern vector x, σ is the smoothing parameter x_{ij} is the neuron vector. The summation layer of pattern x being classified in C_i.

Figure 4. Standardized electrode placement scheme (Li & Li, 2013)

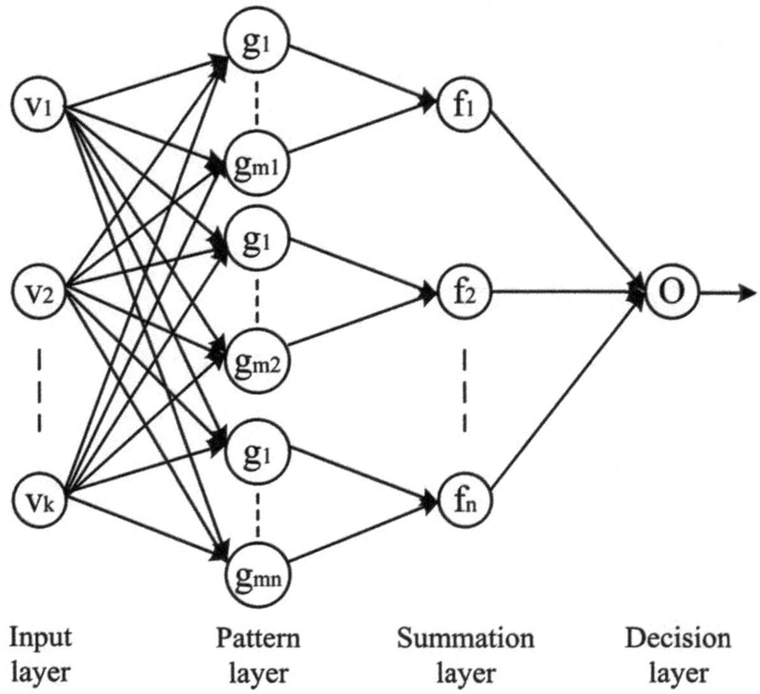

Recurrent Neural Networks (RNN)

RNNs are being used for a number of applications ranging from associative memories to generalization of pattern sequences Fully recurrent networks use learning algorithms that are capable of dealing with time varying inputs, or output in non trivial ways Even after several modifications of the learning algorithms to reduce computational cost, fully recurrent networks are still quite complex when dealing with complicated problems (Samanwoy Ghosh et.al., 2007)(Yuedong Song & Pietro Li_o, 2010).

RESULT COMPARISON PARAMETERS

Performance of classifiers is judged on the basis of following parameters:

- **Accuracy:** This is one of the most important metrics to evaluate the effectiveness of a predictive model. It refers to the closeness between the computed outcomes and the diagnosed labels. It can be calculated by equation 12.
- **Specificity:** This metric measures the proportion of negatives that are correctly identified as such. Together with recall, it is considered to be one of the most important metrics in the area of medical image analysis. Mathematical formulation given by equation 14.

Some other parameters like sensitivity, false positive rate and false negative rates are also calculated. Where, sensitivity shows ability to correct detection of disease or true positive rate equation 13, the false positive rate is also known as false alarm rate, is the probability of falsely rejecting the null hypothesis for a particular case given in equation 15, and false negative rate is the rate of result generated by the system negative in case of positive result shown in equation 16.

Multiple parameters have been considered for evaluation of our proposed method, the parameters that were considered are:

$$Accuracy\left(in\ \%\right) = \frac{TP + TN}{TP + TN + FP + FN} *100 \tag{12}$$

$$Sensitivity\left(in\ \%\right) = \frac{TP}{TP + FN} * 100 \tag{13}$$

$$Specificity\left(in\ \%\right) = \frac{TN}{TN + FP} * 100 \tag{14}$$

$$False\,Positive\,Rate\left(FNR\right) = \frac{TP}{TP + FN} \tag{15}$$

$$False\,Negative\,Rate\left(FNR\right) = \frac{TN}{TN + FN} \tag{16}$$

RESULTS AND DISCUSSION

The Back Propagation Algorithm proposed in the current work employs one hidden layer and has been trained with a momentum of 0.9.

The Artificial Neural Network models proposed have been tested by varying the Hidden Neurons from (5-35), Learning Rate from (0.1- 0.5), and Epochs from (500 - 2500). Table 1 shows the performance of various neural network methods on varying learning rate, number of hidden layers and number of epochs.

Further experiments have been performed to evaluate the performance of neural network based classifiers on different parameters shown in table 2.

Graphical representation of comparison of sensitivity, specificity accuracy FPR and FNR is shown in figure 5

Performance of different artificial neural network methods on above dataset are shown in table 3.

Table 1. Experiment with variation of neural network parameters

Method	Learning Rate	Number of Neurons in Hidden Layer	Number of Epochs	Accuracy
BPA	0.1	15	1000	97.5
CL	0.1	20	1000	47.5
LVQ	0.1	15	1000	50.83
PNN	0.1	15	1000	55
RNN	0.1	15	1000	97.5

Table 2. Experiments with variation of neural network parameters

Method	Sensitivity	Specificity	Accuracy	FPR	FNR
BPA	100.0	95.2	97.5	50.0	0.0
CL	33.3	48.7	47.5	95.0	100.0
LVQ	50.9	50.8	50.8	51.7	46.7
PNN	100.0	52.6	55.0	90.0	0.0
RNN	95.2	100.0	97.5	0.0	5.0

Figure 5. Standardized electrode placement scheme

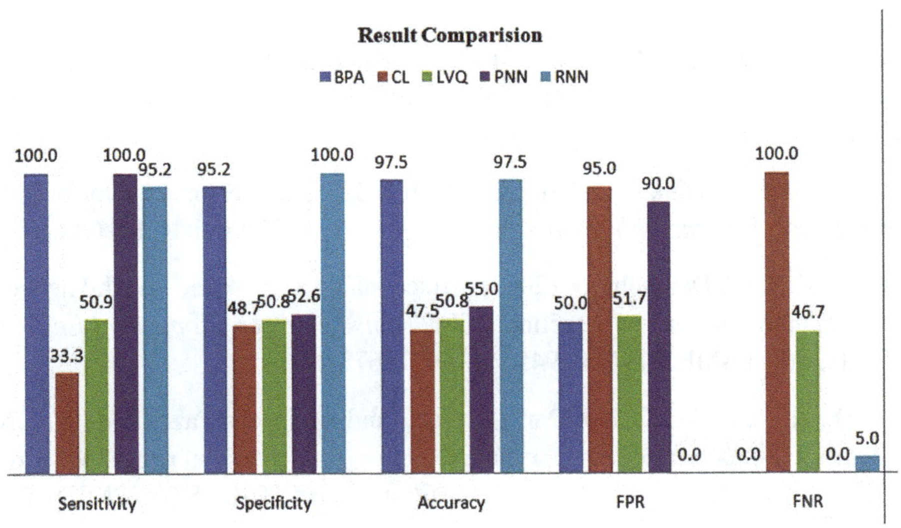

CONCLUSION AND FUTURE WORK

EEG signals can be used to discriminate between normal and epileptic states of the brain. In this work, we have presented an epileptic seizure detection system based on Artificial Neural Networks (ANNs), the ANN models that were implemented were Back Propagation Algorithm (BPA), Competitive Learning (CL), Linear Vector Quantization (LVQ), Probabilistic Neural Networks (PNN) and Recurrent Neural

Table 3. Synopsis of prior research for recognition of normal and epileptic states

Authors	Method Used	Accuracy Achieved
Nigam & Graupe, 2004	Diagnostic Neural Network	97.2
Kannathal et al. 2005	Adaptive Neuro-Fuzzy Inference systems (ANFIS)	92.3
Sadati et al 2006	Adaptive neural fuzzy network	85.9
Subasi et.al. 2007	Mixture expert model (a modular neural network)	94.5
Guo et al. 2010	ANN	95.2
Nigam & Graupe, 2004	Artificial Neural Networks (ANN)	97.5

Networks (RNN). Experiments have shown that the ANN model built on Back Propagation Algorithm (BPA) and Recurrent Neural Networks (RNN) perform the best among the ANN models reported in the study and give an accuracy of 97.5%. Here, experiments also found that learning rate should be set to 0.1 and number of neurons in hidden layer should be 15 for better results. It is also concluded that the Competitive Learning (CL), Linear Vector Quantization (LVQ), Probabilistic Neural Networks (PNN) method does not work well on this database, because accuracy of classification of these methods are near about 50% which is not acceptable for diagnosis purpose.

REFERENCES

Cook, O'Brien, Berkovic, Murphy, Morokof, Fabinyi, … Himes. (2013). Prediction of seizure likelihood with a long-term, implanted seizure advisory system in patients with drug-resistant epilepsy: A first in- man study. *The Lancet Neurology, 12*(6), 563-571.

Gandhi, T., Panigrahi, B. K., Bhatia, M., & Anand, S. (2010). Expert model for detection of epileptic activity in EEG signature. *Expert Systems with Applications, 37*(4), 3513–3520. doi:10.1016/j.eswa.2009.10.036

Ghosh, S., Dastidar, H. A., & Dadmehr, N. (2007). Mixedband wavelet-chaos-neural network methodology for epilepsy and epileptic seizure detection. *IEEE Transactions on Biomedical Engineering, 54*(9), 1545–1551. doi:10.1109/TBME.2007.891945 PMID:17867346

Guo, L., Rivero, D., & Pazos, A. (2010). Daniel Rivero, and Alejandro Pazos. Epileptic seizure detection using multiwavelet transform based approximate entropy and artificial neural networks. *Journal of Neuroscience Methods, 193*(1), 156–163. doi:10.1016/j.jneumeth.2010.08.030 PMID:20817036

Guo, P., Wang, J., Gao, X. Z., & Jarno, M. A. (2012). Epileptic EEG signal classification with marching pursuit based on harmony search method. *Conference Proceedings - IEEE International Conference on Systems, Man and Cybernetics*, 283-288.

Hinton. (1992). How Neural Networks Learn from Experience. *Scientific American, 267*(3), 144-151.

Janghel, Shukla, Tiwari, & Kala. (2010). *Breast Cancer Diagnosis using Artificial Neural Network Models*. Academic Press.

Janghel, R. R., Shukla, A., & Tiwari, R. (2012). Hybrid computing based intelligent system for breast cancer diagnosis. *International Journal of Biomedical Engineering and Technology*, *10*(1), 1–18. doi:10.1504/IJBET.2012.049321

Kannathal, N., & Min Lim Choo, U. (2005). Entropies for detection of epilepsy in EEG. *Computer Methods and Programs in Biomedicine*, *80*(3), 187–194. doi:10.1016/j.cmpb.2005.06.012 PMID:16219385

Kriesel, D. (2005). A Brief Introduction to Neural Networks. Academic Press.

Li & Li. (2013). Online Finger Gesture Recognition Using Surface Electromyography Signals. *Journal of Signal and Information Processing, 4*(2).

Nigam, V. P., & Graupe, D. (2004). A neural-network-based detection of epilepsy. *Neurological Research*, *26*(1), 55–60. doi:10.1179/016164104773026534 PMID:14977058

Polat, K., & Güneş, S. (2007). Classification of epileptiform EEG using a hybrid system based on decision tree classifier and fast Fourier transform. *Applied Mathematics and Computation*, *187*(2), 1017–1026. doi:10.1016/j.amc.2006.09.022

Rahul Kala, R. R. (2011). Diagnosis of breast cancer by modular evolutionary neural networks. *International Journal of Biomedical Engineering and Technology*, *7*(2), 194. doi:10.1504/IJBET.2011.043179

Rajendra Acharya, U., Vinitha Sree, S., & Swapna, G. (2013). Roshan Joy Martis, and Jasjit S. Suri. Automated EEG analysis of epilepsy: A review. *Knowledge-Based Systems*, *45*, 147–165. doi:10.1016/j.knosys.2013.02.014

Ralph, G. (2001). Andrzejak, Klaus Lehnertz, Florian Mormann, Christoph Rieke, Peter David, and Christian E. Elger. Indications of nonlinear deterministic and nite-dimensional structures in time series of brain electrical activity: Dependence on recording region and brain state. *Physical Review. E*, *64*(6), 061907. doi:10.1103/PhysRevE.64.061907

Rivero. (2009). Classification of EEG Signals Using Relative Wavelet Energy and Artificial Neural Networks. Academic Press.

Sadati, N., Mohseni, H. R., & Maghsoudi, A. (2006). Epileptic Seizure Detection Using Neural Fuzzy Networks. *2006 IEEE International Conference on Fuzzy Systems*, 596-600. 10.1109/FUZZY.2006.1681772

Selvan & Srinivasan. (1999). Removal of ocular artifacts from EEG using an efficient neural network based adaptive filtering technique. *IEEE Signal Processing Letters, 6*(12), 330-332.

Song, Y., & Liò, P. (2010). A new approach for epileptic seizure detection: Sample entropy based feature extraction and extreme learning machine. *Journal of Biomedical Science and Engineering*, *03*(06), 556–567. doi:10.4236/jbise.2010.36078

Specht. (1990). Probabilistic neural networks. *Neural Networks, 3*(1), 109-118.

Srinivasan, V., Eswaran, C., & Sriraam, N. (2005). Artificial neural network based epileptic detection using time-domain and frequency-domain features. *Journal of Medical Systems*, *29*(6), 647–660. doi:10.100710916-005-6133-1 PMID:16235818

Subasi, A. (2007). EEG signal classification using wavelet feature extraction and a mixture of expert model. *Expert Systems with Applications*, *32*(4), 1084–1093. doi:10.1016/j.eswa.2006.02.005

Venema, V., Ament, F., & Simmer, C. (2006). A stochastic iterative amplitude adjusted fourier transform algorithm with improved accuracy. *Nonlinear Processes in Geophysics*, *13*(3), 321–328. doi:10.5194/npg-13-321-2006

Zarkogianni, K., Athanasiou, M., Thanopoulou, A. C., & Nikita, K. S. (2017). Comparison of machine learning approaches towards assessing the risk of developing Cardiovascular disease as a long term diabetes complication. *IEEE Journal of Biomedical and Health Informatics*, *2194*(c). PMID:29990007

Zhou, W., & Gotman, J. (2004). Removal of EMG and ECG artifacts from EEG based on wavelet transform and ICA. *26th Annual International Conference of the IEEE Engineering in Medicine and Biology Society*, *1*, 392-395.

Chapter 10
Neurocognitive Mechanisms for Detecting Early Phase of Depressive Disorder:
Analysis of Event-Related Potentials in Human Brain

Shashikanta Tarai
National Institute of Technology Raipur, India

ABSTRACT

This chapter discusses neurocognitive mechanisms in terms of latency and amplitudes of EEG signals in depression that are presented in the form of event-related potentials (ERPs). Reviewing the available literature on depression, this chapter classifies early P100, ERN, N100, N170, P200, N200, and late P300 ERP components in frontal, mid-frontal, temporal, and parietal lobes. Using auditory oddball paradigm, most of the studies testing depressive patients have found robust P300 amplitude reduction. Proposing EEG methods and summarizing behavioral, neuroanatomical, and electrophysiological findings, this chapter discusses how the different tasks, paradigms, and stimuli contribute to the cohesiveness of neural signatures and psychobiological markers for identifying the patients with depression. Existing research gaps are directed to conduct ERP studies following go/no-go, flanker interference, and Stroop tasks on global and local attentional stimuli associated with happy and sad emotions to examine anterior cingulate cortex (ACC) dysfunction in depression.

INTRODUCTION

Depression is an activity of abhorrence with a sad mood that severely affects human personality, behaviour, language, thoughts, emotions and sagacity of well-being (Schnaas, 2003). Studies on cognitive theories of depression posit that depressive disorder patients always suffer from the cognitive dysfunctions and impairments, dysregulation of emotions, inhibitory processing, deficits in working memory, and faster response to negative life events. Patients with depressive disorder are characterized with a sad mood, lack

DOI: 10.4018/978-1-5225-8567-1.ch010

of interests, distrust, destructive belief of self, lack of motivation, communicative passivity, and suicidal thoughts McCabe et al., 2018). They largely show the incompetency to enhance optimistic and positive environmental stimuli for controlling their sad emotion and negative mood. These adverse cognitive and affective syndromes have severe effects on brain activity, leading to neuro-degeneration and disorders. In this regard, a state of mind that is characterized by apprehension, sorrow, grief, irritation, anger, hopeless, and guilty, is called a depressed mood (Rottenberg, 2005). When this type of mood occurs frequently after remission and controls day-to-day activities of the patients, by following a pathological stability at the neurocognitive level, it is categorised as a major depressive disorder (MDD) (Goodwin and Jamison, 2007; Taylor et al., 2007). Therefore, the screening and recognition of pathophysiological symptoms, based on the neurocognitive signatures, are some of the challenges that are not only to trace the origin, progress and recurrence of the depressive disorder, but also to prevent and treat the recurrence of it in a regular interval. The aim of this chapter is to discuss the various symptoms and types of depression, methodological insights and neurocognitive mechanisms to capture the severity of depression.

The course of depressive illness is unpredictable and episodic in nature, even patients feel fine between acute depressive episodes. Most of the cases, the longevity, number and patterns of episodes help to classify different types of depression. Considering the duration or phase of symptomatic mental illness, the depressive disorder is categorised into seven sub-categories such as (i) onset phase with a unipolar and single depressive episode, (Penninx et al., 2011; Spijker et al., 2002), (ii) recurring phase of episodes with major depression (Boschloo et al., 2014; Angst et al., 2009), (iii) chronic phase of episodes with dysthymia (Sansone et al., 2009), (iv) bipolar and manic-depressive disorder (Simon et al., 2008; Baik et al., 2018; Bertolote et al., 2004; Lejoyeux et al., 2010), (v) psychotic and delusional depression (Korn et al., 2014; Tondo et al., 2014; Rapinesi et al., 2015) and (vi) seasonal affective disorder (Winthorst et al., 2017). Before applying any therapeutic solution, patients use to go through the psychometric and neurocognitive diagnostic procedures for classifying these types of depressive disorder. Currently, there is a little explanation and discussion relating to the neural deficit and neurocognitive mechanisms that recognise the different types of depressive disorder.

Neural Deficit and Cognitive Impairments

The neural networking system of MDD is related to the function of multi-domain cognitive damage including working memory function, mental imagery and schema, attention span, executive function, and perceptual speed (Chen et al., 2013; Chen et al., 2015). In this direction, various brain imaging techniques are used to diagnose depression and provide an understanding of the essential underlying mechanisms leading to neural dysfunction and cognitive impairments in human (Christoffel et al., 2011). For example, the dysregulation of synaptic plasticity (Cruz-Martín et al., 2010; Hayashi-Takagi et al., 2010; Penzes et al., 2011), neurological ailments (Akram et al., 2008; Bingol and Sheng, 2011), and cognitive deficiency (Dumitriu et al., 2010) are recognised in different types of psychiatric disorder. The reduction and disruption of spine synapses that connect between neurons, contributes to the depressive vulnerability. Therefore, the disruption in synaptic plasticity, reduction in the volume of hippocampus and activity of brain regions are correlated with the depression in the clinical population (Woolley et al., 1990). Pizzagalli (2014) and Wacker et al., (2009) demonstrated that the reduction of NAc volume and NAc responsiveness to rewarding stimuli are directly linked with anhedonia, which is considered as a core symptom of depression. Anhedonia has also been proposed as a biomarker for the recovery of depression (Hasler et al., 2004). Previous studies have also recognised the regions of the brain such as the prefrontal cortex (PFC), hippocampus, cingulate cortex, amygdala, and basal ganglia that regulate depression and anxiety at the neural level (Savitz et al., 2009. Mayberg et al. 2009). Neural-connection disturbances between PFC and amygdala along with ventral striatum may decrease the motivation, reward and return which are affected by eating and sleeping in depression. Further, it is observed that the reduced volumes of PFC and other mesolimbic regions are responsible for depressive disorder (Koolschijn et al., 2009; Rajkowska et al., 2007; Drevets et al. 2008; MacQueen, 2011). The neuronal atrophy and the loss of brain regions, which control emotion causing disconnection and loss of neural functions, are also contributing to the development of depressive disorder in limbic regions (Duman and Monteggia, 2006). Reduction in neuronal cell body size and glia in PFC are also observed during the post-mortem analysis (Shansky et al., 2009; Liu et al., 2008; McEwen et al., 2012). Overall these studies have perceived the progress of depressed functional circuit of neurons in brain.

An inconsistency debate persists regarding the growth, decline or no change in the volume of amygdala of depressed patients (Lorenzetti et al., 2010; Koolschijn et al., 2009). A study has found that the high blood-flow leads to hyper-excitability in amygdala (Drevets et al., 2008). All these controversial clinical findings are due to either heterogeneous clinical populations or medication effects. Therefore, the functional magnetic resonance imaging (fMRI) data with independent component analysis (ICA) and region-of-interest (ROI) analysis are used to determine the exact functional and structural changes in the brain regions of depressive and mood disorders patients (Fox et al., 2008). So far, neuroimaging studies on major depression (MD) have found the abnormalities in frontal cortex (FC), orbital and medial prefrontal cortex (OMPFC), dorsal medial, anterior parietal, occipital and brainstem regions(Samara et al., 2018). Low connectivity of frontal-limbic circuits is also found in the case of depressed patients, using ROI analysis (Lui et al., 2011). Neural atrophy and damage of synaptic networks in limbic regions are associated with depression. However, more subtle neurocognitive changes in terms of information processing cannot be detected by using the current brain imaging techniques. Therefore, neural processing of information can be captured by conducting behavioural and EEG experiments. The spatiotemporal neural processing, in terms of latency and regions of human brain, can provide evidence on neural disruption towards the medication of depressive disorder. The underlying pathophysiological origin and progress of depression remain obscurity. Therefore, pathophysiological and basic science studies are started to deliver some neural signatures in terms of latency and regions of brain that are involved in depressive disorder. This chapter discusses research gaps along with complicated methodological challenges and clinical findings that are consistent across studies.

RESEARCH ISSUES AND CONTROVERSIES

Both clinical and pre-clinical experimental studies have concentrated on the neural path of depression while analysing the anterior cingulate cortex (ACC), prefrontal cortex (PFC), hippocampus, and amygdala regions (Mayberg, 1997; Harvey et al., 2004). However, it is not clear how these regions process emotional and non-emotional verbal and non-verbal information in terms latency and amplitudes. This research gap addresses the day-to-day problem of MDD patho-physiology and may aid to design a novel EEG experiment, which is not only to locate the regions of brain, but also to capture the processing time of verbal and non-verbal information. This would help for developing antidepressants that might reconnect the disturbed synaptic circuit alternating the neural path of the limbic regions of brain. So far, brain neuroimaging studies have shown only the affected regions of brain in terms of reduction of blood flow and glucose metabolism in PFC and limbic regions, which are attributed to the reduction of the volume of neuronal atrophy in these regions (Kang et al., 2012). Further, the reduction in the size of PFC and hippocampus may contribute to the slow processing of information related to the executive function and memory that are regularly found in the case of MDD patients. Even there is no longitudinal study by which we can track individuals before and after the onset of depression. It is further not clear whether the neurocognitive changes occur due to stressful life events or life-long vulnerabilities of depressive disorder. Within the framework of existing behavioural and neurocognitive methods and paradigms, this chapter explores the neurocognitive mechanisms and signalling pathways that underlie neuronal atrophy of depression in limbic regions of brain. Recognising underlying mechanisms of synaptic adaptation is important for classifying the state of depression and developing the novel therapeutic solution to it. Without the clinical application of neurocognitive mechanisms of depression, the existing treatments clearly show the low and slow rate of response and resistance (Trivedi et al., 2006; Duman, 2014). A major hindrance to the progress of more effective treatments for major depression has been the inadequate understanding of its pathophysiology and neurocognitive mechanisms that may be relevant for experimental efficiency. Longitudinal studies on neuronal dynamics and cognitive plasticity of depressive patients would explore the origin and development of synaptic disruption for improving diagnostic and analytical tools for antidepressants. On the basis of these research gaps, the current chapter examines the neurocognitive mechanisms of early onset and recurrent phase of depression by examining the clinical and pre-clinical event-related potential studies with regards to the processing of emotional verbal and non-verbal stimulus.

BEHAVIOURAL AND NEUROCOGNITIVE METHODS

The popularity of cognitive neuroscience during the past few decades is widespread due to non-invasive electroencephalogram (EEG). EEG offers a temporal measurement of event-related potentials (ERPs) through the recording of the cerebral activity of depressive disorder patients in milliseconds (Boutros et al., 2011) while establishing a correlation between neural activity and stimulus processing (Luck, 2014; Luck and Kappenman, 2012; Jagaroo and Santangelo, 2017). This method directly stimulates the specific region of brain through the stimulus, and records electrical signals by placing electrodes on the surface of the scalp and comparing the electrical voltage fluctuation across regions of brain. Using this EEG technique, ERPs can easily display the topographical representation of brain with quick changes in neural activity involving cognitive process related to the onset of dysfunction (Dennis, 2010; Duncan et al., 2009), which is minor and still not visible at the behavioural level. Most of the cases, the electrical potential activities of brain, with a high spatiotemporal resolution, are compared with behavioural response time and accuracy of the stimulus. Further, it addresses which brain regions tend to be engaged and how much time a particular region takes when patients with depressive disorder and control healthy individuals perform a particular type of cognitive task. Ultimately, the EEG results would be implemented for clinical efforts to diagnose and develop an appropriate intervention strategy for neural impairments of patients. Overall, the cognitive neuroscience methods include the selection of stimuli, participants (patients and control healthy individuals), designing experiments, procedures for conducting EEG experiments, and analysis of behavioural and EEG data.

Norms for Selecting Participants

Considering the subjective reports of insomnia and hypersomnia which are common in bipolar disorder, the participants are usually selected for EEG experiment with different sets of patients. Healthy participants for behavioural and EEG experiments would be adults of same age group as compared to the patients with depressive disorder. The number of participants for one experiment could be around two hundred (control group=100; patient group=100) with an equal proportion of male and female. An equal proportion of female patients (F=100) is to be selected to maintain gender ratio for EEG experiment. For example, on study recruited forty-four patients (N=44) those who were diagnosed with MDD according to the Diagnostic and Statistical Manual of Mental Disorders (Fifth Edition (DSM-5; American Psychiatric Association, 2013; Baik et al., 2018). This gender representation would help the investigator to establish why bipolar depression occurs more in women than men. Patients are grouped based on their developmental cognitive, anxiety and stress-related disorder. The homogeneity in terms of age, class and education is maintained while selecting the participants for the EEG study. Most of the studies kept the aged of participants between 17 and 65 years (18-62 years, Barrick et al., 2018; 20-65 years, Baik et al., 2018; 17-65 years, Bailey et al., 2014; 21-57 years, Bridwell et al., 2015; 18-50 years, Camfield et al., 2018). Patients are not recruited if they have any EEG contraindications, hearing, vision and any other sensory problems or serious medical disease or neurologic maladies such as epilepsy, head trauma with loss of consciousness, alcohol or substance abuse within 6 months preceding the experiment. All the research is monitored and governed according to the ethical guidelines and rules approved by the ethics committee of the Medical Institute/University. Utmost care is taken to guard their personal data, as per the ethical norms and rules prescribed by the Medical institutes and universities.

Stimuli and Experimental Design

Early rapid processing of negative emotional faces as compared to positive emotional face can provide the ERPs evidence on the patient with unipolar and bipolar depression. The stimulus should be randomized to reduce the probability of results that can be influenced by habituation, anticipation, or strategic processing within a block design. This would help the researcher to analyse the accuracy based on the participants' correct or erroneous response. These kinds of experiment will address the degree of severity of depression and classify the patients accordingly. Ultimately, it may lead to address why the patients with bipolar disorder increase the risk of dementia and attempt suicide more frequently than those with unipolar depression. EEG experiments are conducted across patients with unipolar and bipolar disorder. Following a clinical and neurocognitive assessment before and after the EEG experiments, a significant interaction between cognitive flexibility and visual attention towards emotional stimuli are explored in a patient with bipolar depression.

Types of Experimental Tasks and Paradigms

A rapid odd-ball, mismatch, and Stroop dictation paradigm are usually employed to observe the attentional mechanisms towards emotional faces, tones or voice and words. Participants are asked to attend emotion pictures or voice and words whether the respective stimulus is happy or sad/angry. Appropriate timing of the rapid appearance of trail structures (200ms for emotional and attention-related stimulus)

Figure 1. Sample trail structure of the experiment

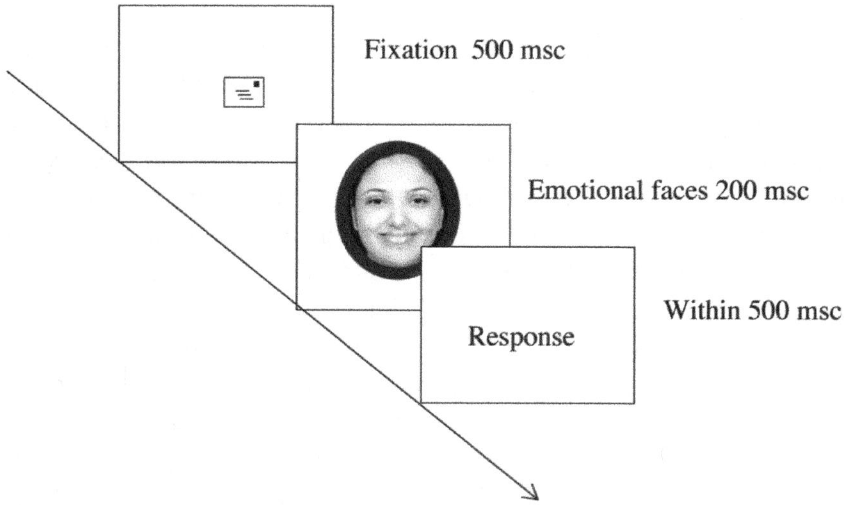

is followed as per the literature related to above said attentional paradigms. An example of the trail structure is as follows (Figure 1).

In this context, patients are usually asked to attend the blank-black screen before and after the eyes-closed resting state condition. Most of these procedures may vary from one study to another, considering the frequent or deviant occurrences of the target and non-target stimulus. Further, studies are also varied on the basis of stimulus duration, interstimulus intervals, and response mode with a basic attentional oddball task.

EEG Recording Procedures

Electrical signals of neurons are recorded in a millisecond timescale during the processing of stimulus in brain. This is done by using electrodes that are extracranially placed on the scalp, so as to record the firing of neurons, based on the experimental stimulus. The EEG signals are usually recorded from a 16-channel or 125 channel maps. Electrode impedance has to be kept below 5KΩ. The EEG signals are usually recorded with an online band-pass filter with pass-band frequency from 0.1 Hz to 100 Hz for emotional dictation. To perceive and expose the effectiveness of rationality, quantifiable EEG (QEEG) data are acquired when participants are seated in an electrically shielded room in a reclining chair, as the step by step procedures for EEG recording and data acquisitions are given in figure 2.

Electrodes are to be placed across the head according to the international 10–20 system arrangement. Left and right hemispheric coherence are measured across electrode pairs Fp1-Fp2, Af1-Af2, F1-F2, F3-F4, T1-T2, C1-C2, P1-P2 and O1-O2 on the left and right hemispheres. EEG signals are filtered with a band-pass (.01–40 Hz) before the elimination of artefacts. Various artifacts such as baseline wandering, ocular and muscular artefacts are manually removed for further post-processing and classification of EEG signals. The source localization technique is to be applied to classify brain regions that are individually associated with unipolar and bipolar depression. Relevant biomarkers can be developed and evaluated by following the region-based diagnostic tool to avoid any overlapping regions between two types of depression.

Figure 2. Procedures for conducting behavioural and EEG experiment

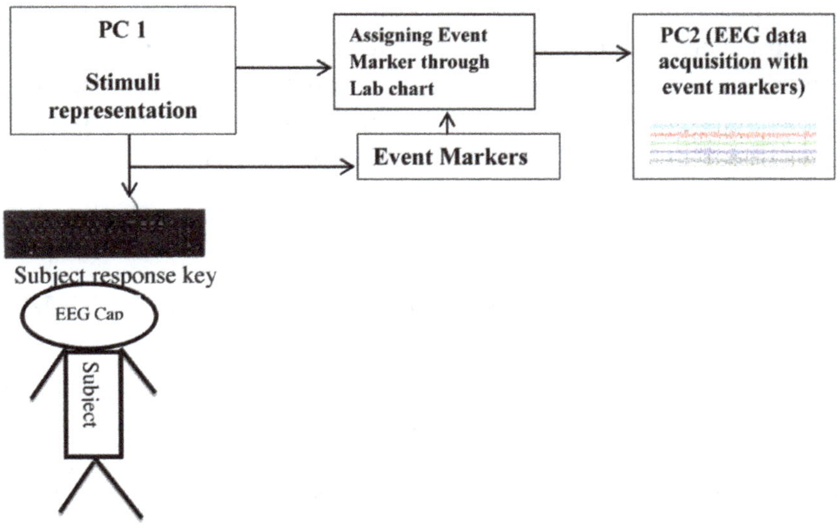

Analysing Amplitudes of ERP Across Windows

Averaged ERPs which are small voltage fluctuations are time-locked by segmenting the target stimulus (Jagaroo and Santangelo, 2017). This procedure is often used to measure cognitive processes in terms of latencies and amplitudes of ERPs (Fichtenholtz et al., 2007). Artefacts-free data are computed by measuring the average amplitudes (100 ms pre-stimulus baseline) in time windows of interest (800 ms post-stimulus time). Baseline-corrected EPR waves are presented to inspect how the variations occur across the scalp of healthy control and patient individuals. Mean amplitudes (μν) are collected across experimental conditions to perform ANOVAs. The observation can be made on ERPs of healthy control and depressive patients, by using a two-way or three-way ANOVA over the mean amplitudes of the left and right hemispheric sides of the central (C), centroparietal (CP), temporal, (T) temporo-parietal (TP), parieto-occipital (PO), and occipital (O) regions. Hemispheric factor (left, right) are also included to perform a three-way ANOVA on the mean amplitudes of ERPs. Tukey *post-hoc* test is used for factorial comparisons, keeping the significance level of alpha =.05.

The observations are made on the modulation of P100 (47-143) and P300 (255-483) amplitudes. For example, the early P1 component is measured between 47 ms and 143 ms, like the time window of P1 in the case of emotion-word processing: Herbert et al., (2008) P1(80-130), Scott et al., (2009) P1(80-120), Kissler et al., (2009) P1(80-130), and Sass et al., (2010) P1(88-128). P300 is measured between 255 ms and 483 ms, like the component reported in Herbert (2006) P3 (250-400) and Scott et al., (2009) P3 (300-450). Within these ranges, average ERP waveforms are usually inspected for the novel P3 (220–375 ms) and target P3 (280–470 ms) stimulus in depressed patients (Friedman et al., 1993). Further, the amplitudes of P300 are reduced by the different phases of depression which are documented as markers for understanding the pathophysiological mechanisms and supporting the analysis, diagnosis and cure of depression of MDD (Karaaslan et al., 2003). Finally, the analysis, which is much closer to the actual firing of neurons, allows the investigator to explore latency (msc) and amplitude (μν) ERPs in different brain regions. For example, occipital regions induce elementary visual hallucination that includes colors, stars, and flickering lights, whereas the superior temporal regions process elementary auditory hallucinations that include ringing, clicking, and buzzing. All these methodological insights of EEG are useful to provide neural correlates of specific cognitive capacities in terms of latency (time-course of processing), amplitudes (μν), polarity (negative and positive deflection), and topography (scalp distribution of effect) (Kemmerer, 2015). Taking together the behavioural and ERP results, this chapter explores the neural mechanisms of depressive disorder by characterizing the cognitive impairments, deficit and underlying neurophysiological mechanisms.

BEHAVIOURAL MECHANISMS: ACCURACY AND REACTION TIME

In this section, the chapter discusses the behavioural and electrophysiological data that are collected from recent studies following the perception, attention, inhibition, and working memory of verbal and non-verbal stimulus (Sternberg, 1969; Delle-Vigne et al., 2014; Ueoka et al., 2011; Lecardeur et al., 2009). Comparing female patients with MDD and anorexia nervosa, the study of Mendlewicz et al., 2005 has found that MDD patients are less accurate to decode anger as compared to happy stimulus. A greater intensity of arousal is required for patients with MDD to recognise happy faces, though the lesser arousal is required for sad than angry faces (Joorman and Gotlib, 2006). The happy expression is less intense than neutral faces for depressed patients (Yoon et al., 2009). Gollan et al., (2010) demonstrate that patients with MDD always recognise neutral faces as sad ones, whereas control participants interpret neutral faces as happy ones. Moreover, the patients with MDD are well-versed with sad and anger faces than positive valences of facial expressions (Gollan et al., 2010; Anderson et al., 2011), as their recurrence of depressive phases is compatible to the increasing accuracy of sad faces. The unipolar depressive (UD) patients show higher response accuracy for sad expressions than happy and neutral expressions (Milders et al., 2010). In recognizing the boundary of the emotional continuum, patients with depression display ultra-rapid response to sad in the happy-sad continuum, whereas they show the quick response to angry in the angry-fearful continuum (Liu et al., 2012). Overall these studies revealed that UD and BD patients are more abnormal than control participants in the facial recognition task, in which patients are more accurate towards negative and unpleasant as compared to positive and pleasant stimulus (Raes et al., 2006). In the priming task, patients with depression recognise positive and negative prime only in the case of sad faces, revealing higher enhancement for the negative stimuli than the positive one (Dai and Feng, 2011). Control subjects have a stronger interference of happy emotion with sad than depressed patients (Lemoult et al., 2012). Further, using a dot-probe task, the study of Joorman and Gotlib (2007) finds that MDD patients allot faster response and higher accuracy for sad than happy faces, suggesting broader attention bias toward negative than positive stimuli. Similarly using classic colour Stroop task and emotional Stroop task, studies have shown that control healthy participants are slower to attend colour of negative words while ignoring the word meaning, whereas patients with MDD and BD display an automatic bias towards naming the colour emotional words (Phaf and Kan, 2007; Kircanski et al., 2012; Dernovsek et al., 2010). Most of these emotional and attentional biases towards negative stimulus are continued during early onset and late bipolar phases.

To examine the working memory vulnerability of depressed patients, Joorman and Gotlib (2008) are asked patients to memorize two different lists of emotional words with some irrelevant words in each list. Depresses patients are very difficult to expel the negative words from their working memory. Further, in comparison to the normal group, the patient group complete the memory task more poorly while memorizing the task-relevant positive words than negative words (Levens and Gotlib, 2009; Joormann and Siemer, 2012; Levens and Phelps, 2008). These results suggest that depressed patients do not prefer to assign the cognitive resources for preserving the positive content of stimuli. As a result, the enhancement of positive words in terms of decoding is paralysed and the content of positive material is never applied to recover the negative mood. Using an emotional 2-back task, the study of Levens and Gotlib (2010) suggests that patients with MDD memorize the sad faces faster than the control group. Considering these behavioural results, it is evident that depression is clearly biased towards preserving the irrelevant negative words, face and voices from the working memory, while erasing and diminishing positive information (Rottenberg et al., 2005). The slower disengagement from sad stimuli confirms the enhanced responses to negative stimulus (Deveney and Deldin 2006).

NEUROCOGNITIVE MECHANISMS: ERPS

Here the neurocognitive mechanisms of depressed patients refer to the perceptual information of sensory, cognitive, and emotional tasks that are represented through neural activity at the cerebral level in terms of latency (msc) and amplitudes (μν) (Friedman, 2000; Olofsson et al., 2008). Potential responses of the neuron are acquired from depressed patients when they perform a specific task while attending emotional and non-emotional stimulus during EEG recording. This type of event-related potential (ERP) effects is categorised in terms of time and the regions of the brain to observe the specific processes and neurophysiological mechanisms that are dysfunctional in depressive disorders. Depressed participants show neural signatures and neurophysiological processes that are related with negatively biased and attention-related behavioural results during the processing of verbal and non-verbal information (Poulsen et al., 2009; Thomas et al., 2007). It is found that attentional biases towards emotional information are key features of bipolar and major depressive disorders (García-Blanco et al., 2014; Disner et al., 2011). Most of these emotional and attentional biases could be tested within psycho-neurocognitive paradigms by classifying the early, fast-automatic, the late-elaborative and flexible ERP windows. Therefore, the following ERP components (P1, N1, N170, N2, early and late P3, a late positive potential (LPP), and N400) are categorized and discussed by considering the pathophysiological aspects of depressed patients.

Early ERP Components: P100, N100 and N170

Behavioural results have previously confirmed the negativity bias in depression. However, it is not clear at the neural level how happy and sad faces, voices and words are processed in depression (Dai et al., 2016). Using a cued target-response task, 22 depressed patients have shown a cognitive bias towards the processing of emotional faces, revealing higher amplitudes of P100 and N170 components for only sad faces, but not for other faces (Zhao et al., 2015). Unlike the N170, the patients with MDD have shown the reduction of early sensory N100 as compared to the healthy individuals when both groups are asked to perform dichotic emotional listening or tone- counting tasks (Burkhart and Thomas, 1993). Further, when the twenty-four healthy and depressive patients performed emotional valence rating tasks, the patient group obtained lesser valence scores, quicker responses, and greater N1 amplitudes for only sad faces, whereas sub-clinical groups showed faster responses and greater P1 amplitudes for all faces but lower valence scores and enhanced P2 amplitudes for happy faces (Dai et al., 2016). A study has also found that both existing and remitted MDD patients modulate P1 amplitudes for negative stimuli in comparison to healthy control groups (Shestyuk and Deldin, 2010). Further, the current MDD group processed detail evaluation of negative stimulus, revealing higher late positive potentials (LPP) as compared to other groups. This result is also consistently appeared when female adolescents comprising patients and healthy control perform the same task. Depressed females exhibit higher P1 and LPP amplitudes in response to negative words than positive words (Auerbach et al., 2015). These findings clearly suggest that the early-sensory cognitive bias towards negative stimulus occur within 100 msec time-windows, in which N100 and N170 are considered as electro-neurophysiological biomarkers for depressive patients (Zhao et al., 2015). However, the presence of LPP component reveals that the early attention towards negative stimuli continues over the larger time course of ERP.

ERP Components: N200/N270 and P200

In a standard bi-tone auditory oddball task, the patients with remitted MD (N=20) obtained reduced N200 amplitudes to relevant tones in frontal, central and parietal regions (Feldmann et al., 2018). However, patients with MD (N=22) showed a reduction in N200 amplitudes to target tones only in the frontal regions as compared to healthy control (N=32). In these cases, the reduction in N2 amplitudes in both rMD and MD represents the auditory attentional bias in stimulus organisation and response choice. These neural signatures are considered as the neurophysiological trait for adolescents' depression (Feldmann et al., 2018). Earlier the reduction of N2 amplitudes is more associated with schizophrenia than other neuropsychiatric disorders (Force et al., 2008). However, the positive deflection of P100 and P200 components were more modulated by sad faces than happy faces, when the patients with MDD (N=24) were asked to judge the intensity of emotional faces (Dai and Feng, 2012). This finding reveals that MMD participants are more interested in negative facial expressions, adding a stable cognitive liability towards reoccurrence of depression with a high chance of suicidal ideation. Further, using the emotional face and word match-mismatch task, the study of Deldin et al., (2000) found a lateralised abnormality of N200 component over the right parietal region of depressed patients (N-19) as compared to healthy controls. Similarly, the amplitudes of N270 were more fluctuated during the colour dot-processing of S1-S2 (stimuli 1 and 2) by depressed patients (N=25) as compared to healthy individuals (N=25) (Mao et al., 2005). In this case, the differential wave analysis revealed the smaller difference in N270 amplitudes in depressed patients compared to control at frontal and parietal regions. This differential result is an indication of cognitive impairment related to stimulus conflict processing connecting with anterior cingulate and dorsal lateral prefrontal cortex (Mao et al., 2005). A study also revealed that the participants with MDD and TBI-MDD showed lessor fronto-central negativity of N2 amplitudes than control groups during the processing of No-Go emotional trails (Baily et al., 2018).

Using auditory Go No-go task, a study observed that the depressed patients (N=16) performed better in go-task than no-go task as compared to control groups. As a result, patients obtained a reduction of N2 latency in frontotemporal regions suggesting a deficit in response inhibition in depression during the processing of the no-go task. This result is consistent with the findings of the electrophysiological study of Huster et al. (2013) in response inhibition of No-go trails that are obtained in frontal-midline N2 (200–400 ms) and P3 (300–600 ms) ERPs. Contrarily to the reduction of N2, some studies have observed the increase of N2 amplitudes in depressed patients as compared to healthy control individuals (Bruder et al., 1998; Giese-Davis et al., 1993). Additionally, there are two sub-components of N2 such as N2a (120–165 ms) and N2b (170–235 ms) that are prominent when depressed patients (N=36) process the mismatch between deviant and frequent stimulus (Ogura et al. 1993). In this study, the N2a amplitudes were reduced during the processing of deviant stimuli as compared to frequent stimuli, whereas the N2b amplitudes were greater for frequent than deviant stimuli in depressed patients in comparison to control individuals (N=36). These findings suggest that the NoGo-N2 along with other associate subcomponents is linked with response execution and inhibition (Donkers and Van Boxtel, 2004; Yeung et al., 2004). In addition to negative deflection of N200, the amplitudes of P200 were reduced when patients with medication-resistant major depression (N-18, F=13) were asked to perform an auditory oddball task (Choi et al., 2015). However, the amplitudes were significantly increased in FP1, FP2, FZ, FCZ, CZ, and PZ channels after 3 weeks of rTMS treatment of MDD patients. This result implies that the rTMS treatment has positive outcome and improvement in brain function in patients MDD using the ERP analysis.

ERP Component: Error Related Negativity (ERN)

The ERN component which is a negative-going brain-potential appears between 50 and 100ms after the erroneous response. Schrijvers et al. (2009) have found that the enhancement of ERN is associated with anhedonia, apathy, and psychomotor problems of depressed patients. This result is consistent as some studies reporting no differences in the amplitudes of ERN between patients and control groups (Ruchsow et al., 2006). Patients with MDD showed the post error negativity increasing the ERNs amplitudes (Chiu and Deldin, 2007). It is also evident that the serotonin transporter gene (5-HTTLRP) is linked with the enhancement of ERN amplitudes (Fallgatter et al., 2004), suggesting high amplitude of ERN is a risk marker of depression. In this regard, Chiu and Deldin (2007) found that depressed group (N=18) showed greater ERN amplitude than controls (N=17) by frontal and front-central regions of brain, by attending flanker task related to punishment and reward conditions. Holmes and Pizzagalli (2008) showed that the depressed patients (N=20) had significantly larger ERN than the control individuals (N=20) at the ACC and medial prefrontal regions. Luu et al. (2004) have found that a larger feedback-related negativity is associated with ERN amplitudes in participants having a major depression as compared to non-depressed controls. So to say, the enhanced ERN always present in depressive disorder. Moreover, studies have shown that depressed patients have poor concentration and retrieval when they are asked to retrieve the meaning of words in memory task (Barrick et al., 2018). Depressed adults display greater left parietal ERPs from 400 to 800 ms and 800–1400 ms which are negatively correlated with sleep disturbance (Barrick et al., 2018). Negative words capture detail processing in the late complete of ERP (380 to 1000 ms) across posterior sites, representing a self-referent negative engagement of neurocognitive depression (Dainer-Best et al., 2017).

ERP Components: P300/P3a/P3b and Mismatch Negativity

Performing the spatial cueing task while processing suicide-relevant and negatively-valence words, the patients with MDD (N=44) modulated P300 amplitudes at the parietal regions (Baik et al., 2018). P300 amplitudes were higher for suicide-relevant words compared to negatively-valence words, suggesting the broad attentional engagement towards sad words. This result suggests that suicide attempters have more difficulty in avoiding the responsibility of reading the suicide-relevant words, demonstrating attentional bias, as opposed to other types of words (Cisler et al., 2009). This kind of attentional bias is considered as key features of mood disordered, as it has been further tested in the case of manic and depressed patients during the processing of emotional words (Szczepan et al., 2015). This study observed that patients with manic episode allocated larger cognitive resources than control groups at an early stage of sensory processing within 100ms after the onset of words, indicating more automatic attention towards emotional words. However, in the later stage of processing i.e., between 200-209 ms, detail valences of emotional words were evaluated by assigning higher response to negative than positive words in manic patients, suggesting cognitive bias towards incongruent stimuli during the lexico-semantic analysis stage (Szczepan and Wyczesany, 2016). Using olfactory pleasant (phenyl-ethyl alcohol = rose) and unpleasant (isobutyraldehyde = rotten butter) task in depressed patients (N=22) and healthy control (N=22), the study of Pause et al. (2003) found the reduced amplitude of P2 and P3 potentials at frontal sites. Here the reduction of olfactory P2 potential represents a deficit in the ability of pre-attentively encoding the pleasantness of odors, whereas the reduced amplitude of early P3 reflects a cognitive evaluative process in depressed patients. This happens because of the synaptic disruption in the amygdala and the orbitofrontal cortex of depressed patients. Further, using the standard oddball task with frequent and deviant appearance of stimuli, the Diner et al. (1985) showed a reduction in P3 amplitudes in depressed patients as compared to controls at Pz electrode sites, revealing the severity of depression associated with smaller P3. Similar results were also found in MDD patients who obtained higher P300 amplitudes with a dot-probe task by replacing a sad than a neutral face, suggesting patients' disengagement towards negative emotional faces (Li et al., 2018). Anticipating the automatic interference of emotion on response inhibition in emotional stop signal task (SST), an experimental study on depressive patients (N=14) and healthy control (N=21) was conducted by using neutral, negative or positive visual images (Camfield et al., 2018). Here the depressed participants showed larger inhibitory processing of positive stimuli than healthy control participants. These results illustrate that ERP components could be applied as tools for early diagnosis of depression, and considered as cognitive and cerebral biomarkers of negativity bias in depression (Dai et al., 2016).

Even subjects with a family history of depression showed the lower amplitude of P300 over temporoparietal regions as compared to subjects without any family history of depression when both groups processed emotional faces (Bruder et al., 2007). This finding suggests that P3 reduction in visual tasks indicates the neurocognitive vulnerability for depressive disorder.

Similarly, patients with depressive comorbid anxiety (N=18) showed a smaller early P3 than healthy controls (N-49) at the front-central regions (Bruder et al., 2002). This effect was also obtained during the processing of visuospatial stimuli using oddball task, in the case of young women with a history of a major depressive episode (N= 29), who showed smaller P3 amplitude than those with no history of depression(N = 101) (Houston et al., 2003). Using auditory-visual unimodal and bi-modal tasks, a study found that patients with depression had lower P300 amplitude and longer latency than controls in the bimodal task (Nan et al., 2018). Bimodal task modulated higher P300 amplitudes than unimodal auditory or visual tasks, suggesting the severity of depression. In emotional face priming task, patients with MDD showed larger P1 and P3 amplitudes for sad faces in the positive priming condition as compared to currently remitted depression (CMD) and healthy control groups (Dai et al., 2011). However, the smaller P3 amplitudes were obtained during the processing of sad faces when these were compared to other faces in negative priming condition, revealing the enhancement of negative emotion that was associated with cognitive risk-factor of depression (Dai et al., 2011). Therefore, the modulations of P3 amplitudes vary from one type of depression to another. For example, patients with psychotic depression demonstrate more reduced form of P3 amplitudes as compared to non-psychotic depression (Karaaslan et al., 2003; Kaustio et al., 2002), adding further reduction of P3 in the case of patients who attempted suicide as compared to non-suicidal patients (Castaneda et al., 2008; Hansenne et al., 1996).

Like the P300, the amplitudes of its subcomponents P3a and P3b were reduced during the processing of emotional stimuli in depressed subjects. Using the visual representation of stimuli within oddball paradigms, patients with depression exhibit maximum amplitudes of P3b representing parietal or temporo-parietal mechanisms related to memory, whereas P3a displays the frontal or frontocentral attentional related-mechanisms (Polich and Criado, 2006; Polich, 2007; Bruder et al., 2009). Some studies also claim that, along with P300 and its subcomponents (P3a and P3b), the mismatch negativity (MMN) which is called as auditory mismatch negativity falls between 100ms and 250 ms after onset of the stimulus at front-central region in depressed patients (Naatanen and Kreegipuu, 2011; Kaur et al., 2011; Takei et al.,2009). Using bi-tone passive oddball paradigms, the study of Naismith et al. (2012) found the decrease MMN in depressed people compared to healthy ones. Within the same paradigm, Mu et al. (2016) found greater MMN amplitudes in patients those who were affected by major depressive disorder as compared to a healthy control-group. All these studies have found that MMNs index emotional tone, voice and music are related to the dysfunctions of neurons in depressed patients (Carlson et al., 2015; Joormann et al., 2012; Troy eta l., 2010). For example, in an emotional prosody recognition task, Pang et al. (2014) found that, in MMN, the sad tones were absent in case of patients with MDD, revealing the impaired capacity of patients to automatically process sad prosody as compared to the healthy group.

Whether this MMN component is associated with pre-attentive negative bias symptoms of depression, Wu et al., (2017) conducted a study by using emotional face match-mismatch oddball paradigm, in which the remitted patients with late-life depression (LLD, N=30) demonstrated a reduced mean amplitude of positive and negative deflection of MMN as compared to normal control (NC, N=30). This MMN component is a biomarker to evaluate cortical signs corresponding to the neurobiology of MDD, as it is shown that patients have enlarged MMN amplitudes (Kahkonen et al., 2007) or reduced and delayed mean auditory MMN amplitudes at temporal and central sites (Naismith et al., 2012; Qiao et al., 2013). These studies argue that MMN, P3, P3a and P3b components sequentially occur when the MDD patients process pre-attentive and attentive information of emotion and attention inference and inhibition. Using the bi-tone auditory paradigm in the form of deviant and frequent appearance of stimuli, Chen et al., (2015) observed that the patients with recurrent major depression (R-MD, N=40) had lower P3 amplitudes and longer P3a latencies compared to healthy control (HC, N= 46), though no differences of P3 amplitude were obtained between patients with R-MD and first episode depression (F-MD, N=45). Further, differences were not found in the amplitudes of MMN that could link with the severity of the depression. However, the sluggish and slow P3a amplitudes were negatively correlated with the severity of depression between F-MD and R-MD (Chen et al., 2015). As a result, the MMN is considered as a stable neural biomarker for the onset arrival stage or appearance of depression, whereas the modulation of P3a amplitudes is used as a potential marker correlated with the recurrence of major depressive disorder (R-MD). All these co-existential ERPs are widely considered to be neurophysiological biomarkers for MDD (Bonetti et al., 2017). Further, the MMN, P3, P3a and P3b amplitudes are related to cognitive and psychosocial function in depression (Hermens et al.,2010; Kaur et al., 2012; Kaur et al.,2011; Naismith et al.,2012).

Late Negative and Positive Components: LPP and N400

A detail comprehensive processing of emotional information, semantic and syntactic violation related to cognitive evaluation and engagement of verbal and nonverbal stimulus such as word, tone, and face always takes place between 300ms and 1000 ms containing the late positive complex (LPP 300-1500),

N400 and P600 components (Hajcak et al., 2013). In this direction, it is reported that the reduction in the amplitudes of LPP occurs due to the presence of depression (Foti et al., 2010; Kayser et al., 2000; Williams et al., 2007). It is also found that the amplitudes of LPP are largely reduced in emotional stimuli as compared to neutral stimuli within the framework of memory task in depression (Deldin et al. 2009; Deveney and Deldin, 2004), suggesting a strong association between LPP component and MDD (Proudfit et al., 2015; Weinberg et al., 2016). Contrarily, a study, using negative emotional words, has found the higher amplitude of LPP in younger female participants with high-risk of depression (N=121 i.e., maternal history of MDD) than the participants with low risk for MDD (Speed et al., 2016). The study of Shestyuk and Deldin (2010) has also found more positive amplitudes in the late positive potential (LPP) for negative stimuli than positive one. Using semantic violation task, a study found that a diminished N400 associated with a stronger self-reference only to negative, but not positive adjectives (Kiang et al., 2017). From the point of view of hemispheric laterality, patients with MDD have an impact on the right parietal regions during the processing of emotional stimuli (Heller, 1993). Applying the magnetic resonance imaging (MRI), Sapolsky (2000) showed that patients having severe and repeated depressive episodes clearly showed the evidence of hippocampal atrophy, which was greater on the left side, than the right side. This hippocampal toxic reduction has been explicitly linked with memory impairments (Sapolsky, 2000; Shah et al., 1998) that occurs in the left parietal region.

TREATMENT METHODS FOR NEURAL AND DEPRESSIVE DISORDER

All these neural signatures in terms of ERPs (P100, ERN, N100, N170, P200, N200 and late P300) can help the mental health practitioner to categorise and classify the patients with major depressive disorder (MDD). Further, these neural biomarkers not only provide the early diagnostic detection of MDD but also assess symptom severity of MDD. Using these markers, the strategic decisions can be taken to choose the treatment settings such as outpatients, day hospital and inpatient setting. Based on the severity of symptoms coupled with neural biomarkers, patients with MDD can avail various types of therapeutic procedures and treatment methods such as electroconvulsive therapy (ECT), light therapy, interpersonal therapy, cognitive and psychotherapy, psychosocial therapy, and the physical, spiritual and social supports (Evans et al., 2006). It is observed that patients with ECT referral demonstrate significant neural plasticity that can enhance their episodic memory (Kalogerakou et al., 2018). Therefore, the intervention of ECT is largely effective to combat MDD. Further, cognitive (CT) and interpersonal psychotherapy (IPT) are widely used as a psychological intervention to combat MDD (Cuijpers et al., 2016; Barth et al., 2016).

Interpersonal and Psychosocial Therapy

Interpersonal problems are usually stated by patients with MDD (Pinkham et al., 2014). However, the treatment procedures to eradicate the interpersonal problems through psychotherapeutic treatment remain in obscurity (McFarquhara et al., 2018). Therefore, interpersonal therapy (IT), as a psychotherapeutic treatment for the patients with a personality disorder (PD) and MDD, is designed to enhance positive emotion and dominance affiliation (Gordon-King et al., 2018; McFarquhara et al., 2018). Most of the effects of PD are correlated with the characteristics of MDD; therefore patients with PD or MDD require the intervention of Cognitive Therapy (CT) and Interpersonal Psychotherapy (IPT) (van Bronswijk et al., 2018). A study has also found the long-term effective treatment for the patients with MDD (n=134), who positively respond to the interference of CT and IPT (Lemmens et al., 2018). The implementation of this therapeutic solution reduces depressive symptoms and improves interpersonal functioning (Bina et al., 2018; Ollila et al., 2016). Family intervention for outpatients' treatment is effective for a young person to recover from a mental disorder. This therapeutic intervention needs a cooperative relationship between a family member (caregivers, siblings) and patients who can then recover from severe and complex depression (Rice et al., 2018). Even the training on social skills which internalises social behaviours such as coping, adjusting, motivating and sharing leads to a better outcome in the case of students having depression (Sang and Tan, 2018; Joo et al., 2016). The effect of rigorous short-term dynamic psychotherapy on the social life of patients improves the social cognition in which patients guard against their sorrow and painful aspects of life, feelings, interpersonal and emotional closeness (Ajilch et al., 2018).

Cognitive and Psychotherapy With Medication

Current pharmacological treatments for MDD contain monoamine oxidase inhibitors (MAOI), tricyclic antidepressants (TCAs), tetracyclic antidepressants (TeCAs), serotonin (SSRI) and serotonin/norepinephrine (SNRI) (Heresco-Levy, 2018). All antidepressants were more effective than placebo (Cipriani et al., 2018). However, these antidepressants have severe side-effect along with 60 - 65% remission or become symptom – free (Heresco-Levy, 2018; Cheung et al., 2018). Thus, antidepressants along with psychotherapy aiming towards depression reduce anxiety symptoms in relation to control conditions (Weitz et al., 2018; Ollila et al., 2016). Further, the mindfulness based-cognitive therapy (MBCT) improves the self-efficacy that is linked with the decline of depressive symptoms (Farb et al., 2018; Segal et al., 2018).

Improving the cognitive dynamics of patients with MDD requires face-to-face psychological treatments. Since it is time, labour and cost consuming, the mental health practitioners have engaged with patients by using internet-supported cognitive-behaviour therapy (ICBT) (Pihlaja et al, 2018; Morgan et al., 2017). It is observed that ICBT stands out as an effective, practical, acceptable and regular mental health-care for MDD (Andrews et al., 2018; Berger et al., 2018; Hadjistavropoulo et al., 2017). Applying cognitive behaviour therapy and schema therapy for depression, a study has shown that patients (n=100) with MDD have improved the verbal learning and memory impairments (Carter et al., 2018). These studies show that ICBT programs which largely attract patients with symptoms of depression and anxiety improve their wellbeing (Morgan et al., 2017). Many employees, after attending the work-focused cognitive behavioural therapy (W-CBT) program, return to their work (Brenninkmeijer et al., 2018). Further, the combination of cognitive-behavioural analysis system of psychotherapy (CBASP) and antidepressant pharmacotherapy is more effective to reduce the depressive symptoms than monotherapies (Furukawa et al., 2018). A meta-analysis study shows that peer, family and other social supports decrease the depressive symptoms of patients (Joo et al., 2018). Therefore, the interventions of social therapy offer a promising treatment to reduce the burden of MDD (Rice et al., 2016).

Yoga and Meditation Therapy

Yoga and mindful-meditation is widely accepted as a therapeutic solution to physical, social, psychological and neuro-cognitive problems that are largely associated with stress and depressive disorders (Yadav, 2016; Dariot's, et al. 2016; Fishbein, et al. 2016). The intervention of Iyengar yoga and coherent breathing reduces depressive symptoms of MDD (Streeter et al., 2017; Nyer et al., 2019). Spiritual therapies such as meditation, tai chi, qigong, and yoga reduce symptoms of depression more than other exercises including cognitive behavioural therapy (Saeed et al., 2010). These findings are clinically supported by many neuroimaging and electrophysiological studies (Davidson, et al. 2003; Davidson, et al. 2012; Pagani, et al. 2008). For example, the reduction of the amygdala and hippocampus volume, which is due to the effect of MDD, is significantly recovered by the intervention of meditation and yoga practices (Gotink et al., 2018). Most of these therapeutic solutions and pharmaceutical medications should be personalised and adopted by mental health physicians and consultants according to the degree of severity of MDD.

SUMMARY AND FUTURE DIRECTIONS

This chapter critically examines the devastating effects of depression while focusing on the behavioural methods and neurocognitive mechanisms to combat the mental illness. It broadly defines the types of depression along with symptoms from the point of view of the method of screening and diagnosis. Emphasising the early screening, diagnosis and identification of pathophysiological symptoms such as cognitive impairments, emotional bias, inhibitory imbalance, insufficiency in working memory, and entangle towards negative life, this chapter explores how these cognitive and affective behavioural syndromes of depression paralyse neural activities and mechanisms leading to synaptic degeneration. Further, it is observed that neural atrophy and disruption in synaptic networks in limbic regions are connected with depression. It further raises the question: how these affected limbic regions of brain process the verbal and non-verbal information. It also points out the obstacle for the advancement of effective treatments for MDD, which is due to the insufficient observation of its pathophysiology and neurocognitive mechanisms. Therefore, at the methodological front, this chapter provides a detailed step towards conducting the behavioural and neurocognitive EEG experiments which include design, selection and rejection norms for patients, paradigms, stimuli, tasks and ERP analysis. All these methodological understandings of EEG are valuable to establish neural correlates of specific cognitive mechanism in terms of latency (time-course of processing), amplitudes ($\mu\nu$), polarity (negative and positive deflection), and topography (scalp distribution of effect). To understand electro-neurophysiological mechanisms and biomarkers, most of the emotional and attentional biases in depression are discussed within psycho-neurocognitive paradigms (i.e, oddball, Stroop, match-mismatch, Flanker, and word priming) by observing ERP components (P1, N1, N170, N2, early and late P300, late positive potential (LPP), and N400). In this sense, these ERP components are considered as recognition tools for early diagnosis of depression and considered as cognitive and cerebral biomarkers for depression.

Both positive and negative early sensory components such as P100, N170, N200 and P200 (within 100ms-200ms) clearly represent enhanced amplitudes, when patients with depression process emotional faces, voices and words. All these sensory components characterize the early recognition of sad stimuli with higher amplitudes than the happy one. This is an important breakthrough for the understanding of pathophysiological and clinical bias towards negation in depressive patients. Except for the previous study of Burkhart and Thomas (1993), most of the recent studies reveal the enhanced amplitude of these early components. Few studies have reported inconsistency in N2 amplitudes which is either decreased or increased in depressed or dysthymic subjects due to the differences in the tasks, medication, EEG montage with limited channels and heterogeneous characteristics of patients. However, most of the studies report that depressed patients have reduced the amplitudes of N2 potentials with short-latency in frontal, central and parietal regions. Here the reduction in N2 represents the processing of negative facial expressions, adding a high chance of suicidal ideation. The future study may be focused on the emotion and action correlation in depression to find out whether patients recognize the match and mismatch between action and emotion in this early component of ERPs. Some studies have revealed that the ERN component is amplified in medial frontal areas or near the ACC in depressed subjects. Here the ERN is considered as a biomarker for evolving depression.

There is a shift of neurocognitive component from MMN to P3a when the first episode of depression changes to recurrence depressive episodes. This change is clearly shown in the early components with higher amplitudes in pre-attentive information processing, and the late reduced amplitudes of P300, P3a and P3b provide a detailed processing of information. These findings provide a solid clinical implication for understanding the recurrence of physiopathologic mechanisms for establishing novel disease treatments for MDD. A thorough analysis reveals that heightened MMN amplitudes signify firm biomarker for the presence of the first episode of depression, whereas the reduction in P3a amplitudes symbolizes a potential biomarker for recurrence of depressive episodes. This chapter also claims that the late reduction of P300 amplitudes including P3a and P3b over the parietal regions is correlated with depressed patients. With little disagreement, scholars have agreed that the reduction in P300 component is one of the neurophysiological biomarkers, which are presented when patients with MDD have attended target visual and auditory affective oddball tasks. Most of the patients show the decrement of P3 at temporoparietal regions. Specifically, the variations in the reduction of P300 are correlated with the clinical variations due to types of depression. For example, patients with psychotic depression indicate a larger reduction of P300 amplitudes than patients with MDD. However, the P3 latency is longer in bipolar disorder than unipolar disorder. After the antidepressant medication, there is an improvised enhancement of P3 amplitudes. Further, the P3a component which is distributed over frontocentral regions is also reduced in depressed patients, but it is increased in patients having an anxiety disorder. Though both the frontal and the anterior cingular cortex (ACC) are responsible for reductions of P300 amplitudes in depression, some studies specify the hippocampus that is linked with the reduction of P3 amplitudes (Kiehl et al., 2001; Knight, 1996). Overall, the P3 reduction is related to the discrepancy and dysfunction of attention to task-irrelevant stimuli over the prefrontal, anterior cingulate, and hippocampal regions. These neural signatures are considered as biomarkers to assess symptom severity of patients with MDD. At the neural and behavioural levels, this diagnostic information is essential prior to initiating and selecting the treatment settings, procedures and methods. As per the severity of symptoms, patients often use to go through interpersonal, psychosocial, behavioural, cognitive, yoga and meditation therapies.

The future research should focus on the cause of P300 deficit in depressed patients. A further study is needed to establish a close and reciprocal relationship between the scope of attention and emotion by using Navon's oddball attention paradigm in depressed patients. This type of experiment may establish whether there is an association between global-local attentions with happy-sad emotions in depressive patients. Future investigation should also be put forth to establish a cross-talk between neurogenetic polymorphisms and neurocognitive mechanisms of depression, thereby increasing our efforts to prevent and treat cognitive dysfunction, and enhancing long-lasting results for those suffering from the depressive disorder. This outcome could expand our knowledge about the nature, scope and magnitude of the vulnerable disease in terms of neurocognitive mechanisms offering theoretical insights into illness, aetiology and pathophysiology of depression.

ACKNOWLEDGMENT

This research was supported by the National Institute of Technology Raipur, India (Grant No. NITRR/SeedGrant/2016- 17/009).

REFERENCES

Ajilchi, B., Kisely, S., Nejati, V., & Frederickson, J. (2018). Effects of intensive short-term dynamic psychotherapy on social cognition in major depression. *Journal of Mental Health (Abingdon, England)*, 1–5. doi:10.1080/09638237.2018.1466035 PMID:29792087

Akram, A., Christoffel, D., Rocher, A. B., Bouras, C., Kövari, E., Perl, D. P., ... Hof, P. R. (2008). Stereologic estimates of total spinophilin-immunoreactive spine number in area 9 and the CA1 field: Relationship with the progression of Alzheimer's disease. *Neurobiology of Aging*, *29*(9), 1296–1307. doi:10.1016/j.neurobiolaging.2007.03.007 PMID:17420070

Anderson, I. M., Shippen, C., Juhasz, G., Chase, D., Thomas, E., Downey, D., ... Deakin, J. W. (2011). State-dependent alteration in face emotion recognition in depression. *The British Journal of Psychiatry*, *198*(4), 302–308. doi:10.1192/bjp.bp.110.078139 PMID:21263011

Andrews, G., Basu, A., Cuijpers, P., Craske, M. G., McEvoy, P., English, C. L., & Newby, J. M. (2018). Computer therapy for the anxiety and depression disorders is effective, acceptable and practical health care: An updated meta-analysis. *Journal of Anxiety Disorders*, *55*, 70–78. doi:10.1016/j.janxdis.2018.01.001 PMID:29422409

Angst, J., Gamma, A., Rössler, W., Ajdacic, V., & Klein, D. N. (2009). Long-term depression versus episodic major depression: Results from the prospective Zurich study of a community sample. *Journal of Affective Disorders*, *115*(1-2), 112–121. doi:10.1016/j.jad.2008.09.023 PMID:18973954

Auerbach, R. P., Stanton, C. H., Proudfit, G. H., & Pizzagalli, D. A. (2015). Self-referential processing in depressed adolescents: A high-density event-related potential study. *Journal of Abnormal Psychology*, *124*(2), 233–245. doi:10.1037/abn0000023 PMID:25643205

Baik, S. Y., Jeong, M., Kim, H. S., & Lee, S. H. (2018). ERP investigation of attentional disengagement from suicide-relevant information in patients with major depressive disorder. *Journal of Affective Disorders*, *225*, 357–364. doi:10.1016/j.jad.2017.08.046 PMID:28846957

Bailey, N., Freedman, G., Raj, K., Sullivan, C., Rogasch, N., Chung, S., ... Fitzgerald, P. (2018). Mindfulness meditators show altered distributions of early and late neural activity markers of attention in a response inhibition task. *bioRxiv*, 396259.

Bailey, N. W., Hoy, K. E., Maller, J. J., Segrave, R. A., Thomson, R., Williams, N., ... Fitzgerald, P. B. (2014). An exploratory analysis of go/nogo event-related potentials in major depression and depression following traumatic brain injury. *Psychiatry Research: Neuroimaging*, *224*(3), 324–334. doi:10.1016/j.pscychresns.2014.09.008 PMID:25452196

Barrick, E. M., & Dillon, D. G. (2018). An ERP study of multidimensional source retrieval in depression. *Biological Psychology, 132*, 176–191. doi:10.1016/j.biopsycho.2018.01.001 PMID:29305874

Barth, J., Munder, T., Gerger, H., Nüesch, E., Trelle, S., Znoj, H., ... Cuijpers, P. (2016). Comparative efficacy of seven psychotherapeutic interventions for patients with depression: A network meta-analysis. *Focus (San Francisco, Calif.), 14*(2), 229–243.

Berger, T., Krieger, T., Sude, K., Meyer, B., & Maercker, A. (2018). Evaluating an e-mental health program ("deprexis") as adjunctive treatment tool in psychotherapy for depression: Results of a pragmatic randomized controlled trial. *Journal of Affective Disorders, 227*, 455–462. doi:10.1016/j.jad.2017.11.021 PMID:29154168

Bertolote, J. M., Fleischmann, A., De Leo, D., & Wasserman, D. (2004). Psychiatric diagnoses and suicide: Revisiting the evidence. *Crisis, 25*(4), 147–155. doi:10.1027/0227-5910.25.4.147 PMID:15580849

Bina, R., Barak, A., Posmontier, B., Glasser, S., & Cinamon, T. (2018). Social workers' perceptions of barriers to interpersonal therapy implementation for treating postpartum depression in a primary care setting in Israel. *Health & Social Care in the Community, 26*(1), e75–e84. doi:10.1111/hsc.12479 PMID:28726342

Bingol, B., & Sheng, M. (2011). Deconstruction for reconstruction: The role of proteolysis in neural plasticity and disease. *Neuron, 69*(1), 22–32. doi:10.1016/j.neuron.2010.11.006 PMID:21220096

Bonetti, L., Haumann, N. T., Vuust, P., Kliuchko, M., & Brattico, E. (2017). Risk of depression enhances auditory Pitch discrimination in the brain as indexed by the mismatch negativity. *Clinical Neurophysiology, 128*(10), 1923–1936. doi:10.1016/j.clinph.2017.07.004 PMID:28826023

Boschloo, L., Schoevers, R. A., Beekman, A. T., Smit, J. H., Van Hemert, A. M., & Penninx, B. W. (2014). The four-year course of major depressive disorder: The role of staging and risk factor determination. *Psychotherapy and Psychosomatics, 83*(5), 279–288. doi:10.1159/000362563 PMID:25116639

Boutros, N. N., Galderisi, S., Pogarell, O., & Riggio, S. (2011). *Standard electroencephalography in clinical psychiatry: a practical handbook.* John Wiley & Sons. doi:10.1002/9780470974612

Brenninkmeijer, V., Lagerveld, S. E., Blonk, R. W., Schaufeli, W. B., & Wijngaards-de Meij, L. D. (2018). Predicting the effectiveness of work-focused CBT for common mental disorders: The influence of baseline self-efficacy, depression and anxiety. *Journal of Occupational Rehabilitation*, 1–11. PMID:29450678

Bridwell, D. A., Steele, V. R., Maurer, J. M., Kiehl, K. A., & Calhoun, V. D. (2015). The relationship between somatic and cognitive-affective depression symptoms and error-related ERPs. *Journal of Affective Disorders, 172*, 89–95. doi:10.1016/j.jad.2014.09.054 PMID:25451400

Bruder, G. E., Kayser, J., Tenke, C. E., Leite, P., Schneier, F. R., Stewart, J. W., & Quitkin, F. M. (2002). Cognitive ERPs in depressive and anxiety disorders during tonal and phonetic oddball tasks. *Clinical EEG (Electroencephalography), 33*(3), 119–124. doi:10.1177/155005940203300308 PMID:12192661

Bruder, G. E., Kroppmann, C. J., Kayser, J., Stewart, J. W., McGrath, P. J., & Tenke, C. E. (2009). Reduced brain responses to novel sound in depression: P3 findings in a novelty oddball task. *Psychiatry Research, 170*(2-3), 218–223. doi:10.1016/j.psychres.2008.10.023 PMID:19900720

Bruder, G. E., Tenke, C. E., Towey, J. P., Leite, P., Fong, R., Stewart, J. E., ... Quitkin, F. M. (1998). Brain ERPs of depressed patients to complex tones in an oddball task: Relation of reduced P3 asymmetry to physical anhedonia. *Psychophysiology*, *35*(1), 54–63. doi:10.1111/1469-8986.3510054 PMID:9499706

Bruder, G. E., Tenke, C. E., Warner, V., & Weissman, M. M. (2007). Grandchildren at high and low risk for depression differ in EEG measures of regional brain asymmetry. *Biological Psychiatry*, *62*(11), 1317–1323. doi:10.1016/j.biopsych.2006.12.006 PMID:17481594

Burkhart, M. A., & Thomas, D. G. (1993). Event-related potential measures of attention in moderately depressed subjects. *Electroencephalography and Clinical Neurophysiology/Evoked Potentials Section*, *88*(1), 42-50.

Camfield, D. A., Burton, T. K., De Blasio, F. M., Barry, R. J., & Croft, R. J. (2018). ERP components associated with an indirect emotional stop signal task in healthy and depressed participants. *International Journal of Psychophysiology*, *124*, 12–25. doi:10.1016/j.ijpsycho.2017.12.008 PMID:29278691

Carlson, J. M., Foti, D., Harmon-Jones, E., & Proudfit, G. H. (2015). Midbrain volume predicts fMRI and ERP measures of reward reactivity. *Brain Structure & Function*, *220*(3), 1861–1866. doi:10.100700429-014-0725-9 PMID:24549705

Carter, J. D., McIntosh, V. V., Jordan, J., Porter, R. J., Douglas, K., Frampton, C. M., & Joyce, P. R. (2018). Patient predictors of response to cognitive behaviour therapy and schema therapy for depression. *The Australian and New Zealand Journal of Psychiatry*. PMID:29325436

Castaneda, A. E., Tuulio-Henriksson, A., Marttunen, M., Suvisaari, J., & Lönnqvist, J. (2008). A review on cognitive impairments in depressive and anxiety disorders with a focus on young adults. *Journal of Affective Disorders*, *106*(1-2), 1–27. doi:10.1016/j.jad.2007.06.006 PMID:17707915

Chen, J., Yang, L. Q., Zhang, Z. J., Ma, W. T., Xing-qu, W., Zhang, X. R., ... Hua, Z. (2013a). The association between the disruption of motor imagery and the number of depressive episodes of major depression. *Journal of Affective Disorders*, *150*(2), 337–343. doi:10.1016/j.jad.2013.04.015 PMID:23684121

Chen, J., Zhang, Y., Wei, D., Wu, X., Fu, Q., Xu, F., ... Zhang, Z. (2015). Neurophysiological handover from MMN to P3a in first-episode and recurrent major depression. *Journal of Affective Disorders*, *174*, 173-179.

Cheung, A. H., Zuckerbrot, R. A., Jensen, P. S., Laraque, D., & Stein, R. E. (2018). Guidelines for adolescent depression in primary care (GLAD-PC): Part II. Treatment and ongoing management. *Pediatrics*, *141*(3). doi:10.1542/peds.2017-4082 PMID:29483201

Chiu, P. H., & Deldin, P. J. (2007). Neural evidence for enhanced error detection in major depressive disorder. *The American Journal of Psychiatry*, *164*(4), 608–616. doi:10.1176/ajp.2007.164.4.608 PMID:17403974

Choi, K. M., Jang, K. I., Huh, H. J., Baek, K. H., Kim, S. Y., Lee, S. M., ... Chae, J. H. (2015). The effects of 3 weeks of rTMS treatment on P200 amplitude in patients with depression. *Brain Stimulation: Basic, Translational, and Clinical Research in Neuromodulation*, *8*(2), 332. doi:10.1016/j.brs.2015.01.076

Christoffel, D. J., Golden, S. A., & Russo, S. J. (2011). Structural and synaptic plasticity in stress-related disorders. *Reviews in the Neurosciences*, *22*(5), 535–549. doi:10.1515/RNS.2011.044 PMID:21967517

Cipriani, A., Furukawa, T. A., Salanti, G., Chaimani, A., Atkinson, L. Z., Ogawa, Y., ... Egger, M. (2018). Comparative efficacy and acceptability of 21 antidepressant drugs for the acute treatment of adults with major depressive disorder: A systematic review and network meta-analysis. *Lancet*, *391*(10128), 1357–1366. doi:10.1016/S0140-6736(17)32802-7 PMID:29477251

Cisler, J. M., Olatunji, B. O., & Lohr, J. M. (2009). Disgust, fear, and anxiety disorders: A critical review. *Clinical Psychology Review*, *29*(1), 34–46. doi:10.1016/j.cpr.2008.09.007 PMID:18977061

Cruz-Martín, A., Crespo, M., & Portera-Cailliau, C. (2010). Delayed stabilization of dendritic spines in fragile X mice. *The Journal of Neuroscience*, *30*(23), 7793–7803. doi:10.1523/JNEUROSCI.0577-10.2010 PMID:20534828

Cuijpers, P., Cristea, I. A., Karyotaki, E., Reijnders, M., & Huibers, M. J. (2016). How effective are cognitive behavior therapies for major depression and anxiety disorders? A meta-analytic update of the evidence. *World Psychiatry; Official Journal of the World Psychiatric Association (WPA)*, *15*(3), 245–258. doi:10.1002/wps.20346 PMID:27717254

Dai, Q., & Feng, Z. (2011). Deficient interference inhibition for negative stimuli in depression: An event-related potential study. *Clinical Neurophysiology*, *122*(1), 52–61. doi:10.1016/j.clinph.2010.05.025 PMID:20605107

Dai, Q., & Feng, Z. (2012). More excited for negative facial expressions in depression: Evidence from an event-related potential study. *Clinical Neurophysiology*, *123*(11), 2172–2179. doi:10.1016/j.clinph.2012.04.018 PMID:22727714

Dai, Q., Wei, J., Shu, X., & Feng, Z. (2016). Negativity bias for sad faces in depression: An event-related potential study. *Clinical Neurophysiology*, *127*(12), 3552–3560. doi:10.1016/j.clinph.2016.10.003 PMID:27833064

Dainer-Best, J., Trujillo, L. T., Schnyer, D. M., & Beevers, C. G. (2017). Sustained engagement of attention is associated with increased negative self-referent processing in major depressive disorder. *Biological Psychology*, *129*, 231–241. doi:10.1016/j.biopsycho.2017.09.005 PMID:28893596

Dariotis, J. K., Mirabal-Beltran, R., Cluxton-Keller, F., Gould, L. F., Greenberg, M. T., & Mendelson, T. (2016). A Qualitative Evaluation of Student Learning and Skills Use in a School-Based Mindfulness and Yoga Program. *Mindfulness*, *7*(1), 76–89. doi:10.100712671-015-0463-y PMID:26918064

Davidson, R. J., Kabat-Zinn, J., Schumacher, J., Rosenkranz, M., Muller, D., Santorelli, S. F., ... Sheridan, J. F. (2003). Alterations in brain and immune function produced by mindfulness meditation. *Psychosomatic Medicine*, *65*(4), 564–570. doi:10.1097/01.PSY.0000077505.67574.E3 PMID:12883106

Davidson, R. J., & McEwen, B. S. (2012). Social influences on neuroplasticity: Stress and interventions to promote well-being. *Nature Neuroscience*, *15*(5), 689–695. doi:10.1038/nn.3093 PMID:22534579

Deldin, P. J., Keller, J., Gergen, J. A., & Miller, G. A. (2000). Right-posterior face processing anomaly in depression. *Journal of Abnormal Psychology*, *109*(1), 116–121. doi:10.1037/0021-843X.109.1.116 PMID:10740942

Deldin, P. J., Naidu, S. K., Shestyuk, A. Y., & Casas, B. R. (2009). Neurophysiological indices of free recall memory biases in major depression: The impact of stimulus arousal and valence. *Cognition and Emotion*, *23*(5), 1002–1020. doi:10.1080/02699930802273573

Delle-Vigne, D., Wang, W., Kornreich, C., Verbanck, P., & Campanella, S. (2014). Emotional facial expression processing in depression: Data from behavioral and event-related potential studies. *Neurophysiologie Clinique. Clinical Neurophysiology*, *44*(2), 169–187. doi:10.1016/j.neucli.2014.03.003 PMID:24930940

Dennis, T. A. (2010). Neurophysiological markers for child emotion regulation from the perspective of emotion–cognition integration: Current directions and future challenges. *Developmental Neuropsychology*, *35*(2), 212–230. doi:10.1080/87565640903526579 PMID:20390603

Dernovsek, M., Novak, T., & Sprah, L. (2010). PW01-09-Assessment of cognitive functioning within different emotional contexts in the group of euthymic bipolar patients. *European Psychiatry*, *25*, 1425. doi:10.1016/S0924-9338(10)71411-5

Deveney, C. M., & Deldin, P. J. (2004). Memory of faces: A slow wave ERP study of major depression. *Emotion (Washington, D.C.)*, *4*(3), 295–304. doi:10.1037/1528-3542.4.3.295 PMID:15456398

Deveney, C. M., & Deldin, P. J. (2006). A preliminary investigation of cognitive flexibility for emotional information in major depressive disorder and non-psychiatric controls. *Emotion (Washington, D.C.)*, *6*(3), 429–437. doi:10.1037/1528-3542.6.3.429 PMID:16938084

Diner, B. C., Holcomb, P. J., & Dykman, R. A. (1985). P300 in major depressive disorder. *Psychiatry Research*, *15*(3), 175–184. doi:10.1016/0165-1781(85)90074-5 PMID:3862153

Disner, S. G., Beevers, C. G., Haigh, E. A., & Beck, A. T. (2011). Neural mechanisms of the cognitive model of depression. *Nature Reviews. Neuroscience*, *12*(8), 467–477. doi:10.1038/nrn3027 PMID:21731066

Donkers, F. C., Nieuwenhuis, S., & Van Boxtel, G. J. (2005). Mediofrontal negativities in the absence of responding. *Brain Research. Cognitive Brain Research*, *25*(3), 777–787. doi:10.1016/j.cogbrainres.2005.09.007 PMID:16249075

Drevets, W. C., Price, J. L., & Furey, M. L. (2008). Brain structural and functional abnormalities in mood disorders: Implications for neurocircuitry models of depression. *Brain Structure & Function*, *213*(1-2), 93–118. doi:10.100700429-008-0189-x PMID:18704495

Duman, R. S. (2014). Pathophysiology of depression and innovative treatments: Remodelling glutamatergic synaptic connections. *Dialogues in Clinical Neuroscience*, *16*(1), 11. PMID:24733968

Duman, R. S., & Monteggia, L. M. (2006). A neurotrophic model for stress-related mood disorders. *Biological Psychiatry*, *59*(12), 1116–1127. doi:10.1016/j.biopsych.2006.02.013 PMID:16631126

Dumitriu, D., Hao, J., Hara, Y., Kaufmann, J., Janssen, W. G., Lou, W., ... Morrison, J. H. (2010). Selective changes in thin spine density and morphology in monkey prefrontal cortex correlate with ageing-related cognitive impairment. *The Journal of Neuroscience*, *30*(22), 7507–7515. doi:10.1523/JNEUROSCI.6410-09.2010 PMID:20519525

Duncan, C. C., Barry, R. J., Connolly, J. F., Fischer, C., Michie, P. T., Näätänen, R., ... Van Petten, C. (2009). Event-related potentials in clinical research: Guidelines for eliciting, recording, and quantifying mismatch negativity, P300, and N400. *Clinical Neurophysiology*, *120*(11), 1883–1908. doi:10.1016/j.clinph.2009.07.045 PMID:19796989

Evans, D. L., Charney, D. S., & Lewis, L. (2006). *The Physician's Guide to Depression & Bipolar Disorders*. McGraw-Hill Professional.

Fallgatter, A. J., Herrmann, M. J., Roemmler, J., Ehlis, A. C., Wagener, A., Heidrich, A., ... Lesch, K. P. (2004). Allelic variation of serotonin transporter function modulates the brain electrical response for error processing. *Neuropsychopharmacology*, *29*(8), 1506–1511. doi:10.1038j.npp.1300409 PMID:15187981

Farb, N., Anderson, A., Ravindran, A., Hawley, L., Irving, J., Mancuso, E., ... Segal, Z. V. (2018). Prevention of relapse/recurrence in major depressive disorder with either mindfulness-based cognitive therapy or cognitive therapy. *Journal of Consulting and Clinical Psychology*, *86*(2), 200–204. doi:10.1037/ccp0000266 PMID:29265831

Feldmann, L., Piechaczek, C. E., Pehl, V., Bartling, J., Bakos, S., Schulte-Körne, G., & Greimel, E. (2018). State or trait? Auditory event-related potentials in adolescents with current and remitted major depression. *Neuropsychologia*, *113*, 95–103. doi:10.1016/j.neuropsychologia.2018.03.035 PMID:29604322

Fishbein, D., Miller, S., Herman-Stahl, M., Williams, J., Lavery, B., Markovitz, L., ... Johnson, M. (2016). Behavioral and psychophysiological effects of a yoga intervention on high-risk adolescents: A randomized control trial. *Journal of Child and Family Studies*, *25*(2), 518–529. doi:10.100710826-015-0231-6

Force, R. B., Venables, N. C., & Sponheim, S. R. (2008). An auditory processing abnormality specific to liability for schizophrenia. *Schizophrenia Research*, *103*(1-3), 298–310. doi:10.1016/j.schres.2008.04.038 PMID:18571375

Foti, D., Olvet, D. M., Klein, D. N., & Hajcak, G. (2010). Reduced electrocortical response to threatening faces in major depressive disorder. *Depression and Anxiety*, *27*(9), 813–820. doi:10.1002/da.20712 PMID:20577985

Fox, H. C., Hong, K. A., & Sinha, R. (2008). Difficulties in emotion regulation and impulse control in recently abstinent alcoholics compared with social drinkers. *Addictive Behaviors*, *33*(2), 388–3948. doi:10.1016/j.addbeh.2007.10.002 PMID:18023295

Friedman, D., Cycowicz, Y. M., & Gaeta, H. (2001). The novelty P3: An event-related brain potential (ERP) sign of the brain's evaluation of novelty. *Neuroscience and Biobehavioral Reviews*, *25*(4), 355–373. doi:10.1016/S0149-7634(01)00019-7 PMID:11445140

Friedman, D., Simpson, G., & Hamberger, M. (1993). Age-related changes in scalp topography to novel and target stimuli. *Psychophysiology*, *30*(4), 383–396. doi:10.1111/j.1469-8986.1993.tb02060.x PMID:8327624

Furukawa, T. A., Efthimiou, O., Weitz, E. S., Cipriani, A., Keller, M. B., Kocsis, J. H., ... Schramm, E. (2018). Cognitive-Behavioral Analysis System of Psychotherapy, Drug, or Their Combination for Persistent Depressive Disorder: Personalizing the Treatment Choice Using Individual Participant Data Network Metaregression. *Psychotherapy and Psychosomatics*, *87*(3), 140–153. doi:10.1159/000489227 PMID:29847831

García-Blanco, A., Salmerón, L., Perea, M., & Livianos, L. (2014). Attentional biases toward emotional images in the different episodes of bipolar disorder: An eye-tracking study. *Psychiatry Research*, *215*(3), 628–633. doi:10.1016/j.psychres.2013.12.039 PMID:24439518

Giese-Davis, J., Sephton, S. E., Abercrombie, H. C., Durán, R. E., & Spiegel, D. (2004). Repression and high anxiety are associated with aberrant diurnal cortisol rhythms in women with metastatic breast cancer. *Health Psychology*, *23*(6), 645–650. doi:10.1037/0278-6133.23.6.645 PMID:15546233

Gollan, J. K., McCloskey, M., Hoxha, D., & Coccaro, E. F. (2010). How do depressed and healthy adults interpret nuanced facial expressions? *Journal of Abnormal Psychology*, *119*(4), 804–810. doi:10.1037/a0020234 PMID:20939654

Goodwin, F. K., & Jamison, K. R. (2007). *Manic-depressive illness: bipolar disorders and recurrent depression* (Vol. 1). Oxford University Press.

Gordon-King, K., Schweitzer, R. D., & Dimaggio, G. (2018). Metacognitive interpersonal therapy for personality disorders featuring emotional inhibition: A multiple baseline case series. *The Journal of Nervous and Mental Disease*, *206*(4), 263–269. PMID:29377848

Gotink, R. A., Vernooij, M. W., Ikram, M. A., Niessen, W. J., Krestin, G. P., Hofman, A., ... Hunink, M. M. (2018). Meditation and yoga practice are associated with smaller right amygdala volume: The Rotterdam study. *Brain Imaging and Behavior*, 1–9. PMID:29417491

Hadjistavropoulos, H. D., Schneider, L. H., Edmonds, M., Karin, E., Nugent, M. N., Dirkse, D., ... Titov, N. (2017). Randomized controlled trial of internet-delivered cognitive behaviour therapy comparing standard weekly versus optional weekly therapist support. *Journal of Anxiety Disorders*, *52*, 15–24. doi:10.1016/j.janxdis.2017.09.006 PMID:28964994

Hansenne, M., Pitchot, W., Moreno, A. G., Zaldua, I. U., & Ansseau, M. (1996). Suicidal behavior in depressive disorder: An event-related potential study. *Biological Psychiatry*, *40*(2), 116–122. doi:10.1016/0006-3223(95)00372-X PMID:8793043

Harvey, J. A., Quinn, J. L., Liu, R., Aloyo, V. J., & Romano, A. G. (2004). Selective remodelling of rabbit frontal cortex: Relationship between 5-HT 2A receptor density and associative learning. *Psychopharmacology*, *172*(4), 435–442. doi:10.100700213-003-1687-4 PMID:14685644

Hasler, G., Drevets, W. C., Manji, H. K., & Charney, D. S. (2004). Discovering endophenotypes for major depression. *Neuropsychopharmacology*, *29*(10), 1765–1781. doi:10.1038j.npp.1300506 PMID:15213704

Hayashi-Takagi, A., & Sawa, A. (2010). Disturbed synaptic connectivity in schizophrenia: Convergence of genetic risk factors during neurodevelopment. *Brain Research Bulletin*, *83*(3-4), 140–146. doi:10.1016/j.brainresbull.2010.04.007 PMID:20433911

Heller, W. (1993). Neuropsychological mechanisms of individual differences in emotion, personality, and arousal. *Neuropsychology*, *7*(4), 476–489. doi:10.1037/0894-4105.7.4.476

Herbert, C., Kissler, J., Junghöfer, M., Peyk, P., & Rockstroh, B. (2006). Processing of emotional adjectives: Evidence from startle EMG and ERPs. *Psychophysiology*, *43*(2), 197–206. doi:10.1111/j.1469-8986.2006.00385.x PMID:16712590

Heresco-Levy, U., & Javitt, D. (2018). *U.S. Patent Application No. 15/729,692*. Washington, DC: US Patent Office.

Hermens, D. F., Ward, P. B., Hodge, M. A. R., Kaur, M., Naismith, S. L., & Hickie, I. B. (2010). Impaired MMN/P3a complex in first-episode psychosis: Cognitive and psychosocial associations. *Progress in Neuro-Psychopharmacology & Biological Psychiatry*, *34*(6), 822–829. doi:10.1016/j.pnpbp.2010.03.019 PMID:20302901

Holmes, A. J., & Pizzagalli, D. A. (2008). Spatiotemporal dynamics of error processing dysfunctions in major depressive disorder. *Archives of General Psychiatry*, *65*(2), 179–188. doi:10.1001/archgenpsychiatry.2007.19 PMID:18250256

Houston, R. J., Bauer, L. O., & Hesselbrock, V. M. (2003). Depression and familial risk for substance dependence: A P300 study of young women. *Psychiatry Research: Neuroimaging*, *124*(1), 49–62. doi:10.1016/S0925-4927(03)00074-X PMID:14511795

Huster, R. J., Enriquez-Geppert, S., Lavallee, C. F., Falkenstein, M., & Herrmann, C. S. (2013). Electroencephalography of response inhibition tasks: Functional networks and cognitive contributions. *International Journal of Psychophysiology*, *87*(3), 217–233. doi:10.1016/j.ijpsycho.2012.08.001 PMID:22906815

Jagaroo, V., & Santangelo, S. L. (2017). Erratum to: Neurophenotypes. *Neurophenotypes*, *12*(193), 296.

Jennifer. (2013). Sleep Awake Disorder. In W. E. Craighead, D. J. Miklowitz, & L. W. Craighead (Eds.), Psychopathology: History, diagnosis, and empirical foundations. Academic Press.

Joo, J. H., Hwang, S., Abu, H., & Gallo, J. J. (2016). An innovative model of depression care delivery: Peer mentors in collaboration with a mental health professional to relieve depression in older adults. *The American Journal of Geriatric Psychiatry*, *24*(5), 407–416. doi:10.1016/j.jagp.2016.02.002 PMID:27066731

Joo, J. H., Hwang, S., Gallo, J. J., & Roter, D. L. (2018). The impact of peer mentor communication with older adults on depressive symptoms and working alliance: A pilot study. *Patient Education and Counseling*, *101*(4), 665–671. doi:10.1016/j.pec.2017.10.012 PMID:29128295

Joormann, J., Cooney, R. E., Henry, M. L., & Gotlib, I. H. (2012). Neural correlates of automatic mood regulation in girls at high risk for depression. *Journal of Abnormal Psychology*, *121*(1), 61–72. doi:10.1037/a0025294 PMID:21895344

Joormann, J., & Gotlib, I. H. (2006). Is this happiness I see? Biases in the identification of emotional facial expressions in depression and social phobia. *Journal of Abnormal Psychology*, *115*(4), 705–714. doi:10.1037/0021-843X.115.4.705 PMID:17100528

Joormann, J., & Gotlib, I. H. (2007). Selective attention to emotional faces following recovery from depression. *Journal of Abnormal Psychology*, *116*(1), 80–85. doi:10.1037/0021-843X.116.1.80 PMID:17324018

Joormann, J., & Gotlib, I. H. (2008). Updating the contents of working memory in depression: Interference from irrelevant negative material. *Journal of Abnormal Psychology, 117*(1), 182–192. doi:10.1037/0021-843X.117.1.182 PMID:18266496

Kähkönen, S., Yamashita, H., Rytsälä, H., Suominen, K., Ahveninen, J., & Isometsä, E. (2007). Dysfunction in early auditory processing in major depressive disorder revealed by combined MEG and EEG. *Journal of psychiatry & neuroscience. JPN, 32*(5), 316. PMID:17823647

Kalogerakou, S., Tsaltas, E., Anyfandi, E., Papakosta, V. M., Kontis, D., Angelopoulos, E., ... Zervas, I. M. (2018). Neuropsychological profile as a marker of major depressive disorder subtypes: contribution to treatment strategy formulation. *Dialogues in Clinical Neuroscience & Mental Health, 1.*

Kang, H. J., Voleti, B., Hajszan, T., Rajkowska, G., Stockmeier, C. A., Licznerski, P., ... Son, H. (2012). Decreased expression of synapse-related genes and loss of synapses in major depressive disorder. *Nature Medicine, 18*(9), 1413–1417. doi:10.1038/nm.2886 PMID:22885997

Karaaslan, F., Gonul, A. S., Oguz, A., Erdinc, E., & Esel, E. (2003). P300 changes in major depressive disorders with and without psychotic features. *Journal of Affective Disorders, 73*(3), 283–287. doi:10.1016/S0165-0327(01)00477-3 PMID:12547298

Kaur, M., Battisti, R. A., Lagopoulos, J., Ward, P. B., Hickie, I. B., & Hermens, D. F. (2012). Neurophysiological biomarkers support bipolar-spectrum disorders within psychosis cluster. *Journal of psychiatry & neuroscience. JPN, 37*(5), 313–321. doi:10.1503/jpn.110081 PMID:22469054

Kaur, M., Battisti, R. A., Ward, P. B., Ahmed, A., Hickie, I. B., & Hermens, D. F. (2011). MMN/P3a deficits in first episode psychosis: Comparing schizophrenia-spectrum and affective-spectrum subgroups. *Schizophrenia Research, 130*(1-3), 203–209. doi:10.1016/j.schres.2011.03.025 PMID:21550211

Kaustio, O., Partanen, J., Valkonen-Korhonen, M., Viinamäki, H., & Lehtonen, J. (2002). Affective and psychotic symptoms relate to different types of P300 alteration in depressive disorder. *Journal of Affective Disorders, 71*(1-3), 43–50. doi:10.1016/S0165-0327(01)00410-4 PMID:12167500

Kemmerer, D. (2015). *Cognitive neuroscience of language.* Psychology Press.

Kiang, M., Farzan, F., Blumberger, D. M., Kutas, M., McKinnon, M. C., Kansal, V., ... Daskalakis, Z. J. (2017). Abnormal self-schema in semantic memory in major depressive disorder: Evidence from event-related brain potentials. *Biological Psychology, 126,* 41–47. doi:10.1016/j.biopsycho.2017.04.003 PMID:28385626

Kiehl, K. A., & Liddle, P. F. (2001). An event-related functional magnetic resonance imaging study of an auditory oddball task in schizophrenia. *Schizophrenia Research, 48*(2-3), 159–171. doi:10.1016/S0920-9964(00)00117-1 PMID:11295369

Kircanski, K., Joormann, J., & Gotlib, I. H. (2012). Cognitive aspects of depression. *Wiley Interdisciplinary Reviews: Cognitive Science, 3*(3), 301–313. doi:10.1002/wcs.1177 PMID:23240069

Kissler, J., Herbert, C., Winkler, I., & Junghofer, M. (2009). Emotion and attention in visual word processing—An ERP study. *Biological Psychology, 80*(1), 75-83.

Knight, R. T. (1996). Contribution of human hippocampal region to novelty detection. *Nature*, *383*(6597), 256–259. doi:10.1038/383256a0 PMID:8805701

Koolschijn, P. C. M., van Haren, N. E., Lensvelt-Mulders, G. J., Hulshoff Pol, H. E., & Kahn, R. S. (2009). Brain volume abnormalities in major depressive disorder: A meta-analysis of magnetic resonance imaging studies. *Human Brain Mapping*, *30*(11), 3719–3735. doi:10.1002/hbm.20801 PMID:19441021

Korn, C. W., Sharot, T., Walter, H., Heekeren, H. R., & Dolan, R. J. (2014). Depression is related to an absence of optimistically biased belief updating about future life events. *Psychological Medicine*, *44*(3), 579–592. doi:10.1017/S0033291713001074 PMID:23672737

Lecardeur, L., Briand, C., Prouteau, A., Lalonde, P., Nicole, L., Lesage, A., & Stip, E. (2009). Preserved awareness of their cognitive deficits in patients with schizophrenia: Convergent validity of the SSTICS. *Schizophrenia Research*, *107*(2-3), 303–306. doi:10.1016/j.schres.2008.09.003 PMID:18835134

Lejoyeux, M., & Lehert, P. (2010). Alcohol-use disorders and depression: Results from individual patient data meta-analysis of the acamprosate-controlled studies. *Alcohol and Alcoholism (Oxford, Oxfordshire)*, *46*(1), 61–67. doi:10.1093/alcalc/agq077 PMID:21118900

Lemmens, L. H., van Bronswijk, S. C., Peeters, F., Arntz, A., Hollon, S. D., & Huibers, M. J. (2018). Long-term outcomes of acute treatment with cognitive therapy v. interpersonal psychotherapy for adult depression: Follow-up of a randomized controlled trial. *Psychological Medicine*, 1–9. PMID:29792234

LeMoult, J., Yoon, K. L., & Joormann, J. (2012). Affective priming in major depressive disorder. *Frontiers in Integrative Neuroscience*, *6*, 76. doi:10.3389/fnint.2012.00076 PMID:23060758

Levens, S. M., & Gotlib, I. H. (2009). Impaired selection of relevant positive information in depression. *Depression and Anxiety*, *26*(5), 403–410. doi:10.1002/da.20565 PMID:19347861

Levens, S. M., & Gotlib, I. H. (2010). Updating positive and negative stimuli in working memory in depression. *Journal of Experimental Psychology. General*, *139*(4), 654–664. doi:10.1037/a0020283 PMID:21038984

Levens, S. M., & Phelps, E. A. (2008). Emotion processing effects on interference resolution in working memory. *Emotion (Washington, D.C.)*, *8*(2), 267–280. doi:10.1037/1528-3542.8.2.267 PMID:18410200

Li, B. J., Friston, K., Mody, M., Wang, H. N., Lu, H. B., & Hu, D. W. (2018). A brain network model for depression: From symptom understanding to disease intervention. *CNS Neuroscience & Therapeutics*, *24*(11), 1004–1019. doi:10.1111/cns.12998 PMID:29931740

Liu, R. J., & Aghajanian, G. K. (2008). Stress blunts serotonin-and hypocretin-evoked EPSCs in prefrontal cortex: Role of corticosterone-mediated apical dendritic atrophy. *Proceedings of the National Academy of Sciences of the United States of America*, *105*(1), 359–364. doi:10.1073/pnas.0706679105 PMID:18172209

Liu, W. H., Huang, J., Wang, L. Z., Gong, Q. Y., & Chan, R. C. (2012). Facial perception bias in patients with major depression. *Psychiatry Research*, *197*(3), 217–220. doi:10.1016/j.psychres.2011.09.021 PMID:22357354

Liu, Y., Spulber, G., Lehtimäki, K. K., Könönen, M., Hallikainen, I., Gröhn, H., ... Soininen, H. (2011). Diffusion tensor imaging and tract-based spatial statistics in Alzheimer's disease and mild cognitive impairment. *Neurobiology of Aging*, *32*(9), 1558–1571. doi:10.1016/j.neurobiolaging.2009.10.006 PMID:19913331

Lorenzetti, V., Allen, N. B., Whittle, S., & Yücel, M. (2010). Amygdala volumes in a sample of current depressed and remitted depressed patients and healthy controls. *Journal of Affective Disorders*, *120*(1-3), 112–119. doi:10.1016/j.jad.2009.04.021 PMID:19464062

Luck, S. J. (2014). *An introduction to the event-related potential technique*. MIT Press.

Luck, S. J., & Kappenman, E. S. (Eds.). (2011). *The Oxford handbook of event-related potential components*. Oxford University Press.

Luu, P., Tucker, D. M., & Makeig, S. (2004). Frontal midline theta and the error-related negativity: Neurophysiological mechanisms of action regulation. *Clinical Neurophysiology*, *115*(8), 1821–1835. doi:10.1016/j.clinph.2004.03.031 PMID:15261861

MacQueen, G., & Frodl, T. (2011). The hippocampus in major depression: Evidence for the convergence of the bench and bedside in psychiatric research? *Molecular Psychiatry*, *16*(3), 252–264. doi:10.1038/mp.2010.80 PMID:20661246

Mao, W., Wang, Y., & Wang, D. (2005). Cognitive impairment in major depressive disorder revealed by event-related potential N270. *Clinical EEG and Neuroscience*, *36*(1), 9–14. doi:10.1177/155005940503600104 PMID:15683192

Mayberg, H. S. (1997). Limbic-cortical dysregulation: A proposed model of depression. *The Journal of Neuropsychiatry and Clinical Neurosciences*, *9*, 471–481. PubMed

Mayberg, H. S. (2009). Targeted electrode-based modulation of neural circuits for depression. *The Journal of Clinical Investigation*, *119*(4), 717–725. doi:10.1172/JCI38454 PMID:19339763

McCabe, R., Garside, R., Backhouse, A., & Xanthopoulou, P. (2018). Effectiveness of brief psychological interventions for suicidal presentations: A systematic review. *BMC Psychiatry*, *18*(1), 120. doi:10.118612888-018-1663-5 PMID:29724203

McEwen, B. S. (2012). The ever-changing brain: Cellular and molecular mechanisms for the effects of stressful experiences. *Developmental Neurobiology*, *72*(6), 878–890. doi:10.1002/dneu.20968 PMID:21898852

McFarquhar, T., Luyten, P., & Fonagy, P. (2018). Changes in interpersonal problems in the psychotherapeutic treatment of depression as measured by the Inventory of Interpersonal Problems: A systematic review and meta-analysis. *Journal of Affective Disorders*, *226*, 108–123. doi:10.1016/j.jad.2017.09.036 PMID:28968563

Mendlewicz, L., Linkowski, P., Bazelmans, C., & Philippot, P. (2005). Decoding emotional facial expressions in depressed and anorexic patients. *Journal of Affective Disorders*, *89*(1-3), 195–199. doi:10.1016/j.jad.2005.07.010 PMID:16256204

Milders, M., Bell, S., Platt, J., Serrano, R., & Runcie, O. (2010). Stable expression recognition abnormalities in unipolar depression. *Psychiatry Research*, *179*(1), 38–42. doi:10.1016/j.psychres.2009.05.015 PMID:20478626

Morgan, C., Mason, E., Newby, J. M., Mahoney, A. E., Hobbs, M. J., McAloon, J., & Andrews, G. (2017). The effectiveness of unguided internet cognitive behavioural therapy for mixed anxiety and depression. *Internet Interventions*, *10*, 47–53. doi:10.1016/j.invent.2017.10.003 PMID:30135752

Mu, Z., Chang, Y., Xu, J., Pang, X., Zhang, H., Liu, X., ... Wan, Y. (2016). Pre-attentive dysfunction of musical processing in major depressive disorder: A mismatch negativity study. *Journal of Affective Disorders*, *194*, 50–56. doi:10.1016/j.jad.2016.01.028 PMID:26802507

Näätänen, R., & Kreegipuu, K. (2011). The Mismatch negativity (MMN). In S. Kappenman & S. J. Luck (Eds.), The Oxford Handbook of Event-Related Potential Components (pp. 143-158). Oxford University Press.

Näätänen, R., Kujala, T., Kreegipuu, K., Carlson, S., Escera, C., Baldeweg, T., & Ponton, C. (2011). The mismatch negativity: An index of cognitive decline in neuropsychiatric and neurological diseases and in ageing. *Brain*, *134*(12), 3435–3453. doi:10.1093/brain/awr064 PMID:21624926

Naismith, S. L., Mowszowski, L., Ward, P. B., Diamond, K., Paradise, M., Kaur, M., ... Hermens, D. F. (2012). Reduced temporal mismatch negativity in late-life depression: An event-related potential index of cognitive deficit and functional disability? *Journal of Affective Disorders*, *138*(1-2), 71–78. doi:10.1016/j.jad.2011.12.028 PMID:22301116

Nan, C., Wang, G., Wang, H., Wang, X., Liu, Z., Xiao, L., ... Wu, S. (2018). The P300 component decreases in a bimodal oddball task in individuals with depression: An event-related potentials study. *Clinical Neurophysiology*, *129*(12), 2525–2533. doi:10.1016/j.clinph.2018.09.012 PMID:30366168

Nyer, M., Roberg, R., Nauphal, M., & Streeter, C. C. (2019). Yoga as a Treatment for Depression. In *The Massachusetts General Hospital Guide to Depression* (pp. 223–231). Cham: Humana Press. doi:10.1007/978-3-319-97241-1_17

Ogura, C., Nageishi, Y., Omura, F., Fukao, K., Ohta, H., Kishimoto, A., & Matsubayashi, M. (1993). N200 component of event-related potentials in depression. *Biological Psychiatry*, *33*(10), 720–726. doi:10.1016/0006-3223(93)90122-T PMID:8353167

Ollila, P., Knekt, P., Heinonen, E., & Lindfors, O. (2016). Patients' pre-treatment interpersonal problems as predictors of therapeutic alliance in long-term psychodynamic psychotherapy. *Psychiatry Research*, *241*, 110–117. doi:10.1016/j.psychres.2016.04.093 PMID:27173654

Olofsson, J. K., Nordin, S., Sequeira, H., & Polich, J. (2008). Affective picture processing: An integrative review of ERP findings. *Biological Psychology*, *77*(3), 247–265. doi:10.1016/j.biopsycho.2007.11.006 PMID:18164800

Pagani, G., Cekic, M., & Guo, Y. (2008). "Thinking about not thinking": Neural correlates of conceptual processing during Zen meditation. *PLoS One*, *3*(9), e3083. doi:10.1371/journal.pone.0003083 PMID:18769538

Pang, X., Xu, J., Chang, Y., Tang, D., Zheng, Y., Liu, Y., & Sun, Y. (2014). Mismatch negativity of sad syllables is absent in patients with major depressive disorder. *PLoS One*, *9*(3), e91995. doi:10.1371/journal.pone.0091995 PMID:24658084

Pause, B. M., Raack, N., Sojka, B., Göder, R., Aldenhoff, J. B., & Ferstl, R. (2003). Convergent and divergent effects of odors and emotions in depression. *Psychophysiology*, *40*(2), 209–225. doi:10.1111/1469-8986.00023 PMID:12820862

Penninx, B. W., Nolen, W. A., Lamers, F., Zitman, F. G., Smit, J. H., Spinhoven, P., ... Verhaak, P. (2011). Two-year course of depressive and anxiety disorders: Results from the Netherlands Study of Depression and Anxiety (NESDA). *Journal of Affective Disorders*, *133*(1-2), 76–85. doi:10.1016/j.jad.2011.03.027 PMID:21496929

Penzes, P., & VanLeeuwen, J. E. (2011). Impaired regulation of synaptic actin cytoskeleton in Alzheimer's disease. *Brain Research. Brain Research Reviews*, *67*(1-2), 184–192. doi:10.1016/j.brainresrev.2011.01.003 PMID:21276817

Phaf, R. H., & Kan, K. J. (2007). The automaticity of emotional Stroop: A meta-analysis. *Journal of Behavior Therapy and Experimental Psychiatry*, *38*(2), 184–199. doi:10.1016/j.jbtep.2006.10.008 PMID:17112461

Pihlaja, S., Stenberg, J. H., Joutsenniemi, K., Mehik, H., Ritola, V., & Joffe, G. (2018). Therapeutic alliance in guided internet therapy programs for depression and anxiety disorders–a systematic review. *Internet Interventions, 11*, 1-10.

Pinkham, A. E. (2014). Social cognition in schizophrenia. *The Journal of Clinical Psychiatry*, *75*(suppl 2), 14–19. doi:10.4088/JCP.13065su1.04 PMID:24919166

Pizzagalli, D. A. (2014). Depression, stress, and anhedonia: Toward a synthesis and integrated model. *Annual Review of Clinical Psychology*, *10*(1), 393–423. doi:10.1146/annurev-clinpsy-050212-185606 PMID:24471371

Polich, J. (2007). Updating P300: An integrative theory of P3a and P3b. *Clinical Neurophysiology*, *118*(10), 2128–2148. doi:10.1016/j.clinph.2007.04.019 PMID:17573239

Polich, J., & Criado, J. R. (2006). Neuropsychology and neuropharmacology of P3a and P3b. *International Journal of Psychophysiology*, *60*(2), 172–185. doi:10.1016/j.ijpsycho.2005.12.012 PMID:16510201

Proudfit, G. H., Bress, J. N., Foti, D., Kujawa, A., & Klein, D. N. (2015). Depression and event-related potentials: Emotional disengagement and reward insensitivity. *Current Opinion in Psychology*, *4*, 110–113. doi:10.1016/j.copsyc.2014.12.018 PMID:26462292

Qiao, Z., Yu, Y., Wang, L., Yang, X., Qiu, X., Zhang, C., ... Liu, J. (2013). Impaired pre-attentive change detection in major depressive disorder patients revealed by auditory mismatch negativity. *Psychiatry Research: Neuroimaging*, *211*(1), 78–84. doi:10.1016/j.pscychresns.2012.07.006 PMID:23149029

Raes, F., Hermans, D., & Williams, J. M. G. (2006). Negative bias in the perception of others' facial emotional expressions in major depression: The role of depressive rumination. *The Journal of Nervous and Mental Disease*, *194*(10), 796–799. doi:10.1097/01.nmd.0000240187.80270.bb PMID:17041294

Rajkowska, G., Miguel-Hidalgo, J. J., & Wei, J. (1999). Morphometric evidencenfor neuronal and glial prefrontal cell pathology in major depression. *Biological Psychiatry*, *45*, 1085–1098. doi:10.1016/S0006-3223(99)00041-4 PMID:10331101

Rapinesi, C., Bersani, F. S., Kotzalidis, G. D., Imperatori, C., Del Casale, A., Di Pietro, S., ... Angeletti, G. (2015). Maintenance deep transcranial magnetic stimulation sessions are associated with reduced depressive relapses in patients with unipolar or bipolar depression. *Frontiers in Neurology*, *6*, 16. doi:10.3389/fneur.2015.00016 PMID:25709596

Rice, S., Gleeson, J., Davey, C., Hetrick, S., Parker, A., Lederman, R., ... Russon, P. (2018). Moderated online social therapy for depression relapse prevention in young people: Pilot study of a 'next generation'online intervention. *Early Intervention in Psychiatry*, *12*(4), 613–625. doi:10.1111/eip.12354 PMID:27311581

Rice, S., Robinson, J., Bendall, S., Hetrick, S., Cox, G., Bailey, E., ... Alvarez-Jimenez, M. (2016). Online and social media suicide prevention interventions for young people: A focus on implementation and moderation. *Journal of the Canadian Academy of Child and Adolescent Psychiatry*, *25*(2), 80. PMID:27274743

Rottenberg, J. (2005). Mood and emotion in major depression. *Current Directions in Psychological Science*, *14*(3), 167–170. doi:10.1111/j.0963-7214.2005.00354.x

Ruchsow, M., Herrnberger, B., Beschoner, P., Grön, G., Spitzer, M., & Kiefer, M. (2006). Error processing in major depressive disorder: Evidence from event-related potentials. *Journal of Psychiatric Research*, *40*(1), 37–46. doi:10.1016/j.jpsychires.2005.02.002 PMID:15882872

Saeed, S. A., Antonacci, D. J., & Bloch, R. M. (2010). Exercise, yoga, and meditation for depressive and anxiety disorders. *American Family Physician*, *81*(8). PMID:20387774

Samara, Z., Evers, E. A., Peeters, F., Uylings, H. B., Rajkowska, G., Ramaekers, J. G., & Stiers, P. (2018). Orbital and medial prefrontal cortex functional connectivity of major depression vulnerability and disease. *Biological Psychiatry: Cognitive Neuroscience and Neuroimaging*, *3*(4), 348–357. PMID:29628067

Sang, H., & Tan, D. (2018). Internalizing behavior disorders symptoms reduction by a social skills training program among Chinese students: A randomized controlled trial. *NeuroQuantology: An Interdisciplinary Journal of Neuroscience and Quantum Physics*, *16*(5). doi:10.14704/nq.2018.16.5.1312

Sansone, R. A., & Sansone, L. A. (2009). Dysthymic disorder: Forlorn and overlooked? *Psychiatry (Edgmont)*, *6*(5), 46. PMID:19724735

Sapolsky, R. M. (2000). Glucocorticoids and hippocampal atrophy in neuropsychiatric disorders. *Archives of General Psychiatry*, *57*(10), 925–935. doi:10.1001/archpsyc.57.10.925 PMID:11015810

Sass, S. M., Heller, W., Stewart, J. L., Silton, R. L., Edgar, J. C., Fisher, J. E., & Miller, G. A. (2010). Time course of attentional bias in anxiety: Emotion and gender specificity. *Psychophysiology*, *47*(2), 247–259. doi:10.1111/j.1469-8986.2009.00926.x PMID:19863758

Savitz, J., & Drevets, W. C. (2009). Bipolar and major depressive disorder: Neuroimaging the developmental-degenerative divide. *Neuroscience and Biobehavioral Reviews*, *33*(5), 699–771. doi:10.1016/j.neubiorev.2009.01.004 PMID:19428491

Schnaas, F. J. (2003). Handbook of depression. *The Journal of Clinical Psychiatry*, *64*(12), 1523–1524. doi:10.4088/JCP.v64n1218c

Schrijvers, D., De Bruijn, E. R., Maas, Y. J., Vancoillie, P., Hulstijn, W., & Sabbe, B. G. (2009). Action monitoring and depressive symptom reduction in major depressive disorder. *International Journal of Psychophysiology*, *71*(3), 218–224. doi:10.1016/j.ijpsycho.2008.09.005 PMID:18926863

Scott, G. G., O'Donnell, P. J., Leuthold, H., & Sereno, S. C. (2009). Early emotion word processing: Evidence from event-related potentials. *Biological Psychology*, *80*(1), 95–104. doi:10.1016/j.biopsycho.2008.03.010 PMID:18440691

Segal, Z. V., Williams, M., & Teasdale, J. (2018). *Mindfulness-based cognitive therapy for depression*. Guilford Publications.

Shah, P. J., Ebmeier, K. P., Glabus, M. F., & Goodwin, G. M. (1998). Cortical grey matter reductions associated with treatment-resistant chronic unipolar depression: Controlled magnetic resonance imaging study. *The British Journal of Psychiatry*, *172*(6), 527–532. doi:10.1192/bjp.172.6.527 PMID:9828995

Shansky, R. M., & Morrison, J. H. (2009). Stress-induced dendritic remodeling in the medial prefrontal cortex: Effects of circuit, hormones and rest. *Brain Research*, *1293*, 108–113. doi:10.1016/j.brainres.2009.03.062 PMID:19361488

Shestyuk, A. Y., & Deldin, P. J. (2010). Automatic and strategic representation of the self in major depression: trait and state abnormalities. *The American Journal of Psychiatry*, *167*(5), 536–544. doi:10.1176/appi.ajp.2009.06091444 PMID:20360316

Simon, N. M., McNamara, K., Chow, C. W., Maser, R. S., Papakostas, G. I., Pollack, M. H., ... Wong, K. K. (2008). A detailed examination of cytokine abnormalities in Major Depressive Disorder. *European Neuropsychopharmacology*, *18*(3), 230–233. doi:10.1016/j.euroneuro.2007.06.004 PMID:17681762

Speed, B. C., Nelson, B. D., Auerbach, R. P., Klein, D. N., & Hajcak, G. (2016). Depression risk and electrocortical reactivity during self-referential emotional processing in 8 to 14 year-old girls. *Journal of Abnormal Psychology*, *125*(5), 607–619. doi:10.1037/abn0000173 PMID:27175985

Spijker, J. A. N., De Graaf, R., Bijl, R. V., Beekman, A. T., Ormel, J., & Nolen, W. A. (2002). Duration of major depressive episodes in the general population: Results from The Netherlands Mental Health Survey and Incidence Study (NEMESIS). *The British Journal of Psychiatry*, *181*(3), 208–213. doi:10.1192/bjp.181.3.208 PMID:12204924

Sternberg, S. (1969). The discovery of processing stages: Extensions of Donders' method. *Acta Psychologica*, *30*, 276–315. doi:10.1016/0001-6918(69)90055-9

Streeter, C. C., Gerbarg, P. L., Whitfield, T. H., Owen, L., Johnston, J., Silveri, M. M., ... Hernon, A. M. (2017). Treatment of major depressive disorder with Iyengar yoga and coherent breathing: A randomized controlled dosing study. *Journal of Alternative and Complementary Medicine (New York, N.Y.)*, *23*(3), 201–207. doi:10.1089/acm.2016.0140 PMID:28296480

Takei, Y., Kumano, S., Hattori, S., Uehara, T., Kawakubo, Y., Kasai, K., ... Mikuni, M. (2009). Preattentive dysfunction in major depression: A magnetoencephalography study using auditory mismatch negativity. *Psychophysiology*, *46*(1), 52–61. doi:10.1111/j.1469-8986.2008.00748.x PMID:19055502

Taylor, W. D., MacFall, J. R., Gerig, G., & Krishnan, R. R. (2007). Structural integrity of the uncinate fasciculus in geriatric depression: Relationship with age of onset. *Neuropsychiatric Disease and Treatment*, *3*(5), 669. PMID:19300596

Tondo, L., Visioli, C., Preti, A., & Baldessarini, R. J. (2014). Bipolar disorders following initial depression: Modeling predictive clinical factors. *Journal of Affective Disorders*, *167*, 44–49. doi:10.1016/j.jad.2014.05.043 PMID:25082113

Trivedi, M. H., Rush, A. J., Wisniewski, S. R., Nierenberg, A. A., Warden, D., Ritz, L., ... Shores-Wilson, K. (2006). Evaluation of outcomes with citalopram for depression using measurement-based care in STAR* D: Implications for clinical practice. *The American Journal of Psychiatry*, *163*(1), 28–40. doi:10.1176/appi.ajp.163.1.28 PMID:16390886

Troy, A. S., Wilhelm, F. H., Shallcross, A. J., & Mauss, I. B. (2010). Seeing the silver lining: Cognitive reappraisal ability moderates the relationship between stress and depressive symptoms. *Emotion (Washington, D.C.)*, *10*(6), 783–795. doi:10.1037/a0020262 PMID:21058843

Ueoka, Y., Tomotake, M., Tanaka, T., Kaneda, Y., Taniguchi, K., Nakataki, M., ... Ohmori, T. (2011). Quality of life and cognitive dysfunction in people with schizophrenia. *Progress in Neuro-Psychopharmacology & Biological Psychiatry*, *35*(1), 53–59. doi:10.1016/j.pnpbp.2010.08.018 PMID:20804809

van Bronswijk, S. C., Lemmens, L. H., Keefe, J. R., Huibers, M. J., DeRubeis, R. J., & Peeters, F. P. (2018). A prognostic index for long-term outcome after successful acute phase cognitive therapy and interpersonal psychotherapy for major depressive disorder. *Depression and Anxiety*. doi:10.1002/da.22868 PMID:30516871

Wacker, J., Dillon, D. G., & Pizzagalli, D. A. (2009). The role of the nucleus accumbens and rostral anterior cingulate cortex in anhedonia: Integration of resting EEG, fMRI, and volumetric techniques. *NeuroImage*, *46*(1), 327–337. doi:10.1016/j.neuroimage.2009.01.058 PMID:19457367

Weinberg, A., Perlman, G., Kotov, R., & Hajcak, G. (2016). Depression and reduced neural response to emotional images: Distinction from anxiety, and importance of symptom dimensions and age of onset. *Journal of Abnormal Psychology*, *125*(1), 26–39. doi:10.1037/abn0000118 PMID:26726817

Weitz, E., Kleiboer, A., van Straten, A., & Cuijpers, P. (2018). The effects of psychotherapy for depression on anxiety symptoms: A meta-analysis. *Psychological Medicine*, 1–13. PMID:29361995

Winthorst, W. H., Roest, A. M., Bos, E. H., Meesters, Y., Penninx, B. W., Nolen, W. A., & de Jonge, P. (2017). Seasonal affective disorder and non-seasonal affective disorders: results from the NESDA study. *BJPsych Open, 3*(4), 196-203.

Woolley, C. S., Gould, E., Frankfurt, M., & McEwen, B. S. (1990). Naturally occurring fluctuation in dendritic spine density on adult hippocampal pyramidal neurons. *The Journal of Neuroscience*, *10*(12), 4035–4039. doi:10.1523/JNEUROSCI.10-12-04035.1990 PMID:2269895

Wu, Z., Zhong, X., Peng, Q., Chen, B., Mai, N., & Ning, Y. (2017). Negative bias in expression-related mismatch negativity (MMN) in remitted late-life depression: An event-related potential study. *Journal of Psychiatric Research*, *95*, 224–230. doi:10.1016/j.jpsychires.2017.08.019 PMID:28892767

Wyczesany, M., Ligeza, T. S., & Grzybowski, S. J. (2015). Effective connectivity during visual processing is affected by emotional state. *Brain Imaging and Behavior*, *9*(4), 717–728. doi:10.100711682-014-9326-8 PMID:25339066

Yadav, G., & Mutha, P. K. (2016). Deep Breathing Practice9 Facilitates Retention of Newly Learned Motor Skills. *Scientific Reports*, *6*(1), 37069. doi:10.1038rep37069 PMID:27841345

Yeung, N., Botvinick, M. M., & Cohen, J. D. (2004). The neural basis of error detection: Conflict monitoring and the error-related negativity. *Psychological Review*, *111*(4), 931–959. doi:10.1037/0033-295X.111.4.931 PMID:15482068

Yoon, K. L., Joormann, J., & Gotlib, I. H. (2009). Judging the intensity of facial expressions of emotion: Depression-related biases in the processing of positive affect. *Journal of Abnormal Psychology*, *118*(1), 223–228. doi:10.1037/a0014658 PMID:19222328

Zhao, Q., Tang, Y., Chen, S., Lyu, Y., Curtin, A., Wang, J., ... Tong, S. (2015). Early perceptual anomaly of negative facial expression in depression: An event-related potential study. *Neurophysiologie Clinique. Clinical Neurophysiology*, *45*(6), 435–443. doi:10.1016/j.neucli.2015.09.011 PMID:26602972

Chapter 11
Social Media Analytics to Predict Depression Level in the Users

Mohammad Shahid Husain
https://orcid.org/0000-0003-4864-9485
Ibri College of Applied Sciences, Oman

ABSTRACT

As people around the world are spending increasing amounts of time online, the question of how online experiences are linked to health and wellbeing is essential. Depression has become a public health concern around the world. Traditional methods for detecting depression rely on self-report techniques, which suffer from inefficient data collection and processing. Research shows that symptoms linked to mental illness are detectable on social media like Twitter, Facebook, and web forums, and automatic methods are more and more able to locate inactivity and other mental disease. The pattern of social media usage can be very helpful to predict the mental state of a user. This chapter also presents how activities on Facebook are associated with the depressive states of users. Based on online logs, we can predict the mental state of users.

INTRODUCTION

This chapter also presents how activities on Facebook are associated with the depressive states of users. Based on online logs, we can predict the mental state of users. For example depressed individuals reported smaller involvement on social networks regarding comments and likes, the two popular forms of interactions. In contrast to the decreased level of interactions, depressed individuals showed an increase in the wall post rates and were active online during odd times of the day, which can be interpreted as an endemic behavior linked to the perceived degree of loneliness among young adults who are avid users of social media.

DOI: 10.4018/978-1-5225-8567-1.ch011

In this chapter, I will discuss these findings from theoretical, empirical, and subjective perspectives. In this chapter, I proposed a classifier that could differentiate between depressed and non-depressed users on Facebook. The results of the proposed system corroborates the idea that it may indeed be possible to differentiate between depressed and non-depressed Facebook users based on subtle linguistic and behavioral cues. My research could also benefit those who are struggling with other mental illnesses.

BACKGROUND

Depression is a common mental disorder, characterized by persistent sadness and a loss of interest in activities that you normally enjoy, accompanied by an inability to carry out daily activities, for at least two weeks.

Depression is a common chronic disorder with adverse effects for well-being and daily functioning. people with depression normally have several of the following: a loss of energy; a change in appetite; sleeping more or less; anxiety; reduced concentration; indecisiveness; restlessness; feelings of worthlessness, guilt, or hopelessness; and thoughts of self-harm or suicide. One of the most common depression types is major depression disorder (MDD) with patients having symptoms like depressive mood accompanied by low self-esteem, laziness and lack of pleasure:

The number of patients diagnosed with depression increases by 20% every year ranking it as the leading cause of disability worldwide and is a major contributor to the overall global burden of disease. (World Health Organization, 2018)

Depression may become a serious health condition. It can cause the affected person to suffer greatly and function poorly at work, at school and in the family. At its worst, depression can lead to suicide. A study conducted in 2012 shows that depression causes one death every 40 seconds worldwide (World Health Organization, n.d.). Close to 800,000 people die due to suicide every year and suicide is the second leading cause of death in 15-29-year-olds (World Health Organization, n.d.).

Depression has severe effects on individuals as well as society because it can lead to a suicide as well as other mental disorders.

According to WHO, approx. 5 crore people suffer from Depression. The WHO report estimates that about 322 million people worldwide suffered from depression over in 2015 (World Health Organization (World Health Organization, 2017b). In 2012 Lancet report revealed that "A Student Commit Suicide Every Hour in India" (Bhardwa, 2017). WHO in his report "Depression and other common Mental Disorders-Global Health Estimates" mentioned that overall 7, 88,000 commit suicide and the number of suicides of students is approx. 8934 in 2015 (World Health Organization, 2017a).

In the leading five years 39775 students killed themselves and many of the suicides are unreported. Depression accounts for more disability-adjusted life years (DALYs) than all other mental disorders, and it is becoming the main reason of disability in high-income countries (World Health Organization, 2017a).

Early detection of depression can help in providing required treatment like educating family members so that they provide support for stress relief, Psychotherapy such as cognitive behavioural therapy (CBT), interpersonal psychotherapy and drug treatment.

Miserably, traditional detection methods demand access to and desire to express using a psychologist and rely chiefly over annotation created at some stage in short sessions. Subsequently, circumstances leading to preventable suicides pot usually no longer hold correctly diagnosed (World Health Organization, 2017b). Without Identifying physical symptoms, diagnosing of depression is a challenging issue (Lin et al., 2016). Various studies shows mixed results related to depression, and all of them concluded that by applying various methods and techniques it is possible to predict mental state of a user.

Social Networking sites like Facebook and Twitter are now become popular in every one's life, over 90% people using social media every day for sharing their sentiments, opinions etc. (Suhara, Xu, & Pentland, 2017).

According to statistics of Social Media the overall World population is 7.6 billion and internet possesses 3.5 billion users and 3.03 billion active social media users (Hassan & Hijazi, 2018). Facebook has its own 2.072 billon users and it adds 500,000 users every day and Twitter has330 million users (Statista, n.d.). Facebook Messenger and WhatsApp handle 60 million messages a day (Goode, 2016).

It is possible that social networking sites provide a sense of security and belonging which allow users to disclose thoughts and feelings that are normally hidden to other people in other forms of communication. These seemingly private thoughts and feelings can then be used by the concerns with help of social media analytical tools to detect subclinical depression and suggest remedies to the users.

The analysis of data gathered from the social media can help effectively in predicting the mental state of a user. Like the content a user posts on social media, the contents liked or disliked by the users, the geographic locations tagged by the users and the time of a day user is more active on social media.

Symptoms of Depression

In general, different patients suffering from depression exhibits different symptoms based on their condition and severity. According to the recommendations of the Diagnostic and Statistical Manual 4th ed. (DSM-IV) that to be diagnosed with major depressive disorder, a patient must exhibit five or more of the following symptoms:

- Having depressed mood most of the time almost every day.
- Their interest or pleasure diminishes in all or almost all activities day by day.
- Substantial weight loss or gain
- Unintentional increase/decrease in appetite.
- Affected with sleeplessness or oversleeping.
- Noticeable psychomotor agitation or retardation nearly every day.
- Lethargies or loss of energy.
- Feelings of worthlessness.
- Either excessive or inappropriate guilt.
- Diminished ability to think, concentrate, or make decisions nearly every day.
- Recurrent thoughts of death
- No desire to live, recurrent suicidal ideation without a specific plan, or a suicide attempt and specific plan

Significance

A report published in November 2017 states that "according to the Centers for Disease Control and Prevention (CDC), 7.6 percent of people over the age of 12 have depression in any 2-week period" (Chang, 2018). This is substantial and shows the scale of the issue.

In 2012 Lancet report revealed that "A Student Commit Suicide Every Hour in India". WHO in his report "Depression and other common Mental Disorders-Global Health Estimates" mentioned that overall 7, 88,000 commit suicide and the number of suicides of students is approx. 8934 in 2015 (World Health Organization, 2017a).

It is important to monitor user's psychological states such as anxiety disorders, insomnia, and depression. With the rapid spread of social networks, researches on using social media data for physical and mental healthcare are also increasingly growing. Among them, depression is currently one of the most commonly diagnosed mental disorder around the world. And, depression has severe effects on individuals as well as society because it can lead to a suicide as well as other mental disorders.

Some Statistics

1. Around 6.7% persons have serious problems with depression.
2. Depression is more in women compared to men.
3. The prevalence of adults with a major depressive episode is highest among individuals between 18 and 25.

PREDICTION OF DEPRESSION

Prediction Based on Survey Responses

In psychological and epidemiological research, self-report surveys are second only to clinical interviews. Psychometric self-report surveys for mental illness have a high degree of validity and reliability. In this approach, data collected from various sources is analysed against some set of benchmarks to predict or classify whether a user is suffering from depression or not and its severity. Commonly used standards by researchers for this purpose to score the level of depression are:

1. Center for Epidemiologic Studies Depression Scale Revised (CESD-R).
2. Beck's Depression Inventory (BDI).

Center for Epidemiologic Studies Depression Scale developed in 1977 is the most widely used method in the field of psychiatric epidemiology. This survey has 20 questions to measure the depression symptoms divided into in 9 categories. For each question, user must give his response ranging from 0-3, based on his feeling. The total score is calculated as the sum of all the responses.

Beck's Depression Inventory consists of 21 items to measure the symptoms of depression in a person above the age of 13. It's a multiple-choice format where each item has four responses with severity ranging from 0-3.

Figure 1. (Source: National Institute of Mental Health (NIMH) report, 2015)

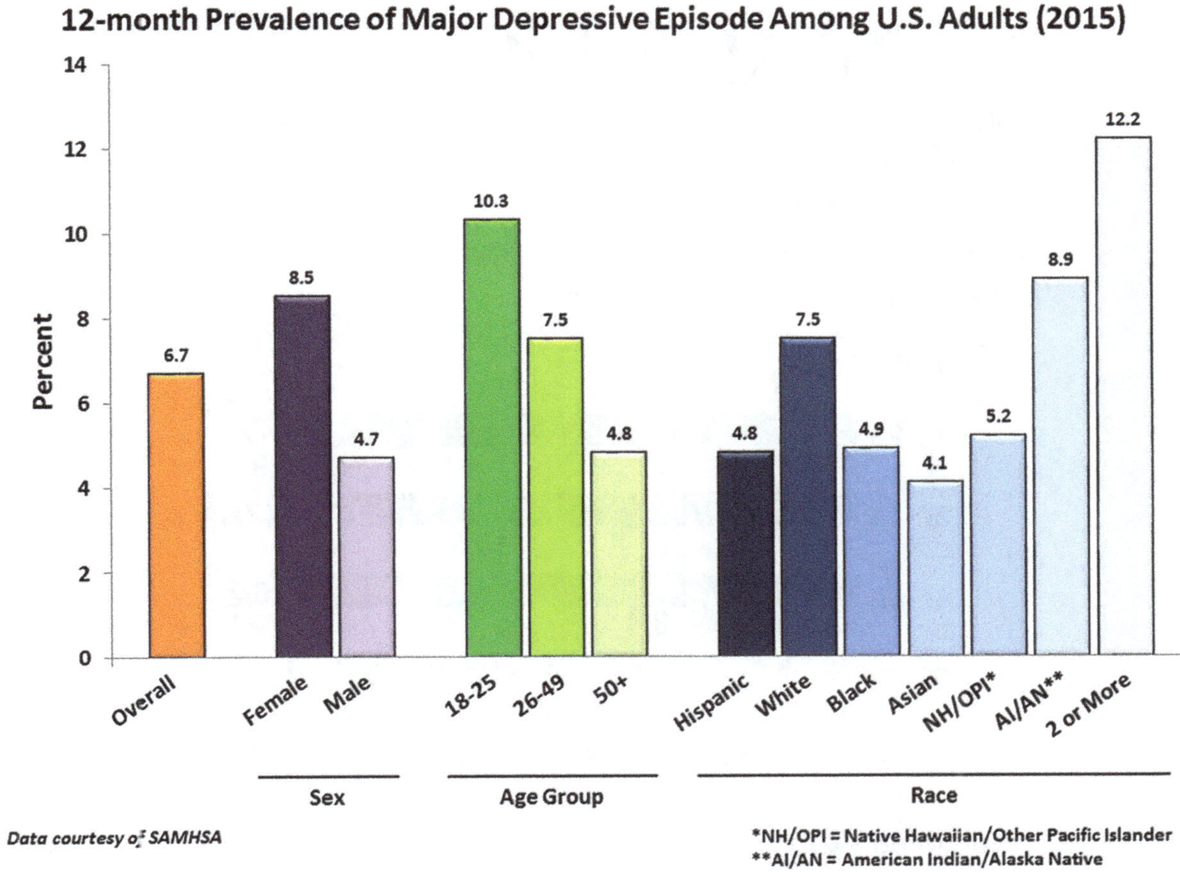

Prediction Based on Self-Declared Mental Health Status

Several studies use publicly accessible data. 'Self-declared' mental illness diagnosis on Twitter (identified through statements such as 'I was diagnosed with depression today') is one such source of publicly-available data. We review seven studies of this kind. Helping to facilitate studies of this kind, a Computational Linguistics and Clinical Psychology (CLPsych) workshop was started in 2014 to foster cooperation between clinical psychologists and computer scientists.

Prediction Based on Forum Membership

Online forums and discussion websites are a second source of publicly-available text related to mental health. They offer a space in which users can ask for advice, receive and provide emotional support, and generally discuss stigmatized mental health problems openly.

Figure 2. Suicide rate in India (2014)

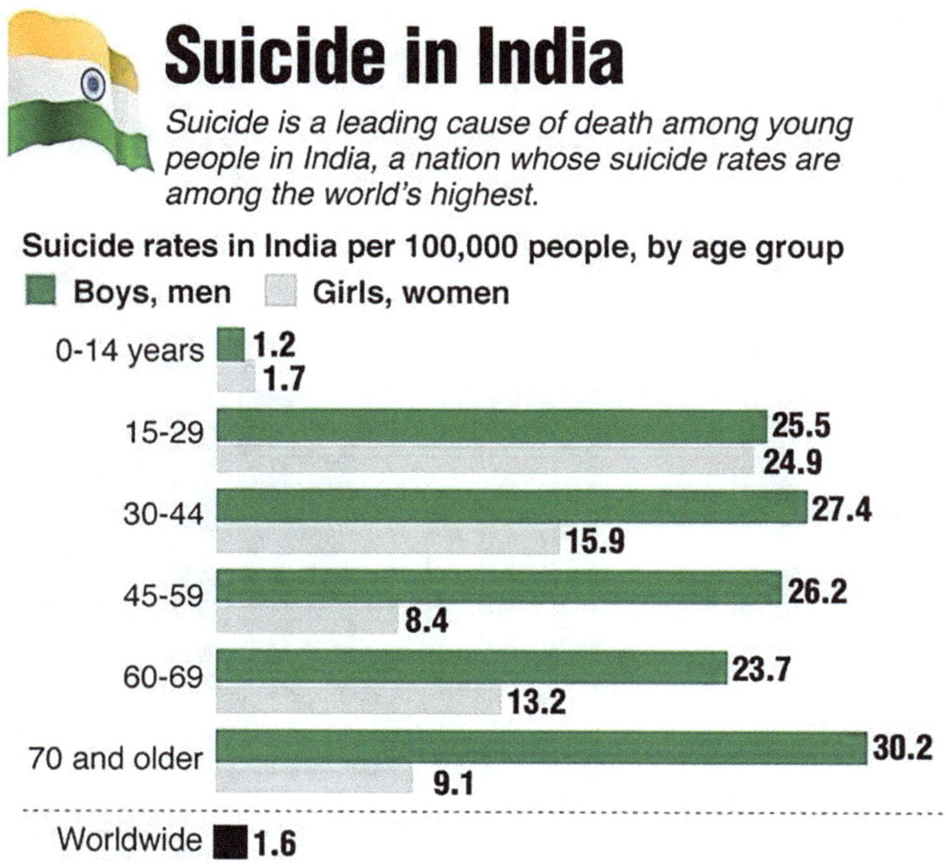

Figure 3. Suicide rate in students over the years (source: The Telegraph India, 2018)

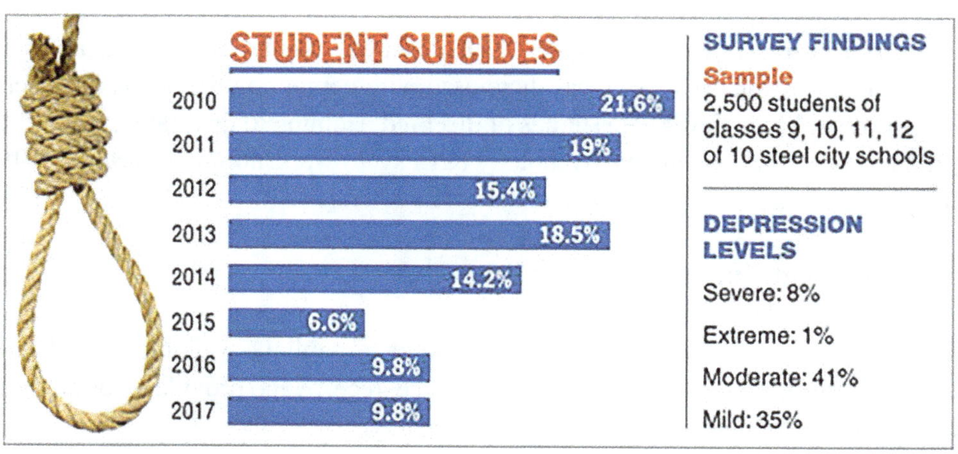

Prediction Based on Annotated Posts

A third source of publicly-available text involves manually examining and annotating Tweets that contain mental health keywords. Annotators code social media posts according to pre-established (a priori, theory-driven) or bottom-up (determined from the data) classifications; annotations can be predicted from the language of posts. Big data in the behavioural sciences that is, not using cross-validation.

Current Opinion in Behavioural Sciences, most annotation studies on depression focus on identifying posts in which users are discussing their own experience with depression.

Annotators are provided with guidelines on how to recognize a broad range of symptoms of depression that are derived from clinical assessment manuals such as the DSM-5, or a reduced set of symptoms, such as depressed mood, disturbed sleep and fatigue.

Annotation has also been used to differentiate between mentions of mental illness for the purpose of stigmatization or insult as opposed to voicing support or sharing useful information with those suffering from a mental illness.

In general, annotations of posts are a complementary (but labour-intensive) method that can reveal life circumstances associated with mental illness (e.g. occupational and educational problems, or the weather not captured by traditional depression diagnostic criteria. Questionnaire (PHQ) and Hospital Anxiety and Depression Scale (HADS) obtain high AUCs of around .90 against structured clinical interviews.

MENTAL STATE ANALYTICS USING SOCIAL MEDIA

Supervised Models

Most of the work on predicting latent user attributes in social media apply supervised models – Support Vector Machines (SVM) for binary classification e.g., gender and regression for continuous categorical attributes e.g., age with lexical bag-of-word features for predicting user gender or political orientation. work on adding socio-linguistic features to improve user attribute prediction, show that incorporating stylistic and syntactic information to the bag-of-word features improves classification performance.

Unsupervised Models

Other works for personal analytics exploit unsupervised approaches show that large-scale clustering of user names in Twitter improves gender, ethnicity and location classification performance.

STATE OF THE ART

Peter Burnap et.al Created a new human-annotated dataset to help identify features of suicidal ideation, creating a set of benchmark experimental results for machine learning approaches to the classification of suicidal ideation, and developing a machine classifier capable of distinguishing between worrying language such as suicidal ideation, and implant references to suicide, awareness raising about suicide and reports of suicide. They collected user posts from four known Web sites identified by experts in the field Then they collected data from micro blogging site Tumbler specifically, content containing self-classified suicidal ideation then they applied Term Frequency / inverse document frequency (TF. IDF) method to the corpus of annotated documents in order to identify terms that appear frequently in the suicidal ideation class but appear with less frequency in the non-ideation class. They use Stanford parts of speech for feature extraction, Linguistic Inquiry and Word Count LIWC text analysis software to extract more specific labels representing a effective emotions and feelings within the text. Applied Principal Component Analysis (PCA) as a dimension reduction procedure to convert the set of all possibly correlated variables within the combined set into a new set of linearly uncorrelated features (called principal components). Weka machine learning libraries-to conduct baseline experiments most popular classifiers- for classification Support Vector Machine (SVM), Rule Based (we used Decision Trees (DT)), Naive Bayes (NB) used as a probabilistic approachJ48 decision tree (C4.5) to perform rule-based experiments Rotation Forest (RF), which splits the feature set into a number of smaller sets the results are calculated by taking the mean accuracy across all models . From this analysis we observed that word-lists and regular expressions (regex) extracted from online suicide-related discussion fora and other micro blogging Web sites appear capable of capturing relevant language `clues', both in terms of single words, n-grams (word-lists) and more complex patterns.

Keumhee Kang et al. proposed an approach to identify users with the depressive moods from their daily tweets. For this, they develop a multimodal analysis using texts, emoticons, and images. Theyuse Sentistrength: considers texts and emoticons to understand the mood of short informal texts, F1-score: the harmonic mean of precision and recall. Color compositions (CCs) and SIFT as visual features to describe the images. (1)A learning-based analysis is performed for the texts, which considers the forms and structures of a sentence as well as the words related to the human moods; (2) for the emoticon, they build a new lexicon that includes 136 negatives and 66 positives and perform the word-based analysis; (3) the images belong to a tweet is analyzed by SVM-based learning. Color-based descriptors (color compositions) demonstrate the strong relationship between visual features, such as colors and shapes, and human moods. They SIFT descriptors for images. K-means clustering- for building a vocabulary tree WorldNet 2.1 parser, they identify each word's parts of speech (POS) in a sentence. The radial basis functions- for mood prediction LIWC- for comparing the obtained results. Results confirmed that the proposed multimodal analysis method has the higher accuracy than existing methods and it can predict individuals' moods more efficiently.

Elvis Saravia et al. proposed a novel data collection mechanism and build predictive models that leverage language and behavioral patterns, used particularly on Twitter, to determine whether a user is suffering from a mental disorder. By utilizing users Twitter feed, they design a system; MIDAS that automatically performs a mental health checkup. This is beneficial for the patients that are physically or mentally unable to partake in traditional screening tests. TF-IDF - to model the linguist features of patients. Pattern of Life Features (PLF) - adopted from the work of Coppersmith et al., is used to model the behavioral style of patients. They built an online system that allows for the exploration of various properties of a user with respect to two particular mental disorders. This system provides minimal results which can be exploited to build more complex systems to better understand a user behavior online. In addition, the system can be used to collect more data of patients through providing a means of returning feedback.

Munmun De Choudhury et al. have demonstrated the potential of using social media as a reliable tool for measuring population-scale depression patterns. The author adopted a crowdsourcing strategy of collecting ground truth data on depression from Twitter, and devised a variety of measures such as language, emotion, style and user engagement to build an SVM classifier. The classifier predicted with high accuracy (73%) whether or not a post on Twitter could be depression-indicative. Thereafter, the trained model was leveraged in a population-scale measurement metric of depression—called the social media depression index. Variety of analyses around geography, gender and time showed that SMDI can closely mirror CDC defined statistics on depression. Using Amazon's Mechanical Turk interface, we designed HITs wherein crowd workers were asked to take a clinical depression survey, followed by self-report seeking questions on their depression history. CES-D (Center for Epidemiologic Studies Depression Scale) questionnaire as the primary tool to determine the depression levels in the crowd workers. Use LIWC to measure the emotional state. They deploy principal component analysis (PCA). The classification algorithm is a standard Support Vector Machine classifier with an RBF kernel, although we experimented with other parametric and non-parametric supervised learning methods. They use five-fold cross validation and conduct 100 randomized experimental runs.

Quan Hu et al. proposed a model to predict user's depression via SinaWeibo data. Specifically, they aimed to build classification models for differentiating participants with high and low scores on self-report depression measurement (CES-D), and train regression models for predicting the CESD score of any individual user. This study only focused on active user's whose Weibo data three steps were followed in this study: (1) Data collection, (2) Features extraction and selection, and (3) Models training and evaluation. And they uses, breadth-first search. - For crawling a particular user's social network., online depression questionnaire CES-D to be filled by users.

In this study, they used Chinese text analysis software "WenXin" to process the text of Weibo posts and extract 88 designed linguistic features Based on the two-dimensional matrix; they can export time series data. In this paper, they define 5 behavior series for each initial dynamic feature. Then, they used Greedy Stepwise (GS) algorithm for features selection, built classification models using Logistic regression. For training classification models, they calculated the mean value and standard deviation of depression scores in each matrix and averaged values of twenty matrices. Besides, they built regression models using linear regression method and run 10-fold cross-validation while training and testing classification and regression models in this paper, they used Precision (P) to evaluate the performance of classification models, and used Pearson's Correlation Coefficient (CC) to evaluate the performance of regression models.

The results indicate that: (1) It is feasible to predict individual user's depression via social media data. (2) There is an effect of hysteresis for predicting depression through social media data.

Pan Liu et al. aimed to examine the relationship between emotional expressions in Facebook status updates and SWB further Data were obtained from the my Personality Facebook application, which has been used by more than six million users to voluntarily take a variety of psychological tests and receive feedback. They used LIWC: a reliable tool for measuring emotional expressions Result: The study reveals the temporal relationship between emotional expressions in Facebook status updates and SWB. It showed that users' negative (but not positive) emotional expressions in Facebook status updates from the past 9–10 months were negatively related to their life satisfaction. The results suggest that both the valence and the time frame of emotional expressions determine whether Facebook status updates can accurately reflect users' subjective well-being. The findings shed light on the characteristics of online social media and improve the understanding of how user-generated contents reflect users' psychological states.

CASE STUDY

System Design

This work aims to determine Mental State of users using Social Media (Facebook) to find out depressed and non-Depressed users. Mentally ill users usually post their sentiments and emotions on Facebook and by applying methods and techniques to find out depressed users. Based on a set of optimized features, our goal was automatic depression recognition which will still be able to correctly classify a person as depressed even if they are trying to hide their depression. Healthy individuals who alter their behavior to appear depressed were not of interest in this study.

The psychological state of an individual is reflected in several day-to-day behavior and activities, including phone call interval and duration, pattern of test messaging through SMS and social network, preferred company and place etc.

We created a Social Networking Platform RapidShot just like a Facebook using Java, and it almost works like a Facebook in which approx. 500 users are registered. They post their status, comments, like other user's posts. In short here Users shows their true emotions and sentiments by posting and liking on Facebook. By creating this platform we collected a real-time data of different users so that we can predict the Mental State of Users.

Data Collection

We registered the users who are willing to use this platform by their own choice, because the traditional methods such as questionnaires are given to the users to predict their mental state by asking questions to them. So in questionnaire system there is not surety that a user is showing their sentiments honestly or not. But my platform uses only real -time data where users post their sentiments honestly. The platform is designed for both desktop computer and mobile environments, and it therefore has two different versions, one for the desktop computer and one for the mobile device. The two versions share the same database.

Figure 4. Dataset of all users in CSV format

	A	B	C	D	E	F	G	H	I	J
1	19	asharr896(	uploadphotos/_2018-05-	I love my Mom and Dad	08:25:13am	2/1/2018	Jankipuram	Lucknow	Uttar Pradesh 226021	India
2	21	asharr896(	uploadphotos/_2018-05-	One of the greatest titles in the world is parent, and on	08:27:42am	2/1/2018	Jankipuram	Lucknow	Uttar Pradesh 226021	India
3	22	asharr896(	uploadphotos/_2018-05-	Enjoy life..Try to Forgive Everyone..	09:01:14am	2/1/2018	Jankipuram	Lucknow	Uttar Pradesh 226021	India
4	23	asharr896(	uploadphotos/_2018-05-	I want to visit this place once in a life..its awesome..	08:47:44am	2/2/2018	Jankipuram	Lucknow	Uttar Pradesh 226022	India
5	24	asharr896(	uploadphotos/_2018-05-	When life puts you in tough situations, dont say, why m	08:52:26am	2/3/2018	Jankipuram	Lucknow	Uttar Pradesh 226023	India
6	25	kashif945:	uploadphotos/_2018-05-	My Life's thought..i do not expect anything from anyo	09:04:38am	2/6/2018	Damana	Bhubaneswar	Odhisa	India
7	26	kashif945:	uploadphotos/_2018-05-	Life is the second name of enjoy...so enjoy every mom	09:12:30am	2/6/2018	Damana	Bhubaneswar	Odhisa	India
8	27	kashif945:	uploadphotos/_2018-05-	Happiness is the best medicine to be healthy.....	09:18:38am	2/6/2018	Damana	Bhubaneswar	Odhisa	India
9	28	kashif945:	uploadphotos/_2018-05-	Always be cool....because nobody knows tomorrow wh	09:22:01am	2/7/2018	Damana	Bhubaneswar	Odhisa	India
10	29	kashif945:	uploadphotos/_2018-05-	Always speak politely to others..first understand and th	09:27:19am	2/8/2018	Damana	Bhubaneswar	Odhisa	India
11	30	artiy@gm	uploadphotos/_2018-05-	I am not alone because loneliness is always with me	09:41:54am	2/11/2018	Kasimkota	Visakhapatnam	Andhra Pradesh	India
12	31	artiy@gm	uploadphotos/_2018-05-	Today I m sad because sometimes people live without	09:47:17am	2/11/2018	Kasimkota	Visakhapatnam	Andhra Pradesh	India
13	32	artiy@gm	uploadphotos/_2018-05-	Its ok to be a little sad sometimes	09:48:39am	2/12/2018	Kasimkota	Visakhapatnam	Andhra Pradesh	India
14	33	artiy@gm	uploadphotos/_2018-05-	Looking into others windows is a sign of extreme loneli	09:50:50am	2/13/2018	Kasimkota	Visakhapatnam	Andhra Pradesh	India
15	34	artiy@gm	uploadphotos/_2018-05-	I cannot prove myself everytime to everyone I m upset	09:56:47am	2/13/2018	Kasimkota	Visakhapatnam	Andhra Pradesh	India
16	35	artiy@gm	uploadphotos/_2018-05-	nothing to say I just want to die	10:07:40am	2/14/2018	Kasimkota	Visakhapatnam	Uttar Pradesh 226021	India
17	36	ayesha@g	uploadphotos/_2018-05-	i never forget you please comeback I cannot live withou	10:13:29am	2/17/2018	Ayojan Nagar	Ahmedabad	Gujarat	India
18	37	ayesha@g	uploadphotos/_2018-05-	I m sad because its nothing to be happy	10:15:09am	2/17/2018	Ayojan Nagar	Ahmedabad	Gujarat	India
19	38	ayesha@g	uploadphotos/_2018-05-	there i no one for whom i can share my pain so i remain	10:16:30am	2/18/2018	Ayojan Nagar	Ahmedabad	Gujarat	India
20	39	ayesha@g	uploadphotos/_2018-05-	Rain is the best partener because it hides my tears and	10:19:19am	2/18/2018	Ayojan Nagar	Ahmedabad	Gujarat	India
21	40	ayesha@g	uploadphotos/_2018-05-	Life hurts alot more than death Istruggled alot in my lif	10:22:23am	2/19/2018	Ayojan Nagar	Ahmedabad	Gujarat	India
22	41	navshad@	uploadphotos/_2018-05-	I hate people who comforts me with a lie i like truth ev	10:48:41am	2/22/2018	Hokka	Itanagar	Arunachal Pradesh	India
23	42	navshad@	uploadphotos/_2018-05-	My Life is hell as life is moving with a time complicatio	10:51:09am	2/22/2018	Hokka	Itanagar	Arunachal Pradesh	India
24	43	navshad@	uploadphotos/_2018-05-	Once if trust is broken then it will never be gain and i m	10:53:39am	2/24/2018	Hokka	Itanagar	Arunachal Pradesh	India
25	44	navshad@	uploadphotos/_2018-05-	U leave me today ur part in my life ends today is the mc	10:55:56am	2/24/2018	Hokka	Itanagar	Arunachal Pradesh	India

file10

About 2000 entries of different users are collect in the Dataset in which each user has different mental condition. Mentally ill users usually post their sentiments and emotions on Facebook.

Data Cleaning

We did a Data Cleaning process in which we remove data of that user which has less than 2 posts or that user who only registered but do not post any posts or like any post.

Creating a Classifier

The procedure to create the classifier, the tool I developed, can be broken down into the three steps. First, I gathered a set of depressed and non-depressed users and their posts, likes. Afterwards, I identified a set of features, characteristics of a user and his or her posts and likes that could be used to differentiate between depressed and non-depressed users. Finally, I used map reduce method to create a classifier to differentiate between depressed and non-depressed users based on these features. To gather a group of depressed users, I searched for Facebook users who discussed their depression online within a 24-hour window. To find a group of non-depressed users, I randomly sampled a set of users within that same 24-hour window. After gathering the depressed and non-depressed users, I obtained the last 2000 public posts. I did this starting from the month of July 2017 and up to the month of April 2018. After gathering the posts and likes of the depressed and non-depressed users, I observed many of their behavioral (how a user interacts with this Social network platform) and linguistic (characteristics of a user's language) features. Behavioral features included how often a user posted each day and how often a user mentioned other users in his or her posts. Linguistic features included characteristics of a user's language on. To put it all together, I used to create a classifier to differentiate between depressed and non-depressed users based on the features I identified. In my thesis, I specifically used a group of machine learning methods called supervised machine learning. These methods work by first providing a computer with many examples of depressed and non-depressed users. The computer analyzes these examples, and then based on what it observes, "learns" a set of rules through which it can classify future users. For example, a computer might decide that a user who references other users in his or her posts is not likely to be depressed, but if that user also uses many terms related to sadness, then the user is very likely to be depressed. A classifier is then created based on this set of rules. I used the February 2016 group of users as the examples, and then tested the resulting classifier by having it classify the April 2016 group of users

There are various aspects through which we can identify that a user is depressed.

- **Negative Emotion:** One Characteristic of the language of depressed users is that depressed individuals tend to use more words that carry negative emotion, such as "hurt" and "useless," than non-depressed individuals. This finding corresponds well with the theory that depressed individuals tend to have a negative cognitive bias—they generally have more negative thoughts than positive thoughts (Beck, 1967).
- **Anxiety:** Depressed individuals also tend to use more words related to feelings of anxiety, such as "afraid" and "confused," than non-depressed individuals. Anxiety is one of the mental disorders that occur most often with depression.

- **Sleep Duration and Quality:** Irregularity in sleep duration and quality is one of the key symptoms of depressive disorder. We can potentially detect depression by monitoring sleep pattern of users.
- **GPS Location:** Our survey outcome depicts that depression creates a significant change in movement pattern of individuals. Most of our survey participants prefer staying at home while depressed, when they were supposed to be at their work place. Our system will be designed and takes the location with a view to identify the change in movement pattern due to depression.
- **Communication Through Social Network:** Depressed individuals largely deviate from their usual social interaction which can be a potential indicator for depression detection.

Classification on the Basis of Keywords

From our Dataset we use keywords that indicate that a user is depressed, and from these keywords we find out both depressed and non-depressed users and classify them as shown in Table 1.

Table 1. Sample of keywords used by users to indicate depression

Keywords	Posts
Sadness	In deep sadness there is no place for sentimentality.
Alone	Pain makes people change, i wants to be alone, i am totally upset
Sad	I am all alone inside and also outside. Alone #loneliness #sad #upset
Death	Life hurts a lot more than death struggled a lot in my life
Die	nothing to say I just want to die
Suicide	I'm broken. There is no reason to alive I am going to attempt suicide
Upset	Pain makes people change, i wants to be alone, i am totally upset
Angry	Time changes everything, nobody supports me when i m in a trouble# angry# sad
Stressed	I really want to be happy, but there is something inside me that screams, you don't deserve it, feeling stressed
Pain	No one commit suicide because they want to die, but because they want to stop the pain.
Loneliness	I am all alone inside and also outside. Alone #loneliness #sad #upset
Painful	Death is easy. To live is the most painful thing I could imagine and I am weak and no longer willing to fight.
Worst	U leave me today your part in my life ends today is the most worst day in my life
Depressed	I am feeling so lonely and depressed, and even more i can't explain my feelings
Depression	Yesterday, I concerned psychiatrist, and i m suffering from Depression
Sick	I die every day. With this damn smile, And I am sick and tired of it already. I am not okay
Lonely	I am so lonely.
Kill	Loneliness doesn't KILL, but sometimes I wish it DID

Classification According to User Behavior

Classification on the Basis of User's Posts Time

We monitor user's sleeping time, and predict the mental state of a user also by monitoring the user's sleep quality. For example if a user posting negative thoughts late at 2 am then we considers that may be user is depressed.

Classification on the Basis of Location

We also classify users on the basis of location, means if a user is staying at home and not wants to go outside and meet anyone, because usually users when they are sad and depressed then they always want to stay at home and do not wants to meet anyone, posting negative posts on Social Networking site.

FINDINGS

Figure 7 shows the negative posts of all the users. Here red color indicates that these users posts more depressed posts indicating that they are depressed.

The Figure 8 represents the results obtained for one particular user discussing all the parameters (no of posts, time, location, likes). The Figure shows the total number of positive and negative posts in 2017. In the figure red color denotes the negative posts by the users, blue color denotes the positive posts by the users and purple color denotes the ratio between the two.

Figure 5. User post at time 2:00 am

381	399	meher@gmail.com	uploadph	When I dont express themselves, i will die one piece at a time	08:21:58am	5/23/2018	Nathnaga	Bhagalpur	West Ben	India
382	400	meher@gmail.com	uploadph	Dont feel bad, I am usually about to die	08:23:01am	5/24/2018	MG Marg	Gangtok	Sikkim	India
383	401	pallavi@gmail.com	uploadph	Depression is like a war. You either win or you die.	12:24:33pm	5/25/2018	MG Marg	Gangtok	Sikkim	India
384	402	pallavi@gmail.com	uploadph	You dont understand how much I hate myself.	11:25:13am	5/26/2018	MG Marg	Gangtok	Sikkim	India
385	403	pallavi@gmail.com	uploadph	I am feeling so lonely and depressed, and even more i cant explain my	08:26:09am	2/1/2018	MG Marg	Gangtok	Sikkim	India
386	404	pallavi@gmail.com	uploadph	Depression is about as close as you get to somewhere between dead	04:26:53pm	2/1/2018	MG Marg	Gangtok	Sikkim	India
387	405	pallavi@gmail.com	uploadph	my depression leads me into darkness. I don't want to meet anyone, I v	02:16:57am	2/1/2018	MG Marg	Gangtok	Sikkim	India
388	406	pallavi@gmail.com	uploadph	I didnt want to wake up. I was having a much better time asleep. And	08:29:46am	2/2/2018	MG Marg	Gangtok	Sikkim	India
389	407	pallavi@gmail.com	uploadph	Please save me, otherwise i will die	05:37:46pm	2/3/2018	Lotus Bak	Geyzing	Sikkim	India
390	408	pallavi@gmail.com	uploadph	when you have been sad for so long that when something bad happens	10:39:36am	2/6/2018	Lotus Bak	Geyzing	Sikkim	India
391	409	pallavi@gmail.com	uploadph	I just wanna disappear, Please kill me	09:40:31am	2/6/2018	Lotus Bak	Geyzing	Sikkim	India
392	410	pallavi@gmail.com	uploadph	That feeling when you are not necessarily sad, but you just feel really e	0346:51pm	2/6/2018	Lotus Bak	Geyzing	Sikkim	India

Figure 6. User post indicating location

381	399	meher@gmail.com	uploadph	When I dont express themselves, i will die one piece at a time	08:21:58am	5/23/2018	Nathnaga	Bhagalpur	West Ben	India
382	400	meher@gmail.com	uploadph	Dont feel bad, I am usually about to die	08:23:01am	5/24/2018	MG Marg	Gangtok	Sikkim	India
383	401	pallavi@gmail.com	uploadph	Depression is like a war. You either win or you die.	12:24:33pm	5/25/2018	MG Marg	Gangtok	Sikkim	India
384	402	pallavi@gmail.com	uploadph	You dont understand how much I hate myself.	11:25:13am	5/26/2018	MG Marg	Gangtok	Sikkim	India
385	403	pallavi@gmail.com	uploadph	I am feeling so lonely and depressed, and even more i cant explain my	08:26:09am	2/1/2018	MG Marg	Gangtok	Sikkim	India
386	404	pallavi@gmail.com	uploadph	Depression is about as close as you get to somewhere between dead	04:26:53pm	2/1/2018	MG Marg	Gangtok	Sikkim	India
387	405	pallavi@gmail.com	uploadph	my depression leads me into darkness. I don't want to meet anyone, I v	02:16:57am	2/1/2018	MG Marg	Gangtok	Sikkim	India
388	406	pallavi@gmail.com	uploadph	I didnt want to wake up. I was having a much better time asleep. And	08:29:46am	2/2/2018	MG Marg	Gangtok	Sikkim	India
389	407	pallavi@gmail.com	uploadph	Please save me, otherwise i will die	05:37:46pm	2/3/2018	Lotus Bak	Geyzing	Sikkim	India
390	408	pallavi@gmail.com	uploadph	when you have been sad for so long that when something bad happens	10:39:36am	2/6/2018	Lotus Bak	Geyzing	Sikkim	India
391	409	pallavi@gmail.com	uploadph	I just wanna disappear, Please kill me	09:40:31am	2/6/2018	Lotus Bak	Geyzing	Sikkim	India
392	410	pallavi@gmail.com	uploadph	That feeling when you are not necessarily sad, but you just feel really e	0346:51pm	2/6/2018	Lotus Bak	Geyzing	Sikkim	India

Figure 7. Graph of total no. of users and their posts

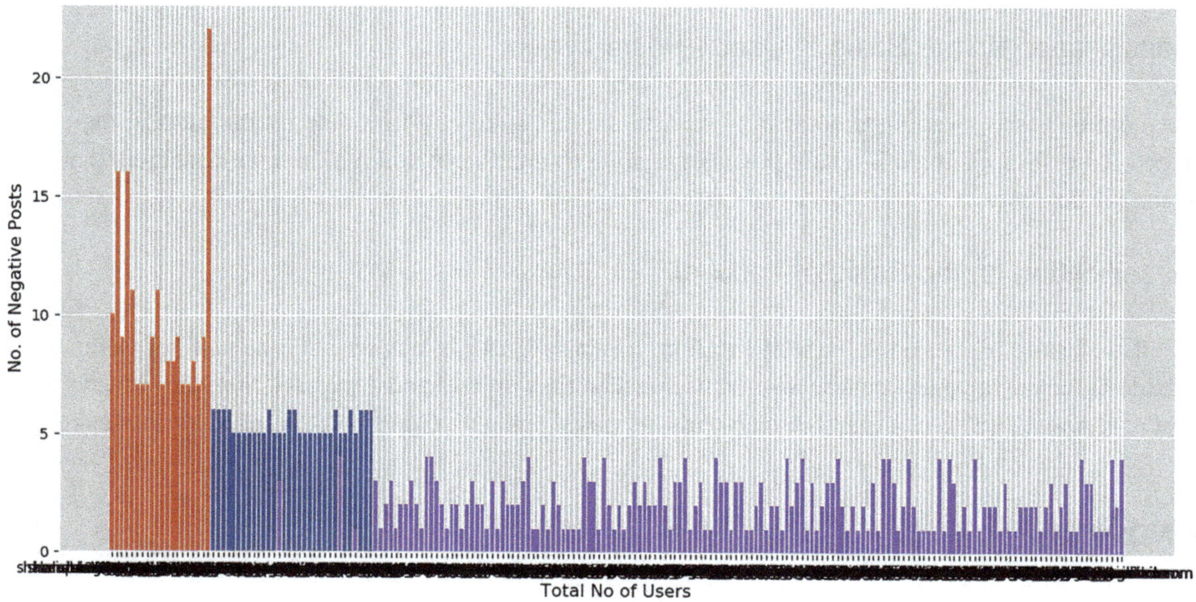

Figure 8. User's mental state in the month of May

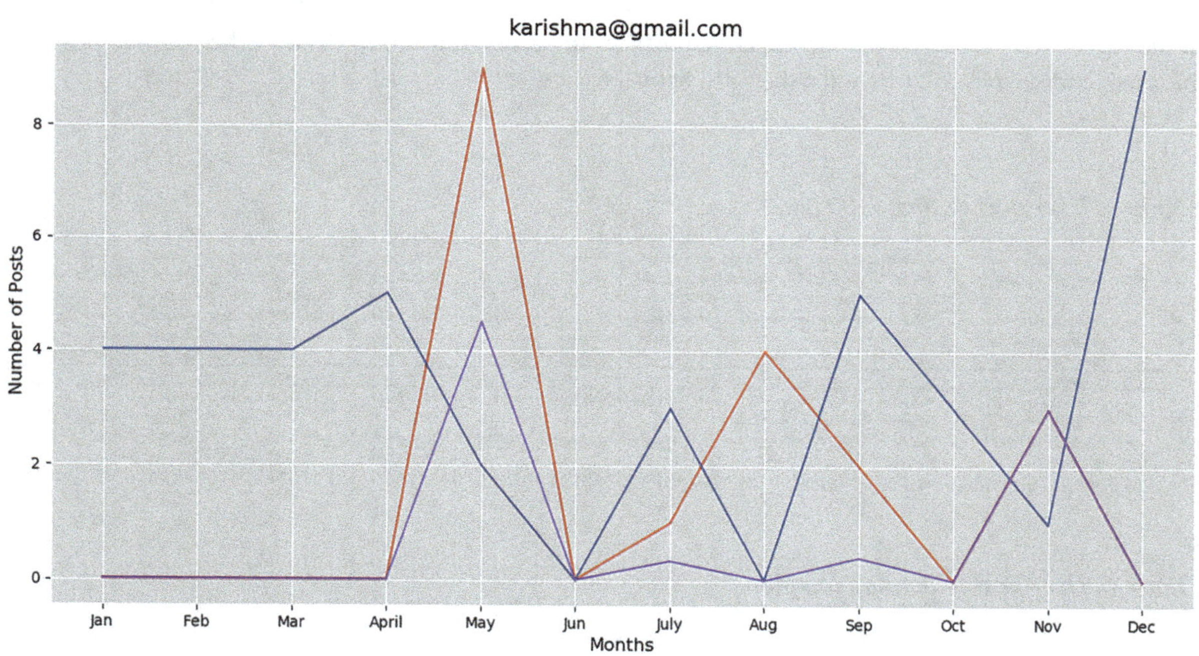

We monitor and analyze the sleeping time and location of the user and results shows that this user posts most of the sad and depressive posts late at night and her location remains constant for a long time. So from this monitoring, our analysis results that the user is critically depressed in the month of May.

CONCLUSION

The emergence of social media services such as Twitter, Google+ and online social networks like Facebook has dramatically influenced peoples' lives over the last decade. These services allow people to share their lives with others by posting updates and pictures online, follow other peoples' posts and stay connected across the world.

In this chapter we have addressed the depression that causes social, economic and health burden all around the globe. We have discussed by using keywords that what type of posts users usually posts that shows depression. We have shown the use of social media and machine learning techniques for developing a system which is capable of predicting depression automatically.

REFERENCES

American Psychiatric Association. (2013). Diagnostic and Statistical Manual of Mental Disorders (DSM-5). American Psychiatric Publishing.

Bagroy, S., Kumaraguru, P., & De Choudhury, M. (2017). A social media based index of mental well-being in college campuses. *Proceedings of the 2017 CHI Conference on Human Factors in Computing Systems*. 10.1145/3025453.3025909

Beck, A.T., Steer, R.A., & Brown, G.K. (1996). Beck depression inventory II. *San Antonio, 78*, 490-498.

Beck, Ward, & Mendelson. (1961). Beck depression inventory (bdi). *Archives of General Psychiatry, 4*(6), 561–571. doi:10.1001/archpsyc.1961.01710120031004 PMID:13688369

Bhardwa, S. (2017). *What do Student Mental Health Services Look Like Around the World*. Retrieved from https://www.timeshighereducation.com/student/blogs/what-do-student-mental-health-services-look-around-world

Cavazos-Rehg, P. A., Krauss, M., Sowles, S., Connolly, S., Rosas, C., Bharadwaj, M., & Bierut, L. (2016). A content analysis of depression-related tweets. *Computers in Human Behavior, 54*, 351–357. doi:10.1016/j.chb.2015.08.023 PMID:26392678

Chang, P. (2018). *What you need to Know About Depression*. Retrieved from https://virginiainfusion-therapies.com/what-you-need-to-know-about-depression/

Charlson, F. J., Baxter, A. J., Cheng, H. G., Shidhaye, R., & Whiteford, H. A. (2016). The burden of mental, neurological, and substance use disorders in China and India: A systematic analysis of community representative epidemiological studies. *Lancet, 388*(10042), 376–389. doi:10.1016/S0140-6736(16)30590-6 PMID:27209143

Ferrari, A. J., Charlson, F. J., Norman, R. E., Patten, S. B., Freedman, G., Murray, C. J. L., ... Whiteford, H. A. (2013). Burden of Depressive Disorders by Country, Sex, Age, and Year: Findings from the Global Burden of Disease Study 2010. *PLoS Medicine*, *10*(11), e1001547. doi:10.1371/journal.pmed.1001547 PMID:24223526

Goode, L. (2016). *Messenger and WhatsApp Process 60 Billion Messages a Day, Three Times More than SMS*. Retrieved from https://www.theverge.com/2016/4/12/11415198/facebook-messenger-whatsapp-number-messages-vs-sms-f8-2016

Hassan, N. A., & Hijazi, R. (2018). *Open Source Intelligence Methods and Tools*. New York: Apress. doi:10.1007/978-1-4842-3213-2

Kessler, R. C., & Bromet, E. J. (2013). The epidemiology of depression across cultures. *Annual Review of Public Health*, *34*(1), 119–138. doi:10.1146/annurev-publhealth-031912-114409 PMID:23514317

Li, J., Ritter, A., & Hovy, E. (2014). Weakly supervised user profile extraction from Twitter. *Proceedings of ACL*. 10.3115/v1/P14-1016

Lin, L. Y., Sidani, J. E., Shensa, A., Radovic, A., Miller, E., Colditz, J. B., ... Primack, B. A. (2016). Association between Social Media use and Depression among U.S. young adults. *Depression and Anxiety*, *33*(4), 323–331. doi:10.1002/da.22466 PMID:26783723

Lowe, B., Kroenke, K., Herzog, W., & Grafe, K. (2004). Measuring depression outcome with a brief self-report instrument: Sensitivity to change of the Patient Health Questionnaire (PHQ-9). *Journal of Affective Disorders*, *81*(1), 61–66. doi:10.1016/S0165-0327(03)00198-8 PMID:15183601

Megan, A. (2011). Feeling bad on Facebook: Depression disclosures by college students on a social networking site. *Depression and Anxiety*, *28*(6), 447–455. doi:10.1002/da.20805 PMID:21400639

National Institute of Mental Health. (2015). Retrieved from https://www.nih.gov/about-nih/what-we-do/nih-almanac/national-institute-mental-health-nimh

Radloff, L. S. (1977). The CES-D scale: A self-report depression scale for research in the general population. *Applied Psychological Measurement*, *1*(3), 385–401. doi:10.1177/014662167700100306

Reece, A.G., Reagan, A.J., Lix, K.L.M., Dodds, P.S., Danforth, C.M., & Langer, E.J. (2016). *Forecasting the Onset and Course of Mental Illness with Twitter Data*. Academic Press.

Reece & Danforth. (2016). *Instagram photos reveal predictive markers of depression*. Academic Press.

Statista. (n.d.). *Number of monthly active Facebook users worldwide as of 4th quarter 2018 (in millions)*. Retrieved from https://www.statista.com/statistics/264810/number-of-monthly-active-facebook-users-worldwide/

Stuart, A. (1979). A new depression scale designed to be sensitive to change. *The British Journal of Psychiatry*, *134*(4), 382–389. doi:10.1192/bjp.134.4.382 PMID:444788

Suhara, Y., Xu, Y., & Pentland, A. S. (2017). *DeepMood: Forecasting Depressed Mood Based on Self-Reported Histories via Recurrent Neural Networks*. Retrieved from http://papers.www2017.com.au.s3-website-ap-southeast-2.amazonaws.com/proceedings/p715.pdf

The Telegraph India. (2018). *Silent tormentor of students: depression.* Retrieved from https://www.telegraphindia.com/states/jharkhand/silent-tormentor-of-students-depression/cid/1373651

Üstün, T. B., Ayuso-Mateos, J. L., Chatterji, S., Mathers, C., & Murray, C. J. L. (2000). Global burden of depressive disorders in the year. *The British Journal of Psychiatry*, *2004*(184), 386–392. PMID:15123501

Woods, H. C., & Scott, H. (2016). #Sleepyteens: Social media use in adolescence is associated with poor sleep quality, anxiety, depression and low self-esteem. *Journal of Adolescence*, *51*, 41–49. doi:10.1016/j.adolescence.2016.05.008 PMID:27294324

World Health Organization. (2017a). *Depression and Other Common Mental Disorders.* Retrieved from https://apps.who.int/iris/bitstream/handle/10665/254610/WHO-MSD-MER-2017.2-eng.pdf;jsessionid=1529C9707E98EA8E0BAA603CF50A1927?sequence=1

World Health Organization. (2017b). *Depression in India Let's talk.* Retrieved from http://www.searo.who.int/india/depression_in_india.pdf

World Health Organization. (2018). *Depression.* Retrieved from https://www.who.int/news-room/fact-sheets/detail/depression

World Health Organization. (n.d.). *Suicide Data.* Retrieved from https://www.who.int/mental_health/prevention/suicide/suicideprevent/en/

Chapter 12
Linguistic Markers in Individuals With Symptoms of Depression in Bi-Multilingual Context

Anbu Savekar
National Institute of Technology Raipur, India

Shashikanta Tarai
National Institute of Technology Raipur, India

Moksha Singh
National Institute of Technology Raipur, India

ABSTRACT

Depression has been identified as the most prevalent mental disorder worldwide. Due to the stigma of mental illness, the population remains unidentified, undiagnosed, and untreated. Various studies have been carried out to detect and track depression following symptoms of dichotomous thinking, absolutist thinking, linguistic markers, and linguistic behavior. However, there is little study focused on the linguistic behavior of bilingual and multilingual with anxiety and depression. This chapter aims to identify the bi-multilingual linguistic markers by analyzing the recorded verbal content of depressive discourse resulting from life situations and stressors causing anxiety, depression, and suicidal ideation. Different contextual domains of word usage, content words, function words (pronouns), and negative valance words have been identified as indicators of psychological process affecting cognitive behavior, emotional health, and mental illness. These findings are discussed within the framework of Beck's model of depression to support the linguistic connection to mental illness-depression.

DOI: 10.4018/978-1-5225-8567-1.ch012

INTRODUCTION

The increasing levels of strain, anxiety and unending pressure of life events, adversities and constant life stress have been identified to be a source and trigger for depression (Fried et al., 2015; Mehl et al., 2017).The consistent source of stressors conjures depression particularly in interpersonal relationships demonstrating the bi-directional link between stress and depression(Hammen, 2015).According to WHO report (2017), depression is a common mental disorder that affects the people of all age group. The mental illness is considered a major cause of neural disability, neurodegenerator and most likely to incur suicide (Tarai et al.,2016). The onset of depression often goes undetected until it erupts into dysfunctional behavior, emotional disability, psychotic episode and even suicidality (Briggs et al., 2018; Stafford, 2018). The cause of depression could be biological, medical, social, situational, relational, or psychological. Most often mental illness remains untreated, undiagnosed and unidentified due to the stigma associated with mental health (Corrigan et al., 2014). A study by Beck and Alford (2009), has provided insights into understanding depression which assists both patients and their caregivers. Beck's study (1979), has established an understanding of depression as a cognitive disorder, whereas depression according to Fossati (2018), is a disorder with both emotional and cognitive symptoms in which cognition is the key element responsible for functional and social outcomes. Both linguists and psychologists agree that language is an effective medium indicating the emotional, psychological states and behavioural changes (Pennebaker & Stone, 2003; Rude et al., 2004; Pennebaker et al., 2003; Chung & Pennebaker, 2007). Language also identifies personality traits and emotional changes which are echoed in not only in the verbal communication of an individual but also in online digital communication between individuals (Boyd & Pennebaker, 2017; De Chaudhary et al., 2013). The key to understanding oneself and others is understanding emotions. Study of language is the most apt mode to understand emotions as language represents emotions and emotions enhance the use of language (Dewaele, 2010; Argaman, 2010; Yule, 2016). The increasing accuracy of emotion detection in text and transcript analysis has paved the way for numerous uses ranging from utilization in the field of Artificial Intelligence (AI) to preventing suicide. As established, at every dimension and structure of language (the syntactic and semantic elements), there is an expression of emotion in the style and content (Jedud, 2018).

Studies have been carried out on the use of language of the depressed and control group on cognitive functions associated with depression and those vulnerable to depression and what emerged was the predominant use of negative valance words and self-focus as in use of first-person pronoun "I" (Rude et al., 2010; Fossati, 2018). Emotional intensity in verbal communication is expressed by the use of intensifiers, the use of emotion words, repetitions, the use of first-person singular pronoun, the use of metaphors, and the use of exclamations (Argaman, 2010). The study of linguistic markers of severely stressed and depressed, can identify one who is on the threshold of chronic state, thereby facilitate early detection, care, handling and treatment. LeMoult and Gotlib (2018), pointed out the need to improve the approach towards the identification, prevention of depression and also refining cognitive models of depression to decrease the prevalence and severity as a debilitating emotional and mental disorder. Past study has identified the linguistic markers in major depressive disorders (Trifu et al., 2017), including bi-lingual context to find out words in use in the depression forums online in English and Spanish (Ramirez et al., 2008). However, the current study intends to identify the Hindi-English linguistic markers in bi-lingual context as prevalent in the state of Chhattisgarh in India.

Prevalence of Depressive Disorder

World Mental health day on October 10, 2018, aimed to bring awareness to a common illness affecting the population world over which nevertheless is marginalized by the society. The growing focus and significant concern have brought depression into a priority zone, and is now covered by WHO's mental health Gap Action Programme (mhGAP) (WHO Global Health estimate report 2017). Depression as a common yet serious mental health issue worldwide has affected and incapacitated a large number of people of all age groups. According to a survey by WHO, more than 322 million suffer and half of the numbers identified as the population suffering from depression, live in the South-East Asia Region and Western Pacific Region, the region which includes India and China (WHO report 2017).

Suicide has been identified as the main reason for deaths of youth every year. The most shocking point emerging is that inaccurate assessment and poor diagnosis of depression are due to a single major reason: the stigma associated with depression. Timely care and effective treatment can be administered provided depression is detected. According to WHO study and report, depressed individuals suffer from anxiety symptoms, poor sleep, poor appetite, low self-worth. It is far more than a mood swing and erratic emotional fluctuations of day to day life which if undiagnosed and untreated, results in disruption of normal functioning of the individual, his social skills and activities, seriously affecting and impacting the individual's life, work and family (WHO report 2017). The severity of depression ranges from mild, moderate to severe; affecting the individuals' routine life, health and family. The prevalence of depression is widespread and researchers are working to identify both clinical and non-clinical markers with better accuracy to facilitate early detection.

Stigma and Its Impact on Depression

Stigma has been identified as a universal phenomenon, with region-based variations relevant to the regional context (Thornicroft, 2006; Koschorke et al., 2017). A study has revealed that mental illness is under greater stigma than other illnesses (Corrigan, 2004). People do not seek treatment or utilize the services offered by healthcare schemes due to the stigma associated with owning the mental ill health (Corrigan & Kosyluk, 2014). The linguistic framing of depression using linguistic cues is a method to shift and shape the way people, situation or an event are perceived, as a drive against stigma and notions of depression (Reali et al., 2016). The stigma of depression has a psychosocial impact not only on the individual but also on the family causing larger levels of psychological suffering and disruption of their lives (Corrigan & Watson, 2002; Corrigan & Kleinlein, 2005). Stigma and depression are interrelated (Lannin et al., 2016; Pearl et al.,2017; Schomerus et al., 2018) as stigma corresponds to the context of the reasons causing, influencing, triggering, worsening the mental health condition. Stigma induces lowered cognitive and emotional functioning due to lower self-esteem, shame, guilt, futility, rumination, sleep disorders, and impairment. Stigmatizing attitudes such as prejudice, discrimination and lack of knowledge have obstructed not only the identification of signs of mental illness but also the pursuit of treatment with primary or specialist caregivers. Rendering support to family members by the community and mental health professionals can counter the negative effect of stigma (van der Sanden et al., 2016). The deliberation on the pros and cons continues whether mental illness requires normalcy (to be treated as one amongst us) or solidarity (where the community extends support) as a proactive measure in the stigma removal effort (Corrigan & Kosyluk, 2014).In the Indian context, definite sources associated with depression and the social stigma are identified with the various kinds of abuse (substance abuse, domestic violence, emotional, physical and sexual abuse); sexual and gender minority (transgender);medical (Tuberculosis, Leprosy, HIV patients, infertility in women) and medical abnormalities; society-based caste and community issues, inter-caste marriage, occupational (prostitution, manual waste scavenging) (Bohra et al., 2015; Verma et al., 2018). The identification of linguistic indicators in the bilingual context can be a very significant in identifying, diagnosing and treating the widely prevalent mental illness along with providing a proper social support system.

Depression: A Major Mental Illness

The reasons for depression, be it temporary or long-term could be social, internal-biological or psychological, medical, life events or even situational affecting the individual and his family. Symptoms of depression are cognitive, emotional, behavioural, physiological and motivational (American Psychiatric Association, 2013). Major Depressive Disorder (MDD) is a debilitating mental illness characterized by phases of depressed mood swings ranging from low mood to loss of interest in preferred activities accompanied by low self-esteem, impaired cognitive functions, disturbed sleep patterns and loss of appetite (Iyer & Khan, 2012; Yusof et al., 2017). The focus of attention is always towards negative thinking and therefore constantly on unhappiness, hopelessness, and a critical approach towards receiving information and interpreting information negatively (Beck, 1979; LeMoult et al., 2017). The symptoms of mental illness also include anxiety, reduced concentration, indecisiveness, restlessness, agitation, anger, guilt, self-harm, suicide ideation, attempting suicide due to chronic pessimistic beliefs (Rude et al., 2004; Otte et al., 2016). The diagnosis of depression is based on a number of indications including linguistic cues and evidence based on the patient's own self-identified experiences, behaviour informed by relatives or friends and clinical screening and examination of mental state. Studies have shown that self-identification induces the need and thereafter the intention to be helped in case of mental disorder (Schomerus et al., 2018). Currently, studies on tracking the social media interactions are being carried out to identify the depression by analysing the text (De Chaudhary et al., 2013). The study of language exposes the emotional, mental, socio-psychological and personality traits.

LANGUAGE CORRELATION BETWEEN ANXIETY, DEPRESSION, AND SUICIDE

Language plays a key role in bringing out the thought patterns and emotional state of the individuals affected by stress, anxiety, depression and suicidal ideation. The sources of stress, anxiety, depression and even suicide are numerous, and the factors leading to mental health issues could be social, personal, medical or biological in nature. The social factors leading to mental health issues can be classified by social bias in gender discrimination, social apathy and intolerance, relationship, professional and work place issues. The personal issues and concerns such as poor self-esteem, guilt, shame, anger, anxiety, substance abuse, sexual abuse, ageing, thwarted desires, the trauma of loss and neglect by family can be a cause of mental ill-health. The medical conditions such as personality disorders- bi-polar, eating disorder, and biological causes such as pre or post-partum depression, pre-menstrual syndrome or post menopause are also factors leading to mental health issues (Borah et al., 2015; Antoniou et al., 2017; Yusof et al., 2017).

Suicide, depression, anxiety and stress are interlinked. The consequence of stigma resulting in social isolation, increased hopelessness and financial burden such as joblessness has also the power to drive the depressed towards suicide ideation and suicide (Rusch et al., 2014). The relationship between mental illness and the identification followed by shame, secrecy, public stigma after disclosure has been the cause of suffering and trauma for the individual. One of the non-clinical and interdisciplinary modes of identifying the mental illness and detecting anxiety, depression and suicide ideation is by the study of the language of the affected individual. Table 1, contains the characteristic symptoms of both anxiety and depression and also the symptoms that are viable to both. The linguistic markers can identify the emotional, cognitive, behavioural and physical symptoms that are affected by stress, anxiety and depression. The study of linguistic markers in English language has recognised the pronounced use of absolute words as specific markers for anxiety, depression and suicide ideation (Rude et al., 2004; Al-Mosaiwi & Johnstone, 2018a). This study aims to explore the use of bilingual absolute words among other linguistic cues, present in the language of the bi-multilinguals.

Cognitive Characteristics Affected by Depression

Understanding the cognitive aspects of depression including language use and processing, relates the emotional and thought states to the phenomenon of depression. The shift towards negative bias in the information processing, perception, interpretation, attention and memory lapses are due to emotional dysregulation (Kircanski et al., 2012) and quite evident in the language of the depressed. Depression is characterized by cognitive biases and deficits in cognitive control (Joorman & Stanton, 2016). The cognitive functions that are affected in the initial phase are attention, learning, memory and executive functions. Cognitive issues causing disruption are likely to be the core features and indicators of the subsequent social and functional behavioral pattern in depressive individuals. It is characterized by negative processing of stimuli and increases the self-focus inclining to an unfavorable view of themselves. The thought patterns of the depressed are different from the normal people. As per the cognitive theory of depression laid by Beck, negative bias driven by negative thinking causes the depressed to perceive themselves, their environment and future in a pessimistic and negative light (Beck, 1979). Previously, the diagnosis was based on emotional changes correlating to depression (consistent sadness, mood fluc-

Table 1. Characteristic Symptoms (Emotional, Cognitive, Behavioral, Physical)

CHARACTERISTIC SYMPTOMS (Emotional, Cognitive, Behavioural, Physical)		
ANXIETY	COMMON SYMPTOMS	DEPRESSION
Indecision, Excessive worry, Difficulty in concentrating, Tense, Nervousness, Fear of social interaction, Irritability, Sleep disturbance, Fear, Weakness, Avoidance, Loss of appetite, Dry mouth, Nausea, Sweating, Nail biting, Lethargy, Introversion, Fidgeting. (American Psychiatric Association,2013; World Health Organisation, 2017)	Restlessness, Agitation, Troubled thinking, Trouble in concentrating, Trouble in decision making, Excessive worry, Tired, Physical symptoms: Stomach aches, Headaches, Cramps, Digestive problems. (American Psychiatric Association, 2013; World Health Organisation, 2017)	Sadness, Anxiety, Guilt, Anger, Mood swings, Irritability, Self-critical, Low memory, Indecisiveness, Confusion, Suicidal ideation, Withdrawal, Neglect of responsibilities, Changes in personal appearance, Chronic fatigue, Lack of energy, Poor Sleep-excess or sleeplessness, Weight gain / loss, Loss of motivation, Substance abuse. (American Psychiatric Association, 2013; World Health Organisation, 2017; Iyer & Khan, 2012)

tuations, anhedonia) (LeMoult & Gotlib, 2018). Subsequent studies concluded that proper diagnosis of any major depressive incidence needs to be based on symptoms related to the emotional, motivational, cognitive and behavioural domains or the clinical interactions with the individual. Cognition, as defined by Fossati refers to several processes and domains including attention, memory, language, executive functions and also the socio-emotional processes. Cognition influences functional and social outcomes (Fossati, 2018).

Linguistic Behavior

Linguistic behavior is the process of building language skills based on learning from the environment. It is a cognitive social behavior that connects people to culture in the field of interpersonal communication, social group communication, management and self-realization. The linguistic behavior of the user is evident in the lexicon. The linguistic behavior of the depressed is reflective of the negative bias in the style of language and in the content where both reflect the emotional state and thinking (Ramos et al., 2008; De Chaudhary et al., 2013). According to Becks cognitive theory of depression, the individual's "negative schemas reflect his negative view of not only himself but the world around him and the future through language" (Beck, 1979). In the current scenario the wide ranges of media communication, social networking and communication reveal and expose the linguistic, cognitive, affective state and behavior of the users. Linguistic behavior of depression is characterized by specific markers.

Absolutist Thinking-Dichotomous Thinking

Absolutist thinking is a cognitive distortion related to anger which leads to anxiety and depression. It promotes expressions of anger when expectations are violated. Although absolute words are interchangeably used with extreme words, the absolutist words are born out of absolutist thinking. One form of absolute thinking is "all-or-nothing", also known as dichotomous thinking (often involves using absolute terms, such as *never* or *every*) (Weishaar & Beck, 1992), and the second form is categorical imperatives (involving a tendency for being rigid towards oneself and others). The words, phrases, ideas and thoughts that imply a totality of a probability or of magnitude are "absolute" words (Rude et al., 2004; Al-Mosaiwi & Johnstone, 2018a, 2018b). Empirical studies have revealed a link between absolute thinking and certain mental disorders like suicide ideation, borderline personality disorder and eating disorder (Antonio et al., 2017). Absolutist thinking, according to a study by Al-Mosaiwi and Tom Johnstone (2018a), is found to be a vulnerable ground for anxiety, depression and suicide. The absolute words used in language are found to be far more prevalent than negative emotion words in identifying the severity of depression (Al-Mosaiwi & Johnstone, 2018a). Dichotomous thinking is characterized by extreme patterns of thought and rigidity. The "all or nothing" patterns of "the black or white, the good or bad, acceptable or totally unacceptable" are reflected in the rigid and extreme thinking (Antoniou et al., 2017).The emotional disturbance and hopelessness arising from dichotomous thinking and poor problem-solving cognitive skills thrust the depressed towards suicide (Weishaar & Beck, 1992).The presence of dichotomous thinking is amply evident in the expression by the use of language -its structure and content. The study on depressed writers compared with the non-depressed provides clear evidence of greater cognitive distortions found to be present in their works and evident in their use of language (Thomas et al., 2007).

Emotion Regulation

Emotion regulation is an essential feature of mental health. The ability to regulate responses to a subjective experience involves thought (cognitive), feelings (affective) and physical (physiological / somatic) response. The cognitive ability is affected by rumination and suppression of emotion, which are evidences of dysfunctional emotion regulation and the underpinning of depression (Compare, 2014). The emotion regulation is dysfunctional and corresponds to the degree of the severity and is linked to other physical illness (Compare et al., 2014). The emotional response to positive or negative situations and to the thoughts is affected by emotions, or biased thoughts affecting emotions, and is displayed visibly through behaviour and language. The dysfunctional emotional regulation of social media users, author and writers who have committed suicide is evident in their works. Self- awareness involves emotion awareness. The inability to self-regulate the negative emotions like sadness, unhappiness leads to hopelessness and futility (Joorman & Stanton, 2016).

Music, Songs, and Poetry Relate to the State of Mind

The broad range of media communication and the wide range in having a choice of music can be considered a suitable platform to identify the mental health (Ramos et al., 2008; Baker & Bor, 2008). Studies suggest that music preferred by individuals is reflective of their emotional vulnerabilities besides relating to their mental health, personality traits and is also indicative of emotional disturbance, self-harm, depression and suicide vulnerabilities. Different genre of music corresponds to specific personality traits. Music is found to be a trigger for memories, emotions and thoughts. Music can either have a trigger effect or be purgative, creating a positive calming effect after the cathartic experience. The trigger can activate negative effect (anti-social behaviour), such as displaying aggressive thoughts or exhibiting negative emotions, prompt aggressive behaviour, deaden reactions to violence, and decrease empathy towards the suffering of the victim. The study brought forth a relevant enquiry to identify the choice of music, its lyrics and preference of the genre as a diagnostic indicator of emotional vulnerability and mental health (Baker& Bor, 2008).

A study carried out on poets who committed suicide and their works, established a link between their language and their emotional and mental health. It is also found that suicidal individuals are detached from others and are preoccupied with self and the linguistic study of their written works highlighted the linguistic predictors of suicide. The language of the depressed writers and authors is found to contain dark imagery, the use of metaphors and personal pronouns. The consistent use of a first-person singular pronoun (I, Me, and Mine) is far more than first-person plural pronoun (We, Ours) (Stirman & Pennebaker, 2001; Ramirez et al., 2008) in the poets who committed suicide. The subconscious use of function words conveys the self-focus attention through the language (style and content) of the depressed writer.

LANGUAGE AS AN INDICATOR OF PERSONALITY, THINKING, AND INTERPERSONAL CONNECTION

There is a strong correlation between personality traits and the development of depressive symptoms. In fact, even the temporary or consistent depressive symptoms are related to the changes in personality (Hakulinen et al., 2015). The deviance in normal behavior, often with symptoms of dysfunctional cognition, low emotional regulation and negative thought bias indicate the disruption of mental health. Numerous studies have established that language can be used as a diagnostic tool to gauge mental and emotional health using quantitative text analysis or statistical text analysis -the use of word count strategies of standard grammatical units (personal pronoun) and psychologically derived linguistic samples of emotion words (Pennebaker & Stone, 2003; Pennebaker et al., 2003). A computer-based text analysis program identifies the "fingerprint" of words used in speech discourse and text. Language contains thoughts and emotions expressed in the text, which identifies the personality and emotional health (Pennebaker & Graybeal, 2001). The style of language function relates to the "how", rather than the "what" of the content. According to Pennebaker language is the way an individual connects to the world. The essential feature of interpersonal connection is interpersonal communication where language is used and the "how" has greater significance than "what". The style of language used is indicative of emotions and thought patterns (Al-Mosaiwi & Johnstone, 2018a, 2018b). Dichotomous thinking contributes to interpersonal problems and to emotional and behavioural instability. The analysis of content of words and frequency identifies the signature pattern of words, which in effect is an insight into their affective (emotional) and cognitive (thinking-thoughts) state. The consistent self-focus and the constant negative bias in thinking are elements that expose the mental health and are amply indicated in the content and style of language.

Linguistic Markers of Depression

Effective tools to detect and track depression ensure prevention of depression and effective treatment by psychologists for the depressive individuals and their caregivers. According to Mehl et al. (2017), people under stress talk less and tend to be self-focused than others and their subconscious use of language reflects their internal mental state. The dysfunctional cognitive, affective and behavioral symptoms and deviations from normal behavior are therefore reflected in language. The signature patterns of words used in natural settings or writing, indicate specific patterns of word use which predict not only mental health but also reflect personality styles (Pennebaker & Graybeal, 2001). Analysis of text or transcripts of oral discourse, using computerized text analysis program for the purpose, are employed for benefit in many domains such as counseling for well-being and health. The common occurrences of negative emotion words, first-person singular pronoun, absolutist words and metaphors are the linguistic markers of depression (Argaman, 2010; Trifu et al., 2017; Al-Mosaiwi & Tombstone, 2018a). Not only can the study of language and linguistic behaviour identify mental disorders, the results of the studies can also pave the way for treatment and care. The linguistic markers of depression along with corresponding psychological and emotional state are illustrated in Table 2.

Negative Content Words in Depression

Words that constitute a major part of the content have lexical meaning which can be modified or changed or by adding new words. The content words comprise of nouns, verbs, adjectives and adverbs. Content and style can be identified as two dimensions of language. The content relates to "what" we express –the meaning or subject matter of statements. The individuals having symptoms of depression use an excessive amount of words conveying negative emotions to describe how they feel, specifically negative adjectives and adverbs – such as *lonely, sad, miserable, bad, sad, helpless, hopeless, aching, lost, worthless, useless, stupid, stuck, untethered, adrift, hurting, alone, afraid, unsure, insecure, despair, black and blue.*

The use of metaphors to express is also an indication of the negative mental state portraying the negative perception of self and the outside world. (Chung & Pennebaker, 2007; Ramirez et al., 2008; Argaman, 2009; Tausczik & Pennebaker, 2010).

Function Words in Depression

Function words include articles, pronouns, conjunctions, prepositions, auxiliary verb, words that cannot be changed or added and though these words have no lexical meaning, they have grammatical significance. The people who are under stress regularly use function words like "*really* or *incredibly*" and although the words don't have any meaning, "they clarify what is going on with the speaker". These words are primarily emotional intensifiers and are used far more automatically than content words like noun and adjectives, which are chosen consciously for their meaning (Mehl et al., 2017).The way function words are used is a representation of the linguistic style and psychological state (Chung & Pennebaker, 2007). The use of pronoun provides an insight into the user's degree of social integration and level of self-focus ("we" and "I") as markers of group versus self-identity and also the extent to which the individual related to others(Tausczik & Pennebaker, 2010; Zimmerman et al., 2013).The function words are referential and have significance as they provide social as well as psychological meaning to both speaker and listener who have to relate to the reference.

Absolutist Words in Depression

Words conveying an extreme absolute such as *always, never, nothing, completely, should, must, every, totally, constantly, entirely, all, definitely, full and one hundred percent,* have been identified as markers, as depressed people do not use 'subtleties' in their expression (Rude et al., 2004).The use of absolutist words is proved to be a definite marker as compared to the pronouns and negative emotion words, as the occurrence of absolutist words is 50% greater in anxiety and depression and 80% greater in suicide ideation (Al-Mosaiwi & Johnstone, 2018a, 2018b).The high occurrence of absolutist words indicates "black and white thinking" where the individual follows the "all or nothing", with no grey areas or a middle ground. This reflects their inability to find balance and adjustment. Life for such individuals is either amazing or terrible, they either hate or love, and they either fail in exams or have perfect scores.

Self-Focus Reflected by Language

The self-focus words and pronouns along with keywords are greatly used in negative memory recall than in positive recall in case of anxiety and depression (Jarrold et al., 2011; Brockmeyer et al., 2015; Trifu et al., 2017). Individuals with symptoms of depression specifically use the first-person singular pronouns ("me", "myself" and "I") far more than second and third-person pronouns ("they", "them" or "she"). This finding suggests that people with depression are more focused on themselves, and less connected with others. Researches have revealed that self-focus pronouns are far more reliable linguistic markers in identifying stress (Mehl et al., 2017) and depression than negative emotion words.

Table 2. Linguistic markers of depression

<table>
<tr><th colspan="4">Linguistic Markers of Depression</th></tr>
<tr><th>Content Words</th><th>Function Words</th><th>Absolute Words</th><th>Negative Emotions</th></tr>
<tr><td rowspan="2">Nouns, Verbs, Adjectives, Adverbs (Chung & Pennebaker, 2007)</td><td>Articles, Pronouns, Conjunctions, Interjections, Prepositions, Auxiliary verbs</td><td>Words that are absolute and cover the magnitude, "all or nothing" thinking</td><td>Words convey negative emotions about self and the future</td></tr>
<tr><td>First person pronouns: I, me, myself; Emotional intensifiers (clarify what the speaker is feeling)- Really, never, the most, Incredibly (Argaman, 2009; Rude et al., 2004; Zimmerman et al.,2013; Al-Mosaiwi & Johnstone, 2018a,2018b)</td><td>always, never, nothing, completely, should, must, every, totally, constantly, entirely, all, definitely, full and one hundred percent (Rude et al.,2004; Al-Mosaiwi & Johnstone, 2018a,2018b)</td><td>low, upset, down, feeling blue, stressed, bad, sad, hopeless, aching, lost, worthless, useless, stupid, stuck, adrift, hurting, alone, lonely, afraid, unsure, insecure, despair, bleak, black (Ramirez et al.,2008; Argaman, 2010; Tausczik & Pennebaker, 2010)</td></tr>
<tr><th colspan="4">Phrases and corresponding Emotion</th></tr>
<tr><td colspan="4">I want to be alone- Isolation / Withdrawal</td></tr>
<tr><td colspan="4">No one cares- Helplessness</td></tr>
<tr><td colspan="4">I don't feel like it- Loss of Interest</td></tr>
<tr><td colspan="4">It is not fun anymore- Loss of interest</td></tr>
<tr><td colspan="4">What's the point- Futility</td></tr>
<tr><td colspan="4">I feel fine- Fear of stigma</td></tr>
<tr><td colspan="4">I am tired- Fatigue /Aches /Pain</td></tr>
<tr><td colspan="4">I am tired of dealing with this- Emotional fatigue / Exhaustion</td></tr>
<tr><td colspan="4">It is all my fault- Guilt/ Self-blame/ Overgeneralization / All or nothing pattern of thinking</td></tr>
<tr><td colspan="4">If I am gone, it will be over for you- Burden / Suicidal thought</td></tr>
<tr><td colspan="4">I can't do this. / I can't feel better. / I can't get my work done. / I can't get out of bed. - Indicating the foreclosure of possibilities</td></tr>
</table>

Depression in Bi-Multilingual Context in India

Study of language and emotions have been carried out to understand the language used by bilinguals and multilinguals (Pavlenko, 2005, 2006; Dewaele, 2010, 2012, 2015).In the case of bilinguals and multilinguals, the expression of emotions and thoughts of depressed individuals could be in a language of his preference, although the preference of the mother tongue for the subjective experience is likely to be dominant (Altarriba & Morier, 2008).It is interesting to follow the findings of yet another study that presents a different view on the choice of language of a bi-multilingual. A study demonstrates that the bilinguals' emotional or subjective experience is based upon the experiences (during the upbringing) that have impacted his way of relating himself emotionally and socially to the world around him (Dewaele, 2010). The choice of language, to respond in a state of anxiety and depression, is therefore based on the role the language plays in his life and his competence in the language. Do the bilinguals in India use their mother tongue predominantly to express their subjective experiences and emotions or choose another language that they feel at ease with, or choose to switch between the known languages? The bilingualism also provides the choice and ease of expressing by language switching (Gutfreund, 1990). A study on the use of language, in online forums, confirms that cross-cultural differences are reflected in the use of language (De Chaudhary et al.,2013). The use of Hindi and English is common, in day to day interpersonal communication predominantly across northern India, even for those who are conversant and fluent in other Indian languages. In light of these studies, the linguistic markers have been analyzed for identifying a correlation between speakers and their depressive condition in bi-multilingual context.

Aaron Beck's Cognitive Theory of Depression

According to Aaron Beck (1979), the dysfunctional beliefs that give rise to negative thoughts are the main source of depression. There is a very definite correlation between the chronicity of negative thoughts and the correspondingly chronic depression, and the increase in the degree of negativity further raises the severity of depression. Beck has identified three main dysfunctional beliefs /schemas that characterise the thinking of the depressed:

1. I am defective or inadequate,
2. All of my experiences result in defeats or failures, and
3. The future is hopeless.

Together, these three themes have been described as Negative Cognitive Triad (NCT).

The depressed people have selective attention to their environment and refuse to perceive anything contrary to their selective beliefs. This occurs due to faulty information processing. Any shift towards the positivity will be countered with their focus on the slightest of negative, thereby sustaining their negative thought patterns and schemas. The tendency to magnify the negative is unconscious and takes place to substantiate their core negative beliefs about everything. (LeMoult & Gotlib, 2018). This indicates that the low self-belief and self -esteem are a precursor to depression in the face of life situations and adversities.

METHOD OF COLLECTION AND COLLATION OF DATA

Participants

The participants chosen for the case study were identified for their issues related to life stresses, relationship issue, and physical health causes and their degree of anxiety and depression ranging from mild to moderate with evidence of suicide ideation. Four individuals were identified for the case study, two were students from an engineering college who had approached the counselor and sought guidance (case study 2 and 3). Two more chosen were identified as individuals with anxiety issue (case study 1) and depression with suicide ideation (case study 4). The inputs from a family member were also taken into consideration in the study, to substantiate additionally, the linguistic evidence of depression recordings. To look further into the thinking and psychological state of the individuals, information about the preference in choice of music was also collected. Two of the individuals (having a very similar background) were also subjected to picture storytelling, to provide insights into their thinking and psychological-emotional processing of information.

Procedure

The participants were made to feel at ease through a few preliminary interactions, to facilitate recording their own inputs about their mental and emotional state. The recording was carried out by a face to face conversation which had a few structured enquiries put forth to the individual. The collection of data was carried out at the college with two individuals, who sought the counseling from an inhouse counselor and from two others in their home along with additional input from their family member. The inputs from a family member of two individuals were also taken. In case study 1, the parent's input of the behavior of the individual (crying and feeling low, having headaches, feeling tired, irritated by the noise and inconsiderate behavior of roommates) was taken. In case study 4, details from the spouse of the depressed individual was obtained which reflected the verbal expression (suicide ideation and expressions of the futility of living under extreme levels of physical pain past emotional trauma) and provided insights to other behavioral symptoms. The inputs from family members in case study 2 and 3 were not taken, as the cause of stress, anxiety, depression was due to the family member itself. In case study 2, the mother and in case study 3 due to both the parents (father and mother). The data collected in the four-case study, is shown in Table 3, with inputs related to social and family background including the linguistic patterns of the chosen candidates with symptoms of anxiety and depression.

Table 3. Case study: background and linguistic markers

CASE 1	
Identity	MS
Gender	*Female*
Age	*19-20*
Occupation	*Student: Creative Arts*
Family	*Single Parent: Mother- Professor*
Issue	*Coping up with people and environment*
Mentor	*Mother*
Clinical Treatment	*n/a*
Personality	*Friendly, Outgoing, Mature*
Hobbies	*Singing, Writing, Sketching, Playing Piano*
Music Preference	*English & Hindi old to new; Pop, Country songs, Bollywood, Gazals*
Language: Bi-Multilingual	*English, Hindi, Tamil*
Dominant language use	*English*
Linguistic Markers: English& Hindi	*"I feel like crying, I have a bad headache, I want to go and sleep. My present and past experiences in life with people is upsetting and makes me feel bad. I am a social being. It is my inability to cope with people. I am not lonely, I am happier by myself also and with people. Some people are sensitive. We feel bad sometimes. The best thing to do is to put yourself to work. You have to calm yourself down. Keep Breathing. Be out in nature"*
Frequently used	*I do get helped, people do support me, I receive help from parent and friends. I feel lighter after overcoming the phase. I feel sad and angry with people. I want to feel detached from pain, want relief.*

Input of family member	*Mother: input from the conversations during the phase of stress felt at having to cope up with people and responsibilities.*
Linguistic Inputs (of the individuals): from natural conversations with family member	*"I don't want to talk about it. I am feeling low. I am crying. I have a headache. I am tired. I had nightmare again. I want to come home. Please come and hug me ".*
CASE 2	
Identity	SJ
Gender	*Male*
Age	*20-21*
Occupation	*Student: Engineering*
Family	*Single Parent: Mother-Government employee*
Issue	*Mother's temperament, behaviour and nature*
Mentor	*Counselor*
Clinical Treatment	*n/a*
Personality	*Quiet, Watchful*
Hobbies	*Sports, Writing, Playing guitar*
Music Preference	*Heavy Metal: Linkin Park, Bullet for my valentine, Piano instrumental*
Language: Bi-Multilingual	*English, Hindi*
Dominant language use	*English & Hindi*
Linguistic Markers: English& Hindi	*"I don't care anymore, Mujhe farak nahin padta.I am now ignoring, sirf sunn leta hun. I plug in my earphones, listen to my music, ignore the non-stop taunts. I listen to violent music on full volume Mein gana chilake gata hun -Linkin Park ke saath gaake, apna gussa nikalta hun.I have detached myself. I don't feel like doing any activity as my mind is not free, Mera mann activity mein nahi lagta. I am rude and aggressive sometimes with my classmates. No one I can talk to or no one to trust. No one cares in my family and now I manage alone, by myself".*
Frequently used	*I am now ignoring. I am now managing my way. I don't trust anyone. Koi support nahi karte hain, behen log bhi nahi.*
Input of family member	*nil*
Linguistic Inputs (of the individuals): from natural conversations with family member	*nil*
CASE 3	
Identity	Ak
Gender	*Female*
Age	*19-20*
Occupation	*Student: Engineering*
Family	*Both Parents: Father - Civil Engineer; Mother - Housewife*
Issue	*Father's alcoholism & domestic fights*
Mentor	*Counselor*
Clinical Treatment	*n/a*

Personality	*Quiet, Shy*
Hobbies	*Painting, Listening to music*
Music Preference	*Hindi: Bollywood - Slow or soothing melodies*
Language: Bi-Multilingual	*English, Hindi*
Dominant language use	*Hindi*
Linguistic Markers: English& Hindi	*"Life mein negativity hai. Apne se problem nahi solve kar sakti hun. Kuch ho hi nahi pata . Pura nahi ho pata padhai. Mann disturb hota hai. I can't do anything. Jaldi nervous ho jati hun ...rasta nahi dikhta hai. Darr lagta hai, ab thoda bol deti hun. Sirf kam ki baat hoti hai ghar mein".*
Frequently used	*Ghar mei achha nahi lagta, mann nahi karta padhne ka. Gahar me jhagda roz hota hai. Papa se darr lagta hai*
Input of family member	*nil*
Linguistic Inputs (of the individuals): from natural conversations with family member	*nil*
CASE 4	
Identity	MG
Gender	*Female*
Age	*26-27*
Occupation	*Housewife (Engineer)*
Family	*Husband: Professor*
Issue	*Childhood trauma-related to family members & rejection and Emotional & Physical pain*
Mentor	*Psychologist and Psychiatrist*
Clinical Treatment	*Yes*
Personality	*Quiet, Selective interaction*
Hobbies	*Singing, Writing, Dancing, Painting, Craft,*
Music Preference	*Old & New Hindi Bollywood songs*
Language: Bi-Multilingual	*English, Hindi*
Dominant language use	*Hindi*
Linguistic Markers: English& Hindi	*"Iss se kya hoga? Mein pehle optimistic thi, ab koi bhi cheez nahi lagti ki kaam karegi. Itna samay ho gaya hai aur taklif abhi bhi hai. Mera vishwas khatam ho gaya...thoda bhi nahi hai, ab aisa lagta hai ki ab kya hoga...poora faith khatam ho gaya.*
Frequently used	*Kuch nahi hoga, Mujh par koi farak nahi padta hai treatment ka -taklif kam nahin ho rahi hai."*
Input of family member	*Husband: inputs from home and mobile text messages*
Linguistic Inputs (of the individuals): from natural conversations with family member	*(During the episode of extreme physical pain). "No one understands my pain. Mujhe koi nahi samajh sakta. No one can ever cure me. Ab koi mujhe thik nahi kar sakta. I have become useless. Mein useless aur bojh ban gayi hun.I should die. Accha hai mei mar jaoun".*

RESULTS

Case Study 1: The participant was articulating in a mature manner. She identified herself as a sensitive natured, friendly and happy go lucky individual. She felt unable to cope with people around in a schedule that is hectic and demanding. Description of her emotional state in the course of conversation and ways of dealing with her discomfort was candid. The individual was not totally self-focused and exhibited self-awareness in describing her mental and emotional state during the phases when she felt low and overwhelmed. Mentoring and guidance from her caregiver would suffice to help her cope with the causes of her stress.

Case Study 2: The participant's conversation revealed emotional suppression in his dealing with the home issues. The effect of the constant pressure of a negative home environment was a major disturbance and cause for him to feel frustration in working out to improving the interpersonal relationship with the parent. The conversation highlighted the disturbance in his life which affected his daily routine and temperament. The counseling from the counselor appeared to be taken lightly. The preference of music for heavy metal also indicated the emotional and psychological state of angst.

Case Study 3: The participant had received counseling and felt some degree of relief in coping with the stress and anxiety of daily domestic disturbance. She had made attempts to increase her resilience, through meditation and counseling, to handle the constant stress at home. The counseling had assisted her to overcome her low self-esteem, bleakness and the hopelessness of her current situation. She gained from her willingness to seek help and receive guidance and this was evident from her conversation.

Case Study 4: The chronic levels of physical pain, along with negative thought bias that had developed in the past, were visible in the conversation with the participant. She had a greater number of absolutist words than other case study participants. Also, the futility of care and treatment along with the mental rejection of treatment was evident in the conversation. The individual needed specialized care from psychiatrist and psychologist to recover from depression. Proper effective counselling was provided to change negative bias and belief patterns of thoughts, negative thinking and suicide ideation.

The four individuals spoke willingly about the reasons for their stress, anxiety, depression and suicide ideation. The style of language and the content of the linguistic expression of all four, is given in Table 4.

Picture Story and Music

In the case study 1 and 2, the participants were shown an image of a bird which was caught in the web of a spider as in Figure 1.

Case Study 1

The visual image spurred the overwhelming feeling, as she identified herself with the bird, and the spider's web to be the complexities of her own life, where she felt trapped and stuck even though she wishes to fly free. The image triggered her memories of growing up as a single child with single parent- working mother, the challenges of studying away from home, living in a hostel and stress of coping with the academic curriculum and people around her. The image was cathartic, she was teary-eyed as she nar-

Table 4. Linguistic markers: bilingual Hindi and English

Linguistic Markers: Bilingual Hindi and English								
	Case 1		Case 2		Case 3		Case 4	
LINGUISTIC MARKERS	**English**	**Hindi**	**English**	**Hindi**	**English**	**Hindi**	**English**	**Hindi**
Content Words	Crying, breathing, bad, low, upset, best, thing, headache, sensitive, social, nature, work, calm, support, cope, hug	nil	ignoring, plug-in, care, violent, trust, listen, alone, talk, manage, aggressive, rude	Farak, chilake	life, solve, nervous, problem	ghar, padhai, rasta, dikhta, jhagda, papa, darr, mann, jaldi	treatment, optimistic, faith,	cheez, khatam, bojh, thoda, taklif, kar
Function Words	I, me, myself, we, you	nil	I, my, myself	mera,mujhe,apna	I	apne se, mera	I	mein, mujhe
Absolute Words	nil	nil	no-one, anymore, full volume, non-stop, by myself	chilake,koi, nahin lahta	can't do anything,	nahin lagta,nahin kar sakti hun,roz,sirf,pura		koi nahin kar sakta, nahin kaam karega, ab koi, nahin hoga,
Self -focus Words	I, me, myself	nil	Myself, I, my	mujhe,mera,apna		apne se	I	mein,mujhe,
Negative Valence Words	bad, angry, low, upset	nil	aggressive, rude, don't care, no-one, violent, alone, don't trust	farak nahi padta	negative, disturb	achha nahin lagta,darr,thoda,kuch,jaldi		thoda bhi,taklif, kya hoga, nahin karega, khatam, mar jaon, bojh, nahin hoga

Figure 1. Picture story

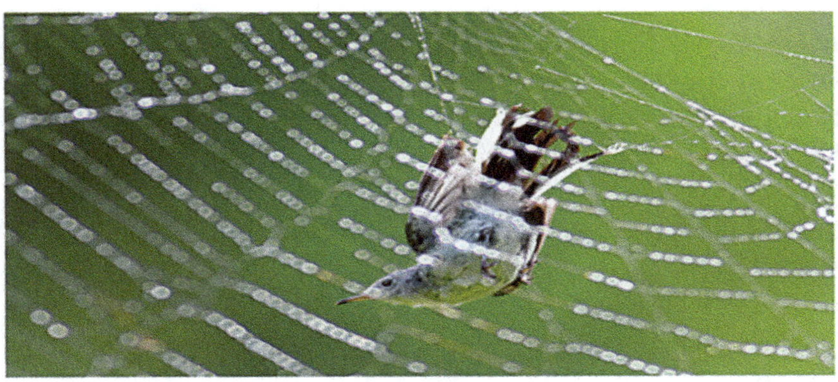

rated her perception. It served to release her suppressed emotions and thoughts. The preferred choice of music of this individual ranged wide from old to contemporary music in Hindi and English. The choice of music indicated her preference for soothing, melodious country music, instrumental and contemporary pop (Don Williams, Adele, Sam Smith, Ed Sheeran, Kishore Kumar, Arjit Singh, Ghulam Ali).

Case Study 2

The boy also had a single parent, was conscious and aware that he faced constant stress due to the over protective and possessive nature of the working mother. The boy was subjected to constant bombardment from the mother right from the morning, and faced constant monitoring over the telephone. He was frustrated as he was constantly under surveillance and not trusted. His counter action to get away from the constant verbal battle and physical assault was to maintain silence and non-responsive behavior at those moments. He admitted to being rude and irritated with his friends and classmates, besides keeping a low profile and having no good friends. In the case study 2, when the participant, was asked to look at the picture of the bird caught in the spider's web, he had similar interpretation. However, he seemed unaffected by the picture of the bird caught in the spider's web. In response to the picture storytelling, he simply stated that the bird was stuck in the web and could escape provided it used the beak to break free. His choice of music in the morning hours during the interaction with the parent at home was heavy metal music by Likin Park (songs: Numb, Waiting for the end, Faint) and heavy metal music bands (like Bullet for my valentine), played out in high volume, accompanied by loud singing to shut out the world, to shout in anger along with the whooping of the singers.

The psychological and emotional states in depression vulnerability, were revealed by the processing of information in the picture interpretation, and choice of music as a clear indication of the emotional vulnerability. The study highlights the language of depressive bilinguals- the linguistic markers in both Hindi and English as clear indicators of thinking patterns, emotional and psychological states, personality and behavioral changes.

For example:

- **Case Study 1:** I feel bad, upsetting, crying, tired, headaches...- behavioral and physical symptoms of depression
- **Case Study 2:** I don't care-detachment, isolation and withdrawal… - emotional and psychological state
- **Case Study 3:** Mann nahi lagta… – (I can't concentrate / focus -on studies)-helplessness and lack of self-motivation. - psychological state.
- **Case Study 4:** Koi farak nahi padta… - (there is no difference)-futility (the sense of hopelessness)-cognitive bias, negative valence, absolutist thinking,

The negative bias of thought as seen in case study 4, follows Beck's cognitive theory of depression (Beck, 1979).

DISCUSSION

The results in this study affirm that the signs and cues of anxiety and depression are visible and evident from the various linguistic indicators. The negative bias of processing, the emotion regulation deficit leading to absolute and dichotomous thinking, the behavioral changes, the vulnerability to suicide ideation are visible not only by the linguistic markers but also in the choice of music and physical symptoms. A holistic approach and referential cognizance of the language content and style, need to be considered to interpret accurately the linguistic markers. The major findings of the case study are the bilinguals' use of content words, function words, self -focus and absolute thinking, to be indicative of their degree of depression and their emotional states and thought patterns. The findings reflect the degree of depression ranging from mild to moderate to suicide ideation, constructed on the observations of emotion regulation deficit, the bias in the processing of information, their absolute thinking, and the self-focus, as evident in the linguistic markers. The past studies have identified young adults as most vulnerable to depression and suicide ideation. The current study has confirmed most vulnerable to depression are primarily in the age bracket of youth -young adults as they go about coping with life events, routine and common stressors. The prevalence of depression is found to be neither gender specific nor background specific.

The use of content words and function words in the four-case study are similar in both English and Hindi. The self-focus in the language-function words (use of the first-person singular pronoun is far more than third-person pronoun), the negative valence words, the absolute thinking reflected by absolute words and the dichotomous thinking of "all or nothing" have been established as various linguistic markers of depression (Pennebaker & Graybeal, 2001; Rude et al., 2004; Brookmeyer et al., 2015; Mehl et al., 2017; Al-Mosaiwi & Johnstone, 2018a).The findings of the four case study even in bilinguals, confirm largely the findings of the previous studies, which have identified linguistic markers in English language. The use of words in Hindi corresponds to the identified English words. The Hindi lexica also convey negative bias of the depressive individual by the use of content words and function words, revealing the absolute and dichotomous thinking patterns.

The preferred language of the four bilinguals is either Hindi or English and a mix of both. The recordings of the case study affirm two approaches to bilingualism: first – bilinguals' preference of mother tongue in case of subjective experiences (Altarriba & Morier, 2008) as in the case study 3 and 4, though both are bilinguals, their preference is clearly Hindi; and second approach, the ease of switching two languages to have better linguistic expression as a bilingual (Gutfreund, 1990), as in the case study 2, switching between English and Hindi. The chosen language in the case study 1, is English which supports the idea that the individual's choice of language is influenced by his comfort and fluency (Dewaele, 2010). Our study reveals that preference of the chosen language by a bilingual is an individuals' subconscious choice which is the comfort of expression and fluency in the language.

Impact of Language in Case of Mental Disorder

Linguistic behavioral study relating to linguistic markers and expressions identifies the mental disorder and also paves the way for treatment and care clinically and non-clinically. Language, as an accurate non-clinical linguistic marker (Al-Mosaiwi & Johnstone, 2018a) signals the emotional, behavioral and psychological changes, and results in identifying mental illness. Language can also be instrumental in combating mental illness by facilitating conducive interpersonal communication with the social support system. As Pennebaker stated, language is not only the way an individual connects to the world, it is also an essential feature of interpersonal communication and interpersonal connection wherein the "how" is far more significant than "what" conveyed.

The subconscious use of function words including first-person pronoun and the use of emotional intensifiers, in addition to self-focus, negative memory recall and negative valence is indicative of social isolation whereas content words are indicative of negative beliefs and perceptions by individuals suffering from mental disorder (Jarrold et al., 2011; Brockmeyer et al., 2015; Trifu et al.,2017; Mehl et al., 2017; Al-Mosaiwi and Johnstone, 2018 a, 2018b). The function words are referential and vital as they provide social as well as psychological meaning wherein both speaker and listener have to relate to the reference (Tausczik & Pennebaker, 2010; Zimmerman et al., 2013). Therefore, the use of a plural pronoun (We, Our) to usher social integration to counter the social isolation and disconnect, arising out of stigma, can be employed. Language as one of the cognition processes, influences emotional, functional and social outcomes (Fossati, 2018). Thus, certain linguistic expressions can be used to shift and influence the way people, situation or an event, are perceived as a counter measure against stigma and notions of depression (Jensen et al., 2013; Reali et al., 2016; Richards, 2018). Specific linguistic cues can be strategically deployed such as linguistic framing, inclusive language, therapeutic writing, positive and prosocial words and empowering language such as "person-first language" to administer care, counseling and treatment by rendering respect, dignity, compassion and empathy (Jensen et al., 2013; Reali et al., 2016; Richards, 2018; Tarai et al., 2018; Tran et al., 2018). Linguistic behavior can be consciously used to empower and reinforce empathy, support, respect, dignity and trust (Richards, 2018), thereby shifting the paradigm. The physicians, caretakers, counselors and social support systems, including online forums (De Choudhury et al., 2013; Eichstaedt et al., 2018), can provide sustenance to the recovery process of mental illness and minimize the trigger effect of certain sources and factors responsible for fermenting mental illness. Just as the trolling online has severe impact on the emotionally vulnerable individuals and pushes them further into depression, the validation and positive words serve to provide relief and sustenance to nurture them in the form of providing social support and acceptance. The online "coming out" of individuals and their acceptance and support online, nurtures their efforts to cope up with their emotional and psychological struggles that could range from stress, anxiety, milder forms of depression to suicide ideation. The health care providers are trained to treat the mental disorder by employing specific linguistic behavior and linguistic markers conducive to treating mental illness (Jensen et al., 2013; Richards 2018). Language can have a significant impact on health and wellbeing. The best way to combat a malady that disrupts life is to identify it and provide an antidote to cure. Interdisciplinary approach by researchers is underway to study, analyze, identify, document and comprehend the impact of language in the domain of mental health care.

CONCLUSION AND FUTURE SCOPE

The study of four cases of mental health reveals that stresses of life routine and relationship issues cause anxiety and can lead to depression. The belief patterns, thinking and emotion regulation are indicated by the language content and style in interpersonal communication. The early identification and detection of mental ill-health is possible with analysis of linguistic markers, inputs by the family, the individual's self- identification and self-awareness. The use of absolute and negative emotion words is more in the case of the individuals with negative thought bias and absolutist thinking. The emotional regulation by self or through guidance and mentoring is of significance and useful in the recovery process as seen in the case study 1 and 3. The linguistic behavior and markers of the four-case study are evident through the dominant language that is preferred by the individuals to convey their emotions and thoughts. As the use of function words is not a conscious choice, rather a subconsciously chosen expression of thoughts and emotions, the four individuals chose either English or Hindi or both as their communication language based on their comfort level in the particular language. The use of content words, absolute words and function words in Hindi correspond to the English lexica that are previously identified and documented as most accurate linguistic markers of depression.

A future longitudinal study of depressive behavior and language used in interpersonal communication in natural surroundings in the presence of family members, co-workers and strangers can be taken up to identify the variations and similarities in the pattern of communication between the depressive individual and others in his life at home, work and social settings. A comparative study on the depressive behavior and the use of language in interpersonal connections in the work place (with superiors, colleagues and subordinates) and personal relationships (parents, spouse, siblings, children or dating partners) can be carried out to trace out the shadows of mild, moderate and severe levels of depression for providing timely care and treatment.

ACKNOWLEDGMENT

This research was supported by the National Institute of Technology Raipur, India (Seed Grant No- NI-TRR/SeedGrant/2016- 17/009)

REFERENCES

Al-Mosaiwi, M., & Johnstone, T. (2018a). In an absolute state: Elevated use of absolutist words is a marker specific to anxiety, depression, and suicidal ideation. *Clinical Psychological Science*.

Al-Mosaiwi, M., & Johnstone, T. (2018b). Linguistic markers of moderate and absolute natural language. *Personality and Individual Differences*, *134*, 119–124. doi:10.1016/j.paid.2018.06.004 PMID:30393418

Altarriba, J., & Morier, R. G. (2008). 10 Bilingualism: Language, Emotion, and Mental Health. The handbook of bilingualism, 8, 250.

American Psychiatric Association. (2013). *Diagnostic and statistical manual of mental disorders (DSM-5®)*. American Psychiatric Pub.

Antoniou, E. E., Bongers, P., & Jansen, A. (2017). The mediating role of dichotomous thinking and emotional eating in the relationship between depression and BMI. *Eating Behaviors*, *26*, 55–60. doi:10.1016/j.eatbeh.2017.01.007 PMID:28135621

Argaman, O. (2010). Linguistic markers and emotional intensity. *Journal of Psycholinguistic Research*, *39*(2), 89–99. doi:10.100710936-009-9127-1 PMID:19644755

Baker, F., & Bor, W. (2008). Can music preference indicate mental health status in young people? *Australasian Psychiatry*, *16*(4), 284–288. doi:10.1080/10398560701879589 PMID:18608148

Beck, A. T. (Ed.). (1979). *Cognitive therapy of depression*. Guilford Press.

Beck, A. T., & Alford, B. A. (2009). *Depression: Causes and treatment*. University of Pennsylvania Press.

Bohra, N., Srivastava, S., & Bhatia, M. S. (2015). Depression in women in Indian context. *Indian Journal of Psychiatry*, *57*(6Suppl 2), S239. doi:10.4103/0019-5545.161485 PMID:26330641

Boyd, R. L., & Pennebaker, J. W. (2017). Language-based personality: A new approach to personality in a digital world. *Current Opinion in Behavioral Sciences*, *18*, 63–68. doi:10.1016/j.cobeha.2017.07.017

Briggs, R., Tobin, K., Kenny, R. A., & Kennelly, S. P. (2018). What is the prevalence of untreated depression and death ideation in older people? Data from the Irish Longitudinal Study on Aging. *International Psychogeriatrics*, 1–9. PMID:29335038

Brockmeyer, T., Zimmermann, J., Kulessa, D., Hautzinger, M., Bents, H., Friederichs, H. C., ... Backenstrass, M. (2015). Me, myself, and I: Self-referent word use as an indicator of self-focused attention in relation to depression and anxiety. *Frontiers in Psychology*, *6*, 1564. doi:10.3389/fpsyg.2015.01564 PMID:26500601

Chung, C., & Pennebaker, J. W. (2007). The psychological functions of function words. *Social Communication, 1*, 343-359.

Compare, A., Zarbo, C., Shonin, E., Van Gordon, W., & Marconi, C. (2014). Emotional regulation and depression: A potential mediator between heart and mind. *Cardiovascular Psychiatry and Neurology*. PMID:25050177

Corrigan, P. W., Druss, B. G., & Perlick, D. A. (2014). The impact of mental illness stigma on seeking and participating in mental health care. *Psychological Science in the Public Interest*, *15*(2), 37–70. doi:10.1177/1529100614531398 PMID:26171956

Corrigan, P. W., &Kleinlein, P. (2005). *The impact of mental illness stigma*. Academic Press.

Corrigan, P. W., &Kosyluk, K. A. (2014). *Mental illness stigma: Types, constructs, and vehicles for change*. Academic Press.

Corrigan, P. W., & Watson, A. C. (2002). The paradox of self-stigma and mental illness. *Clinical Psychology: Science and Practice*, *9*(1), 35–53. doi:10.1093/clipsy.9.1.35

De Choudhury, M., Gamon, M., Counts, S., & Horvitz, E. (2013). Predicting depression via social media. *ICWSM*, *13*, 1–10.

Dewaele, J. M. (2010). *Emotions in multiple languages*. London: Palgrave. doi:10.1057/9780230289505

Dewaele, J. M. (2012). Multilingualism and emotions. The Encyclopedia of Applied Linguistics.

Dewaele, J. M. (2015). Bilingualism and multilingualism. *The international encyclopedia of language and social interaction*, 1-11.

Eichstaedt, J. C., Smith, R. J., Merchant, R. M., Ungar, L. H., Crutchley, P., Preoţiuc-Pietro, D., ... Schwartz, H. A. (2018). Facebook language predicts depression in medical records. *Proceedings of the National Academy of Sciences of the United States of America*, *115*(44), 11203–11208. doi:10.1073/pnas.1802331115 PMID:30322910

Fossati, P. (2018). Is major depression a cognitive disorder? *Revue Neurologique*, *174*(4), 212–215. doi:10.1016/j.neurol.2018.01.365 PMID:29618408

Fried, E. I., Nesse, R. M., Guille, C., & Sen, S. (2015). The differential influence of life stress on individual symptoms of depression. *Acta Psychiatrica Scandinavica*, *131*(6), 465–471. doi:10.1111/acps.12395 PMID:25650176

Guttfreund, D. G. (1990). Effects of language usage on the emotional experience of Spanish-English and English-Spanish bilinguals. *Journal of Consulting and Clinical Psychology*, *58*(5), 604–607. doi:10.1037/0022-006X.58.5.604 PMID:2254507

Hakulinen, C., Elovainio, M., Pulkki-Råback, L., Virtanen, M., Kivimäki, M., & Jokela, M. (2015). Personality and depressive symptoms: Individual participant meta-analysis of 10 cohort studies. *Depression and Anxiety*, *32*(7), 461–470. doi:10.1002/da.22376 PMID:26014798

Hammen, C. L. (2015). Stress and depression: Old questions, new approaches. *Current Opinion in Psychology*, *4*, 80–85. doi:10.1016/j.copsyc.2014.12.024

Iyer, K., & Khan, Z. A. (2012). Depression–A Review. *Research Journal of Recent Sciences*, *1*(4), 79-87.

Jarrold, W., Javitz, H. S., Krasnow, R., Peintner, B., Yeh, E., Swan, G. E., & Mehl, M. (2011). Depression and self-focused language in structured interviews with older men. *Psychological Reports*, *109*(2), 686–700. doi:10.2466/02.09.21.28.PR0.109.5.686-700 PMID:22238866

Jeđud, I. (2018). *Interdisciplinary Approach to Emotion Detection from Text*. Academic Press.

Jensen, M. E., Pease, E. A., Lambert, K., Hickman, D. R., Robinson, O., McCoy, K. T., ... Ramirez, J. (2013). Championing person-first language: A call to psychiatric mental health nurses. *Journal of the American Psychiatric Nurses Association*, *19*(3), 146–151. doi:10.1177/1078390313489729 PMID:23698977

Joormann, J., & Stanton, C. H. (2016). Examining emotion regulation in depression: A review and future directions. *Behaviour Research and Therapy*, *86*, 35–49. doi:10.1016/j.brat.2016.07.007 PMID:27492851

Kircanski, K., Joormann, J., & Gotlib, I. H. (2012). Cognitive aspects of depression. *Wiley Interdisciplinary Reviews: Cognitive Science*, *3*(3), 301–313. doi:10.1002/wcs.1177 PMID:23240069

Koschorke, M., Evans-Lacko, S., Sartorius, N., & Thornicroft, G. (2017). Stigma in different cultures. In The Stigma of Mental Illness-End of the Story? (pp. 67-82). Springer. doi:10.1007/978-3-319-27839-1_4

Lannin, D. G., Vogel, D. L., Brenner, R. E., Abraham, W. T., & Heath, P. J. (2016). Does self-stigma reduce the probability of seeking mental health information? *Journal of Counseling Psychology*, *63*(3), 351–358. doi:10.1037/cou0000108 PMID:26323042

LeMoult, J., & Gotlib, I. H. (2018). Depression: A cognitive perspective. *Clinical Psychology Review*. doi:10.1016/j.cpr.2018.06.008 PMID:29961601

LeMoult, J., Kircanski, K., Prasad, G., & Gotlib, I. H. (2017). Negative self-referential processing predicts the recurrence of major depressive episodes. *Clinical Psychological Science*, *5*(1), 174–181. doi:10.1177/2167702616654898 PMID:28286705

Mehl, M. R., Raison, C. L., Pace, T. W., Arevalo, J. M., & Cole, S. W. (2017). Natural language indicators of differential gene regulation in the human immune system. *Proceedings of the National Academy of Sciences of the United States of America*, *114*(47), 12554–12559. doi:10.1073/pnas.1707373114 PMID:29109260

Otte, C., Gold, S. M., Penninx, B. W., Pariante, C. M., Etkin, A., Fava, M., ... Schatzberg, A. F. (2016). Major depressive disorder. *Nature Reviews. Disease Primers*, *2*, 16065. doi:10.1038/nrdp.2016.65 PMID:27629598

Pavlenko, A. (2005). *Emotions and multilingualism*. Cambridge, UK: Cambridge University Press.

Pavlenko, A. (2006). *Bilingual minds: Emotional experience, expression, and representation*. New York: Multilingual Matters. doi:10.21832/9781853598746

Pearl, R. L., Forgeard, M. J., Rifkin, L., Beard, C., & Björgvinsson, T. (2017). Internalized stigma of mental illness: Changes and associations with treatment outcomes. *Stigma and Health*, *2*(1), 2–15. doi:10.1037ah0000036

Pennebaker, J. W., & Graybeal, A. (2001). Patterns of natural language use: Disclosure, personality, and social integration. *Current Directions in Psychological Science*, *10*(3), 90–93. doi:10.1111/1467-8721.00123

Pennebaker, J. W., Mehl, M. R., & Niederhoffer, K. G. (2003). Psychological aspects of natural language use: Our words, our selves. *Annual Review of Psychology*, *54*(1), 547–577. doi:10.1146/annurev.psych.54.101601.145041 PMID:12185209

Pennebaker, J. W., & Stone, L. D. (2003). Words of wisdom: Language use over the life span. *Journal of Personality and Social Psychology*, *85*(2), 291–301. doi:10.1037/0022-3514.85.2.291 PMID:12916571

Ramirez-Esparza, N., Chung, C. K., Kacewicz, E., & Pennebaker, J. W. (2008, March). *The Psychology of Word Use in Depression Forums in English and in Spanish: Texting Two Text Analytic Approaches*. ICWSM.

Reali, F., Soriano, T., & Rodríguez, D. (2016). How we think about depression: The role of linguistic framing. *Revista Latinoamericana de Psicología*, *48*(2), 127–136. doi:10.1016/j.rlp.2015.09.004

Richards, V. (2018). The importance of language in mental health care. *The Lancet. Psychiatry*, *5*(6), 460–461. doi:10.1016/S2215-0366(18)30042-7 PMID:29482994

Rude, S., Gortner, E. M., & Pennebaker, J. (2004). Language use of depressed and depression-vulnerable college students. *Cognition and Emotion*, *18*(8), 1121–1133. doi:10.1080/02699930441000030

Rüsch, N., Zlati, A., Black, G., & Thornicroft, G. (2014). Does the stigma of mental illness contribute to suicidality? *The British Journal of Psychiatry*, *205*(4), 257–259. doi:10.1192/bjp.bp.114.145755 PMID:25274313

Schomerus, G., Stolzenburg, S., Freitag, S., Speerforck, S., Janowitz, D., Evans-Lacko, S., ... Schmidt, S. (2018). Stigma as a barrier to recognizing personal mental illness and seeking help: A prospective study among untreated persons with mental illness. *European Archives of Psychiatry and Clinical Neuroscience*, 1–11. PMID:29679153

Stafford, M. (2018). Psychotic depression: How to diagnose this often undetected—and hidden—condition. *The Brown University Child and Adolescent Behavior Letter*, *34*(4), 1–7. doi:10.1002/cbl.30284

Stirman, S. W., & Pennebaker, J. W. (2001). Word use in the poetry of suicidal and non-suicidal poets. *Psychosomatic Medicine*, *63*(4), 517–522. doi:10.1097/00006842-200107000-00001 PMID:11485104

Tarai, S., Bit, A., dos Reis, H. J., Palotás, A., Rizvanov, A., & Bissoyi, A. (2016). Stratifying Heterogeneous Dimension of Neurodegenerative Diseases: Intervention for Stipulating Epigenetic Factors to Combat Oxidative Stress in Human Brain. *BioNanoScience*, *6*(4), 411–422. doi:10.100712668-016-0240-y

Tarai, S., Mukherjee, R., Qurratul, Q. A., Singh, B. K., & Bit, A. (2018). Use of Prosocial Word Enhances the Processing of Language: Frequency Domain Analysis of Human EEG. *Journal of Psycholinguistic Research*, 1–17. PMID:30043323

Tausczik, Y. R., & Pennebaker, J. W. (2010). The psychological meaning of words: LIWC and computerized text analysis methods. *Journal of Language and Social Psychology*, *29*(1), 24–54. doi:10.1177/0261927X09351676

Thomas, K. M., & Duke, M. (2007). Depressed writing: Cognitive distortions in the works of depressed and nondepressed poets and writers. *Psychology of Aesthetics, Creativity, and the Arts*, *1*(4), 204–218. doi:10.1037/1931-3896.1.4.204

Thornicroft, G. (2006). *Shunned: discrimination against people with mental illness* (Vol. 399). Oxford, UK: Oxford University Press.

Tran, N. T., Baggio, S., Dawson, A., O'Moore, É., Williams, B., Bedell, P., ... Wolff, H. (2018). Words matter: A call for humanizing and respectful language to describe people who experience incarceration. *BMC International Health and Human Rights*, *18*(1), 41. doi:10.118612914-018-0180-4 PMID:30445949

Trifu, R. N., Nemeş, B., Bodea-Haţegan, C., & Cozman, D. (2017). Linguistic indicators of language in major depressive disorder (MDD). An evidence-based research. *Journal of Evidence-Based Psychotherapies*, *17*(1), 105–128. doi:10.24193/jebp.2017.1.7

van der Sanden, R. L., Pryor, J. B., Stutterheim, S. E., Kok, G., & Bos, A. E. (2016). Stigma by association and family burden among family members of people with mental illness: The mediating role of coping. *Social Psychiatry and Psychiatric Epidemiology*, *51*(9), 1233–1245. doi:10.100700127-016-1256-x PMID:27357819

Verma, S. K., Bharti, P., & Singh, T. (2018). Does stigma always have negative consequences? *Journal of Community & Applied Social Psychology*, *28*(6), 495–507. doi:10.1002/casp.2382

Weishaar, M. E., & Beck, A. T. (1992). Hopelessness and suicide. *International Review of Psychiatry (Abingdon, England)*, *4*(2), 177–184. doi:10.3109/09540269209066315

World Health Organization. (2017). *Depression and other common mental disorders: global health estimates*. WHO.

Yule, G. (2016). *The study of language*. Cambridge University Press.

Yusof, N. F. A., Lin, C., & Guerin, F. (2017). Analysing the causes of depressed mood from depression vulnerable individuals. In *Proceedings of the International Workshop on Digital Disease Detection using Social Media 2017 (DDDSM-2017)* (pp. 9-17). Academic Press.

Zimmermann, J., Wolf, M., Bock, A., Peham, D., & Benecke, C. (2013). The way we refer to ourselves reflects how we relate to others: Associations between first-person pronoun use and interpersonal problems. *Journal of Research in Personality*, *47*(3), 218–225. doi:10.1016/j.jrp.2013.01.008

Chapter 13
Motor Imagery Classification Using EEG Signals for Brain–Computer Interface Applications

Subrota Mazumdar
Kalinga Institute of Industrial Technology University, India

Rohit Chaudhary
Kalinga Institute of Industrial Technology University, India

Suruchi Suruchi
Kalinga Institute of Industrial Technology University, India

Suman Mohanty
Kalinga Institute of Industrial Technology University, India

Divya Kumari
Kalinga Institute of Industrial Technology University, India

Aleena Swetapadma
Kalinga Institute of Industrial Technology University, India

ABSTRACT

In this chapter, a nearest neighbor (k-NN)-based method for efficient classification of motor imagery using EEG for brain-computer interfacing (BCI) applications has been proposed. Electroencephalogram (EEG) signals are obtained from multiple channels from brain. These EEG signals are taken as input features and given to the k-NN-based classifier to classify motor imagery. More specifically, the chapter gives an outline of the Berlin brain-computer interface that can be operated with minimal subject change. All the design and simulation works are carried out with MATLAB software. k-NN-based classifier is trained with data from continuous signals of EEG channels. After the network is trained, it is tested with various test cases. Performance of the network is checked in terms of percentage accuracy, which is found to be 99.25%. The result suggested that the proposed method is accurate for BCI applications.

DOI: 10.4018/978-1-5225-8567-1.ch013

INTRODUCTION

Until now, health research in developing countries like India has focused on highly pervasive infectious diseases and malnutrition. But, it is becoming increasingly important to study brain disorders as well, says an international team of neuroscientist. Types of brain imaging techniques prevalent now are fMRI, CT, PET, EEG etc. EEG is used to show brain activity in certain psychological states, such as alertness or drowsiness. It is useful in the diagnosis of seizures and other medical problems that involve an overabundance or lack of activity in certain parts of the brain. It can also be used for brain computer interface applications mostly helpful for paralyzed persons. Various methods have been suggested for motor imagery classification some of which are discussed below.

In Qin, Ding, and He (2005), source analysis methods such as dipole localization and cortical imaging have been applied to classification of motor imagery tasks for BCI applications. A combination of source analysis approach with signal pre-processing for classification of motor imagery tasks has been used which has classification rate of about 80%. In Sitaram et al. (2007), multichannel near-infrared spectroscopy (NIR) is studied for the development of BCI. Support vector machines (SVM) and hidden Markov model (HMM) are the pattern recognition algorithms which are used here for classification purpose. The result shows that the classification of left-hand imagery from right-hand imagery is done by SVM with an average accuracy of 73%. In Leuthardt, Schalk, Wolpaw, Ojemann, and Moran (2004), it has been shown that electrocorticographic (ECoG) based BCI is better than electroencephalographic (EEG) based BCI. It discusses that EEG based BCI works from the scalp or a single-neuron activity from within the brain is used. But both methods have disadvantages as EEG is inefficient and needs extensive training whereas the method involving single neuron can cause clinical risks.

In Wairagkar (2014), non linear artificial neural network (ANN) classifiers are combined with the signal processing techniques for classifying motor imagery for BCI. The communication with external devices such as computers can be done directly by brain with the help of BCI without using any motor pathways. The classification of the rest state, the right hand imagery and the left hand imagery could be done by BCI by using artificial neural network. Various features are classified into two classes using the non-liner radial basis function based (ANN) classifiers. The result for classifying imaginary hand movements of 16 different subjects shows 80% accuracy. In Batres-Mendoza et al. (2017), one of the most important phases in systems using BCI devices has been discussed which is feature extraction. Quaternion-based signal analysis (QSA) has been presented in this work with improved version called iQSA method. It is used in EEG signal feature extraction for real time which involves mental tasks using motor imagery. The results for QSA shows 3.31% to 40.82% without sampling window and from 33.44% to 41.07% with sampling window. iQSA method has 82.3% accuracy rate for 0.5 s sample and 73.16% accuracy rate for 3s sample.

In Millán, Renkens, Mouriño, and Gerstner (2003), a method had been proposed based on the recent experiments which show that the movement of robotics and prosthetic devices can be controlled by the use of brain electrical activity. A portable non-invasive BCI has been used which can control a mobile robot in home like environment. Advanced robotics, protocol for the analysis of online EEG signal and machine learning algorithms to report first results of a brain-actuated mobile robot by means of a portable non-invasive BCI. Various classification algorithms used to design BCI systems based on EEG are reviewed in Lotte, Congedo, Lsecuyer, Lamarche, and Arnaldi (2007) which focus on five different categories of classification algorithms such as linear classifiers, neural networks, non-linear bayesian classifiers, nearest neighbor classifiers and combination of classifiers. The most frequently used neural networks for BCI is multilayer perceptron (MLP). Gaussian neural network has been specifically created for BCI. According to the recent trend, various classifiers are combined together and used efficiently for BCI.

In Ang, Chin, Wang, Guanand, and Zhang (2012), a filter bank common spatial pattern algorithm to optimize the subject-specific frequency band on datasets 2a and 2b of the BCI competition IV has been proposed. In Nicolas-Alonso, Corralejo, Gomes-Pilar, Álvarez, and Hornero (2015), a method had been proposed for motor imagery by combining information coming from multiple sources and reducing the existing uncertainty in EEG signals using stack generalization. In Zhang, Chin, Ang, Guan, and Wang (2011) a spatio-spectral filtering network has been proposed for BCI to classify motor imagery. In Ghandi, Prasad, Coyle, Behera, and McGinnity (2014) a recurrent quantum neural network filtering procedure has been applied to filter EEG signals before feature extraction and classification to increase signal separability for motor imagery classification. In Fok et al. (2011), an EEG-based brain computer interface for rehabilitation and restoration of hand control following stroke using ipsilateral cortical physiology has been proposed. In Onose et al. (2012), a clinical test and long-term post-trial follow-up on the feasibility of using motor imagery EEG-based brain-computer interface in chronic tetraplegics for assistive robotic arm control has been suggested. In Frolov et al. (2013), principles of neuro-rehabilitation based on the brain computer interface and biologically adequate control of the exoskeleton has been discussed.

Above suggested methods have certain drawbacks such as accuracy is very less. Hence in this work, a k-NN based method has been suggested for increasing the performance in classifying the motor imagery using the EEG signals from multiple channels. The work is organized as follows - section II describes nearest neighbor algorithm, section III contains proposed method, section IV contains the results and section V contains the conclusion of the work.

NEAREST NEIGHBOR ALGORITHM

In pattern recognition, the k-nearest neighbor algorithm (k-NN) is a non-parametric method used for classification and regression. In both cases, the input consists of the k closest training examples in the feature space. The output depends on whether k-NN is used for classification or regression Bermejo and Cabestany (2000). In k-NN classification, the output is a class membership. An object is classified by a majority vote of its neighbors, with the object being assigned to the class most common among its k nearest neighbors (k is a positive integer, typically small). If k = 1, then the object is simply assigned to the class of that single nearest neighbor (Cover & Hart, 1967). A small example of K-NN algorithm is shown in Figure 1.

In k-NN regression, the output is the property value for the object. This value is the average of the values of its k nearest neighbors (Dudani, 1967). k-NN is a type of instance-based learning, or lazy learning, where the function is only approximated locally and all computation is deferred until classification. The k-NN algorithm is among the simplest of all machine learning algorithm. Various types of distance metrics such as Euclidian distance, city block distance, chebysev distance and Minkowski distance, has been used. Minkowski distance can be defined as given in (1),

Figure 1. K-NN classifier

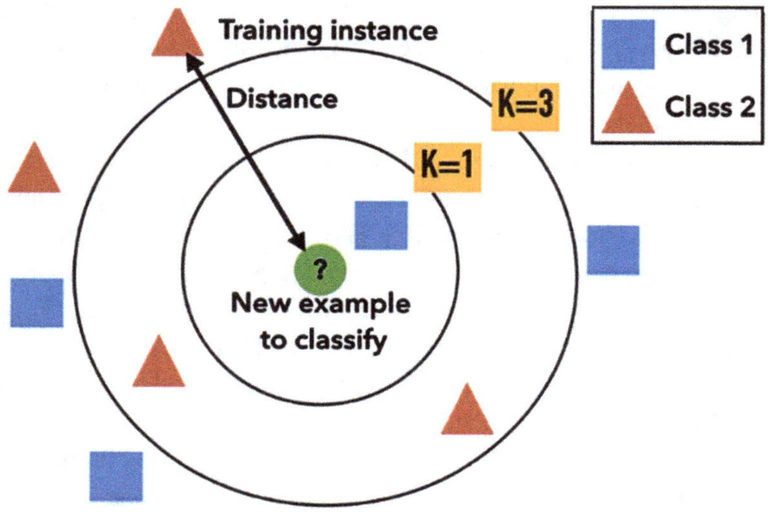

$$M_{ab} = \sqrt[p]{\sum_{j=1}^{n} \left| x_{aj} - y_{bj} \right|^{p}} \tag{1}$$

where M_{ab} = distance between vectors a and b, p = positive integer.

Euclidian distance can be defined as given in (2),

$$M_{ab}^{2} = \left(x_{a} - y_{j}\right)\left(x_{b} - y_{j}\right)' \tag{2}$$

City block distance can be defined as given in (3),

$$M_{ab} = \sum_{j=1}^{n} \left| x_{aj} - y_{bj} \right|^{p} \tag{3}$$

Chebysev distance can be defined as given in (4),

$$M_{ab} = max_{j} \left\{ \left| x_{aj} - y_{bj} \right| \right\} \left(4\right)$$

In this work k-NN is chosen over recurrent neural network (RNN) due to its various advantages. k-NN is much simpler algorithm in comparison to RNN. k-NN determines the class based on nearest distance where as RNN follows complex procedures. Other than that there are no definite criteria to design the RNN network and the training procedure is time taking. In this work k-NN has been used as a pattern classifier to classify the motor imagery from multiple channels of EEG signals which will be discussed in the section below.

PROPOSED METHOD

Most demonstrations of algorithms on BCI data are evaluating classification of EEG trials, i.e., windowed EEG signals for fixed length, where each trial corresponds to a specific mental state. Proposed method has various steps which are shown in the flowchart in Figure 2.

Features Used

These data sets were recorded from seven healthy subjects. In the whole session motor imagery was performed without feedback (BBCI, n.d.). Without feedback means the subject's hands did not move at all throughout the whole session although a subject performed motor imagery according to cues. For each subject two classes of motor imagery were selected from the three classes left hand, right hand, and foot (side chosen by the subject; optionally also both feet). To prepare for an EEG, electrodes are placed on the face and scalp. After placing each electrode in the right position, the electrical potential of each electrode can be measured. According to a person's state (waking, sleeping, etc.), both the frequency and the form of the EEG signal differ. For implementing the proposed method Berlin brain- computer interface data set IV has been used (BBCI, n.d.).

The recording was made using BrainAmp MR plus amplifiers and Ag/AgCl electrode cap. Signals from 59 EEG positions were measured that were most densely distributed over sensorimotor areas. Signals were band-pass filtered between 0.05 and 200 Hz and then digitized at 1000 Hz with 16 bit (0.1 uV) accuracy. A version of the data are also provided that is down sampled at 100 Hz (first low-pass filtering the original data with Chebyshev Type II filter of order 10 with stop band ripple 50dB down and stop band edge frequency 49Hz and then calculating the mean of blocks of 10 samples). Figure 3 shows the EEG signals of three of the channels out of 59 channels. Two sessions are performed for calibration data and four sessions are performed for evaluation data. The calibration data are used for train the network and the evaluation data are used to test the network.

Figure 2. Flowchart of the proposed scheme

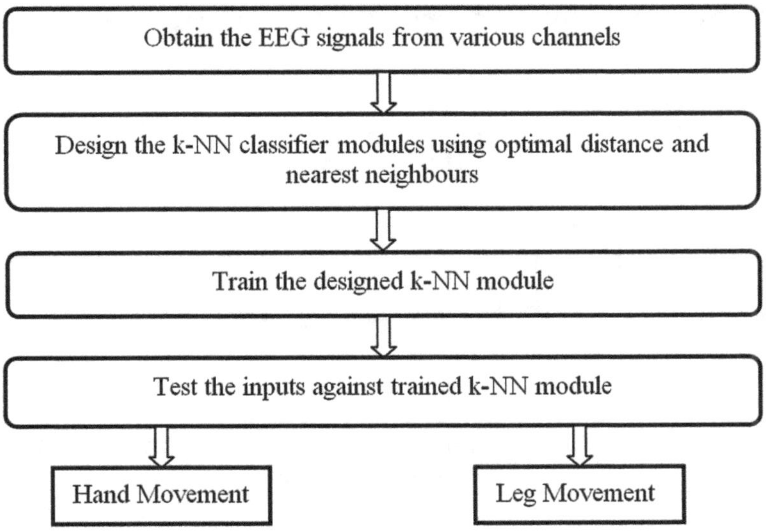

To generate calibration data, arrows pointing left, right, or down were presented as visual cues on a computer screen. Cues were displayed for a period of 4s during which the subject was instructed to perform the cued motor imagery task. These periods were interleaved with 2s of blank screen and 2s with a fixation cross shown in the centre of the screen. The fixation cross was superimposed on the cues, i.e. it was shown for 6s. These data sets are provided with complete marker information.

Evaluation data which are used for evaluating the submissions to the competitions. The motor imagery tasks were cued by soft acoustic stimuli (words left, right, and foot) for periods of varying length between 1.5 and 8 seconds. The end of the motor imagery period was indicated by the word stop. Intermitting periods had also a varying duration of 1.5 to 8s.

Design of the Proposed Method

Proposed method classifies the motor imagery using k-NN algorithm. All the algorithm design and simulation work has been done using MATLAB (2016). The submissions are evaluated in view of a one

Figure 3. EEG signals obtained from three channels (a) Channel 1 (b) Channel 2 (c) Channel 3

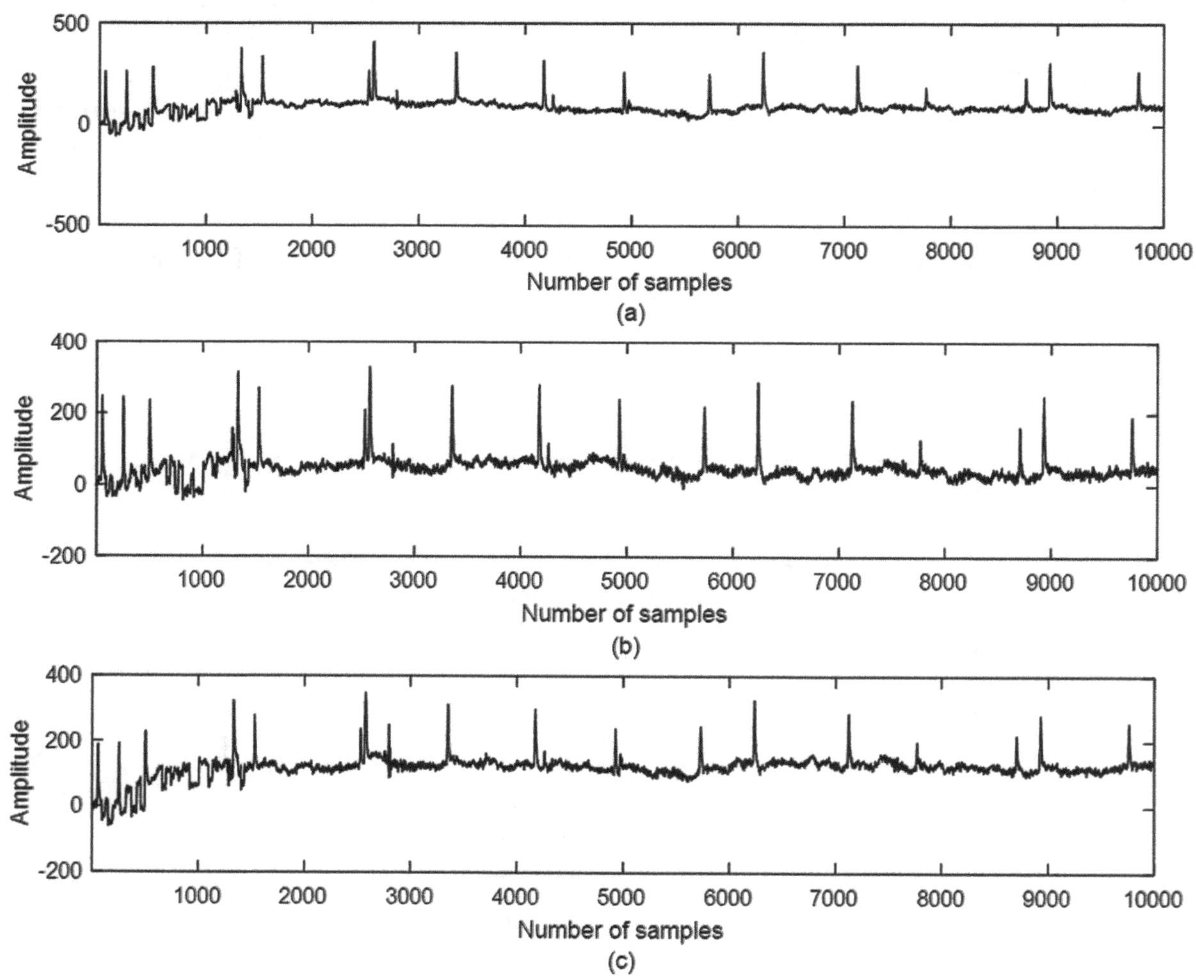

dimensional cursor control application with range from -1 to 1. The mental state of class one is used to position the cursor at -1, and the mental state of class two is used to position the cursor near 1. In the absence of those mental states (intermitting intervals) the cursor should be at position 0. After many hit and trial it can be observed that the accuracy of the proposed method is better with 3 fold validation, number of neighbours is 3 and cosine distance matrix. The results of the proposed method are discussed in the next section.

RESULTS

Proposed method using k-NN is evaluated with various test cases to check the performance of the method varying fold of cross validation, number of nearest neighbor, distance matrices etc. The performance of the network is evaluated in terms of %accuracy. Some of the test results are discussed in the section below.

Performance Varying Fold of Validation

In k-fold cross-validation, the original sample is randomly partitioned into k equal sized sub-samples. Of the k subsamples, a single subsample is retained as the validation data for testing the model, and the remaining k − 1 sub samples are used as training data. The cross-validation process is then repeated k times (the folds), with each of the k subsamples used exactly once as the validation data. The k results from the folds can then be averaged to produce a single estimation. The advantage of this method over repeated random sub-sampling is that all observations are used for both training and validation, and each observation is used for validation exactly once. Table 1 shows some of the results for varying K Folds. From Table 1 it can be observed that %accuracy of the method is highest for 3 Folds. Hence the optimal number of folds is chosen as 3.

Performance Varying Number of Neighbour

The principle behind nearest neighbor methods is to find a predefined number of training samples closest in distance to the new point, and predict the label from these. The number of samples can be a user-defined constant (k-nearest neighbor learning), or vary based on the local density of points (radius-based neighbor learning). Table 2 shows some of the results for varying number of neighbors. From Table 2 it can be observed that %accuracy of the method is highest for 3. Hence the optimal number of number of neighbor is chosen as 3.

Table 1. Performance varying fold of validation

Fold	Profit	Loss	%Accuracy
6	98.81	1.19	98.81
5	98.76	1.24	98.76
4	98.70	1.30	98.70
3	99.25	0.75	99.25
2	98.26	1.74	98.26

Table 2. Performance varying number of neighbors

Number of Neighbors	Profit	Loss	%Accuracy
6	98.42	1.58	98.42
5	98.62	1.38	98.62
4	98.61	1.39	98.61
3	99.25	0.75	99.25
2	98.66	1.34	98.66

Performance Varying Distance

To classify an unknown instance represented by some feature vectors as a point in the feature space, the k-NN classifier calculates the distances between the point and points in the training data set. Table 3 shows some of the results for varying Distance. From Table 3 it can be observed that %accuracy of the method is highest for Cosine Distance. Hence the optimal distance of k-NN is chosen as cosine for the proposed method.

Comparison With Other Method

The proposed method has been compared to various other earlier methods based on datasets used, algorithms used, fold of cross validation and %accuracy. The comparison with other suggested methods has been shown in Table 4. From Table 4 it can be observed that proposed method is better than all the other suggested method.

CONCLUSION

In this work, a k-NN based method is proposed for classification of motor imagery from EEG signals for performance enhancement of BCI applications. Proposed method classifies the tasks such as if person is moving left hand, right hand, or foot. Input features used for proposed method are the EEG signals obtained from 59 channels of the brain. The signals are then filtered with low-pass filtering Chebyshev

Table 3. Performance varying distance metrics

Distance	Profit	Loss	%Accuracy
Cosine	99.25	0.75	99.25
Euclidean	98.86	1.14	98.86
Hamming	55.66	44.3	55.66
Minkowski	98.78	1.22	98.78
Chebychev	99.09	0.91	99.09

Table 4. Comparison of other methods

Suggested By	Dataset Used	Algorithms used	Accuracy
Ang et al [8]	BCI competition IV Datasets 2a and 2b.	Filter bank common spatial pattern	Accuracy obtained using 10 fold cross validation
Nicolas-Alonso et al [9]	BCI Competition IV dataset 2a	Stacked Regularised Linear Discriminant Analysis	Accuracy obtained using 5 fold cross validation (kappa value 0.74)
Zhang et al [10]	BCI Competition IV dataset-I	Optimum Spatio-Spectral Filtering Network for Brain–Computer Interface	Accuracy obtained using 10 fold cross validation (89.9%)
Gandhi et al [11]	BCI competition IV data set 2a	Recurrent quantum neural network	Accuracy obtained using 10 fold cross validation.
Proposed Method	BCI competition dataset I	k-NN classifier	Accuracy obtained using 3 fold cross validation (99.25% accuracy)

Type II filter of order 10 with stop band ripple 50dB down and stop band edge frequency 49Hz. Then mean of blocks of 10 samples are calculated which are then given as input to the k-NN based classifier for motor imagery classification. Accuracy in classifying the motor imagery is up to 99.25% after 10 fold cross validation. Results of the proposed method suggest that it can be used efficiently for classification of motor imagery for BCI applications. The future scope of the work is to use test sample estimate instead of cross validation to reduce the error during real time applications.

REFERENCES

Ang, K., Chin, Z., Wang, C., Guanand, C., & Zhang, H. (2012). Filterbank common spatial pattern algorithm on BCI competition IV Datasets2a and 2b. *Frontiers in Neuroscience*, *6*(39), 1–9. PMID:22479236

Batres-Mendoza, P., Ibarra-Manzano, M., Guerra-Hernandez, E., Almanza-Ojeda, D., Montoro-Sanjose, C., Romero-Troncoso, R., & Rostro-Gonzalez, H. (2017). Improving EEG-Based Motor Imagery Classification for Real-Time Applications Using the QSA Method. *Computational Intelligence and Neuroscience*, *2017*, 1–16. doi:10.1155/2017/9817305 PMID:29348744

BBCI. (n.d.). *BCI Competition IV*. Retrieved from http://www.bbci.de/competition/iv/#dataset1

Bermejo, S., & Cabestany, J. (2000). Adaptive soft k-nearest-neighbour classifiers. *Pattern Recognition*, *33*(12), 1999–2005. doi:10.1016/S0031-3203(99)00186-7

Cover, T., & Hart, P. (1967). Nearest neighbor pattern classification. *IEEE Transactions on Information Theory*, *13*(1), 21–27. doi:10.1109/TIT.1967.1053964

Dudani, S. (1967). The distance-weighted k-nearest-neighbor rule. *IEEE Transactions on Systems, Man, and Cybernetics*, *6*, 325–327.

Fok, S., Schwartz, R., Ronkiewicz, M., Holmes, C., Zhang, J., Somers, T., ... Leuthardt, E. (2011). An EEG-based brain computer interface for rehabilitation and restoration of hand control following stroke using ipsilateral cortical physiology. *33rd Annual International Conf. of the IEEE EMBS*. 10.1109/IEMBS.2011.6091549

Frolov, A., Biryukova, E., Bobrov, P., Mokienko, O., Platonov, A., Pryanichnikov, V., & Chernikova, L. (2013). Principles of Neurorehabilitation Based on the Brain Computer Interface and Biologically Adequate Control of the Exoskeleton. *Human Physiology*, *39*(2), 196–208. doi:10.1134/S0362119713020035

Gandhi, V., Prasad, G., Coyle, D., Behera, L., & McGinnity, T. (2014). Quantum Neural Network-Based EEG Filtering for a Brain–Computer Interface. *IEEE Transactions on Neural Networks and Learning Systems*, *25*(2), 278–288. doi:10.1109/TNNLS.2013.2274436 PMID:24807028

Leuthardt, E., Schalk, G., Wolpaw, J., Ojemann, J., & Moran, D. (2004). A brain–computer interface using electrocorticographic signals in humans. *Journal of Neural Engineering*, *1*(2), 63–71. doi:10.1088/1741-2560/1/2/001 PMID:15876624

Lotte, F., Congedo, M., Lsecuyer, A., Lamarche, F., & Arnaldi, B. (2007). A Review of Classification Algorithms for EEG-based Brain-Computer Interfaces. *Journal of Neural Engineering*, *4*(2), 1–13. doi:10.1088/1741-2560/4/2/R01 PMID:17409472

MATLAB User's Guide: R2016a Documentation. (2016). Natick, MA: MathWorks Inc.

Millán, J., Renkens, F., Mouriño, J., & Gerstner, W. (2003). Non-Invasive Brain-Actuated Control of a Mobile Robot. *Proceedings of the 18th International Joint Conference on Artificial Intelligence*.

Nicolas-Alonso, L., Corralejo, R., Gomez-Pilar, J., Álvarez, D., & Hornero, R. (2015). Adaptive Stacked Generalization for Multiclass Motor Imagery-Based Brain Computer Interfaces. *IEEE Transactions on Neural Systems and Rehabilitation Engineering*, *23*(4), 702–712. doi:10.1109/TNSRE.2015.2398573 PMID:25680208

Onose, G., Grozea, C., Anghelescu, A., Daia, C., Sinescu, C., Ciurea, A., ... Popescu, F. (2012). On the feasibility of using motor imagery EEG-based brain-computer interface in chronic tetraplegics for assistive robotic arm control: A clinical test and long-term post-trial follow-up. *Spinal Cord*, *50*(8), 599–608. doi:10.1038c.2012.14 PMID:22410845

Qin, L., Ding, L., & He, B. (2005). Motor imagery classification by means of source analysis for brain–computer interface applications. *Journal of Neural Engineering*, *2*(4), 65–72. doi:10.1088/1741-2560/2/4/001 PMID:16317229

Sitaram, R., Zhang, H., Guan, C., Thulasidas, M., Hoshi, Y., Ishikawa, A., ... Birbaumer, N. (2007). Temporal classification of multichannel near-infrared spectroscopy signals of motor imagery for developing a brain–computer interface. *NeuroImage*, *34*(4), 1416–1427. doi:10.1016/j.neuroimage.2006.11.005 PMID:17196832

Wairagkar, M. (2014). Motor Imagery based Brain Computer Interface (BCI) using Artificial Neural Network Classifiers. *Proceedings of the British Conference of Undergraduate Research.*

Zhang, H., Chin, Z., Ang, K., Guan, C., & Wang, C. (2011). Optimum Spatio-Spectral Filtering Network for Brain–Computer Interface. *IEEE Transactions on Neural Networks*, *22*(1), 52–63. doi:10.1109/TNN.2010.2084099 PMID:21216696

Chapter 14
Intelligent Big Data Analytics in Health

Ebru Aydindag Bayrak
Istanbul University – Cerrahpaşa, Turkey

Pinar Kirci
Istanbul University – Cerrahpaşa, Turkey

ABSTRACT

Intelligent big data analytics and machine learning systems have been introduced to explain for the early diagnosis of neurological disorders. A number of scholarly researches about intelligent big data analytics in healthcare and machine learning system used in the healthcare system have been mentioned. The authors have explained the definition of big data, big data samples, and big data analytics. But the main goal is helping researchers or specialists in providing opinion about diagnosing or predicting neurological disorders using intelligent big data analytics and machine learning. Therefore, they focused on the healthcare systems using these innovative ways in particular. The information of platform and tools about big data analytics in healthcare is investigated. Numerous academic studies based on the detection of neurological disorders using both machine learning methods and big data analytics have been reviewed.

INTRODUCTION

The concept of big data was first used by Michael Cox and David Ellsworth at Proceedings of the 8th Conference on Visualization held in 1997, entitled "Application Controlled Demand Paging for Out-of-core Visualization". In the same study, it was mentioned that the datasets were too big and the computer system filled up the memory, disks and even external disks, and this problem was called "Big Data Problem" (Aktan, 2018).

The term big data was used for using larger volumes of scientific data for visualization. Although there are a large number of definitions of big data in the literature, the most popular definition comes from IBM. Big data could be characterized by any or all of three "V" words as suggested by IBM. V means that volume, variety, and velocity (O'Leary, 2013).

DOI: 10.4018/978-1-5225-8567-1.ch014

2.5 quintillion bytes of data was created by people, that is to say ninety percent of data (%90) has just been created in the last two years. This data is generated social media posts, videos, cell phone GPS signals or sensors. Here it is, this data is called Big Data (IBM, n.d.a.).

According to Gartner Incorporation "Big data is high-volume, high-variety and/or high-velocity information assets that demand cost-effective, innovative forms of information processing that enable enhanced insight, decision making, and process automation" (Gartner IT Glossary, n.d.).

The concept of big data; can be defined as a problem that occurs when traditional database management systems are inadequate when the data is stored, analyzed and managed (Sağıroğlu, 2017).

Big data indicate to growing dataset that involves unstructured, structured and semi-structured data by contrast with traditional data. The term big data was defined using the three main characteristics (3V) by most scientists and experts (Oussous, Benjelloun, Lahcen and Belfkih, 2017).

- Volume: It means the size of data which is varying from different data unit (terabyte, petabyte). Digital devices and applications (smartphones, IoT, social networks, logs,...) are generate big volumes of digital data. According to the report of International Data Corporation (IDC) the volume of data will increase from 898 exabytes to 6.6 zettabytes between 2012 and 2020. In other words, data will grow more than % 25 per a year.
- Variety: Big data is a variety of different formats (logs, videos, sensors,...) and sources. So it means the diversity of datasets.
- Velocity: Data is generated in a fast way that is means speed of data change.

The three components of big data can be summarized as in Figure 1. In addition to the three 3V's, other dimensions of big data have also been mentioned. These include (Gandomi and Haider, 2015):

- Veracity: This concept was coined by IBM to represent the uncertainty in some sources of data. We can give example such as customer sentiments in social media that are uncertain and include personal opinion. Even so they are valuable for analyzing information.
- Variability: It refers to the variation in the data flow rates, was introduced by SAS (Statistical Analysis Software).
- Value: It is defined by Oracle to define attribute of big data. Clearly it can be explained creating a value to organizations using big data analysis in the decision-making.

When research is done in both academic and business literature Big Data has been identified four key themes to which refers: Information, Technologies, Methods and Impact (De Mauro, Greco & Grimaldi, 2015).

The evaluation of big data is explained that it is equivalent to the oil of 20th century and is the gold mine of the 21th century. It is valuable for organization, government and individual (Sun, 2017).

BACKGROUND

O'Leary (2013) have focused on some of the basic concern and uses of artificial intelligence for big data. About the integration of artificial intelligence and big data case studies were presented. As what is big data, the application of mapreduce and hadoop, the significance of structured data topics were explained. In the end of study, it is accepted that machine learning and artificial intelligence have a key role for providing enterprise with intelligent analysis of big data.

Ward and Barker (2013) have studied a survey of big data definitions between academia, industry and media. Definitions made by Gartner, IBM, Oracle, Intel and Microsoft etc. are included. Additionally the importance of big data and its progress were remarked and the concept of big data was defined following words: Big data is a term describing the storage and analysis of large and or complex data sets using a series of techniques including, but not limited to: NoSQL, MapReduce and Machine Learning.

Sagiroglu and Sinanc (2013) have reviewed an overview of big data's content, scope, samples, methods, advantages and handicap and discusses about the principle of privacy. They explained that have useful information is gained from big data analysis, take advantages for companies or organizations.

De Mauro et al. (2015) have reviewed the existing literature on big data and analyzed its previous definition. They have made out two suggestions about big data. Firstly, they offered a summary of the main research areas related to the concept of big data, trending and opportunities for future development. Secondly, they have provide a general definition for big data to synthesize common themes of previous definitions.

Yoo, Ramirez & Liuzzi (2014) have introduced modern statistical machine learning using big data analysis in medicine. Clinical, genomic and environmental datasets were collected from biomedical science that is too much and complex. To analyze these datasets, regression analysis and modern statistical model can be used. They have explained Linear and Logistic Regression and Bayesian Networks to analyze biomedical datasets. Bayesian Networks used big data sets that are more complicated data, have different type of huge data from clinical genomic and environmental data.

X. Wu, Zhu, G. Wu & Ding (2014) have studied data mining with big data sets. They have presented HACE theorem that models the key characteristics of the big data. This acronym means that huge with Heterogeneous and diverse data, Autonomous with distributed and decentralized control, Complex and Evolving relationships. Also data mining challenges with big data as data accessing, semantic and domain knowledge for different big data applications, algorithm designs were explained.

Singh and Reddy (2015) have studied a survey that is about different platforms for big data analytics, explains advantages and obstacle of data processing platforms. They have asserted a comparison of different platforms using rating, using parametrics for rating are scalability, data input/output performance, fault tolerance, real time processing, data size supported and iterative task support. Data size, speed and model development are specified important factors to choose platform for application.

Gandomi and Haider (2015) have worked on big data concepts, definitions of big data, using methods and big data analytics especially focused on analytics methods used for big data. Big data analytics were explained for using analyze and acquire intelligence from big data. They have reviewed analytics techniques for text, audio, video, social media and predictive analytics.

Özköse, Arı & Gencer (2015) have explained characteristic and classification of big data, big data process, usage areas of big data and methods used in big data in their study. In addition all these, they have mentioned yesterday, today and tomorrow of big data with some studies on big data in Turkey and all over the word.

Xu, Yue, L. Guo, Y. Guo & Fang (2015) have carried out privacy-preserving machine learning algorithms for big data systems. They have proposed a framework based on MapReduce to analyze big data. Additionally they have focused on support vector machines and explained two schemes for vertically and horizontally partitioned training data sets. The breast cancer data set, the Higgs bosons presence dataset and optical character recognition of handwritten digits dataset were used to test performance of their scheme.

Qui, Wu, Ding, Xu & Feng (2016) have presented a survey of machine learning for big data processing. They have reviewed advanced machine learning techniques such as representation learning, deep learning, distributed and parallel learning, transfer learning, active learning and kernel-based learning. The first purpose of their work is explaining current research efforts any challenges of big data. The other purpose is to analyze interaction between machine learning and modern signal processing for big data. In addition to these, different critical issues for machine learning applications on big data are explained.

Atalay and Çelik (2017) have discussed the use of artificial intelligence and machine learning technique in big data analysis. The general information about artificial intelligence and machine learning methods were given and some applications of these methods have been explained. They have suggested that artificial intelligence will be much more important in the future by means of technological developments.

Balasupramanian, Ephrem & Al-Barwani (2017) have purposed framework that is used big data analytics and machine learning technique to prevent online fraud detection before it happens.

Oussous et al. (2017) have prepared a survey about recent technologies developed for big data. They have explained big data definitions, applications and challenges in their study as the main title. Also they have studied different big data technologies and these technologies have been compared by capabilities and limits.

Zhou, Pan, Wang & Vasilakos (2017) have introduced a framework of Machine Learning on Big Data (MLBID). They have prepared an overview of opportunities and challenges of machine learning on big data. Big data, user, domain and system are components of MLBID framework. Also they have summarized open research issues in MLBID according to components of framework. At the end of study they have referred that machine learning is valuable for insights from big data.

BIG DATA SAMPLES

We can use and find big data examples in the literature or different working areas. These areas can be sorted by respectively; astronomy, atmospheric science, genomics, biological science, natural science, health records, scientific research, private sector, military surveillance, financial services, retail. In addition, mobile phones, social networks, call detail records, web logs, photography-audio-video, click streams, search indexing, POS information, radio frequency identification (RFID) and sensor networks can be counted big data samples (Sagiroglu and Sinanc, 2013).

According to "Data Never Sleeps 6.0" project was prepared by Domo (2018), % 90 per of all data today has been created in the last two years. That means 2.5 quintillion bytes of data per a day. For example; approximately more than 4 million video views on YouTube, 2.083.333 snaps sharing on Snapchat, and users post 49.380 photos on Instagram. When we analyzed global internet population growth 2012-2017, the global internet population has grown 3.8 billion people as of 2017 (Domo, n.d.). If the growing continues at this rate, it is clear that the amount of data will continue to increase (Figure 2).

Big data samples can be grouped under three main headings: structural, semi-structural and non-structural data (Aktan, 2018):

Figure 1. The three components of big data (Adapted from Russom, 2011).

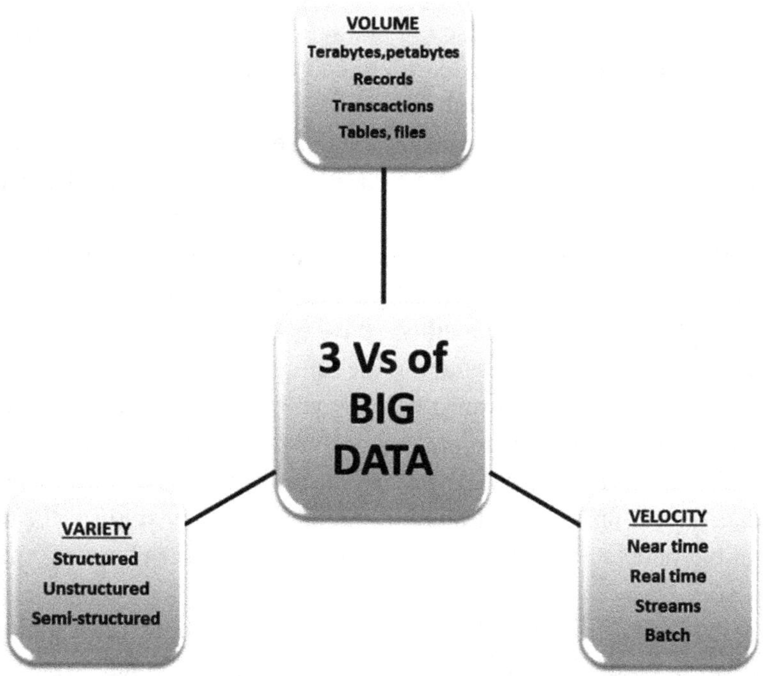

1. **Structured Data:** Is expressed all data types that are easy for modeling, insertion as input, storage, interrogation, processing and visualizing.
2. **Semi-Structured Data:** Has various meta-models, such as tags and markers used to define certain items and hierarchical representations of different fields on the data, as well as models that define the structure data.
3. **Non-Structural Data:** Are types of records that are presented and stored and stored outside of defined format.

Big data is used many different working fields. Some of them are can be listed below (Özköse et al., 2015);

- High technology and industry,
- Medical field,
- Travel and transport sector,
- Education and research,
- Media and show business,
- Automotive industry,
- Financial services,
- Customer relationship management.

Figure 2. A striking picture is shown related to the speed of the data. How much data is generated for every minute in 2018? (Adapted from Domo, n.d.).

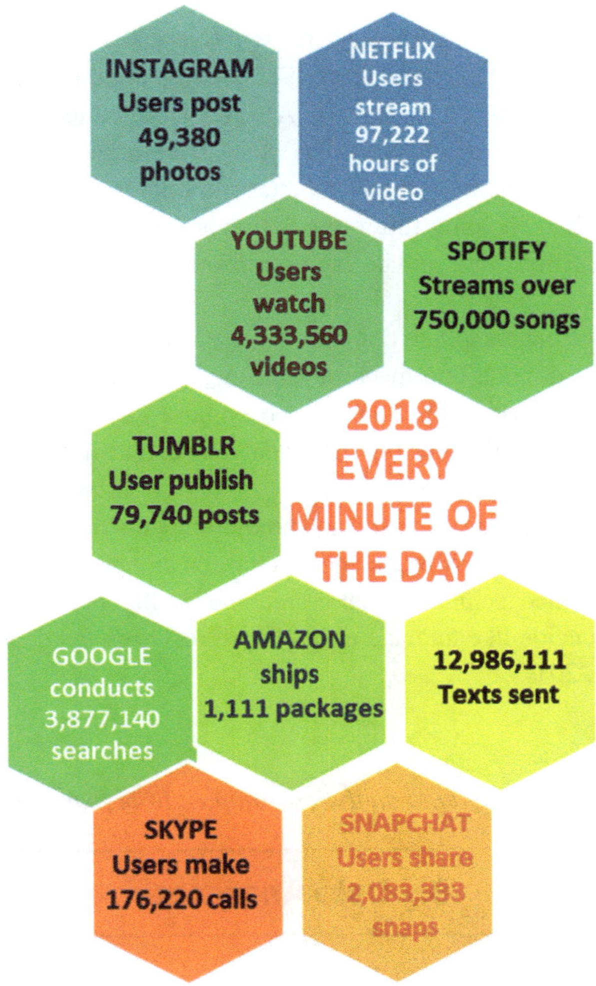

BIG DATA ANALYTICS

With the development of technology, the increasing number of smart devices, producing real-time log records via the help of sensors, increasing mobility and internet access social networks are becoming a part of our daily life have been increased the diversity, speed and volume of data surrounded. This situation brings with it the problems of obtaining, storing and processing big data. At this point, big data analytics provides access to information through selection, storage and processing of structured data (for example: corporate data) and unstructured data (for example: video, audio, text files, etc.) (Aktan, 2018).

Big Data Analytics can be described simply that using advanced analytic techniques operate on big data (Russom, 2011). In other words big data analytics is basically described as the process of collecting, structuring, analyzing and evaluating big datasets. The first goal is to find patterns and other hidden information from large data. Big data analytics assists to make sense of the data that is more significant for making decision and the business (Balasupramanian et al., 2017).

Big Data Analytics is an emerging science and technology involving multidisciplinary state-of-art information and communication technology, mathematics, operations research, machine learning and decision sciences for big data. Three main components of big data analytics include big data descriptive analytics, big data predictive analytics and big data prescriptive analytics (Z. Sun, L. Sun & Strang, 2018)

Big Data Analytics is described as the process of collecting, organizing, analyzing huge datasets to discover useful information and different patterns. Also it is formed techniques and technologies that require new forms of integration to disclose hidden values from large datasets. It is mainly focused on solving new problems or old problems with much better and impressive ways. The main goal of the big data analytics is sorted such as, helping future prediction and making better decision to organization, analyze organization transactions and update the organization data (Verma, Agrawal, B. Patel & A. Patel, 2016).

Technical components of big data analytics can be presented in Figure 3 that it is total of data warehouse, data mining, statistical modelling machine learning, visualization and optimization. Intelligent big data analytics is the core of data science and can be explained by the addition of the intelligent term to previous mention components. Besides big data, analytics and artificial intelligence are inseparable whole (Sun,2017).

Big data analysis can give much more reason and prediction with the use of artificial neural networks, deep learning, natural language processing, image recognition and personalization technologies. On the other hand, artificial intelligence techniques that imitate the intelligent behaviours of living beings, create models that think and decide like human, are preferred resulting from gain advantages on big data analysis (Atalay and Çelik, 2017).

Figure 3. The interrelationship of big data analytics (Adapted from Sun et al, 2018).

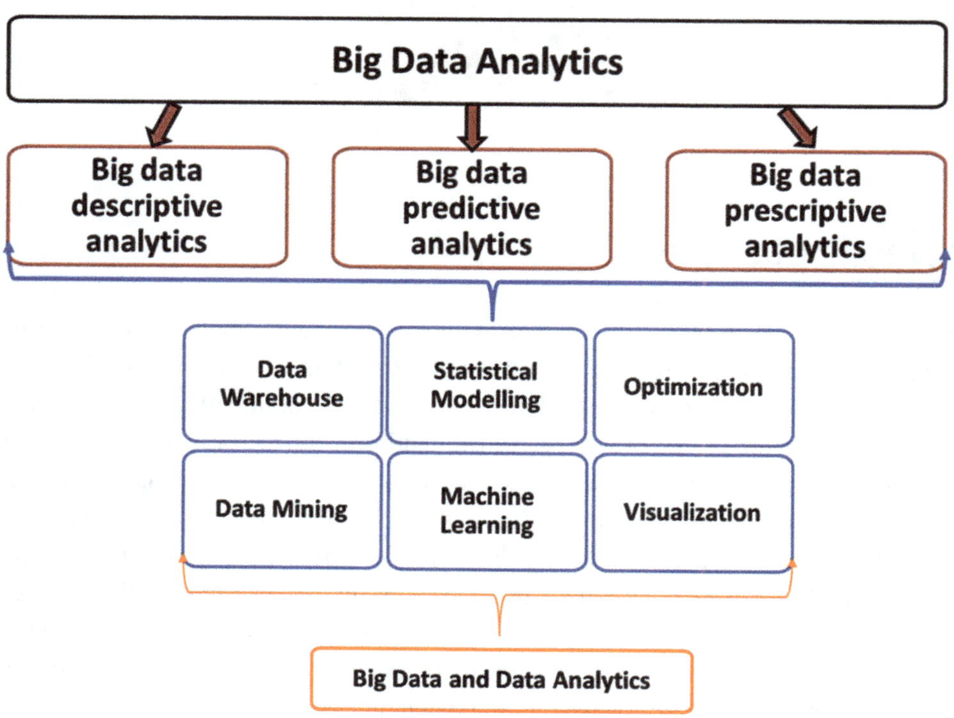

Big data analytics tools aim to obtain worthful information from data through analysis structured, semi-structured and non-structural data that are difficult to process using with traditional database techniques (Aktan, 2018).

Big data analytics is a technique used in the big datasets and can be viewed as a sub-process in the overall process of information extraction from big data. Big data analytics process can be explained five stages in the following words. The first three steps are called data management, while the last two steps are called analytics (Gandomi and Haider);

1. Data acquisition
2. Information extraction
3. Integration
4. Modeling and analysis
5. Interpretation

Transforming Data With Intelligence (TDWI) has asked many user organizations "In your organization, is big data considered mostly a problem or mostly an opportunity. Thirty percent of them said that they consider big data as a problem. The rest of organizations (%70) said that they consider big data an opportunity. The analyses of big data provide new facts to organizations about their customers, markets, partners, costs, and operations and then they can use these information for business advantage (Russom, 2011).

BIG DATA ANALYTICS IN HEALTHCARE SYSTEMS

The role of big data in the healthcare system is to guide datasets related to healthcare which are complicated and hard to manage using current management tools, software and hardware (Kumar and Singh, 2019).

The impact of big data on the healthcare system was defined in five pathways as following (Groves, Kayyali, Knott & Van Kuiken, 2013):

1. **Right Living:** Refers to living more healthier life for patients.
2. **Right Care:** Refers to having convenient treatment for patiens and is obtained same data and objectives.
3. **Right Provider:** Refers to provide better treatment options for patients using health data.
4. **Right Value:** Refers to increase the quality and value of health-related services.
5. **Right Innovation:** Refers to research and development activities about health as recognize new treatments and new medicine.

The process of big data analytic tool can be defined a data flow that provide worthful information from large dataset for decision making as following (Sahu, Jacintha & Singh, 2017);

- Collection of data
- Storage of data
- Processing
- Visualizing

The big health data sources are; Electronic Healthcare Records (EHRs), Biomedical images, Sensing data, Biomedical signals, Genomic data, Clinical text and Social media. EHRs refers a copy of patient's medical history. Biomedical images refers clinical imaging modalities as Magnetic Resonance Imaging (MRI), Positron Emission Tomography (PET), ultrasound, Computed Tomography (CT), etc. Sensing data refers such as Electrocardiogram (ECG) and Electroencephalogram (EEG) signals. Biomedical signals refers as blood pressure, brain activity, oxygen saturation levels etc. many sources. Genomic data refers relationships between genetic markers, mutations and disease. Clinical text refers clinical notes which are stored unstructured data. Social network refers various collected social media resources as Facebook, Twitter, web logs and social network sites (Ta, Liu & Nkabinde, 2016).

Wang, Kung & Byrd (2018) have aimed to identify big data analytics capabilities and explore the potential benefits of big data analytics in healthcare system in the study. They have explained the history of big data analytics from past to today, architecture of its in healthcare and the strategies for success with big data analytics.

Praveena and Bharathi (2017) have prepared a survey paper about big data analytics. They have examined various big data analytics and its operations, infrastructure, challenges and analysis algorithms of big data. Also they have investigated few of big data management tools which are used for different purpose.

Athmaja, Hanumanthappa & Kavitha (2017) have worked on advanced machine learning algorithms and techniques which are used to have solutions to big data analytic problems. They have analyzed some studies that is about different machine learning techniques and prepared literature survey.

Siuly and Zhang (2016) have reviewed medical big data analysis on neurological disease diagnosis. The difficulty of obtaining medical big data, medical big data analysis and computer aid diagnosis systems (CAD) have been explained on study. Also, they have surveyed developing CAD system for automatical diagnosis of neurological diseases.

Sun and Reddy (2013) have studied on big data analytics for healthcare. They have explained predictive models for clinical data analysis, scalable healthcare analytics platform and genetic data analysis. The overall goals of big data analytics in health have been mentioned.

The challenges of Big Data and Analytical process have been grouped as main topics; storage, data representation, the management of data life cycle, data confidentiality, data analysis, data reporting, energy management, redundancy reduction and data compression, expendability and scalability, cooperation and dimensionality reduction of big data (Praveena and Bharathi, 2017).

Platforms or Tools for Big Data Analytics in Healthcare

Apache Hadoop

Hadoop is an open source and parallel computing platform or tool that stores and process big data. The main component of Hadoop can be summarized as firstly, Hadoop Distributed File System (HDFS) secondly MapReduce and thirdly YARN. HDFS is file system distributed on cluster and has storage devices. MapReduce process the data that is stored on HDFS clusters. It has two steps on data. Map step is about divide of data into smaller, Reduce step is about produce a solution. As for, YARN is a resource management (Harerimana, Jang, Kim & Park, 2018).

A more general definition of the Hadoop ecosystem and framework is open source tools, methodologies and libraries for "big data" analysis in which lots of data sets are obtained from different sources (Kumar and Singh, 2019).

It is flexible and user friendly platform working with different data sources to use machine learning process (Praveena and Bharathi, 2017).

MapReduce

MapReduce is explained that is the heart of Apache Hadoop by IBM. It is programming paradigm that allow massive scalability between lots of server in Hadoop cluster. MapReduce term refers to have two different task in Hadoop program as map and reduce. The map task converts dataset into another set of data. The reduce task takes outputs from map and combines them to have reduced tuples (IBM, n.d.b.).

Apache Mahout

Mahout is another Apache project for generating free applications of distributed and scalable machine learning and data mining algorithms. It is used for big data analytics on the Hadoop platform (W. Raghupathi and V. Raghupathi, 2014).

Apache Pig

Apache Pig is open-source platforms for analyzing big data sets. It consists of high level language for identification of data analysis programs and it's infrastructure evaluates analysis programs. The most remarkable feature of Pig structure is that allows to handle very large data sets with parallelization (Apache Pig, n.d.).

Apache Hive

The Apache Hive is data warehouse software facilitates on Hadoop about reading, writing, and managing large datasets in distributed storage using SQL-like language (Apache Hive, n.d.).

Apache Spark

Spark is an open source and parallel computing platform for big data sources as Hadoop and also provides scalable data analytics paltform with in memory computing. When it was compared wih Hadoop, computing power is more power than Hadoop. Spark is planned for machine learning and natural language processing (Patel and Sharma, 2014).

It is programmed in Scala and programmable in Scala or Python. Spark's specific functionalities can be sorted as machine learning, graph analysis and data-streaming (Berral-Garcia, 2016). Spark is a heavily used platform for healthcare big data analytics because of performing more fast analysis using its stream computing capabilities (Harerimana et al., 2018).

MACHINE LEARNING SYSTEM

One of today's the fastest developing technical fields is machine learning and it is at the core of artificial intelligence and data science and also lying at the intersection of computer science and statistics. The study about mmachine learning is focused on the question about how to build computers that improve automatically through experience (Jordan and Mitchell, 2015).

Machine learning has been used both scientific and business study field to extract useful information from hidden pattern. Because it is not possible to analyze and process the data in very large quantities in the traditional way. For this reason, machine learning methods have been developed to analyze big data. This methods use old data to solve problem and predict the future. In addition to these advantages, machine learning methods contribute to decision making mechanism. Machine learning makes inference from the data using mathematical and statistical methods (Diri, n.d.).

Machine learning is defined by (Mithcell, 2006) as follows:" We say that a machine learns with respect to a particular task T, performance metric P, and type of experience E, if the system reliably improves its performance P at task T, following experience E".

For machine learning application generally dataset is divided into two groups and they called trainings set and testing set. The training set is used to teach for algorithm and discover the underlying structure in data. The testing set is used to calculate model accuracy (Altındal, 2006).

Machine learning has a significant role in big data systems due to discovering important knowledge and hidden information (Xu et al., 2015).

The some application of machine learning can sorted as pattern recognition, optical character recognition (OCR), face recognition, medical diagnosis, speech recognition, natural language processing, biometrics, knowledge detection and outlier detection (Alpaydın, 2014).

Especially along with the rising of big data, machine learning has become a key technique for solving problems in different areas; such as computational finance, energy production, automotive, aerospace and manufacturing (Mathworks, n.d.).

Machine learning is the one of most effective method used in big data analytics to predict with some models and algorithms. These analytical models give us a chance to produce reliable and acceptable results. In addition, machine learning algorithms allow to discover some hidden pattern and trends from big data (Angra and Ahuja, 2017).

The critical issue of machine learning for big data have been explained by Qui et al. (2016) with five different perspectives as below:

1. Learning for huge scale of data.
2. Learning for various types of data.
3. Learning for high speed of data stream
4. Learning for ambiguous and missing data.
5. Learning for data with low value density and meaning density.

Machine Learning Methods

The machine Learning methods aim to find the most suitable model for new data available by using the past data. To make this, two different methods are used as to be classification and clustering. Classification is used mostly as a supervised learning, while clustering is used for unsupervised learning.

But some clustering models are used for both supervised and unsupervised learning. Classification is purposed predictive, while clustering is descriptive (Rokach and Maimon, 2005).

Machine learning methods can be divided into three groups; they are called, supervised learning, unsupervised learning and reinforcement learning. In a few words, if we want to explain subdomains of the field of machine learning: Supervised learning requires training with labeled data which has inputs and expected outputs. Unsupervised learning does not require labeled training data and it only use inputs for training. Reinforcement learning provides learning from feedback (reward-penalty) via interactions with enviroment. The supervised and unsupervised learning techniques are preferred for data analysis process whereas reinforcement techniques are preferred for decision making process (Oiu et al., 2016).

Supervised Learning

Supervised learning is a machine learning technique which is used a function matching between preferred output and labelled data. When making a function it use training datasets. Function can be determined with classification and regression algorithms (Uzun, 2016).

It is known that input value corresponds to which output in supervised learning (Kartal, 2015).

Supervised learning is learned from our data when we determine a target variable. We approach to target variable as two cases: The first situation explains when the target variable can take only nominal or categorical values and this situation is called classification. For the second situation, the target variable can take infinite number of numeric and is called regression (Harrington, 2012).

Both of classification and regression are supervised learning problems that learning is carried out mapping from input to output. For example credit scoring, this is an example of classification problem because there are two classes: high risk customers and low risk customers. The customer information has been used an input to classify which customer is belong one of the two classes. The predict of car prices problem is regression problem which the output is numeric (Alpaydın, 2014).

The mostly used supervised learning methods in machine learning are explained as the following, e.g. support vector machines, artificial neural networks, decision trees, k-nearest neighbour, naive bayes classifier, random forest, linear regression, logistic regression and deep learning.

Support Vector Machines

The Support Vector Machines (SVM) is firstly called by Vapnik (1995). SVM is a machine learning method that tries to find optimal hyperplane to separate the classes by using support vectors, can be used for classification and regression. This technique aims to find optimal hyperplane to separate two classes of data. Two classes are to be separated when the margin between them is maximized as in Figure 4. If the problems cannot be separated a simple hyper-plane, the data is transferred to a new space which is higher dimensional space. And it aims to find hyperplane to separate data. (Burakgazi, 2017)

SVM is divided into two groups according to linear separation and non-linear separation dataset. The dataset can not be separated linearly, it can separate applying with kernel function. The most used kernel functions are; linear, polynomial, radial basis function and sigmoid function (Yahyaoui, 2017).

Figure 4. Architecture of support vector machine, using separate two classes with optimum hyperplane (Adapted from Alpaydın, 2014).

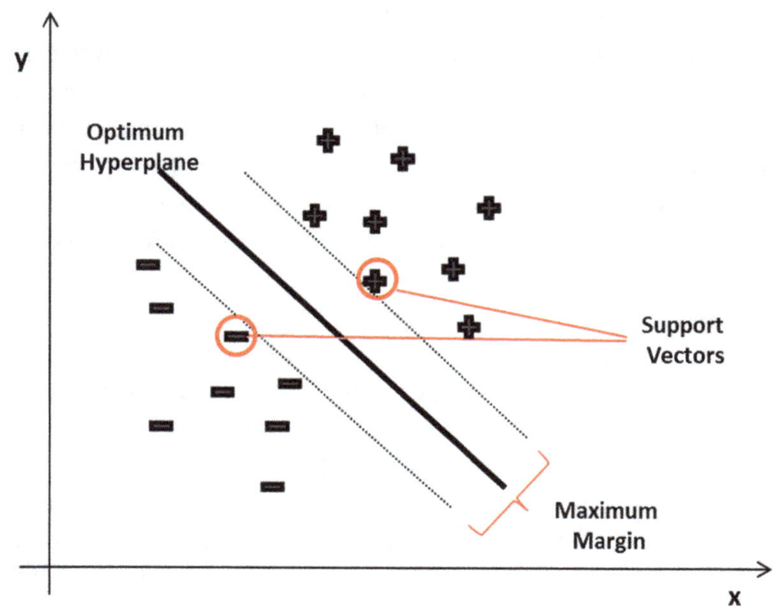

Artificial Neural Networks

Artificial neural networks (ANN) are trying to modelling of the human brain. It is aimed to training, learning and make a decision of machines by means of artificial neural networks (Kızrak, n.d.).

In engineering studies, the goal is not to model neural networks only in the brain. It is beneficial for us to make better computers using artificial neural networks. The brain is more than an engineering product in terms of its abilities such as image, speech, learning and recognition. These capabilities are crucial to implement artificial intelligence networks on computers (Alpaydın, 2013).

The main structure of ANN can be described basically as to be input, hidden and output layers in Figure 5.

Decision Trees

The decision trees method is based on divide and rule strategy. It has a hierarchical structure consisting of decision nodes and leaves (Alpaydın, 2014).

To apply decision tree method, firstly you must make decision which feature is used to divide data. For the best results, every feature and measure should try and then you can split the datasets into subsets in Figure 6. The methods steps can be summarized as the followings: (Harrington,2012)

1. Firstly all of the dataset is used.
2. Dataset divided into two subsets according to value of a feature (the best feature that split).
3. The same procedure is applied for each subset until all of the feature are in same class. Otherwise you need to the splitting process.

Figure 5. The basic structure of artificial neural networks (Adapted from [Atalay and Çelik, 2017]).

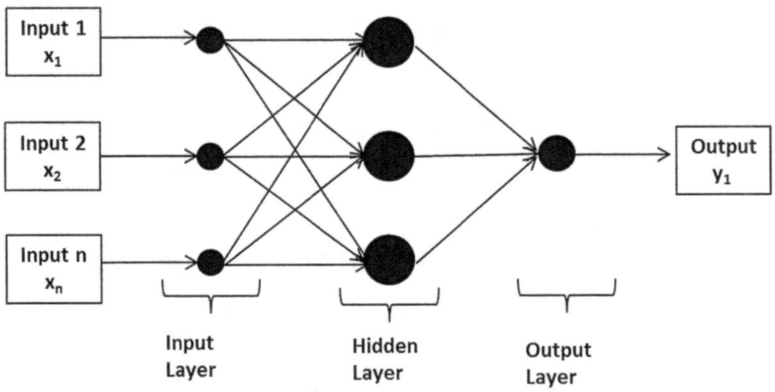

Figure 6. The process of decision is represented by a tree structure (Adapted from Alpaydın, 2014).

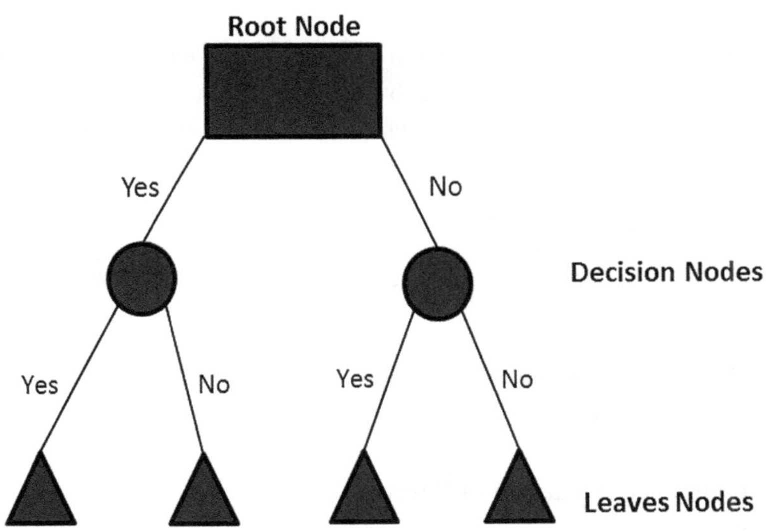

K Nearest Neighbour

The k-Nearest Neighbours (kNN) algorithm is a simple and effective but at the same time is powerful classification method. It uses the concept of distance measurement of classify items in Figure 7. kNN is a supervised learning methods so we have labels for all data and know what class each piece of the data should fall into. When we are given a new piece of data without a label, the classification steps can be summarized as follows (Harrington, 2012):

1. k parameter is determined. k is the number of neigbours closest to new data.
2. The distances between new data (testing) and existing data (training) are calculated.
3. The most closest distance values are selected (find the nearest neigbour)
4. New data falls into which class have highest number of similar data.

Figure 7. The architecture of k nearest neigbours algorithm. For k=1 new data (red circle) belongs to triangle class (right). For k=2 red circle belongs to square class, because two of the three nearest neighbours belong to the square class (Adapted from Ruan et al., 2017).

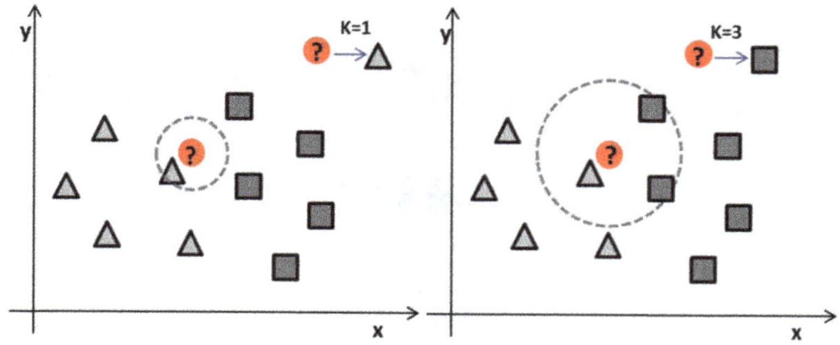

Naive Bayes Classifier

Naive Bayes Classifier is one of the most popular classification methods that based on the Bayesian theorem. Naive Bayes is very simple method, such that just small amount training data can be classify the given examples. The naive bayes algorithm which is used to calculate present and past frequency occurrences, can explain as follows (Umadevi and Marseline, 2017):

$$P(A \setminus B) = P(B \setminus A) * P(A) / P(B)$$

- Where P(A) is the prior probability of A. It counts only the occurrences of A.
- P(A\B) is the conditional probability of A, given B. It is also called as posterior probability which means A is derived from B.
- P(B\A) is the conditional probability of B, given A.
- P(B) is the prior probability of B.

Random Forest

The technique of Random Forest has been firstly improved by Leo Breiman in 2001. It is a classifier that is consisting of lots of tree-structure. Random forests are a combination of tree predictors and each tree depends on the values of a random vector. The classification is used the most popular or the best class according to input. At each node it selects the best of the randomly retrieved qualities and separates all nodes into branches (Breiman, 2001).

The method of Random Forest is based on a recursive approach in Figure 8. For every iteration, one random sample is chosen from sample size of N from data with replacement and another random sample is chosen from the predictors no replacement. After, acquired dataset is partitioned. The out-of-bag data is dropped and steps are repeated depending on how many trees we need. The classification is realized using majority vote over the decision trees (Bazazeh and Shubair, 2016).

Figure 8. The diagram showing how random forest works (Adapted from Bazazeh and Shubair, 2016).

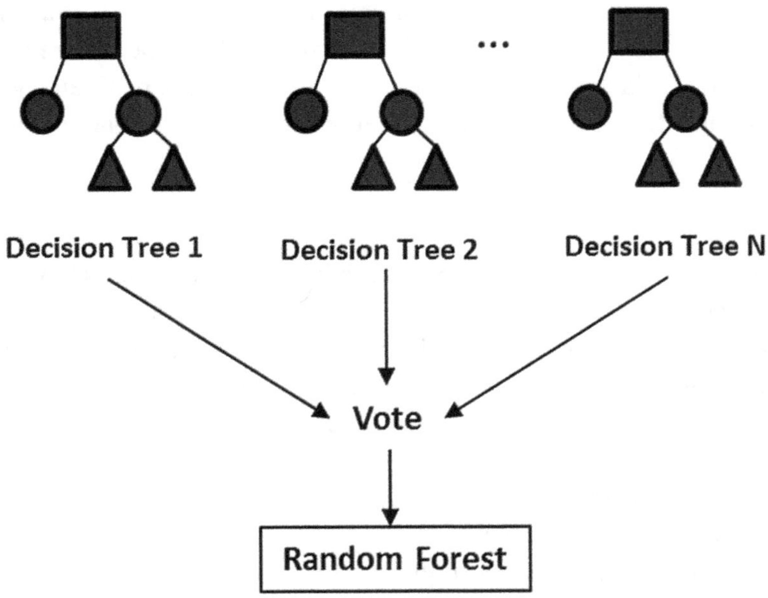

Linear Regression

Linear regression is a statistical method for modeling the relationship between a dependent variable and one or more independent variables. According to method, it supposes that outcome can be estimated via weighted sums of input variables (Yoo et al., 2014).

The linear regression model is represented by this formula:

$$Y = \beta_0 + \beta_1 X_1 + \beta_2 X_2 + \cdots + \beta_n X_n$$

where Y is dependent variable and $X_i, \mathrm{i} = 1, 2, \ldots \mathrm{n},$ are independent variables and $\beta_j, j = 1, 2, \ldots, n$ are regression parameters. The equation enables us to predict the value of dependent variable Y from the independent variable X. The slope of equation is β_j where is called regression coefficent, R^2 is defined the coefficient of determination and is a measure of how well the regression model describes the observed data (Saritha and Abraham, 2017).

Logistic Regression

The Logistic Regression provides the relationship between the predictive attributes (independent variables) and the target attribute (dependent variable) if the target attribute is a categorical variable (Kartal, 2015).

Logistic regression has similarity in many aspects to linear regression, but actually they are very different due to one critical aspect (Figure 9). Logistic regression explains output can be expressed through weighted sum that is special mathematical transformation which is called logit. This transformation allows all weighted sum to be take a value in between 0 and 1 (Yoo et al., 2014).

The purpose of the logistic regression is to establish a model that can be identified the relationship between dependent variables and independent variables as having the best fit using the least variant. The most distinctive feature that separates the logistic regression from the linear regression is the result variable is binary or multiple in the logistics regression. This difference between logistic regression and linear regression have effected both parametric model selection and assumptions (Bircan, 2004).

Deep Learning

Machine learning systems are used to transcribe speech into text, match news items, identify objects in images, posts or products with users interests. In the wake of technical developments, these applications make use of a class of techniques that is called deep learning (LeCun, Bengio & Hinton, 2015).

In 2006, deep learning has arisen as new field of machine learning research that uses multiple layers of information-processing in a hierarchical architecture for pattern classification and representation learning. The main advantage of deep learning can be explained as increasing chip processing abilities, having the much lower cost of computing hardware and the development in machine learning (Al-Jarrah, Yoo, Muhaidat, Karagiannidis & Taha, 2015).

Recently deep learning is one of the most attractive research interest in machine learning (Figure 10). It is different from most traditional learning techniques because of using shallow structured learning architectures. Deep learning can use together both supervised and unsupervised strategies in deep architectures to automatically learn hierarchical representations (Oui et al., 2016).

Unsupervised Learning

Unsupervised learning is a machine learning technique which use a function to predict unknown pattern through unlabeled data. In this method there is no training data. The algorithms group data and new data can be incorporated into the most suitable group (Uzun, 2016).

Figure 9. The figure of linear regression and logistic regression model (Adapted from [Sayad, n.d.b.]).

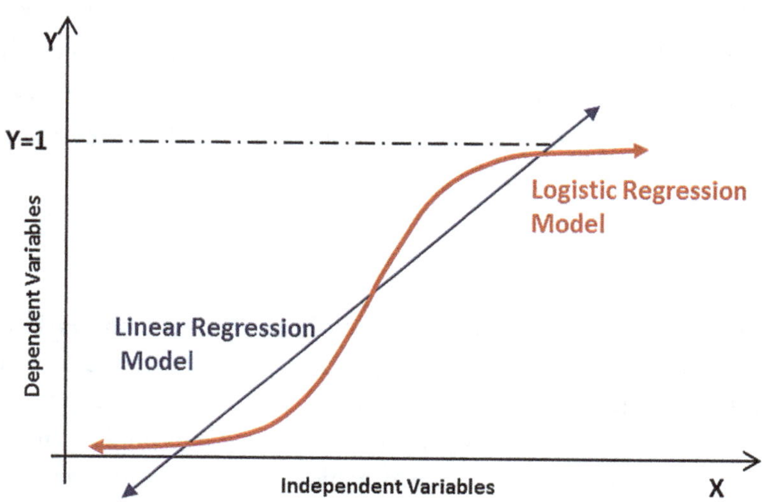

Figure 10. The relationship between deep learning, machine learning and artificial learning (Adapted from [Shorten, 2018]).

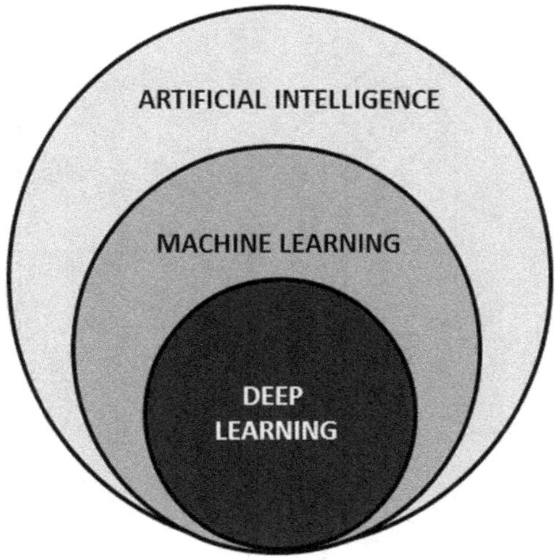

Bishop (2006) has explained unsupervised learning where the training data consist of input data without no mapping target values. The goal of unsupervised learning is to find groups of similar cluster within the data which is called clustering or see the distribution of data, known as density estimation, or reduce high dimension for visualization (Bishop, 2006).

In supervised learning, we do not have supervisor and we only have input data. The purpose is to find the pattern or regularities in the input data. The clustering purpose is to find clusters of input data. The customer segmentation is the best example for understanding clustering method. A company using demographic information and past transactions, can see the distribution of the customer profile and make customer grouping. Thus the company can manage customer relationship management better quality and could make better decide strategies, about services and products for different groups (Alpaydın, 2014).

The unsupervised learning is opposite of supervised learning, we do not have label or target value for given data. We can group similar items together which it is known clustering methods. In statistic, we can want to find values to describe data where it is called density estimation. As the other task, unsupervised learning is used for reducing dimensionality of data (Harrington, 2012).

If we need to give an example about unsupervised learning, we can say human and animal learning is largely unsupervised. The people discover the structure of the world by observing it, not by being told the name of every object (LeCun et al., 2015).

Hierarchical Clustering (HC)

The clusters are composed by iteratively dividing the patterns using bottom up or top-down approach in hierarchical clustering methods. As to be agglomerative and divise hierarchical clustering, hierarchical methods are subdivided two forms in Figure 11. The agglomerative hierarchical clustering is based on the bottom-up paradigm which clusters start with single object and then clusters merge larger clusters. Until all of the objects are lying in a single cluster, this process continue. The divise hierarchical clustering is based on top-down paradigm which firstly all of the objects belongs to only one cluster and then breaks up cluster as to be all objects will be smaller clusters (Saxena et al., 2017).

Figure 11. The hierarchical clustering dendogram (Adapted from Janssen, Walther & Lüdeke, 2012)

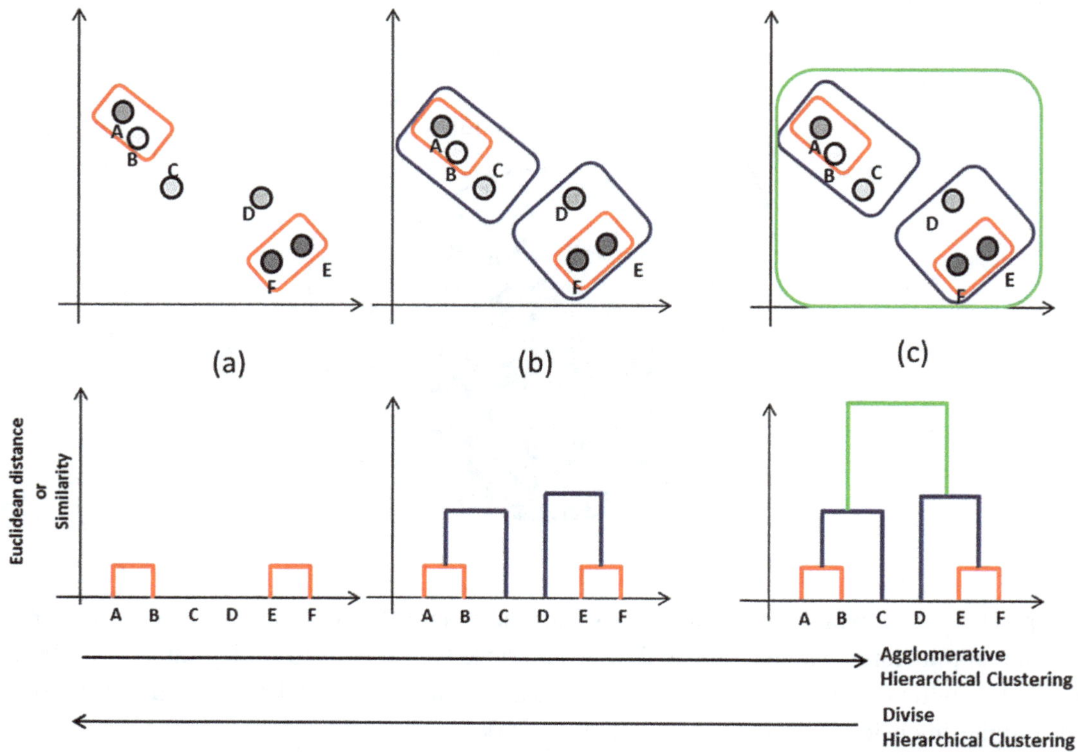

The hierarchical clustering methods can be divided into three groups according to similarity measures as following (Rokach and Maimon, 2005):

- **Single-Linkage Clustering:** Is also known as the connectedness or the neighbour method. In this method, two clusters are combined according to the distance or similarities between two cluster. The distance is defined that is shortest distances from any member of one cluster to any member of the other cluster.
- **Complete-Link Clustering:** Is also known as the diameter or the furthest neighbour method. The distance is the longest distance from any member of one cluster to any member of the other cluster. According to distance, clustering process is applied.
- **Average-Link Clustering:** Is also known as minimum variance method. According to this method, the distance between two clusters is determined by average distance from any member of one cluster to any member of the other cluster.

K-Means

K-Means is for finding the cluster inside the data. The clusters are represented by their corresponding centroids of origin. This process can also be used as a preprocessing step prior to the classification or regression (Alpaydın, 2013).

The K-Means algorithm partitions a set of n objects k cluster that is input parameter. As a result of partitioning intracluster, similarity is high but the intercluster similarity is low. Cluster similarity is measured in regard to the mean value of the objects in a cluster. The center of each cluster is represented by the mean value of the objects in the cluster. The algorithm proceeds can be explained as follows: (Han and Kamber, 2001). The summary of K-Means in Figure 12;

1. Firstly k is choosen randomly from dataset as the initial cluster centroid.
2. Each object is assigned to the cluster which the object is the most similar based on the mean values.
3. The mean value of the objects is updated for each cluster.
4. If the centroids change, 2 and 3 steps are repeated. Else, the process is terminated.

Self Organizing Maps

Around 1981–82 Teuvo Kohonen introduced a new non-linearly projecting mapping and he was called the Self-Organizing Map (SOM). The SOM models are identify with regular nodes such as two-dimensional grid. The SOM algorithm constructs the models like that: More similar models will be correlated nodes

Figure 12. K-means clustering algorithm (Adapted from Chris Piech, n.d.)

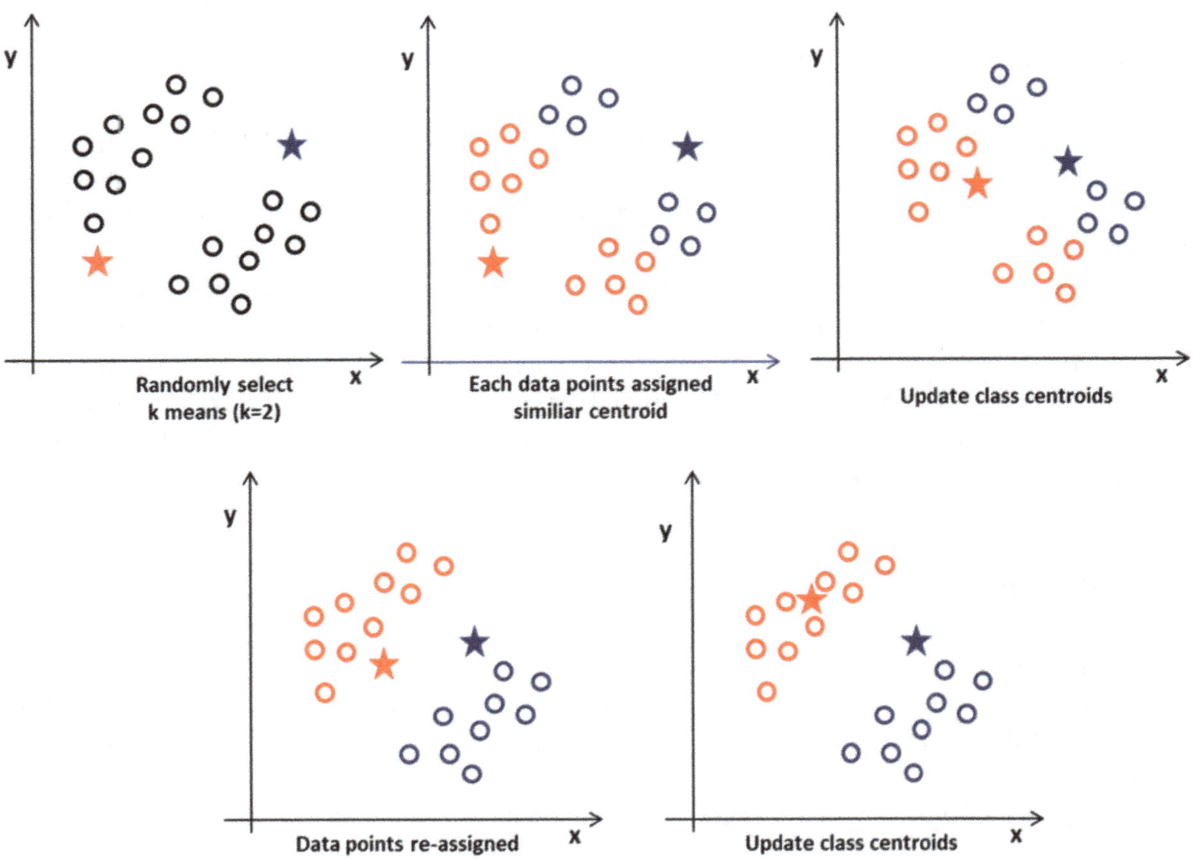

that are closer in the grid, on the contrary less similar models will be associated with nodes that are gradually farther away in the grid. The learning principles and mathematics of the SOM can be explain basically. Every input data unit will select the model that is best matching with input unit and this model, should be modified for much better matching (Kohonen, 2013).

Self-Organizing Map (SOM) is an unsupervised learning algorithm, and does not require a output vector since it learns to classify data without supervised. It is used for analysis of high-dimensional datasets and their visualization. SOM make easier the presentation of high dimensional datasets into lower dimensional ones. With using SOM, higher dimensional dataset can be reduced to two dimensional map. SOM is formed from a grid of nodes to which the input are presented. The algorithm process can be explained at below (Sayad, n.d.b.):

1. Initialization of each node's weights randomly between 0 and 1.
2. Choose a random input vector.
3. Calculate the Best Matching Unit (BMU) between input and weights nodes using Euclidean distance.
4. Calculate the size of the neighbourhood around the BMU.
5. Update nodes' weights of the BMU and neighboring nodes.
6. Repeat from step 2 for enough iterations for convergence.

The Self-Organizing Map was intended as a convenient alternative to more traditional neural network architectures. It has been used for tasks similar to those to which other more traditional neural networks have been applied: pattern recognition, process control, robotics and semantic processing (Kohonen, 1990).

Principal Component Analysis

Principal Components Analysis (PCA) is an unsupervised method because of no using the output information. In this method, main criterion is to be maximized is the variance and we aim to find a mapping from the inputs in the original space to a new lower dimensional space, with minimum loss of information (Alpaydın, 2014).

The Principal Component Analysis (PCA) is a method for dimensionality reduction as given in Figure 13. In PCA, the dataset is transfered from its original coordinate system to a new coordinate system. The new coordinate system is selected by using the data itself. The first new axis is chosen according to obtaining the most variance in the data. The second axis is orthogonal to the first axis and it is chosen by the largest variance. This procedure is iterated for as many features in dataset. Finally, we will see that the majority of the variance is contained in the first few axes. Therefore, we can keep out the rest of the axes, and we can reduce the dimensionality of dataset (Harrington, 2012).

Reinforcement Learning

In some applications, the output of the system is a sequence of actions and single action is not important. The first goal is to reach achievement. In this situation these systems learn from past action sequences which are called reinforcement learning. If we want to clarify what reinforcement learning is, we can give a good example as game playing. In playing, just a single move by itself is not that important; but it is the sequence of right moves that is good and important (Alpaydın, 2014).

Figure 13. The principal component analysis (Adapted from Harrington, 2012)

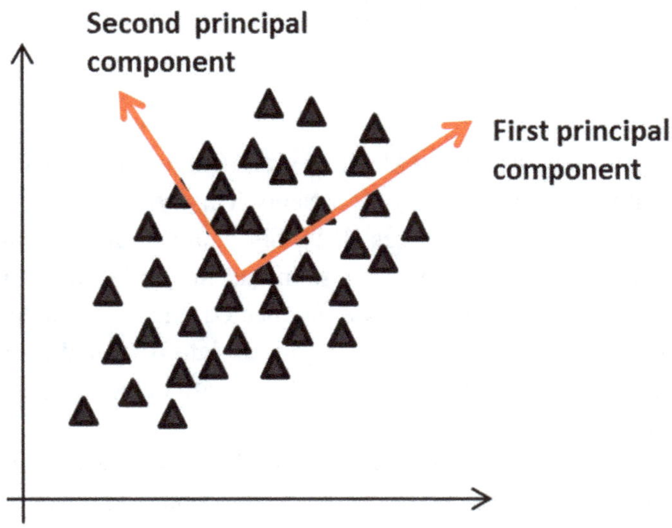

Reinforcement Learning roots has based on control theory. It has a dynamic environment that results of state-action-reward triples as the data as shown in Figure 14. The strategy of learning algorithm must be determined so as to maximize expectation of reward. The most important point of reinforcement learning is to learn what to do in order to maximize a given reward, namely how we can plan situations according to actions (Camastra and Vinciarelli, 2008).

Reinforcement Learning has focused on the question of how an autonomous agent can learn to choose optimal actions to achieve with using senses and acts in its environment. According to the principle of working, trainer may give a reward or penalty to indicate the desirability of the resulting state that is true or not (Mitchell, 1997).

Figure 14. The summary of reinforcement learning (Adapted from Wang et al., 2012).

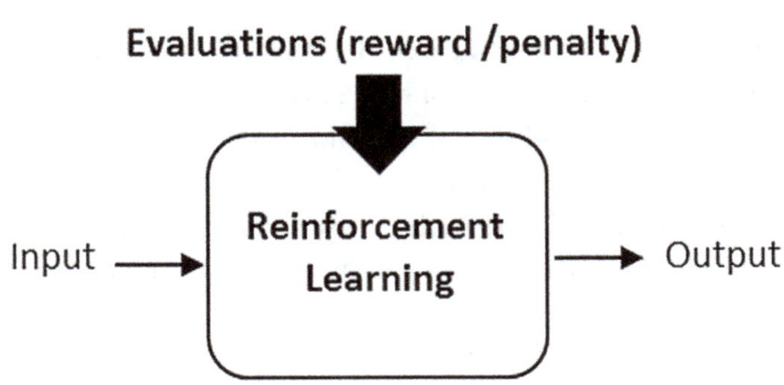

EARLY DETECTION OF NEUROLOGICAL DISORDERS USING MACHINE LEARNING SYSTEMS

Alzheimer Disease

Zhang, Wang & Mao (2018) have designed Alzheimer's Artificial Intelligence Technologies (AAIT) system to improve the quality lives of Alzheimer's patients. This system is consisted of lastest information technologies as Internet of Things services (IoT), big data and artificial intelligence. They have explained the solution architecture of the AAIT system and the designing and deployment of AAIT prototype system. Three categories of big data were collected, the first category of data is related to information of Alzheimer's patients, the second category of data is related to movement behaviour of patients and third category of data is consist of interactions with caregivers, control command for the IoT devices and triggering events.

Maity and Das (2017) were used Bayesian Inference to diagnose Alzheimer's disease based on historical patient data, cognitive test results and risk factors. They obtained historical patient data from the National Alzheimer's Coordinate Center, University of Washington. In the end of study approximately 80% accuracy has been obtained in the Bayesian inference model used to diagnose Alzheimer's disease.

Liu et al. (2014) have studied on early diagnosis of Alzheimer's disease and mild cognitive impairment with using deep learning because at the early stage the accurate diagnosis has important effect for on treatment. They have built a deep learning architecture with stacked auto enconders and a softmax regression on Matlab. Single and multi kernel support vector machine methods were chosen to compare their applied method.

Khedher et al. (2015) computer aided diagnosis for detection of early stages of Alzheimer's Disease. They analyzed tissue segmented brain images from Alzheimer's Disease Neuroimaging Initiative database (188 Alzheimer's disease patients, 401 Mild cognitive impairment patients and 229 Control subjects). For feature selection principal component analysis and partial least squares methods were used, for classification support vector machines with linear and radial basis function kernels were used.

Parkinson's Disease

Lahmiri, Dawson & Shmuel (2018) have compared the performance of machine learning methods to diagnosis Parkinson's Disease (PD) based on dysphonia symptoms in their study. They have studied on 195 voice records (147 PD patient, 48 healthy control) and Support Vector Machine (SVM), Linear Discriminant Analysis (LDA), Naive Bayes, Radical Basis Function Neural Network (RBFNN), Regression Trees (RT), k-Nearest Neighbours (kNN) and Mahalanobis Distance Classifier (MDC) were applied as machine learning methods. Their results have shown that SVM has the best performance compared to other machine learning classifiers.

Alhussein (2017) have studied on a Parkinson's Disease (PD) monitoring framework for using in smart cities. The speech signals from clients that is captured from various sensors were used. They have used two voice sample database from the University of California Irvine (UCI) Machine Learning Repository and Faculty of Medicine in İstanbul University. The proposed framework was based on clouds system for PD detection and its components are smart home, smart city, the cloud system, the doctors and the clients. Support Vector Machine (SVM), Extreme Learning Machine (ELM), Gaussian Mixture Model

(GMM) and Random Forest tree algorithms were used. The best accuracy detection of PD was obtained with the combining ELM and SVM classifiers.

Sonu, Prakash, Ranjan & Saritha (2017) have proposed to predict Parkinson's disease from patients voice recording datasets using data mining algorithm. They have suggested that this system can bu used for early diagnosis of Parkinsons's disease and its early treatment. They have written a javascript program to analyze record voice of patients. Decision Trees, Naive Bayes, Support Vector Machines, Logistic Regression, Linear Discriminant Analysis and k-Nearest Neighbours were used in this study, but they have been more focused on decision tree algorithm. With feature selection and pruning, decision tree algorithm has give accuracy ratio 88% and 94% respectively.

Dinov et al. (2016) used model based and model free approaches for predictive analytics on Parkinson's disease data that is obtained from Parkinson's Progression Markers Initiative (PPMI). AdaBoost, Support Vector Machine (SVM), Naive Bayes, Decision Tree, k-Nearest Neighbour (kNN) and K-Means classifiers were used as model-free approaches. AdaBoost and SVM methods with high accuracy and precision have showed best performances.

Nilashi, Ibrahim & Ahani (2016) have proposed a new hbyrid intelligent system for the prediction of Parkinson's Disease (PD) using machine learning methods and they have studied on prediction techniques for PD progression. The dataset was obtained from Data Mining Repository of the University of California, Irvine (UCI) machine learning repository. Support Vector Regression (SVR) that is an extension of the support vector classifier and Adaptive Neuro-Fuzzy Inference System (ANFIS) are applied this dataset to predict of PD progression. Also, for data clustering Expectation Maximization (EM) was chosen and Principal Component Analysis (PCA) was used for dimensionality reduction and to solve multi-collinearity problem.

Schizophrenia

Madsen, Krohne, Cai, Wang & Chan (2018) have aimed to explain classification of machine learning methods on schizotypy research using Functional Magnetic Resonance Imagining data (fMRI), because these methods can be important for early diagnosis of disease process. They have described as statistical parametric mapping, seed-based analysis, complex network analysis and decomposition methods as feature extraction, also support vector classification and deep learning were focused on in their study.

Winterburn et al. (2017) have researched the accuracy of machine learning methods used in magnetic resonance images of schizophrenia patients and healthy controls classification studies They have used on three independently collected datasets that were used cortical thickness and two estimates of tissue density. These datasets are obtained from Centre for Addiction and Mental Health, Northwestern University Schizophrenia Data and Software Tool and National Institute of Neurology and Neurosurgery. The Logistic Regression, Support Vector Machines (SVM) and Linear Discriminant Analysis have been applied on three independently collected datasets. All machine learning analysis has performed R software. The best performance has gained with % 73.5 SVM on cortical thickness data.

Vyškovský, Schwarz, Janoušová & Kašpárek, (2016) have studied to make an improvement on computer-aided schizophrenia diagnosis, they have combined the classifier in ensembles. They have used random subspace enseble method and combined support vector machines and multi-layer perceptron. The magnetic resonance imaging (MRI) data of 52 schizophrenia patients and 52 healthy control subject were analyzed. They have gained that the performance accuracy of ensemble methods was not much quite a change from the accuracy of single classifier with high dimension feature vectors.

Depression

Mumtaz, Ali, Yasin & Malik (2018) have remarked accurate and early diagnosis of depression can be difficult in their study. They have aimed a machine learning framework involving electroencephalogram (EEG) based synchronization likelihood to diagnose major depressive disorder. They have used Naive Bayes, Logistic Regression and Support Vector Machine as classification methods to determine a model between EEG features and dataset (Major depressive disorder patient and health control). Classification accuracy, specificity, sensitivity and the F-measures have been calculated as classification performance metrics. The highest classification performance were provided by support vector machine as compared using other machine learning methods.

Sadeque, Xu & Bethard (2017) have presented a study that is the techniques employed for the University Arizone team's participations for early depression detection. For dataset, they used the user posts in Reddit website. They applied support vector machine and recurrent neural network these data. Also they have used ensemble methods to strengthen the best of each model. They have asserted that ensemble model is more better than individual models.

Schnyer, Clasen, Gonzalez & Beevers (2017) have applied support vector machine to magnetic resonance images of brain white matter to classify major depressive disorder patients and healthy controls. Fractional Anisotropy, Mean Diffusivity, Axial Diffusivity and Radial Diffusivity maps have been used for diffusion tensor processing. For the all brain fractional anisotropy mapping total classification accuracy has been calculated 70% with sensitivity of 68% and specificity of 80%. Total classification accuracy has been calculated 74% with sensitivity of 76% and specificity of 68%.

Stroke

Park, Chang & Nam (2017) have aimed to develop a Pronator Drift Test (PDT) tool using machine learning classifier. Signal processing and feature selection were applied to PDT features for classification of stroke patients. Also, Support Vector Machine, Random Forest and Radial Basis Function Network were performed to classify stroke patient from healthy controls. They have demonstrated that applying methods based on machine learning were classified with accuracy of 92.3% in PDT cases.

Arslan, Colak & Sarihan (2016) have studied medical data mining techniques to extract pattern from huge datasets. Different medical data mining approaches were examined for prediction of ischemic stroke patients data that is included 80 ischemic stroke patients and 112 healthy individuals. Support Vector Machines, Stochastic Gradient Boosting and Penalized Logistic Regression were used and they were compared based on some performance metrics. According to accuracy and area under the curve, support vector machine have showed the best performance for prediction. They have asserted that all the performance metrics of methods were high and could use for the classification of ischemic stroke.

Colak, Karaman & Turtay (2015) have made a study about application of knowledge discovery process on the prediction of stroke. They have performed Artificial Neural Network (ANN) and Support Vector Machine (SVM) methods for extracting pattern from dataset. The dataset is consist of 297 people that 130 of them are stroke patients and 167 of them are healthy individuals. Feature selection was applied and data was standardized before applying machine learning methods. ANN model is better than SVM for stroke diagnosis as compared to parametry of accuracy and area under the curve.

Cognitive Impairment

El-Gamal et al. (2018) have aimed to present a local based early diagnosis of Mild Cognitive Impairment (MCI). A set of PIB-PET scans that were collected from Alzheimer's Disease Neuroimaging Initiative (ADNI) database, have been used to exercise. They have discussed a personalize MCI diagnosis system. Support Vector Machine and a probabilistic version of SVM (pSVM) were used as two decision making levels. They have used linear-linear SVM based on classifier to build the computer aid diagnosis because of the best results in generally.

Khazaee, Ebrahimzadeh & Babajani-Feremi (2016) have studied to combine a graph theoretical approach with machine learning methods for mild cognitive impairment. They have exercised totaly 168 people who are Alzheimer disease (AD), mild cognitive impairment (MCI) and healthy controls, also the dataset is obtained from Alzheimer's Disease Neuroimaging Initiative (ADNI). The Support Vector Machines, k-Nearest Neighbour, Naive Bayes, Fisher Linear, Linear Discriminant, Quadratic Classifier and Decision Tree were used to classify and they compared them according to classification metrics. They have explained that the recommended method in their study that is about combining graph theory approach with machine learning had high accuracy to classify AD, MCI and healthy controls.

Seixas, Zadrozny, Laks, Conci & Saade (2014) have proposed a Bayesian network decision model to diagnose Mild Cognitive Impairment (MCI), Alzheimer's disease (AD) and Dementia. They have used Expectation maximization supervised learning algorithm on a dataset which includes patients and normal control from Duke University Medical Center and the Center for Alzheimer's Disease and Related Disorders. Five Bayesian Networks (BN) have been designed for classification in their study. They have explained that their aim is to develop a decision model for clinical diagnosis using BN. Besides, they have showed that the results of BN is better than other classification methods for diagnosing MCI, AD and dementia.

Stroke Rehabilitation

Lo and Tseng (2017) have purposed to study the relevance between power of rehabilitation and recurrence of stroke and set a model about stroke recurrence prediction using machine learning approach to help making decisions. They have performed classification methods so as C4.5 and CART Decision Trees and Logistic Regression to classify risk groups of stroke rehabilitation patients in Weka software. The C4.5 methods have been explained the best classifier for stroke recurrrence between the patients with and without stroke recurrence chance.

Yang et al. (2017) have introduced IoT- enabled stroke rehabilitation system based on smart wearable armband and machine learning algorithms. The algorithm of machine learning were used to analyze and determine different hand movements. Linear discriminant analysis, Multi Layer Perceptron and Support Vector Machine algorithms were compared.

Harris et al. (2016) have proposed to explain a fall recognition system that is called mStroke, using wearable technologies and machine learning algorithms. mStroke is real time and mobile health system for stroke recovery and rehabilitation. The system design has been consisted of three wearable sensor and IOS applications. Random Forest, Linear Support Vector Machine, Logistic Regression and k-Nearest Neighbour algorithms were applied for fall recognition. Different machine learning methods applied in the study have achieved high accuracy approximately above 90%.

Stroke Management

Feng, Badgeley, Mocco & Oermann (2018) have reviewed deep learning based stroke management on clinical applications. They have explained which areas deep learning can be applied to stroke management. These areas have been sorted image segmentation, automated featurization and multi-model prognostication. They have asserted that deep learning tools could be used as customized medical process for patients with stroke.

Lee, Y. H., Kim, N., Kim & Kang (2017) have focused on artificial intelligence in stroke imagining and offered its technical principles, clinical application and future perspectives. They have explained that the analysis of stroke imagining must have been sufficent for correct store management. The development in both artificial intelligence techniques and big data can be hopeful in stroke disease were explained.

Medical Imaging and Signal Processing

De Bruijne (2016) has explained some machine learning approaches that are increasingly successful in medical imaging, diagnosis and prognosis and risk assessment. Also he has expressed three main challenges about machine learning techniques in medical imaging. They can be sorted varying imaging protocols, weak labels and interpretation and evaluation of results.

Gait Cycle Impairment

Carnevale et al. (2018) have studied on an alternative approach based on big data analytics using robotic rehabilitation devices to improve the patient's therapy. They have analyzed big data coming from sensors installed in Lokomat and proposed to find the best personalized treatment therapy. Lokomat is the most known advanced robotic technology available for gait training and neurological re-patterning. The used dataset is rehabilitation treatments performed in the period from 2012-2016 and is total 179 patients. The dataset has been analyzed with Python packages.

Shirakawa, Sugiyama, Sato, Sakurai & Sato (2017) have performed gait analysis on 113 young and healthy subjects in normal walking that are taken from National Defense Academy of Japan (NDA). They have aimed to classify walking pattern using machine learning classification techniques. The gait pattern were analyzed according to the accelerometry for pelvic movements of the subjects in normal walking. For classification, they have used cluster analysis and principal component analysis and the both of measurements were performed based on eight parameters. They have found no important difference between male and female subjects, also the correlation with age, training period, body height and body weight of subjects have not been determined for all parameter.

Mannini, Trojaniello, Cereatti & Sabatini (2016) have purposed a machine learning framework for gait classification. They have defined classification framework three steps, firstly is feature extraction using Hidden Markov Models, secondly is classification with Support Vector Machine and thirdly is majority voting classification was applied for summarizing the result of second step. Using leave-one-subject-out cross validation and majority voting the 90.5% of subjects have been classified.

Neurorehabilitation

Deng et al. (2018) have studied on comprehensive review about advances in automation technologies for lower extremity neurorehabilitation. They have examined last technological advances in wearable sensors, assistive robots and biofeedback devices. Also network technologies for the Wireless Body Area Network (WBAN) have been compared according to timing performance, reliability, scalability, privacy and security.

Lledo et al. (2015) have presented Adaptive Resonance Therapy (ART) that is based on neural networks combined with Fuzzy Logic systems, have classified user physiological reactions during rehabilitation therapied by a robot-assisted. This neuro-fuzzy method was called Supervised and Dynamic Fuzzy Adaptive System ART (S-dFasArt) by researchers. Although they have used nine machine learning algorithms, S-dFasArt approach has been obtained accuracy of 92.38 compared with other methods. The second highest accuracy 91.43% has been found out support vector machine with radial basis function kernel.

Motor Function Disorder

Crippa et al. (2015) have developed a machine learning method to determine between 15 pre-school children with Autism Spectrum Disorder (ASD) and 15 typically developing (TD) children. The machine learning method has been applied two steps, first step was feature selection and second step was classification process that separate ASD and TD children datasets from each other. For classification algorithm, support vector machine was used. The classification accuracy has been calculated 96.7%, furthermore the specificity and sensitivity have been achieved respectively 93.8% and 100%.

Stem Cells

Joutsijoki, Haponen, Rasku, Aalto-Setälä & Juhola (2016) have studied on automated identification of the quality of human Induced Pluripotent Stem Cell (iPSC) colony images. To solve the monitoring problem of iPSC colonies, they have asserted to use machine learning methods so as k-Nearest Neighbour (kNN) and Multiclass Support Vector Machines. Also they have used other classification methods as Classification Tree, Naive Bayes variant, Multinomial Logistic Regression and Linear Discriminant Analysis. Scaled Invariant Feature Transformation (SIFT) have been used for feature extraction. The best accuracy of 62.4% has been calculated by kNN method with Euclidean measure.

Shouval et al. (2014) have reviewed data mining approach in hematopoietic stem cell transplantation. They have examined some application of machine learning algorithms for clinical predictive modeling. When they prepare this study, they have aimed to increase data mining and machine learning studies in the field of stem cell transplantation. They have mentioned that better experience based on high technologies could improve patient and donor selection, advance transplantation outcome and decrease transplant-related mortality.

Drug Delivery

Bernick (2015) have studied about the role of machine learning in drug design and delivery system. Some machine learning applications in drug design and delivery have been discussed in the study. Especially, it have been explained that machine learning has several advantages in drug design. Furthermore, it have been highlighted, the importance of machine learning algorithms used in the design and optimization of the preformulation and formulation drug delivery system.

Li, Lenaghan & Zhang (2012) have developed a framework that is data driven predictive system for drug delivery using machine learning methods. This framework have been modelled in reference to the drug-pathogen dynamics. Fuzzy C-Mean clustering algorithm has been used to categorize the drug-pathogen interactions into a discrete set. They have explained that the framework could predict drug-pathogen dynamics according to observations, furthermore experimental training data has been used to determine efficiency on drug delivery method.

Epilepsy

Shen et al. (2013) have studied on the classification of Electroencephalography (EEG) signals for the diagnosis epilepsy. They have explained an EEG analysis systems of seizure detection which is based on cascade wavelet-approximate entropy for feature selection. Support Vector Machines (SVMs), k-Nearest Neighbour (kNN) and Radial Basis Function Neural Network (RBFNN) were used for classification and the results of classification methods were compared. For open source data, the overall accuracy has been achieved 99.97%. In addition, the performance of the system has been tested on clinical EEG data.

Siuly, Li & Wen (2011) have introduced feature extraction by sampling techniques from Electroencephalogram (EEG) signals. The EEG recording of healthy volunteers and the EEG record of epileptic patients during epileptic seizure activity were used for dataset in this study. Least Square Support Vector Machine (LS-SVM) toolbox was applied for classification of the EEG signals in Matlab. LS-SVM classifier has been achieved the accuracy of 80.31% for training data, while the accuracy of 80.05% for the testing data.

Autism

Heinsfeld, Franco, Craddock, Buchweitz & Meneguzzi (2018) have presented to apply deep learning algorithms for identification of autism disorder spectrum. The large brain imaging dataset has been obtained from multi-site database known as ABIDE (Autism Brain İmaging Data Exchange). In addition, Deep Learning, Support Vector Machine and Random Forest classifiers were used and all of the classifiers were compared with the results of accuracy, sensitivity and specificity.

Alhaddad et al. (2012) have studied on diagnosis of autism by Fisher Linear Discriminant Analysis (FLDA) based on autistic children Electroencephalogram (EEG) signal. They have used different preprocessing techniques, different ensemble averages and different feature extraction techniques. The average accuracy rate was calculated 90%.

Bosl, Tierney, Tager-Flusberg & Nelson (2011) have focused on showing Electroencephalogram (EEG) data can be used a biomarker for brain development using Modified Multiscale Entropy (mMSE). Multiclass Support Vector Machine was used for classification of control and High-Rish Autism (HRA). In addition, the classification by gender and age k-Nearest Neighbour, Support Vector Machine and Naive Bayes methods were used and compared. Infants were classified with over 80% accuracy into control and HRA groups at age 9 months with mMSE feature vector.

FUTURE RESEARCH DIRECTIONS

To be more useful for Alzheimer's patients, the Alzheimer's Artificial Intelligence Technologies (AAIT) system can be improved and applied to embedded system as wearable device for future (Zhang et al., 2018).

The division of patients according to pathologies will be analyzed for the improvement of customization therapy. Analytical models will be applied such as deep artificial neural networks for making statistical big data analysis (Carnevale et al., 2018).

Nilashi et al. (2018) have best result support vector regression (SVR)method on Parkinson's disease For reducing the computation time, they have plan to use incremental SVR. Furthermore, they have aimed to develop methods for incremental learning and apply them on big data sets.

Wang et al. (2018) have mentioned that future scientific studies should focused on efficient unstructured data analytical algorithms and major technological progression.

Crippa et al (2015) have explained that they will have work on neurodevelopmental conditions to verify autism spectrum disorder for their next research.

Any development in big data processing for bioinformatics, health informatics imaging and sensing will have show big effect on next clinical research (Perez et al., 2015).

Sexias et al. (2014) have expressed that they propose to revise Bayesian Network on more complete patients dataset comprising neuropsychological test in their future work.

Li et al. (2012) will have use Markov Decision Process on their machine learning framework to separate the dose into discrete actions based on pathogen population and it's effect. This system can be planned for determination of dosage.

CONCLUSION

In this chapter, big data analytics and machine learning systems have been introduced to explain for the early diagnosis of neurological disorders. A number of scholarly researches on big data about intelligent big data analytics in healthcare and machine learning system were used in healthcare system have been mentioned.

This work provides an opinion of how medical big data can be used by intelligent big data analytics and machine learning methods in neurological disorder diagnosis. The main aim behind this study is to assist the researchers or experts to provide an idea and understanding about intelligent big data analytics and machine learning methods in the diagnosis of neurological disorders.

In this survey, the researches about neurological disorder as Alzheimer's Disease, Parkinson's Disease, Schizophrenia, Depression, Stroke, Cognitive Impairment, Stroke Rehabilitation, Stroke Management, Medical Imaging and Signal Processing, Gait Cycle Impairment, Neurorehabilitation, Motor Function Disorder, Stem Cells, Drug Delivery, Epilepsy and Autism were summarized.

The intelligent big data analytics for healthcare system is in the early stage of development, similarly machine learning. Therefore, some challenges and problems can occurred in application areas. Any improvement of machine learning algorithms and big data analytics can be much better for good classification or diagnosis of disorders.

REFERENCES

Akın, M. (2012). *Kanserli hücrelerin mikroarray gen ifadelerinin incelenmesi ve veri madenciliği yöntemleri kullanarak sınıflandırılması*. Gazi Üniversitesi, Fen Bilimleri Enstitüsü, Yüksek Lisans Tezi,Temmuz.

Aktan, E. (2018). Büyük Veri: Uygulama Alanları, Analitiği ve Güvenlik Boyutu. *Bilgi Yönetimi, 1*(1), 1–22.

Al-Jarrah, O. Y., Yoo, P. D., Muhaidat, S., Karagiannidis, G. K., & Taha, K. (2015). Efficient machine learning for big data: A review. *Big Data Research, 2*(3), 87–93. doi:10.1016/j.bdr.2015.04.001

Alhaddad, M. J., Kamel, M. I., Malibary, H. M., Alsaggaf, E. A., Thabit, K., Dahlwi, F., & Hadi, A. A. (2012). Diagnosis autism by fisher linear discriminant analysis FLDA via EEG. *International Journal of Bio-Science and Bio-Technology, 4*(2), 45–54.

Alhussein, M. (2017). Monitoring Parkinson's Disease in Smart Cities. *IEEE Access: Practical Innovations, Open Solutions, 5*, 19835–19841. doi:10.1109/ACCESS.2017.2748561

Alpaydın, E. (2013). *Yapay öğrenme, 2*. Baskı, Boğaziçi Üniversitesi Yayınevi.

Alpaydın, E. (2014). *Introduction to Machine Learning*. MIT Press.

Altındal, T. (2006). *Machine Learning Algorithms in Classification and Diagnostic Prediction of Cancers using Gene Expression Profilling* (Master Dissertation). Ulusal Tez Merkezi. (No. 181232)

Angra, S., & Ahuja, S. (2017, March). Machine learning and its applications: a review. In *Big Data Analytics and Computational Intelligence (ICBDAC), 2017 International Conference on* (pp. 57-60). IEEE. 10.1109/ICBDACI.2017.8070809

Apache Hive. (n.d.). Retrieved December 23, 2018, from https://hive.apache.org/

Apache Pig. (n.d.). Retrieved December 23, 2018, from https://pig.apache.org/

Arslan, A. K., Colak, C., & Sarihan, M. E. (2016). Different medical data mining approaches based prediction of ischemic stroke. *Computer Methods and Programs in Biomedicine, 130*, 87–92. doi:10.1016/j.cmpb.2016.03.022 PMID:27208524

Atalay, M., & Çelik, Ö. G. E. (2017). Artificial Intelligence and Machine Learning Applications in Big Data Analysis. *Mehmet Akif Ersoy University Journal of Social Sciences Institute, 9*(22), 155–172.

Athmaja, S., Hanumanthappa, M., & Kavitha, V. (2017, March). A survey of machine learning algorithms for big data analytics. In *Innovations in Information, Embedded and Communication Systems (ICIIECS), 2017 International Conference on* (pp. 1-4). IEEE. 10.1109/ICIIECS.2017.8276028

Balasupramanian, N., Ephrem, B. G., & Al-Barwani, I. S. (2017, July). User pattern based online fraud detection and prevention using big data analytics and self organizing maps. In *Intelligent Computing, Instrumentation and Control Technologies (ICICICT), 2017 International Conference on* (pp. 691-694). IEEE. 10.1109/ICICICT1.2017.8342647

Bazazeh, D., & Shubair, R. (2016, December). Comparative study of machine learning algorithms for breast cancer detection and diagnosis. In *Electronic Devices, Systems and Applications (ICEDSA), 2016 5th International Conference on* (pp. 1-4). IEEE. 10.1109/ICEDSA.2016.7818560

Bernick, J. P. (2015). The Role of Machine Learning in Drug Design and Delivery. *Journal of Develop Drugs*, *4*(03), E143. doi:10.4172/2329-6631.1000e143

Berral García, J. L. (2016). A quick view on current techniques and machine learning algorithms for big data analytics. In *Proceedings of the 18th International Conference on Transparent Optical Networks (ICTON)* (pp. 1-4). Institute of Electrical and Electronics Engineers (IEEE). 10.1109/ICTON.2016.7550517

Bircan, H. (2004). Lojistik regresyon analizi: Tıp verileri üzerine bir uygulama. *Kocaeli Üniversitesi Sosyal Bilimler Enstitüsü Dergisi*, (8), 185-208.

Bishop, C. M. (2006). Pattern recognition and machine learning (information science and statistics). Academic Press.

Bosl, W., Tierney, A., Tager-Flusberg, H., & Nelson, C. (2011). EEG complexity as a biomarker for autism spectrum disorder risk. *BMC Medicine*, *9*(1), 18. doi:10.1186/1741-7015-9-18 PMID:21342500

Breiman, L. (2001). Random forests. *Machine Learning*, *45*(1), 5–32. doi:10.1023/A:1010933404324

Burakgazi, Y. (2017). *Identification of Breast Cancer Sub-types by Using Machine Learning Techniques* (Master Dissertation). Ulusal Tez Merkezi. (No. 459190)

Camastra, F., & Vinciarelli, A. (2008). *Machine Learning for Audio, Image and Video Analysis*. London: Springer. doi:10.1007/978-1-84800-007-0

Carnevale, L., Calabrò, R. S., Celesti, A., Leo, A., Fazio, M., Bramanti, P., & Villari, M. (2018). *Towards Improving Robotic-Assisted Gait Training: Can Big Data Analysis Help us? IEEE Internet of Things Journal.*

Carnevale, L., Calabrò, R. S., Celesti, A., Leo, A., Fazio, M., Bramanti, P., & Villari, M. (2018). *Towards Improving Robotic-Assisted Gait Training: Can Big Data Analysis Help us? IEEE Internet of Things Journal.*

Colak, C., Karaman, E., & Turtay, M. G. (2015). Application of knowledge discovery process on the prediction of stroke. *Computer Methods and Programs in Biomedicine*, *119*(3), 181–185. doi:10.1016/j.cmpb.2015.03.002 PMID:25827533

Crippa, A., Salvatore, C., Perego, P., Forti, S., Nobile, M., Molteni, M., & Castiglioni, I. (2015). Use of machine learning to identify children with autism and their motor abnormalities. *Journal of Autism and Developmental Disorders*, *45*(7), 2146–2156. doi:10.100710803-015-2379-8 PMID:25652603

De Bruijne, M. (2016). *Machine learning approaches in medical image analysis: From detection to diagnosis*. Academic Press.

De Mauro, A., Greco, M., & Grimaldi, M. (2015, February). What is big data? A consensual definition and a review of key research topics. In AIP conference proceedings: Vol. 1644. *No. 1* (pp. 97–104). AIP. doi:10.1063/1.4907823

Deng, W., Papavasileiou, I., Qiao, Z., Zhang, W., Lam, K. Y., & Song, H. (2018). Advances in Automation Technologies for Lower-extremity Neurorehabilitation: A Review and Future Challenges. *IEEE Reviews in Biomedical Engineering*, *11*, 289–305. doi:10.1109/RBME.2018.2830805 PMID:29994006

Dinov, I. D., Heavner, B., Tang, M., Glusman, G., Chard, K., Darcy, M., ... Foster, I. (2016). Predictive big data analytics: A study of Parkinson's disease using large, complex, heterogeneous, incongruent, multi-source and incomplete observations. *PLoS One*, *11*(8), e0157077. doi:10.1371/journal.pone.0157077 PMID:27494614

Diri, B. (n.d.). *Makine Öğrenmesine Giriş*. Retrieved from Lecture Notes Online Web site: https://www.ce.yildiz.edu.tr/personal/banud/file/2634/Makine+Ogrenmesi-ML-10.pdf

Domo. (n.d.). *Data Never Sleeps 6.0*. Retrieved January 1, 2019, from https://www.domo.com/learn/data-never-sleeps-6

El-Gamal, F. E., Elmogy, M. M., Ghazal, M., Atwan, A., Casanova, M. F., Barnes, G. N., ... Khalil, A. (2018). A Novel Early Diagnosis System for Mild Cognitive Impairment Based on Local Region Analysis: A Pilot Study. *Frontiers in Human Neuroscience*, *11*, 643. doi:10.3389/fnhum.2017.00643 PMID:29375343

Feng, R., Badgeley, M., Mocco, J., & Oermann, E. K. (2018). Deep learning guided stroke management: A review of clinical applications. *Journal of Neurointerventional Surgery*, *10*(4), 358–362. doi:10.1136/neurintsurg-2017-013355 PMID:28954825

Gandomi, A., & Haider, M. (2015). Beyond the hype: Big data concepts, methods, and analytics. *International Journal of Information Management*, *35*(2), 137–144. doi:10.1016/j.ijinfomgt.2014.10.007

Gartner I. T. Glossary. (n.d.) *Big data*. Retrieved December 12, 2018, from https://www.gartner.com/it-glossary/big-data

Groves, P., Kayyali, B., Knott, D., & Van Kuiken, S. (2013). The 'big data'revolution in healthcare. *The McKinsey Quarterly*, *2*(3).

Han, J., & Kamber, M. (2001). *Data Mining Concepts and Techniques* (2nd ed.). Morgan Kauffmann Publishers Inc.

Harerimana, G., Jang, B., Kim, J. W., & Park, H. K. (2018). Health Big Data Analytics: A Technology Survey. *IEEE Access: Practical Innovations, Open Solutions*, *6*, 65661–65678. doi:10.1109/ACCESS.2018.2878254

Harrington, P. (2012). *Machine learning in Action* (Vol. 5). Greenwich, CT: Manning.

Harris, A., True, H., Hu, Z., Cho, J., Fell, N., & Sartipi, M. (2016, December). Fall recognition using wearable technologies and machine learning algorithms. In *Big Data (Big Data), 2016 IEEE International Conference on* (pp. 3974-3976). IEEE. 10.1109/BigData.2016.7841080

Heinsfeld, A. S., Franco, A. R., Craddock, R. C., Buchweitz, A., & Meneguzzi, F. (2018). Identification of autism spectrum disorder using deep learning and the ABIDE dataset. *NeuroImage. Clinical*, *17*, 16–23. doi:10.1016/j.nicl.2017.08.017 PMID:29034163

IBM. (n.d.a). *What is big data? Bringing big data to the enterprise.* Retrieved May 5, 2018, from http://www-01.ibm.com/software/data/bigdata/

IBM. (n.d.b.). *What is MapReduce?* Retrieved December 22, 2018, from https://www.ibm.com/analytics/hadoop/mapreduce

Janssen, P., Walther, C., & Lüdeke, M. (2012). *Cluster analysis to understand socio-ecological systems: a guideline*. Potsdam-Institut für Klimafolgenforschung.

Jordan, M. I., & Mitchell, T. M. (2015). Machine learning: Trends, perspectives, and prospects. *Science*, *349*(6245), 255–260. doi:10.1126cience.aaa8415 PMID:26185243

Joutsijoki, H., Haponen, M., Rasku, J., Aalto-Setälä, K., & Juhola, M. (2016). Machine learning approach to automated quality identification of human induced pluripotent stem cell colony images. *Computational and Mathematical Methods in Medicine*, *2016*, 1–15. doi:10.1155/2016/3091039 PMID:27493680

Kartal, E. (2015). *Sınıflandırmaya Dayalı Makine Öğrenmesi Teknikleri ve Kardiyolojik Risk Değerlendirmesine İlişkin Bir Uygulama* (Doctoral Dissertation). Ulusal Tez Merkezi. (No.394514)

Khazaee, A., Ebrahimzadeh, A., & Babajani-Feremi, A. (2016). Application of advanced machine learning methods on resting-state fMRI network for identification of mild cognitive impairment and Alzheimer's disease. *Brain Imaging and Behavior*, *10*(3), 799–817. doi:10.100711682-015-9448-7 PMID:26363784

Khedher, L., Ramírez, J., Górriz, J. M., Brahim, A., & Segovia, F. (2015). Early diagnosis of Alzheimer' s disease based on partial least squares, principal component analysis and support vector machine using segmented MRI images. *Neurocomputing*, *151*, 139–150. doi:10.1016/j.neucom.2014.09.072

Kızrak, A. (n.d.). *Yapay Sinir Ağı Nedir?* Retrieved January 9, 2018, from https://medium.com/deep-learning-turkiye/%C5%9Fu-kara-kutuyu-a%C3%A7alim-yapay-sinir-a%C4%9Flar%C4%B1-7b65c6a5264a

Kohonen, T. (1990). The self-organizing map. *Proceedings of the IEEE*, *78*(9), 1464–1480. doi:10.1109/5.58325

Kohonen, T. (2013). Essentials of the self-organizing map. *Neural Networks*, *37*, 52–65. doi:10.1016/j.neunet.2012.09.018 PMID:23067803

Kumar, S., & Singh, M. (2019). Big data analytics for healthcare industry: Impact, applications, and tools. *Big Data Mining and Analytics*, *2*(1), 48–57. doi:10.26599/BDMA.2018.9020031

Lahmiri, S., Dawson, D. A., & Shmuel, A. (2018). Performance of machine learning methods in diagnosing Parkinson's disease based on dysphonia measures. *Biomedical Engineering Letters*, *8*(1), 29–39. doi:10.100713534-017-0051-2 PMID:30603188

LeCun, Y., Bengio, Y., & Hinton, G. (2015). Deep Learning. *Nature*, *521*(7553), 436–444. doi:10.1038/nature14539 PMID:26017442

Lee, E. J., Kim, Y. H., Kim, N., & Kang, D. W. (2017). Deep into the brain: Artificial intelligence in stroke imaging. *Journal of Stroke*, *19*(3), 277–285. doi:10.5853/jos.2017.02054 PMID:29037014

Li, Y., Lenaghan, S. C., & Zhang, M. (2012). A data-driven predictive approach for drug delivery using machine learning techniques. *PLoS One*, *7*(2), e31724. doi:10.1371/journal.pone.0031724 PMID:22384063

Liu, S., Liu, S., Cai, W., Pujol, S., Kikinis, R., & Feng, D. (2014, April). Early diagnosis of Alzheimer's disease with deep learning. In *Biomedical Imaging (ISBI), 2014 IEEE 11th International Symposium on* (pp. 1015-1018). IEEE. 10.1109/ISBI.2014.6868045

Lledó, L. D., Badesa, F. J., Almonacid, M., Cano-Izquierdo, J. M., Sabater-Navarro, J. M., Fernández, E., & Garcia-Aracil, N. (2015). Supervised and dynamic neuro-fuzzy systems to classify physiological responses in robot-assisted neurorehabilitation. *PLoS One*, *10*(5), e0127777. doi:10.1371/journal.pone.0127777 PMID:26001214

Lo, C. L., & Tseng, H. T. (2017). Predicting rehabilitation treatment helpfulness to stroke patients: A supervised learning approach. *Artificial Intelligence Review*, *6*(2), 1. doi:10.5430/air.v6n2p1

Madsen, K. H., Krohne, L. G., Cai, X. L., Wang, Y., & Chan, R. C. (2018). Perspectives on Machine Learning for Classification of Schizotypy Using fMRI Data. *Schizophrenia Bulletin*, *44*(suppl_2), S480–S490. doi:10.1093chbulby026 PMID:29554367

Maity, N. G., & Das, S. (2017, March). Machine learning for improved diagnosis and prognosis in healthcare. In *Aerospace Conference, 2017 IEEE* (pp. 1-9). IEEE. 10.1109/AERO.2017.7943950

Mannini, A., Trojaniello, D., Cereatti, A., & Sabatini, A. M. (2016). A machine learning framework for gait classification using inertial sensors: Application to elderly, post-stroke and huntington's disease patients. *Sensors (Basel)*, *16*(1), 134. doi:10.339016010134 PMID:26805847

Mathworks. (n.d.). *What is Machine Learning?* Retrieved May 6, 2018, from https://www.mathworks.com/discovery/machine-learning.html

Mitchell, T. M. (1997). Machine learning. Burr Ridge, IL: McGraw Hill.

Mitchell, T. M. (2006). *The discipline of machine learning* (Vol. 9). Pittsburgh, PA: Carnegie Mellon University, School of Computer Science, Machine Learning Department.

Mumtaz, W., Ali, S. S. A., Yasin, M. A. M., & Malik, A. S. (2018). A machine learning framework involving EEG-based functional connectivity to diagnose major depressive disorder (MDD). *Medical & Biological Engineering & Computing*, *56*(2), 233–246. doi:10.100711517-017-1685-z PMID:28702811

Nilashi, M., Ibrahim, O., & Ahani, A. (2016). Accuracy improvement for predicting Parkinson's disease progression. *Scientific Reports*, *6*(1), 34181. doi:10.1038rep34181 PMID:27686748

O'Leary, D. E. (2013). Artificial intelligence and big data. *IEEE Intelligent Systems*, *28*(2), 96–99. doi:10.1109/MIS.2013.39 PMID:25505373

Oussous, A., Benjelloun, F. Z., Lahcen, A. A., & Belfkih, S. (2018). Big Data technologies: A survey. *Journal of King Saud University-Computer and Information Sciences*, *30*(4), 431–448. doi:10.1016/j.jksuci.2017.06.001

Özköse, H., Arı, E. S., & Gencer, C. (2015). Yesterday, today and tomorrow of big data. *Procedia: Social and Behavioral Sciences*, *195*, 1042–1050. doi:10.1016/j.sbspro.2015.06.147

Park, E., Chang, H. J., & Nam, H. S. (2017). Use of Machine Learning Classifiers and Sensor Data to Detect Neurological Deficit in Stroke Patients. *Journal of Medical Internet Research, 19*(4), e120. doi:10.2196/jmir.7092 PMID:28420599

Patel, J. A., & Sharma, P. (2014, August). Big data for better health planning. In *2014 International Conference on Advances in Engineering and Technology Research (ICAETR)* (pp. 1-5). Unnao: IEEE.

Piech, C. (n.d.). *K-Means.* Retrieved from Lecture Notes from Web site http://stanford.edu/~cpiech/cs221/handouts/kmeans.html

Praveena, M. A., & Bharathi, B. (2017, February). A survey paper on big data analytics. In *Information Communication and Embedded Systems (ICICES), 2017 International Conference on* (pp. 1-9). IEEE. 10.1109/ICICES.2017.8070723

Qiu, J., Wu, Q., Ding, G., Xu, Y., & Feng, S. (2016). A survey of machine learning for big data processing. *EURASIP Journal on Advances in Signal Processing, 2016*(1), 67. doi:10.118613634-016-0355-x

Raghupathi, W., & Raghupathi, V. (2014). Big data analytics in healthcare: promise and potential. *Health Information Science and Systems, 2*(1), 3.

Rokach, L., & Maimon, O. (2005). Clustering methods. In *Data mining and knowledge discovery handbook* (pp. 321–352). Boston, MA: Springer. doi:10.1007/0-387-25465-X_15

Ruan, Y., Xue, X., Liu, H., Tan, J., & Li, X. (2017). Quantum algorithm for k-nearest neighbors classification based on the metric of hamming distance. *International Journal of Theoretical Physics, 56*(11), 3496–3507. doi:10.100710773-017-3514-4

Russom, P. (2011). Big data analytics. *TDWI Best Practices Report, 19*(4), 1-34.

Sadeque, F., Xu, D., & Bethard, S. (2017, September). Uarizona at the CLEF erisk 2017 pilot task: Linear and recurrent models for early depression detection. In *CEUR workshop proceedings* (Vol. 1866). NIH Public Access.

Sağıroğlu, Ş. (2017). *Büyük Veri ve Açık Veri Analitiği: Yöntemler ve Uygulamalar* (Ş. Sağıroğlu & O. Koç, Eds.). Ankara: Grafiker Yayınları.

Sagiroglu, Ş., & Sinanc, D. (2013, May). Big data: A review. In *Collaboration Technologies and Systems (CTS), 2013 International Conference on* (pp. 42-47). Academic Press. 10.1109/CTS.2013.6567202

Sahu, S. K., Jacintha, M. M., & Singh, A. P. (2017, May). Comparative study of tools for big data analytics: An analytical study. In *Computing, Communication and Automation (ICCCA), 2017 International Conference on* (pp. 37-41). IEEE.

Saritha, K., & Abraham, S. (2017, July). Prediction with partitioning: Big data analytics using regression techniques. In *Networks & Advances in Computational Technologies (NetACT), 2017 International Conference on* (pp. 208-214). IEEE.

Saxena, A., Prasad, M., Gupta, A., Bharill, N., Patel, O. P., Tiwari, A., ... Lin, C. T. (2017). A review of clustering techniques and developments. *Neurocomputing, 267*, 664–681. doi:10.1016/j.neucom.2017.06.053

Sayad, S. (n.d.a). *Logistic Regression.* Retrieved May 9, 2018, from, http://www.saedsayad.com/logistic_regression.htm

Sayad, S. (n.d.b). *Self Organizing Map*. Retrieved May 7, 2018, from, http://www.saedsayad.com/clustering_som.htm

Schnyer, D. M., Clasen, P. C., Gonzalez, C., & Beevers, C. G. (2017). Evaluating the diagnostic utility of applying a machine learning algorithm to diffusion tensor MRI measures in individuals with major depressive disorder. *Psychiatry Research: Neuroimaging, 264*, 1–9. doi:10.1016/j.pscychresns.2017.03.003 PMID:28388468

Seixas, F. L., Zadrozny, B., Laks, J., Conci, A., & Saade, D. C. M. (2014). A Bayesian network decision model for supporting the diagnosis of dementia, Alzheimer′ s disease and mild cognitive impairment. *Computers in Biology and Medicine, 51*, 140–158. doi:10.1016/j.compbiomed.2014.04.010 PMID:24946259

Shen, C. P., Chen, C. C., Hsieh, S. L., Chen, W. H., Chen, J. M., Chen, C. M., ... Chiu, M. J. (2013). High-performance seizure detection system using a wavelet-approximate entropy-fSVM cascade with clinical validation. *Clinical EEG and Neuroscience, 44*(4), 247–256. doi:10.1177/1550059413483451 PMID:23610456

Shirakawa, T., Sugiyama, N., Sato, H., Sakurai, K., & Sato, E. (2017). Gait analysis and machine learning classification on healthy subjects in normal walking. *International Journal of Parallel Emergent and Distributed Systems, 32*(2), 185–194. doi:10.1080/17445760.2015.1044007

Shorten, C. (2018). *Machine Learning vs. Deep Learning*. Retrieved July 20, 2018, from https://towardsdatascience.com/machine-learning-vs-deep-learning-62137a1c9842

Shouval, R., Bondi, O., Mishan, H., Shimoni, A., Unger, R., & Nagler, A. (2014). Application of machine learning algorithms for clinical predictive modeling: A data-mining approach in SCT. *Bone Marrow Transplantation, 49*(3), 332–337. doi:10.1038/bmt.2013.146 PMID:24096823

Singh, D., & Reddy, C. K. (2015). A survey on platforms for big data analytics. *Journal of Big Data, 2*(1), 8.

Siuly, L., Li, Y., & Wen, P. (2011). EEG signal classification based on simple random sampling technique with least square support vector machine. *International Journal of Biomedical Engineering and Technology, 7*(4), 390–409. doi:10.1504/IJBET.2011.044417

Siuly, S., & Zhang, Y. (2016). Medical big data: Neurological diseases diagnosis through medical data analysis. *Data Science and Engineering, 1*(2), 54–64. doi:10.100741019-016-0011-3

Sonu, S. R., Prakash, V., Ranjan, R., & Saritha, K. (2017, August). Prediction of Parkinson's disease using data mining. In *2017 International Conference on Energy, Communication, Data Analytics and Soft Computing (ICECDS)* (pp. 1082-1085). IEEE. 10.1109/ICECDS.2017.8389605

Sun, J., & Reddy, C. K. (2013, August). Big data analytics for healthcare. In *Proceedings of the 19th ACM SIGKDD international conference on Knowledge discovery and data mining* (pp. 1525-1525). ACM.

Sun, Z. (2017). *Big Data Analytics and Artificial Intelligence*. UNITECH Research Committee Seminar, No. 7, PNG University of Technology.

Sun, Z., Sun, L., & Strang, K. (2018). Big data analytics services for enhancing business intelligence. *Journal of Computer Information Systems*, *58*(2), 162–169. doi:10.1080/08874417.2016.1220239

Ta, V. D., Liu, C. M., & Nkabinde, G. W. (2016, July). Big data stream computing in healthcare real-time analytics. In *Cloud Computing and Big Data Analysis (ICCCBDA), 2016 IEEE International Conference on* (pp. 37-42). IEEE.

Umadevi, S., & Marseline, K. J. (2017, July). A survey on data mining classification algorithms. In *Signal Processing and Communication (ICSPC), 2017 International Conference on* (pp. 264-268). IEEE. 10.1109/CSPC.2017.8305851

Uzun, E. (2016). *Supervised ve Unsupervised Learning*. Retrieved January 01, 2018, from, https://www.e-adys.com/makine_ogrenmesi/hangisini-secmeliyim-supervised-ve-unsupervised-learning/

Verma, J. P., Agrawal, S., Patel, B., & Patel, A. (2016). Big data analytics: Challenges and applications for text, audio, video, and social media data. *International Journal on Soft Computing, Artificial Intelligence and Applications, 5*(1).

Vyškovský, R., Schwarz, D., Janoušová, E., & Kašpárek, T. (2016). Random subspace ensemble artificial neural networks for first-episode Schizophrenia classification. In *Computer Science and Information Systems (FedCSIS), 2016 Federated Conference on* (pp. 317-321). IEEE.

Wang, S., Chaovalitwongse, W., & Babuska, R. (2012). Machine learning algorithms in bipedal robot control. *IEEE Transactions on Systems, Man and Cybernetics. Part C, Applications and Reviews*, *42*(5), 728–743. doi:10.1109/TSMCC.2012.2186565

Wang, Y., Kung, L., & Byrd, T. A. (2018). Big data analytics: Understanding its capabilities and potential benefits for healthcare organizations. *Technological Forecasting and Social Change*, *126*, 3–13. doi:10.1016/j.techfore.2015.12.019

Ward, J. S., & Barker, A. (2013). *Undefined by data: a survey of big data definitions.* arXiv preprint arXiv:1309.5821

Winterburn, J. L., Voineskos, A. N., Devenyi, G. A., Plitman, E., de la Fuente-Sandoval, C., Bhagwat, N., ... Chakravarty, M. M. (2017). Can we accurately classify schizophrenia patients from healthy controls using magnetic resonance imaging and machine learning? A multi-method and multi-dataset study. *Schizophrenia Research.* doi:10.1016/j.schres.2017.11.038 PMID:29274736

Wu, X., Zhu, X., Wu, G. Q., & Ding, W. (2014). Data mining with big data. *IEEE Transactions on Knowledge and Data Engineering*, *26*(1), 97–107. doi:10.1109/TKDE.2013.109

Xu, K., Yue, H., Guo, L., Guo, Y., & Fang, Y. (2015, June). Privacy-preserving machine learning algorithms for big data systems. In *Distributed Computing Systems (ICDCS), 2015 IEEE 35th International Conference on* (pp. 318-327). IEEE. 10.1109/ICDCS.2015.40

Yahyaouı, A. (2017). *Göğüs Hastalıklarının Teşhis Edilmesinde Makine Öğrenmesi Algoritmalarının Kullanılması* (Doctoral Dissertation). Ulusal Tez Merkezi. (No. 462917)

Yang, G., Deng, J., Pang, G., Zhang, H., Li, J., Deng, B., ... Xie, H. (2018). An IoT-Enabled Stroke Rehabilitation System Based on Smart Wearable Armband and Machine Learning. *IEEE Journal of Translational Engineering in Health and Medicine, 6*, 1–10. doi:10.1109/JTEHM.2018.2879085 PMID:29805919

Yoo, C., Ramirez, L., & Liuzzi, J. (2014). Big data analysis using modern statistical and machine learning methods in medicine. *International Neurourology Journal, 18*(2), 50. doi:10.5213/inj.2014.18.2.50 PMID:24987556

Zhang, A., Wang, K. J., & Mao, Z. H. (2018, August). Design and Realization of Alzheimer. In *2018 IEEE 6th International Conference on Future Internet of Things and Cloud (FiCloud)* (pp. 141-148). IEEE.

Zhou, L., Pan, S., Wang, J., & Vasilakos, A. V. (2017). Machine learning on big data: Opportunities and challenges. *Neurocomputing, 237*, 350–361. doi:10.1016/j.neucom.2017.01.026

ADDITIONAL READING

Andreu-Perez, J., Poon, C. C., Merrifield, R. D., Wong, S. T., & Yang, G. Z. (2015). Big data for health. *IEEE Journal of Biomedical and Health Informatics, 19*(4), 1193–1208. doi:10.1109/JBHI.2015.2450362 PMID:26173222

Belle, A., Thiagarajan, R., Soroushmehr, S. M., Navidi, F., Beard, D. A., & Najarian, K. (2015). Big data analytics in healthcare. *BioMed Research International*. PMID:26229957

Bhardwaj, R., Nambiar, A. R., & Dutta, D. (2017, July). A Study of Machine Learning in Healthcare. In *Computer Software and Applications Conference (COMPSAC), 2017 IEEE 41st Annual* (Vol. 2, pp. 236-241). IEEE. 10.1109/COMPSAC.2017.164

Bzdok, D., & Yeo, B. T. (2017). Inference in the age of big data: Future perspectives on neuroscience. *NeuroImage, 155*, 549–564. doi:10.1016/j.neuroimage.2017.04.061 PMID:28456584

Chen, H., Chiang, R. H., & Storey, V. C. (2012). Business intelligence and analytics: From big data to big impact. *Management Information Systems Quarterly, 36*(4), 1165–1188. doi:10.2307/41703503

Chen, M., Mao, S., Zhang, Y., & Leung, V. C. (2014). Big data: related technologies, challenges and future prospects. Springer Briefs in Computer Science, Springer, 2014. doi:10.1007/978-3-319-06245-7

Jatrniko, W., Arsa, D. M. S., Wisesa, H., Jati, G., & Ma'sum, M. A. (2016, October). A review of big data analytics in the biomedical field. In *Big Data and Information Security (IWBIS), International Workshop on* (pp. 31-41). IEEE.

Manyika, J., Chui, M., Brown, B., Bughin, J., Dobbs, R., Roxburgh, C., & Byers, A. H. (2011). *Big data: The next frontier for innovation, competition, and productivity*. McKinsey Global Institue. Retrieved from https://www.mckinsey.com/business-functions/digital-mckinsey/our-insights/big-data-the-next-frontier-for-innovation

Rahman, F., Slepian, M., & Mitra, A. (2016, December). A novel big-data processing framework for healthcare applications: Big-data-healthcare-in-a-box. In *Big Data (Big Data), 2016 IEEE International Conference on* (pp. 3548-3555). IEEE.

Ramesh, D., Suraj, P., & Saini, L. (2016, January). Big data analytics in healthcare: A survey approach. In *Microelectronics, Computing and Communications (MicroCom), 2016 International Conference on* (pp. 1-6). IEEE. 10.1109/MicroCom.2016.7522520

Reddy, A. R., & Kumar, P. S. (2016, February). Predictive big data analytics in healthcare. In *Computational Intelligence & Communication Technology (CICT), 2016 Second International Conference on* (pp. 623-626). IEEE. 10.1109/CICT.2016.129

KEY TERMS AND DEFINITIONS

Alzheimer's Disease Neuroimaging Initiative (ADNI): Provides database to researchers about the patient of Alzheimer's disease. The biomarkers are collected and analyzed for early diagnose and following the progression of Alzheimer's.

Big Data: Can be described large volume of data that are structural, semi-structural, and non-structural, and it provides valuable information for lots of research areas. It is often characterized by the 3V (volume, variety, and velocity), but it has continued to grow up with other characteristic components.

Big Data Analytics: Can be defined basically using analytics techniques on big data to explore worthful information. The analyzing of big data is pretty important for both prediction of future and decision making in all working areas.

Big Data Samples: Can be counted as social networks, health records, web logs, mobile phones, academic studies, sensors, and call records that surround us.

Machine Learning: Basically refers to the techniques for extracting useful information from hidden patterns. It can be defined a system consist of many methods that learn and improve from data.

Machine Learning Methods: Can be grouped as supervised learning, unsupervised learning, and reinforcement learning.

Neurological Disorder: Refers to any disorder on the nervous system. Alzheimer's disease, Parkinson's disease, autism, stroke, etc. are some neurological disorders explained in this study.

Chapter 15
Medical Image Segmentation:
An Advanced Approach

Ramgopal Kashyap
https://orcid.org/0000-0002-5352-1286
Amity University Chhattisgarh, India

Surendra Rahamatkar
Amity University Chhattisgarh, India

ABSTRACT

Today, IoT in therapeutic administrations has ended up being more productive in light of the fact that the correspondence among authorities and patients has been improved with versatile applications. These applications are made by the associations with the objective that the pros can screen the patient's prosperity. If any issue has hopped out at the patient, by then the authority approaches the patient and gives the correct treatment. In this proposition, particular focus is given to infant human administrations, in light of the fact that the greatest fear of gatekeepers is that they would lose their infant kids at whatever point. Therefore, in this part, a business contraption has been recognized which screens the consistent information about the infant's heart rate, oxygen levels, resting position. In case anything happens to the tyke, the information will get to the adaptable application, which has been made by an association and is mechanically available by finishing a representation field test for the kid; the information is recorded and examined.

INTRODUCTION

The rapidly expanding field of picture investigation examination has started to accept a vital part in the headway of human administrations practices and research. It has offered gadgets to gather, supervise, analyze, and retain significant volumes of disparate, sorted out, and unstructured data conveyed by current human administrations systems. Colossal data examination has been starting late associated with supporting the technique of care transport and sickness examination. Regardless, the assignment rate and research change in this space are still forestal by some significant issues trademark inside the

DOI: 10.4018/978-1-5225-8567-1.ch015

picture investigation perspective (Cruz-Cunha, Simoes, Varajão and Miranda, 2014). Potential zones of research inside this field which can give noteworthy impact on restorative administrations movement are moreover broke down. "Image examination" isn't new; anyway the manner in which is described ceaselessly developing. Distinctive undertakings at describing picture examination depict it as a social occasion of data segments whose size, speed, type remembering the real objective to store viable, look at, and envision the data. Human administrations are a prime instance of how the three data, the speed of period of data, collection, and volume are a unique piece of the data it produces. This data spread among different restorative administrations structures, prosperity back up plans, examiners.

Despite the underlying complexities of therapeutic social data, there is potential and favorable position in making and completing picture investigation courses of action inside this space (Mutula, 2009) 66% of the regard would be through diminishing the US human administrations utilization. Bonafide approaches to managing therapeutic research have all things considered fixated on the examination of disease states in light of the modifications in physiology as a confined viewpoint of the particular specific strategy of data. Disregarding the way that along these lines to manage understanding ailments are central, asks about at this level calms the assortment and interconnectedness that portray the certifiable concealed restorative instruments. Following a long time of creative slump, the field of pharmaceutical has begun to adjust to the present modernized data age. New advances make it possible to get large measures of information about each patient over a significant timescale. Regardless, paying little mind to the happening to remedial equipment, the data got and gathered from these patients has remained hugely underutilized and like this misused. Fundamental physiological and pathophysiological wonders are at the same time appeared as changes over different clinical streams (Gan and Dai, 2014). Along these lines, understanding and foreseeing infirmities require a gathered approach where sorted out and unstructured data beginning from a stack of clinical and nonclinical modalities utilized for a more exhaustive perspective of the sickness states. A piece of human administrations ask about that has started late grabbed balance is in keeping an eye on a segment of the creating torments in exhibiting thoughts of picture investigation examination to the drug. Authorities are analyzing the beautiful idea of human administrations data to the extent the two characteristics of the data itself and the logical grouping of examination that can genuinely perform on them.

Image Processing

Helpful pictures are a fundamental wellspring of data routinely used for discovering, treatment assessment and orchestrating. Computed tomography (CT), Magnetic Resonance Imaging (MRI), is a portion of the cases of imaging systems, restorative picture data can go wherever (Cai, Zhou, Liao and Tan, 2017) from two or three megabytes for a lone report e.g., histology pictures to numerous megabytes per mull over e.g., thin-cut CT analyzes including up to 2500+ yields for each examination. Such data requires broad limit limits if set away for the whole deal. It moreover asks for snappy and exact figurings if any decision helping robotization were to be performed using the data. Also, if different wellsprings of data picked up for each patient are in the like manner utilized in the midst of the judgments, representation, and treatment frames, by then the issue of giving solid accumulating and making effective systems fit for typifying the vast extent of data transforms into a test.

Flag Processing

Like restorative pictures, remedial banners in like manner pose volume and speed impediments especially in the midst of consistent, high-assurance anchoring and limit from countless related with each patient. In any case, despite the data measure issues, physiological banners in a like manner act multi-faceted nature of a spatiotemporal sort (Cohen, Heiman, Carmi, Hadar and Cohen, 2015). In any case, such uncompounded procedures towards change and use of alert structures tend to be tricky, and their sheer numbers could cause "ready shortcoming" for both parental figures and patients. In this setting, the ability to discover new remedial data is constrained by before realizing that has regularly come up short concerning maximally utilizing high-dimensional time course of action data. The reason that these alert instruments tend to fail is mainly in light of the way that these structures tend to rely upon only wellsprings of information while lacking setting of the patients' certain physiological conditions from a broader and more exhaustive point of view. Like this, there is a need to make upgraded and more expansive methodologies towards looking at affiliations and connections among multimodal clinical time course of action data. I am basically in light of the way that audits continue demonstrating that individuals are poor in contemplating changes impacting more than two signs.

Genomics

The cost to game plan the human genome (joining 30,000 to 35,000 characteristics) is rapidly lessening with the progression of high-throughput sequencing advancement. With recommendations for current general prosperity courses of action and transport of care, researching genome-scale data for making important proposition is a massive test to the field of computational science cost and time to pass on proposals are fundamental in a clinical setting ("Genetics: Genome made rapidly sans preparation," 2009). Exercises taking care of this remarkable issue join following of 100,000 subjects more than 20 to 30 years using the insightful, preventive, participatory, and modified prosperity, alluded to pharmaceutical perspective. The action is using a system approach for (i) analyzing genome-scale datasets to choose disease states, (ii) moving towards blood-based demonstrative devices for relentless checking of a subject, (iii) researching better approaches to manage quiet target divulgence, making instruments to oversee enormous data challenges of getting, supporting, securing, mining, planning, ultimately (iv) showing data for each. Finally, recognizing important recommendations at the clinical level remains a breathtaking test for this field. Utilizing such high thickness data for examination, revelation, and clinical elucidation demands novel tremendous data methodologies and analysis.

Despite the monstrous utilization eaten up by the present human administration's systems, clinical outcomes stay defective, particularly in the USA, where 96 people for each stunning from conditions thought about treatable. A key factor attributed to such inefficient perspectives is the inability to effectively gather, offer, and use information in a more intensive manner inside the social protection systems. It is an open entryway for picture examination to expect a more critical part in supporting the examination and disclosure process, upgrading the transport of care, arranging and plan human administrations course of action, giving an approach to thoroughly evaluating, and surveying the ensnared and convoluted social protection data. More fundamentally, choice of bits of learning got from picture examination can save lives, upgrade mind movement, stretch out access to restorative administrations, alter portion to execution, and help control the vexing advancement of human administrations costs.

BACKGROUND

Helpful imaging gives necessary information on life frameworks and organ work despite perceiving contaminations states (Miles-Tribble, 2017). Additionally, it is utilized for organ delineation, regarding tumors in lungs, spinal distortion discovering, passage stenosis disclosure, aneurysm area, and so forth. In these applications, picture taking care of systems, for instance, change, division, and denoising despite machine learning methods are used. As the size and dimensionality of data increase, understanding the conditions among the data and arranging useful, correct, and computationally fruitful methodologies ask for new PC vision helped strategies and stages as appeared in figure 1.

In the going with, data made by imaging methods has kept an eye on and uses of therapeutic imaging from a unique data point of view are discussed.

Data Produced by Imaging Techniques

Restorative imaging wraps an extensive variety of different picture getting strategies usually utilized for a collection of clinical applications (Chung, 2017). For example, envisioning vein structure can be performed using appealing resonation imaging, enlisted tomography, ultrasound, and photoacoustic imaging. From a data estimation viewpoint, helpful pictures may have 2, 3, and four estimations. PET, CT, 3D ultrasound, and useful MRI considered as multidimensional therapeutic data. Show day remedial picture progressions can make high-assurance pictures, for instance, breath related or "four-dimensional" computed tomography (4D CT). Higher assurance and estimations of these pictures make immense volumes of data requiring predominant figuring and advanced investigative procedures. For instance, small ranges of a human cerebrum with high assurance can need 66TB of storage space. Regardless of

Figure 1. Challenge by expanding the span of information

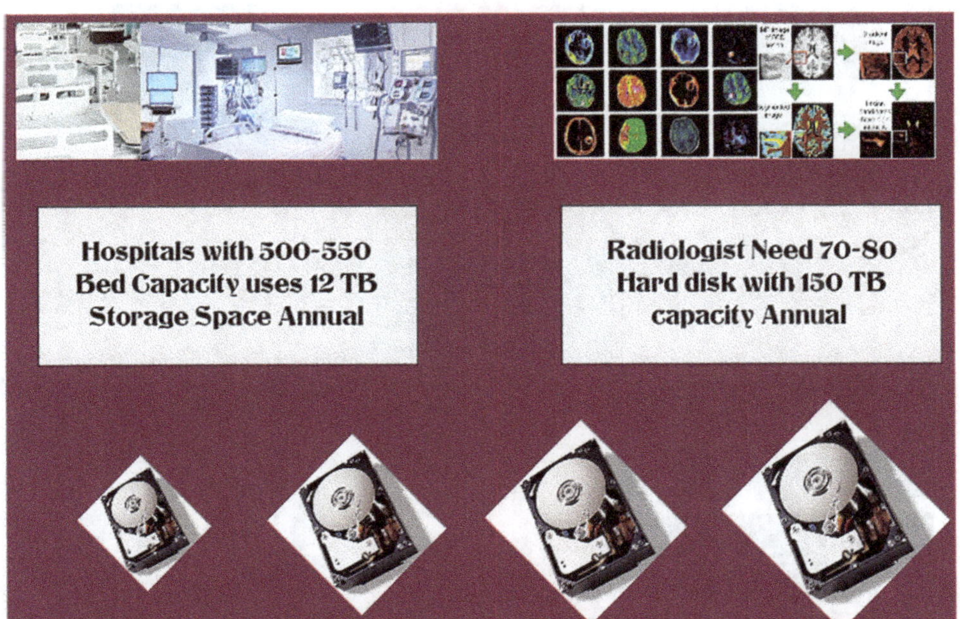

the way that the volume and variety of therapeutic data make its examination a noteworthy test, drives in therapeutic imaging could make individualized care more practical and give quantitative information in the arrangement of usages, for instance, ailment stratification, farsighted illustrating, and central administration systems. In the going with we imply two remedial imaging methodologies and one of their related challenges.

The fast improvement in the amount of human administrations affiliations and furthermore the amount of patients has realized the more conspicuous use of modernized helpful diagnostics and decision sincerely robust systems in clinical settings. Various zones in human administrations, for instance, assurance, perception, and screening can be improved by utilizing computational knowledge (Cresswell and Sheik, 2012). The mix of PC examination with appropriate care can empower clinicians to upgrade symptomatic accuracy. Figure 2 is demonstrating the blend of restorative pictures with various sorts of personal electronic record (EHR) data and genomic data can in like manner upgrade the precision and decline the time taken for a conclusion.

Microwave imaging is a creating system that could make a guide of electromagnetic wave spreading rising out of the separation in the dielectric properties of different tissues (Fromenteze, Decroze, Abid and Yurduseven, 2018). It has both useful and physiological information encoded in the dielectric properties which can encourage independent and depict unmistakable tissues and additionally pathologies. In any case, microwaves have scattering conduct that makes recuperation of information a testing undertaking. The joining of pictures from different modalities and other clinical and physiological information could improve the precision of finding and result from an estimate of ailment. For this kind of disease, the electroanatomic mapping can help in recognizing the subendocardial expansion of infarct. The piece

Figure 2. Compositions of medical data

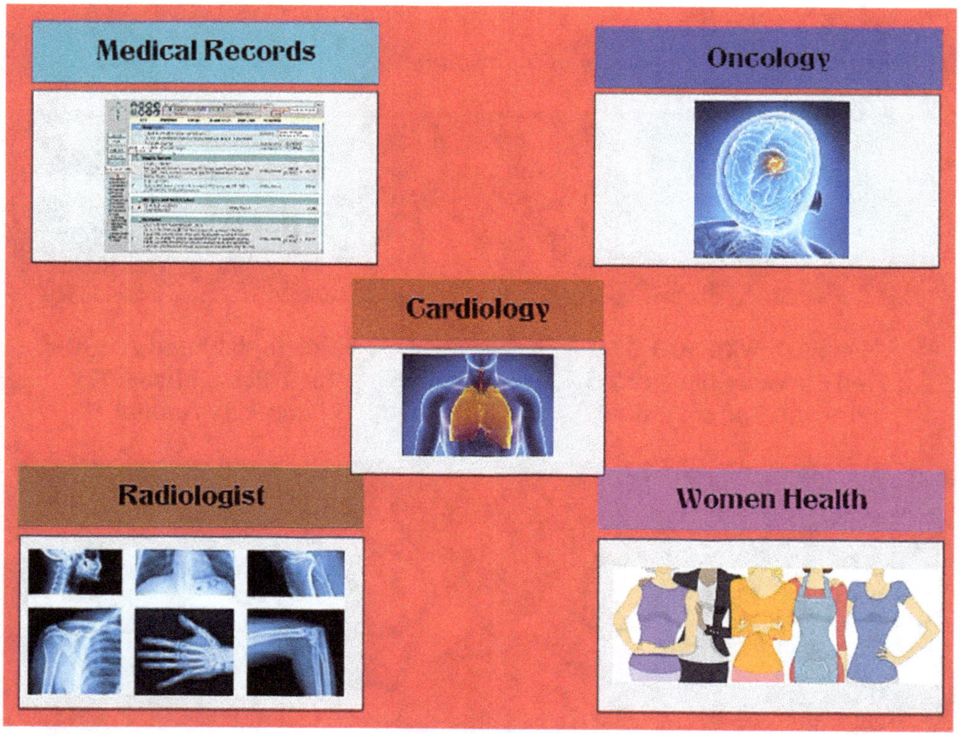

of evaluating both MRI and CT pictures to fabricate the precision of conclusion in recognition of the closeness of deteriorations and osteophytes in the temporomandibular joint (TMJ) has been looked into ("Fusion of MRI and CT Images of Brain Tumor – Comprehensive Survey", 2018), according to this examination simultaneous appraisal of all the available imaging strategies is a disregarded need. Other than the vast space required for securing each one of the data and their analysis, finding the guide and conditions among different data composes are challenges for which there is no perfect plan yet.

Procedures

The volume of remedial pictures is growing exponentially for instance; Image helpful picture dataset contained around 66,000 photos in the region of 2005 and 2007 while just in the season of 2013 around 300,000 views were secured, general. Despite the creating volume of images, they change in procedure, assurance, estimation, and quality which display new challenges, for instance, data coordination and mining especially if diverse datasets are incorporated (Mi, Petitjean, Vera and Ruan, 2015). Appeared differently about the volume of research that exists on single secluded helpful picture examination, there is the widely lesser number of research exercises on multimodal picture examination. While utilizing data at an area/institutional level, an essential piece of an investigation wander is on how the made structure is surveyed and affirmed. Having remarked on data or a composed methodology to clear up new data is an official test. It ends up being impressively all the more troublesome when immense scale data blend from various establishments considered. For example, for related applications and a comparable approach (e.g., CT), unmistakable foundations may use different settings in picture acquisitions, it hard to make bound together remark or investigative systems for such data. To benefit the multimodal pictures and their joining with other helpful data, new descriptive systems with endless plausibility and versatility are required. In the going with we look at interpretive systems that course of action with a couple of parts of picture examination.

Difficulties in Healthcare

The limit of the social protection industry to open of the capacity of picture examination depends upon the manner in which restorative administrations affiliations execute great data game plans spread out the methods fundamental for the productive utilization of picture investigation answers for providers. Human administration's industry is setting its sights on using large data to change quality care through examination that gives steady help to provide, see designs among masses, empower research to widen its compass and exhort central authority by government authorities and workplaces. At its most basic, providers will benefit most inside and out from extensive data, yet the level of this preferred standpoint will depend upon how well their affiliations manage and join their prosperity information systems. "Once Big Data administered and facilitated, affiliations can apply examination to all the more likely grasp the clinical and operational states of their business in light of recorded and current examples and envision what may happen later on with a trusted in the level of immovable quality (Dalessandro, Perlich and Raeder, 2014),".

As demonstrated by the makers, the productive execution of picture investigation courses of action depends upon affiliations following four significant advances:

1. Set up data organization, portray data goals: Implementing real data courses of work begins with setting up the perfect people. With an official leading body of senior people set up, an affiliation would then have the capacity to continue forward to pondering how and why it will utilize picture examination. The remarkable idea must be given to the new automated methods, deducing, estimations, and checking devices gave by Big Data game plans (Hoskins, 2014). Courses of action and frameworks will moreover necessitate that manage the use of data, portray the required exercises and quality control shapes, and streamline, secure, and utilize information as an undertaking asset by altering the goals of various limits.
2. Recognize data and information necessities: Big data is about the data dependent upon the measure of an affiliation, its data could be spread out among an assortment of structures and settings (Kashyap and Piersson, 2018a). Also, data exist in different formations, and some of the most basic information is unstructured, e.g., free substance, imaging. Affiliations should first see the current state of their data and suspect future changes to the manner in which information is getting (Zhu, Lee, and Rosenthal, 2016). "Affiliations need to fathom what data they will use today, and any potential data that they may need to get to later on," the makers clear up. "Affiliations will in like manner need to set up a data acquisition direct in light of business and examination needs."
3. Institutionalize, fuse, and organize large data courses of action: Normalizing a database requires prosperity IT specialists to perceive potential redundancies and conditions in their data fields and tables (Rey-del-Castillo and Cardeñosa, 2016). "Affiliations need to appreciate what data they will use today, and any potential data that they may need to get to later on," the makers elucidate. "Affiliations will in like manner need to set up a data obtainment direct in light of business and examination needs."
4. Guarantee security and assurance of picture examination: In the human administration's industry, insurance and security are enormous stresses for providers and patients. Accumulating all the more before extensive identifiable information and offering it to a broad variety of affiliations and associations adds to these stresses. The makers recommend the following best practice while advancing toward these issues (Recio, 2017). The best way to deal with address security concerns or necessities is for Big Data answers for encouraging FIPPs. FIPPs are industry-pragmatist, important information security decides that can control the thorny exchanges that may be required when deliberate assignments cross ventures, data sources, and data compose. Despite whether picture investigation decidedly influences human administrations will come down to how well social protection affiliations and prosperity IT specialists prepare it and what measures they take to shield the security of patients and the respectability of these data. Data from complex heterogeneous patient sources using the patient/data connections in longitudinal records, understanding unstructured clinical notes in the right setting (Fatt and Ramadas, 2018). Examining genomic data is a computationally focused endeavor and joining with standard clinical data incorporates additional layers of dispersing quality; the most significant test is to discover bits of knowledge and proof as appeared in figure 3.

Catching the patient's conduct data through a couple of sensors; their diverse social participation's and exchanges.

Figure 3. Challenges in healthcare

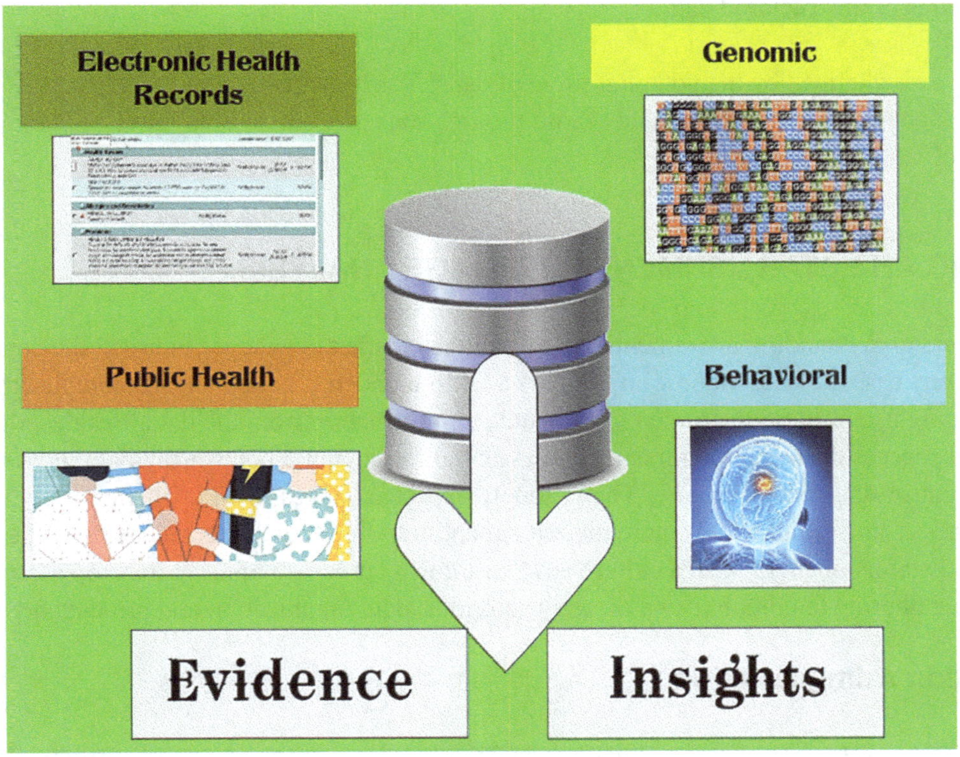

Establishment for Overseeing Image Analysis in Medicinal Services

It is evident in the present human administration's industry that large data is ending up something past a prevalent articulation. As shown by IBM, 90 percent of the information on the planet today has made over the latest two years alone. Despite whether that claim is correct, the measure of data we create both sorted out and unstructured is animating rapidly. The human administration's industry is in the thick of this data impact. We can characteristic a part of the plenitude of data to the HITECH Act, and EHR Incentive Programs, i.e., meaningful use, yet various segments contribute likewise (Palojoki, Pajunen, Saranto and Lehtonen, 2016). Consider these examples that should show to make picture investigation impressively all the more real in social protection:

- Increasingly separated clinical documentation will be required to get correct codification from the expanded ICD-10 investigation codes;
- Continued expansion of biomedical, bedside and adaptable development devices will achieve growing measures of spouting data;
- Recent advances in remedial and human innate characteristics, foundation objects for modified medicine and where genomic sequencing will associate with the helpful care of individual patients will achieve colossal measures of sequenced data;
- Natural Language Processing (NLP) and other development movements are making even the talked word getting as a data asset;

- Secure clinician to clinicians educating and among clinicians and patients will continue creating measures of unstructured data.

Feeling overwhelmed by the potential surge of data? The best approach to managing this tsunami is to develop a course of action proactively those progressions this pile of data into a sensible and viable crucial asset.

BUILDING AN ESTABLISHMENT FOR IMAGE ANALYSIS

New business understanding instruments are entering the market to enhance to use of the creating surge of data. In any case, devices alone won't impact a BI to broaden productively. Accomplishment lies in the convincing use of these instruments to get unique information from the data. Besides, this requires culture and process change. One fundamental essential to moving a noteworthy data movement is the establishment of data-driven culture. The routinely expects changes to an affiliation's key targets and focus business frames, and what's more the critical aptitudes required by its delegates (Skiera and Ringel, 2017). Establishment of such a culture is a "best down" process requiring nonstop assistance from the official gathering to complete two primary activities: data organization and pro data organization.

Information Administration

Data Governance sets up the parts, obligations, and work process for managing an affiliation's endeavor full data. A convincing data organization framework consigns commitment to particular data for no less than one sort of expert data (Naimur Rahman, Esmailpour and Zhao, 2016). Data stewards are then settled to help data proprietors by arranging definitions and estimations used to regulate and measure data quality and execution. Appropriate data organization ensures the consistency of an affiliation's data definitions, opinions, and execution markers a basic essential in the organization of information as a critical corporate asset. Data organization gives accomplices trust in the data that they would then have the capacity to rely upon to settle on more taught decisions.

Ace Information Administration

Pro data organization is the specific structure for data organization; It engages data proprietors and stewards to keep up the affiliation's master data assets easily. Without expert data organization method, various data organization exercises disregard to achieve their objectives. Why? Since without pro data organization the sheer measure of effort required to keep up the expert data is unnecessarily unimaginable. Huge data circumstances are as subject to pro data as large business data stockrooms or data stores (Tian and Peng, 2011). A single wellspring of truth for patient and provider data is similarly as fundamental in a unique data condition and data organization. The pro data organization give the underlying progressive structure, work process, and gadgets if restorative administrations in the United States were to use picture investigation in an original and gainful route in their undertakings to drive adequacy and quality, we could make more than $300 billion in regard every year. 66% of this regard would be seen in a standard 8 percent diminishment when all said in done restorative administrations employments.

That is an essential outcome for the various leveled effort required to set up a data-driven culture.

The human administration's industry, perhaps more than some other, is on the shaky edge of a necessary change utilizing advanced examination and picture investigation propels. In this segment, noteworthy data slants in therapeutic administrations given.

Solutions

A target of current restorative administrations systems is to give perfect human administrations through the massive usage of prosperity information advancement with a particular ultimate objective to:

- Improve human administrations quality and coordination, so comes about are solid with current master data
- Reduce social protection costs; reduce avoidable mishandle
- Provide reinforce for enhanced portion structures

Security net suppliers and general prosperity structures, e.g., Medicare and Medicaid are in the first place times of moving from cost for-advantage pay to regard based data driven inspirations that reward splendid, fiscally wise calm care and show extensive use of electronic human records (Phone, 2018). This approach requires significant updates in declaring, claims dealing with, data organization, and process computerization. The consideration of regard based care contrasts and an extended focus on patient-driven care by using development and focusing human administrations shapes on patient outcomes. A continuum of care, experts, specialist's offices, and medicinal scope need to work with each other to redo mind that is capable and taken a toll aware, direct in its transport and charging, and evaluated in perspective of patient satisfaction. Like this, the target presently is to begin to move more convincingly a long way from the long-standing charge for-advantage sharpen by which portions made to providers. In a general sense, providers get paid for seeing and treating patients. There is alongside zero rewards when and if providers upgrade the nature of organizations, help patient outcomes, or lessening costs. Charge for-advantage has been a critical boundary in plans or needs to place assets into automated responses for, say, improves determined outcomes if the providers can't recoup their endeavors. Current thinking around long-standing, huge portion sharpens beginning to change, preparing for a free propelled change of human administrations.

The Healthcare Internet of Things (IoT)

In like manner called the Industrial Internet, these terms imply the rapidly growing number of smart, interconnected contraptions and sensors and the tidal volumes of data they will deliver and move among devices, and finally to people. Spending on human administrations IoT could top $120 billion in just four years, by a couple of assessments (Blake, 2015). Also, most of the data made by the restorative administrations IoT is of the unstructured variety, making a significant part for Hadoop and advanced gigantic data examination working inside the Hadoop framework. Today, a collection of contraptions screens every sort of patient lead from glucose screens to fetal monitors to electrocardiograms to beat. Countless estimation requires a consequent visit with a specialist. Regardless, more clever watching devices talking with other patient devices could phenomenally refine this system, possibly decreasing the necessities to organize a specialist intervention and maybe supplanting it with a phone call from a therapeutic guardian. Other sharp devices are starting if pharmaceuticals are being taken reliably at home from keen wholesalers and if not; they can begin a call or other contact from providers to get patients adequately restored. The possible results offered by the social protection IoT to cut down costs and improve patient care are moderately limitless.

Prescient Analytics to Improve Outcomes

Exercises, for instance, noteworthy use are animating the allotment of EHR, and the volume and detail of patient information are increasing. The flood in the creation and increasing use for EHR was headed to some degree by a $30 billion government shock, provided by the Health Information Technology for Economic and Clinical Health (HITECH) Act. The Act was formed primarily to offer inspirations to get EHR and after that stimulate the sharing of patient information by clinicians wherever endeavoring to cut down costs, speed finding, and upgrade tireless outcomes (Fife and Eckert, 2017). Having the ability to unite and dismember a variety of sorted out and unstructured data over various data sources helps in the precision of diagnosing understanding conditions, organizing pharmaceuticals with comes about, and anticipating patients in threat for infection or readmission. Farsighted showing over data got from EHRs is being used for early assurance and is diminishing passing rates from issues, for instance, congestive heart dissatisfaction and sepsis. Congestive Heart Failure (CHF) speaks to the most human administrations spending. The earlier it is broke down, the better it can be managed, avoiding expensive challenges; anyway, early signs can be scarcely perceptible by specialists. A machine taking in the event that from Georgia Tech displayed that machine learning computations could look at various a more noteworthy number of components in patients' blueprints than authorities, and by including additional features, there was a huge augmentation in the limit of the model to perceive people who have CHF from people who don't. Insightful exhibiting and machine learning on large case sizes, with more patient data, can uncover nuances and illustrations that couldn't think as of now revealed. Optum Labs has assembled EHRs of more than 30 million patients to make a database for insightful examination gadgets that will empower pros to settle on large data taught decisions to upgrade patients' treatment.

Constant Monitoring of Patients

Restorative administrations workplaces are planning to give more proactive care to their patients by constantly watching quiet central signs. The data from these distinctive screens can be continuously explored and send alerts to mind providers, so they know in a brief moment about changes in a patient's condition. Getting ready steady events with machine learning counts can give specialists bits of information to empower them to settle on lifesaving decisions and mull over efficacious intercessions. Wearable sensors and devices demonstrate the open entryway for gatekeepers to interface with patients in entirely new ways, making human administrations more supportive and decided. Consistent checking changes the specific thought of the relationship in that very close care isn't, for the most part, a need — for example, applications used for remote or in-home checking of patients with the steady obstructive pneumonic disease. Diverse screens track the largeness of patients doing fighting obstructive coronary sickness to distinguish fluid upkeep before hospitalization is required. Still, others follow a child's asthma arrangement use to influence specific home parental figures and relatives to think about what ought to be coordinated, diminishing visits to the ER (Kashyap and Piersson, 2018b). As is so every now and again the case with new data volumes in human administrations, sensor data from wearable screens is unstructured data that regards the data acquisition and limit capacities of Hadoop, and moreover to the power and flexibility of front-line huge data examination.

Machine Learning Revolution for Healthcare Diagnostics

Machine learning could be the best approach to by and large upgrading social protection diagnostics; especially concerning removing most excellent motivator from imaging contemplates. If you are in human administrations, you may have heard the articulation "machine learning" without to a great degree appreciating what it infers. It is not another development, anyway, it is one that has taken great hops forward completed the ongoing years, and it ended up being valuable in social protection. Essentially, machine learning is a sort of fake cognizance that suggests the limit of a PC to recognize and "remember" effectively experienced illustrations and to pick up from new data about those cases and any new cases that are perceived (Chalmers, Altman, McHaffie, Owens and Cooke, 2013). It's a significant advancement in conditions that require examination of a great deal of data or in assignments that cannot react to developing data. It's used as a piece of a full bunch of organizations, empowering PCs to drive cars, run successive development frameworks, fight on Jeopardy and give new encounters from recorded data. In therapeutic administrations, machine learning enables a PC to separate large measures of data and recognize plans in the data. It can be used to empower us to locate an extensive variety of new information. Consider using your therapeutic history and related knick-knacks to associate the probability of a prosperity scene later on. That would be worth knowing, wouldn't it? New bits of information about patient prosperity from documented pictures (Mingle, 2017).

We should take the instance of pictures. Propelled pictures are incorporated cases of pixels. A PC vision can see and react to those illustrations and use figurings to figure or measure the data contained in the circumstances. Mostly, it can recognize the case of pixels in a picture of your spine, for example, measure the physical attributes addressed, and find out whether you are at risk for osteoporosis. In any case, it shouldn't generally be a picture that was made to investigate your threat of osteoporosis (Kashyap and Tiwari, 2018). You have had a chest x-beam, possibly going before a medical procedure, the picture was used to look at your lungs. In any case, it furthermore will contain data about your spine. A computer vision with the benefit examination programming can review that picture and perceive your risk, accepting any, for osteoporosis.

Envision a situation where most of your symptomatic pictures could use for different screening examination despite the disease express that incited the test. That would build the estimation of every representative survey. Observing impressively more remote, think about how conceivable it is that the usage of this discretionary imaging examination could impel your parental figure to orchestrate a genomic focus to redesign the data got from the picture, or if a genomic study could enhance by analysis of past films (Kashyap and Gautam, 2017). It could choose whether you have a tendency to a significant danger or even perceive a potential medicine to address the peril. While this is advanced, the building obstructs for the vision are occurring today.

Mining and Image Information for Bring Down Cost

Characteristic pictures could construct chance screening to recognize people who could benefit from preventive treatment. Is a useful idea, in light of the way that, while everyone that risk screening can be significant; it is furthermore an extra cost and is regularly an extra weight for patients. In this manner, general adherence to various screening programs is low. In case we can look at understanding pictures without requiring additional movement by the patient, we can colossally grow our ability to anticipate prosperity threats. In most original views, there is an existing structure outside the bit of the opinion that the radiologist is evaluating (Kashyap, Gautam and Tiwari, 2018). This life structures may contain data that can be available for assistant disclosures provoking distinctive evidence of asymptomatic affliction, for instance, osteoporosis as I noted beforehand. The typical mending office imaging office has terabytes of data away, and the measure of data is growing exponentially. If we can mine this data, it would help recognize illness extensively earlier, better match treatment with patients who could benefit by it and through early disclosure diminish the impact of a perpetual affliction or balance hospitalization due to the disease.

Machine Vision for Utilization of Enormous Information Files

It is the place machine vision, and machine learning ends up vital when large educational accumulations like this, it takes complex programming and computational vitality to look at thousands, even millions, of pictures and "see" the cases. It's not something a human could do in an advantageous or monetarily smart way. There is necessarily a ton of data there to be significant without examination. While a readied radiologist could find these same cases, it is all the more convincing to save the radiologist's the perfect open door for other work, for instance, making considered significant judgments of final contamination frames, in perspective of a start to finish perception of a patient. Associations are beginning to run machine vision estimations programming that looks for plans against the pixels in early X-beams, CT and MRI ranges to perceive helper variations from the norm that interface with prosperity perils (Kashyap and Gautam, 2016). For example, in a CT scope of the guts, the broadness of the existing frameworks in the picture offers the opportunity to perceive various revelations that show a proclivity for heart illness. Right when this examination joined with other clinical data related to the patient, the mix would more have the capacity to describe the patient's risk clearly.

For example, the mix of blood work with oily liver revelations could in like manner recognize characteristics that are connected with the next progression of cardiovascular illness, allowing a notice signal that could help perceive patients who require preventive treatment (Tiwari S., Gupta R.K., & Kashyap R., 2019). The development to analyze picture data exists now, and we are mostly beginning to see new bits of learning from it. We would now have the capacity to analyze pictures for both osteoporosis and cardiovascular disease peril, and more risk screenings are going ahead of the web within the near future with machine learning advancement, we have the opportunity to make counts that perceive known markers for sickness, and in addition, empower us to recognize new tags. As we relate picture revelations and patient outcomes, there is the probability that examination will find new cases in the pixels that are connected with peril and give us altogether more techniques for perceiving beginning ailment and balancing it.

Restorative Technologies: Robotics Improves Radiology Imaging

As creators make all the more astounding and refined helpful advances, social protection providers complete remote checking instruments, adaptable prosperity applications, wearable devices, telemedicine features, and patient doors with an ultimate objective to upgrade the idea of restorative administrations organizations and people prosperity comes. Nearby the broad grouping of medicinal advancements, mechanical self-governance is accepting a section in affecting understanding thought. For instance, some unusual medical procedures are presently using mechanical self-sufficiency close-by the religious gathering. One captivating robot that has been changing the social protection industry is IBM's Watson. The association proclaimed seven days back that Watson will get a kind of vision by joining its picture examination and mental limits with information and pictures from Merge Healthcare Incorporated's remedial imaging organization structure, as shown by an official proclamation from IBM.

As an exhibited pioneer in passing on restorative administrations answers for over 20 years, Merge is a significant development to the Watson Health arrange. Therapeutic administrations will be one of IBM's most noteworthy advancement zones all through the accompanying ten years, which is the reason we are influencing a vital theory to drive the industry to change and to support a higher nature of care. IBM is planning to secure Merge remembering the real objective to all the more likely serve social protection relationship by offering a more grounded a motivation to therapeutic pictures that would assist specialists with the necessary clinical administration. At the display, Merge is advancing organizations and remedial progressions to more than 7,500 social protection relationships over the United States including pharmaceuticals and clinical research associations (Kashyap and Gautam, 2015). The game plan is for these helpful establishments to utilize Watson's capacities to regulate restorative pictures and increase new bits of learning from electronic patient records, images, therapeutic data, and information from wearable contraptions. "As Watson propels, we are dealing with more awesome and huge issues by ceaselessly evaluating more prominent and furthermore troublesome instructive lists," Kelly continued. "Helpful pictures are without a doubt the most confounded instructive files possible, and there is perhaps no more fundamental domain in which authorities can apply machine learning and mental figuring. That is the bona fide certification of mental figuring and its fake awareness sections making us more worthwhile and to improve the idea of our lives." With the large volumes of pictures that various human administrations specialists must manage on a regular preface, Watson's abilities could exhibit fundamental in diminishing restorative oversights and upgrading the idea of care among the patient base. A couple of radiologists in facility emergency rooms may need to manage upwards of 100,000 remedial pictures for consistently.

Machine Learning: Imaging Analytics Predict Kidney Function

Imaging examination bolstered by machine learning can correctly envision renal survival time in patients with persistent kidney disease. Machine taking in and imaging examination from renal biopsies can envision to what degree a kidney will work tastefully in patients with unremitting kidney hurt, says a questionnaire circulated in Kidney International Reports. Using meaningful learning and neural frameworks, a kind of machine finding that copies the first administration cases of the human identity, researchers found that a movement of new convolutional neural framework counts was correct and exact than standard pathologist-assessed scoring structures while registering kidney diminish. Unending kidney hurt is routinely reviewed semi-quantitatively by scoring the measure of fibrosis, and tubular rot in a renal biopsy test illuminates the investigation bunch from Boston University.

Despite the way that as indicated by ace pathologists can gauge the earnestness of contamination and perceive nuances of histopathology with pivotal exactness, such ability isn't open in all regions, especially at an overall level. In the United States, around 14 percent of the people encounter unending kidney disease, according to the National Institutes of Health. The condition routinely conveys a couple of signs until the point that it is considered best in class, inspiring the importance of standard checking and correct distinctive evidence of how the infection is progressing. Furthermore, there is a genuine need to systematize the assessment of over the top contamination earnestness, to such a degree, to the point that the sufficiency of medicines developed in clinical preliminaries can associate with treat patients with comparably extraordinary sickness in routine practice, the gathering included (Manlhiot, 2018). Artificial intellectual prowess and imaging examination are promising advances for helping pathologists with these endeavors. With the ability to see outlines down to the pixel in multi-gigabyte pictures, AI offers a level of systematic examination for incredibly large volumes of data that human clinicians may primarily be a remarkable match. Early results joining machine learning and imaging data have been enabling and how human services information gathered as appeared in figure 4.

A couple of pilots have recently shown that AI gadgets can be about as exact as human pathologists while in a general sense diminishing the time it takes to dismember necessary measures of data. The count was set up to recognize patients with reasonable renal survival rates of 1, 3, and 5 years. Since the examination used to audit data, the gathering could arrange the figuring's estimates with positive outcomes. The results demonstrated that the CNN exhibit was quantifiably better than anything the pathologist-surveyed scoring system while anticipating renal survival rates over the three target time allotments. The computation was furthermore prepared to more decisively perceive the state of kidney disease for the general population.

Additionally, autonomous restorative assignments of screening, watching, and interminable disease organization can describe. Level managerial endeavors, for instance, resource progression, quality control, adherence to the traditions and treatment plans are similarly to be considered. Summing up the two systems, the objectives of Data Mining (DM) used in pharmaceutical can be summed up into two regular get-togethers: treatment resources improvement (social protection organization zone), and treatment quality change (treatment and research territories).

Figure 4. Healthcare data and sources

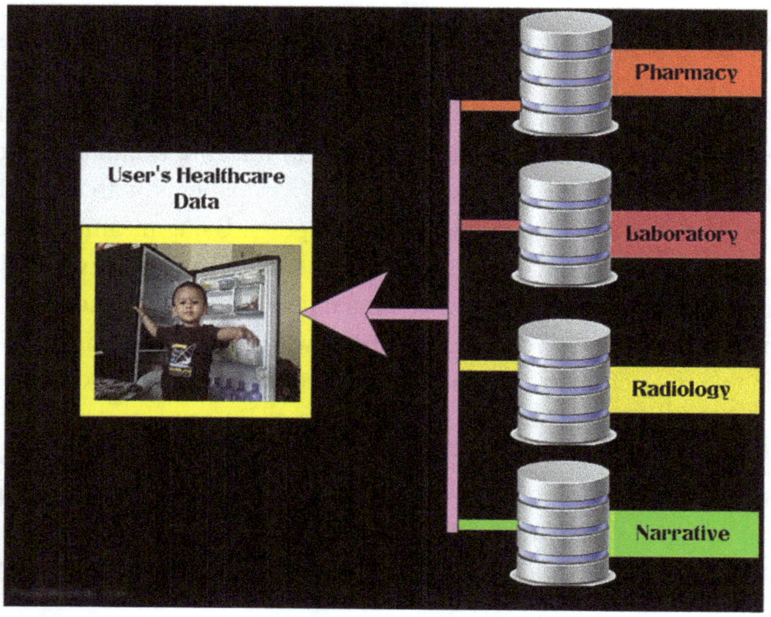

Adventure the broad measures of data and give a valid petition to the right patient at the ideal time. Possibly advantage each one of the sections of a social protection framework Personalized care to the patient. i.e., supplier, payer, patient, and organization.

APPROACHES FOR SOLUTIONS

In the going with, particular troubles and openings discussed as for the usage of Big Information developments in human administrations.

Information Quality

There is a need for reliable and reproducible results particularly in restorative and pharmaceutical inspect where data gathering is to a remarkable degree expensive. Data provenance gives an appreciation of the wellspring of the data how it was accumulated, under which conditions, yet likewise how it was arranged beside, changed before being secured. It is not only for reproducibility of examination and tests yet furthermore to understand the steadfastness of the data that can impact brings about clinical additionally, pharmacological research (Waoo, Kashyap and Jaiswal, 2010). As the versatile nature of exercises creates, with new examination procedures made rapidly, it ends up key to record and fathom the reason for data which thus would altogether be able to affect the conclusion from the examination.

Information

The prosperity division is a data concentrated industry depending upon data and examination to make progress medicines and practices. There has been a massive improvement in the extent of information accumulated, including clinical, inherited, conduct, biological, budgetary, and operational information. Social protection data is creating at staggering rates that have not found previously. There is a need to deal with this vast volume and speed of data to decide critical bits of learning to improve social protection quality and profitability (Kashyap R., 2019a). Affiliations today are gathering a massive amount of data from both elite data sources and open sources, for instance, web-based systems administration and open data. Through a better examination of these large Datasets, there is a significant potential to more readily appreciate accomplice (e.g., constant, clinician) needs, streamline existing things and organizations, and also develop new impetuses.

Multi-Modular Information

In restorative administrations, particular sorts of information are available from different sources, for instance, electronic social protection records, tolerant summaries, genomic and pharmaceutical data, clinical test results, imaging (e.g. x-ray, MRI), assurance claims, basic signs from e.g., telemedicine, adaptable applications, home checking, on-going clinical preliminaries, progressing sensors, and information on flourishing. This data can be both sorted out and unstructured. The mix of human administrations data from various sources could abuse existing helpful energies between data to upgrade clinical decisions and to reveal better approaches to manage treating sicknesses. For instance, the blend of different prosperity data sources could make the examination and association of different phenotypes, e.g. watched verbalization of diseases or danger factors possible that have shown hard to accurately depict from a genomic point of view only, and in this way engage the progression of modified expressive mechanical assemblies and redid tranquilize (Melin and Sánchez, 2017). The blend and examination of multi-secluded data pose a couple of particular challenges related to interoperability, machine learning, and mining.

Information to Getting

Regardless of the way that there is a sentiment of unimaginable open entryways concerning the examination of prosperity data for advancing human administrations, there are primary impediments that purpose of imprisonment the passage and sharing of prosperity data among unmistakable associations and countries. Other than the political concerns, ethics and energetic perspectives have an immense weight around there since people do whatever it takes not to like others profiting from their ailments. Security concerns are a fundamental perspective that prerequisites to be conquered additionally and picture examination process given in figure 5.

There is an abnormal state of crack in the prosperity division: accumulated data isn't shared among associations, even not inside divisions. Bits of information can't get from datasets that withdrawn. Top-down Big Data exercises have not increased much ground as of not long ago, and a while later a couple of undertakings are by and by focusing on a base up approach (Kashyap R., 2019b). By changing the perspective to be steadily arranged, this gives patients a duty regarding data. Patients ought to like this have the ability to get to their data, pick whom to bestow it to, and for what reason. Cases are the casual association which not only empowers patients to coordinate and pick up from different people with comparable conditions, anyway similarly gives an affirmation base of individual data for examination and a phase for interfacing patients with clinical preliminaries.

Figure 5. Effectively data collection and incorporating social insurance information

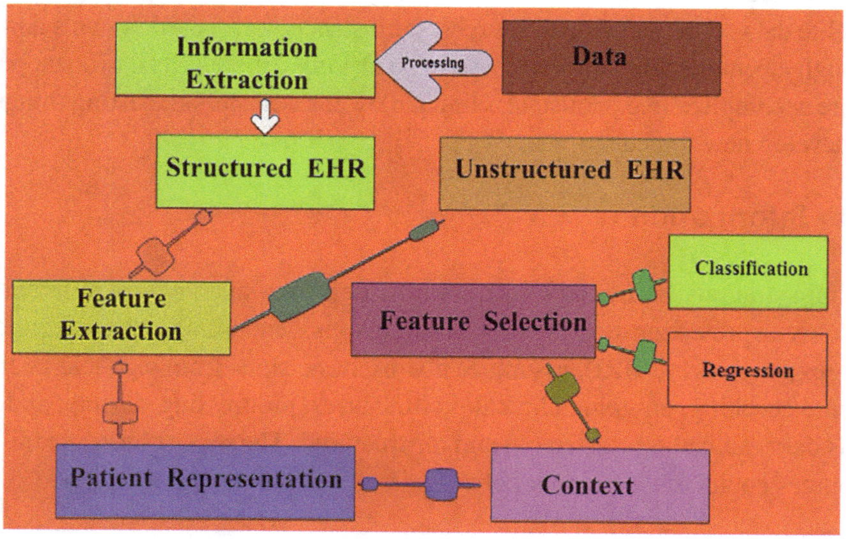

Understanding Produced Information

Understanding generated health data described as "human-related data including prosperity history, signs, biometric data, treatment history, lifestyle choices which made, recorded, gathered, induced by, or from patients/watchmen to help address a prosperity concern." It is isolated from data made in the midst of clinical care since patients are the ones responsible for getting this data and moreover have control over how this data shared. The development of more direct wearable devices, sensors, and advances, for instance, diligent passages to get and transmit, gives an unparalleled opportunity to whole deal, constant. Picture division endures with off-base outcomes, numerous techniques have created for redress comes. However, a few strategies set aside such a significant amount of time for calculation and some approach gives over fragmented outcomes. The all-inclusive ideal geodesic dynamic shape would be one if the best method gave vitality. However, it stuck in nearby minima and gave erroneous issues (Juneja and Kashyap 2016). Here microarray pictures have pulled in much consideration as a result of the powerlessness of making effectively divided spots. Figure 6 indicates a similar investigation of picture division techniques. The test comes about showed that the model had preferred execution over the CV model and LIF display. They affirmed its adequacy in different manufactured pictures and real pictures, and the promising test comes about to show its favorable circumstances concerning precision, capability, and vigor.

Figure 6. Result comparisons of image segmentation methods

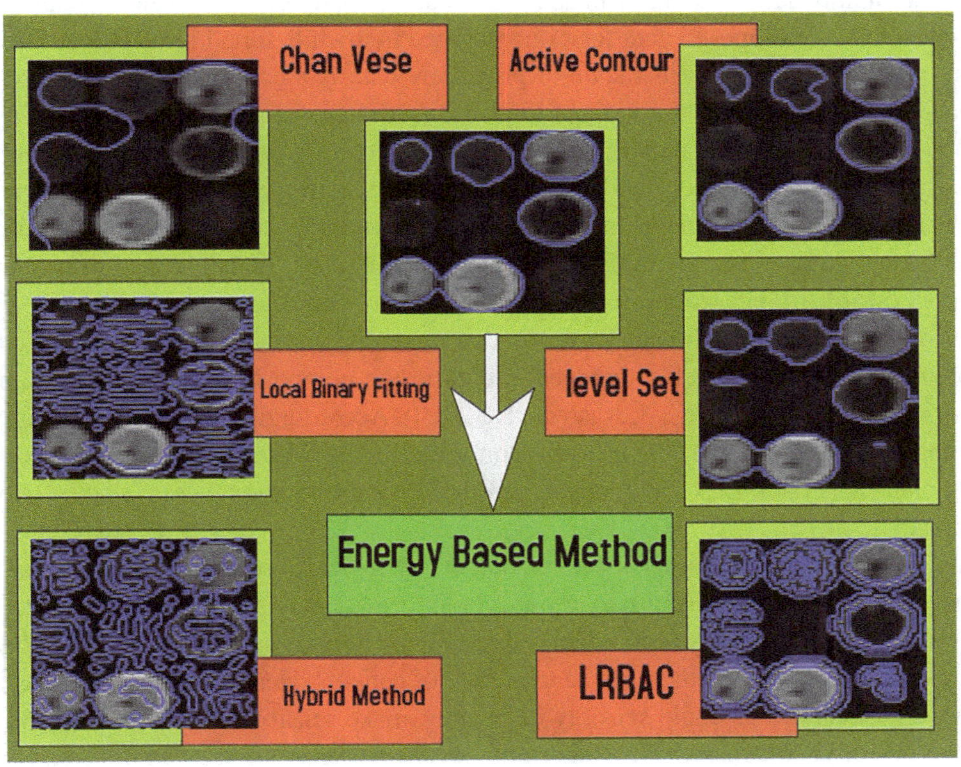

A crisp computerized lung extraction and the edge adjustment strategy composed by Changli Feng incorporate CV display, LBF model the all through the world arched division approach. The analytic precision of the new outskirt location works is significantly more exact than the customary fringe recognition work displays the original division result picture acquired when utilizing the GAC. It will provide wrong issues since it will influence the entire procedure like data extraction, examination, measurement, and assessment of the end is to show signs of improvement and the exact outcome so the accurate survey must produce through division.

INFORMATION ANALYTICS

Restorative research has been continuously data-driven science; with randomized clinical preliminaries being the best quality level all things considered a synopsis of information given in table 2. Nevertheless, on account generally progresses in remedial imaging, expansive electronic human records, and insightful contraptions, therapeutic research and furthermore clinical practice are quickly changing into Big Data-driven fields. Likewise, the therapeutic administrations space by and large experts, patients, organization, assurance, and legislative issues can very primary level advantage from current advances in Big Data progressions, and particularly from examination.

There are particular challenges and requirements to make specific strategies and techniques for Big Information examination in human administrations. These include:

- **Multi-particular data:** Optimally in data examination, there is a game plan of all around curated, systematized, and composed data for example once in a while found in electronic prosperity records. In any case, an abnormal state of prosperity data is a combination of unstructured data. A considerable measure of it comes in kinds of continuous sensor readings, for instance, ECG estimations in real care, content data in clinical reports by pros, remedial writing in trademark lingo, imaging data, or omics data in tweaked tranquilize. It is essential to get gaining from that information. The target should be to get valuable information from such heterogeneous data, make such information open to clinicians, and join learning into the clinical history of patients.
- **Complex establishment learning:** Medical data needs to portray to a high degree complex wonders; from staggered patient data on restorative treatment and philosophy, lifestyle information, the broad measure of available therapeutic data in the composition, bio-banks, or preliminary stores (Shukla R., Gupta R.K., & Kashyap R., 2019). Accordingly, corrective data regularly goes with complex metadata that ought to be considered with a particular true objective to preferably separate the data, make judgments, and find appropriate hypotheses, also, support clinical decisions.
- **Highly qualified end-customers:** End-customers of logical instruments in the pharmaceutical, for instance, pros, clinical investigators and bioinformaticians are significantly qualified. They moreover have a high obligation, which takes after elite necessities on the idea of examination instruments before trusting them in the treatment of patients. Hence, a perfectly logical approach should, anyway much as could sensibly be healthy, make sensible illustrations remembering the ultimate objective to consider cross-checking occurs and enabling trust in the courses of action. It ought to in like manner enable ace driven self-advantage examination to allow the champion to control the examination methodology.

- **Supporting complex decision:** The investigation of imaging data, pathology, good care checking, or the treatment of multi-morbidities are instances of locales in which important decisions must take from noisy data, in complex conditions, and with possibly missing information (Liu, Liang, and Xu, 2011). Neither individuals nor estimations may be guaranteed to pass on a perfect game plan reliably, yet they may be required to take necessary decisions or demonstrate choices in unnecessary time. Another zone of restorative decision help with conceivably high future impact is sharp associates for patients that make use of mobile phones and new wearable contraptions and sensor progressions to empower patients to administer diseases and have more valuable presences.
- **Security:** Medical data is outstandingly unstable information that is guaranteed by strong, legitimate shields at the European level. An adequate right blue framework to enable the examination of such data, and the headway of tasteful security ensuring intelligent gadgets to execute this structure, is of high centrality for the sober-minded relevance and impact of data-driven pharmaceutical and restorative administrations. Approaches to managing address data examination under the up to determined troubles will show in the accompanying.

Propelled Machine Learning and Reinforcement Learning

Various social protection applications would out and out benefit by the getting ready and examination of multimodal data, for instance, pictures, signals, video, 3D models, genomic progressions, reports, et cetera. Advanced machine learning frameworks can be used to take in and relate information from different sources and associations not obvious while pondering only a solitary wellspring of data. For instance, joining features from pictures, e.g., CT compasses, radiographs, and substance, e.g., clinical reports can substantially improve the execution of game plans. The mix of different prosperity data sources could in like manner engage the examination of phenotypes, e.g., diseases or chance factors that have exhibited hard to depict from a genomic point of view. It will involve the headway of modified scientific gadgets and altered pharmaceutical. This advancement will be necessary to use the highest limit of the different wellsprings of Big Data.

Another perspective is the examination of lifestyle data assembled from applications on mobile phones, and from which may join information about risk factors for sicknesses and contamination organization, for instance, specific hardware, activity information, GPS tracks, and outlook following, which can by and large not continuously accumulated. This information can sed inside recommender structures that help screen patients, raise alerts, or give direction for the better treatment of sickness. Stronghold learning is another particularly promising pushed machine learning procedure which a perspective of learning by experimentation, solely from prizes or teaches. It was viable associated with accomplishment advancement, for instance, AlphaGo course of action of Deep identity that won the Go redirection against the best human player. It can work in like manner associate in the human administration's space, for example, to usually discover and upgrade progressive prescriptions for unremitting and unsafe afflictions.

Information Based Approaches

The happening to the semantic web, delineation bases have ended up being a champion among the most discernible perfect models for learning depiction and considering. In the arrangement, with oncology being an observable driver, the usage of databases created from present-day ontologies has ended up being a fruitful way to deal with express complex restorative learning and reinforce the sorting out, quality organization, and compromise of remedial data. In like manner the mining of other complex data forms, for instance, diagrams and other social structures are influenced by various applications in natural frameworks, for example, pathways or in discretionary structures of macromolecules, for example, RNA and DNA. These and several different occasions of data are rising and creating, and picking up from this kind of complex data can subsequently yield more minimal, semantically rich, illustrative cases in the data which better mirror its trademark properties. Consequently, discovered illustrations ensure more clinical significance.

Profound Learning

Significant adapting ordinarily implies a course of action of machine learning counts that deduce significant different leveled models that catch exceptionally non-coordinate associations of low-level information data to outline abnormal state thoughts. The advantage of significant learning estimations is that they can be parallelized to enable the examination of huge and incredibly complex data, for instance, therapeutic pictures or chronicles, content data, or other unstructured information. For example, there is a need to upgrade capability/precision past what is possible using the current procedure for restorative picture examination. Helpful bosses who depend upon encounters from therapeutic pictures, e.g., radiologists or pathologists, expect support to dismember these pictures (Nind, 2007) quickly. Significant different leveled models are Artificial Neural Networks (ANN) with more than three hidden layers and related systems, for instance, Deep Restricted Boltzmann Machines, Deep Belief Networks, and Deep Convolutional Neural Networks. The present accomplishment of Deep Learning techniques is engaged by advances in computations and tip top handling development, which allow separating the large datasets that have now ended up being open. Since these factors have gotten together, deep learning has given remarkable advances, traversing long-standing execution rooftops in a couple of spaces, including image analysis, speech recognition, and natural language processing.

Ongoing Examination

Specific time-essential human administrations applications expect moves to made agreeable minute that a particular event is recognized (e.g., alerts in ICU). Different surges of heterogeneous data offer the credibility to evacuate bits of learning continuously.

A couple of material, interconnected procedures exist:

- Real-time examination suggests examination procedures, which can analyze and make encounters from each available datum and resources strikingly into a structure.
- Data stream mining implies the ability to separate, and the process is spilling data from the present or then again as it lands, rather than securing the data and recouping it in the long run.
- Complex event acknowledgment implies the disclosure and organization of cases over different data streams, where plans are a strange state, semantically rich, and are made finally legitimate to the customer.

"A basic nature of the examination is that the machine learning development associated with trichrome-recolored histologic pictures of routine kidney biopsy tests with no extraordinary planning or control other than cutting-edge analyzing. the gathering noted, "which empowered us to explicitly consider the eventual outcomes of the machine taking in the examination with those got from the clinical masochist give insights in regards to comparable illustrations (MIYAGI, 2009)." The usage of significant learning methodologies moreover made a more impressive appraisal structure than the pathologist-assessed score, which fundamentally relies upon the level of fibrosis appear in a particular case. "Using chairmen, for instance, convolution, inception, and pooling, setting up a CNN demonstrate incorporates playing out these errands various conditions in a ponder way to change pixel-level information to unusual state features of the data picture," says the examination.

Imaging Analytics and Healthcare

Imaging examination is a rapidly creating bit of prosperity IT, yet providers ought to astutely pick the best instruments and methodology that will empower them to upgrade care and cut costs. Imaging examination helped by artificial mental ability is rapidly becoming inside the prosperity IT circle, anyway providers must assess their affiliations and see decisively how this development will redesign the patient experience and diminishing human administrations costs before making any endeavors. As shown by a present report from ReportBuyer, the overall therapeutic imaging examination market will augmentation to $4.26 billion by 2025 as providers grasp instruments to isolate essential bits of learning from only pictures and moreover grander scale data assets. The rising enthusiasm for examination programming mirrors the business' day off work to regard based care. A present Frost and Sullivan examination communicate that the US restorative imaging market is moving toward an industry driven by quality rather than the sum, with accomplices continuously based on upgrading prosperity, cutting costs, and enhancing work process capability. In any case, completing this change is no straightforward endeavor. Achieving a new system is costly, and it is frequently difficult to know whether new gadgets will convey a landing on theory. Therapeutic imaging tests speak to $10 billion of Medicare spending yearly, and repeated helpful imaging tests significantly add to yearly social protection costs, An ongoing report incorporated that imaging for back torment and cerebral torments were among the best performed low-regard benefits in restorative administrations, costing the business $3.1 million and $3.6 million consistently, independently.

The effect of both inside and outside troubles has formally exacted noteworthy harm on the business. The way for accomplices to address these challenges and additionally succeed will be to use things, organizations sensibly, and game plans that improve the capability of the imaging methodology, diminish expenses and upgrade viability without exchanging off quality. To change from sum to quality in helpful imaging, social protection providers must consider what mechanical game plans will most exactly analyze pictures while decreasing expenses. Electronic thinking, particularly significant learning, has exhibited important certification in upgrading picture examination. Significant taking in, a machine learning framework, duplicates the first administration method of reasoning of the human cerebrum and offers an unyieldingly exact way to deal with arrange messages, pictures, and other clinical data. Specialists and researchers have been showing these capacities through pilots, think about, and use cases that are making astounding results.

For example, researchers at Case Western Reserve University developed a significant learning framework that could perceive the proximity of prominent kinds of chest threat in pathology pictures with 100 percent accuracy, performing better than human pathologists. Late research from Google moreover demonstrated that imaging examination fueled by machine learning computations could perceive metastasized chest danger rates with upgraded precision over other automated methods and pathologists. Our procedure yields best in class affectability on the testing task of recognizing small tumors in gigapixel pathology slides, lessening the false negative rate to a fourth of a pathologist and not as much as half of the past best result," the Google researchers said. "Our methodology could upgrade the exactness and consistency of surveying chest tumor cases, and potentially improve understanding outcomes."

While movements in advancement like AI and significant adjusting hold ensure for the inevitable destiny of imaging examination, providers must consider which systems will best fit their needs and goals before placing assets into cutting-edge gadgets. The rapidly creating therapeutic imaging industry joined with the permanent move to quality-based care, empowers large open entryways for development dealers to make an advantage, and multiple hurries to pitch their things to restorative administrations providers who need to upgrade their affiliations. The US remedial imaging industry is changing itself to address the troubles of the present and the solicitations without limits. This change gives unprecedented opportunities to exhibit individuals to solve the difficulties of care providers and develop new things and plans that help influence the imaging to work process more beneficial. It might be essential for providers to escape with enthusiasm and wants over the capacity of AI gadgets. Anyway, they ought to remember that this development won't mysteriously change the manner in which human administrations is passed on.

Notwithstanding vender enthusiasm, AI is still especially in its beginning times, and providers should consider these instruments clinical help limits rather than machines that can settle on remedial decisions entirely in solitude. Furthermore, affiliations shouldn't ricochet into concurrences with shippers before knowing correct what they're advancing, and more fundamentally, how the development will be used to handle issues. That wasn't the offering point. His pitch was dealing with the problem, and I trust that every now and again gets missed in the development of AI and machine learning. Providers should similarly assess where their affiliation stays similar to data dependability and clinical work forms before passing on new prosperity IT mechanical assemblies. Alliances that make a point by point manage outlining their huge goals will ensure that their original hypotheses will have immediate results. AI instruments should in like manner be significant stress for affiliations. While using AI to settle on clinical decisions, providers must guarantee that they fathom why and how these systems are impacting particular recommendations and relationship, to paying little heed to whether it is troublesome for clinicians to see how estimation limits.

DISCUSSION

AI-based therapeutic applications can be requested by either data genuine or data-driven. The specific data procedures intend to get computational models, removed from the clinical component and experts' understanding, to address thoughts, their relations, and the instruments to engage modified reasoning to help restorative decisions. Not in the slightest degree like data heightened, data-driven strategies, at the point of convergence of the vision of picking up prosperity systems, focus such gaining particularly from the accumulated clinical data. This learning is, for the most part, used to clear up a patient's back and forth movement signs/basic signs and to foresee future disease development of the patient. While various biomedical and therapeutic administrations systems are making an extending measure of data, they have not yet totally picked up by the transformative open entryways that these data give. Applying data-driven procedures to tremendous prosperity data can be of remarkable preferred standpoint in the biomedical and human administrations space, allowing ID and extraction of relevant information and diminishing the time spent by biomedical and therapeutic administrations specialists and masters who are endeavcring to find critical cases and new strings of learning. As one of the world's greatest and speediest creating organizations, therapeutic administrations planning suggests all parts of the expectation, investigation, treatment, and organization of affliction, and what's more the protection and change of physical and mental prosperity and thriving through helpful organizations.

Today, the use of significant advances has been insufficient concerning imaging examination in the radiology field and an extraordinary piece of the study must be done physically. IBM wants to use the Watson Health Cloud to measure helpful pictures among a ton of data including lab comes to fruition, prosperity records, clinical examinations, inherited tests, and other therapeutic information. Human administrations providers would have the ability to consider any current therapeutic pictures against a patient's past photographs and over a patient base of practically identical helpful conditions and symptoms to choose any movements or divergences. Therapeutic imaging developments play a consistently expanding number of fundamental parts not merely in the investigation and treatment of afflictions yet what's more in disease repugnance, prosperity checkup, noteworthy ailment screening, prosperity organization, early conclusion, and contamination earnestness evaluation, choice of treatment procedures, treatment affect appraisal and rebuilding. The status of significant imaging headways has extended interminably in social protection applications. On account of its ability to impact the finding and treatment of disease, to picture guided medical procedure and other helpful associations all the more advantageous, correct, and viable, restorative picture change has transformed into a typical errand. Through conveying unfathomable tissue consistency, propelled many-sided quality, edge change, relic end, sharp hullabaloo diminish, and whatnot, forefront picture redesign helps masters disentangle therapeutic pictures, an earnest foundation for better investigation and treatment.

CONCLUSION

Huge data examination which utilizes multitudes of various sorted out and unstructured data sources will accept a vital part in how social protection is bored later on. One would as of now have the capacity to see a scope of examination utilized, helping in the essential administration and execution of social protection work power and patients. Here we focused on three domains of interest: remedial picture examination, physiological banner planning, and genomic data dealing with — the exponential advancement of the volume of restorative pictures powers computational scientists to consider innovative responses to the process this significant volume of intractable data timescales. The example of determination of computational structures for physiological banner getting ready from both research and sharpening remedial specialists is growing tirelessly with the change of some to great degree imaginative and mind-boggling systems that help save a life. Working up a point by point model of a person by solidifying physiological data and high-throughput "- omics" strategies can enhance our knowledge of infirmity states and help in the progression of blood-based symptomatic instruments. Helpful picture examination, hail treatment of physiological data, and a blend of physiological and "- omics" data stand up to near challenges and openings in overseeing disparate composed and unstructured huge data sources.

Therapeutic picture examination covers various zones, for instance, picture acquirement, advancement/amusement, change, transmission, and weight. New mechanical advances have achieved higher assurance, estimation, and openness of multimodal pictures which provoke the development inexactness of finding and change of treatment. Regardless, consolidating helpful pictures with different modalities or with other therapeutic data is a potential opportunity. New logical frameworks and procedures are required to analyze this data in a clinical setting. These methods address a couple of concerns, openings, and troubles, for instance, features from pictures which can improve the accuracy of finding. The ability to utilize different wellsprings of data to extend the precision of assurance and decreasing expense and upgrade the exactness of getting ready procedures, for instance, significant picture overhaul, enlistment, and division to pass on better recommendations at the clinical level. Despite the way that there are some honest to goodness challenges for hail getting ready of physiological data to oversee, given the rhythmic movement state of data competency and noninstitutionalized structure, there are openings in every movement of the methodology towards giving fundamental changes inside the therapeutic administration's research and practice gatherings. Besides the prominent necessity for furthermore investigate in the zone of data wrangling, accumulating, and arranging interminable and discrete remedial data positions, there is in like manner a proportionate prerequisite for making novel banner taking care of methodology specific towards physiological signs. Research identifying with burrowing for biomarkers and covert cases inside biosignals to understand and envision a disease case has demonstrated potential in giving valuable information. In any case, there are open entryways for making computations to address data isolating, expansion, change, feature extraction, incorporate assurance, and so on. Plus, with the notoriety and change of machine learning estimations, there are openings in improving and making healthy CDSS for clinical desire, drug, and diagnostics.

Regardless of the way that accomplice useful contacts with changes in quality enunciation has propelled, the steady augmentation in available genomic data and its relating effects of the remark of characteristics and bungles from the test and sound practices have to inspect valuable result from high-throughput sequencing strategies a testing undertaking. Redoing of frameworks on the genome-scale is a not very much posed issue. Enthusiastic applications have made for redesigning of metabolic structures and quality managerial frameworks. Limited availability of dynamic constants is a bottleneck, and like this extraordinary models try to crush this repression. There is a divided perception for this broad scale issue as quality control, the effect of different framework plans, and formative results for these frameworks are so far penniless down. To address these stresses, the mix of the attentive arrangement of investigations and model change for redoing of structures will help in saving time and resources spent in building perception of heading in genome-scale structures. The possibility of keeping an eye on the high test requires close interest among experimentalists, computational specialists, and clinicians.

The examination of PC vision, imaging taking care of and case affirmation has increased impressive ground in the midst of the past a significant number of years. Furthermore, remedial imaging has pulled in extending thought starting late in light of its essential part in social protection applications. Inspectors have dispersed an abundance of basic science and data detailing the progress and social protection application on restorative imaging. Since the change of these examination fields has set the clinicians to advance from the seat to the bedside, computer vision strategies for social protection building, and likewise review articles that will energize the procedure with attempts to grasp the problems generally experienced in this field. The result is a gathering of fifteen astounding items set up together by specialists. There is a push toward affirming based medicine, which incorporates making use of every clinical datum available and thinking about that into the clinical and advanced examination. Getting and bringing most of the information about a patient together gives a more aggregate view of comprehension into mind coordination and results-based reimbursement masses prosperity organization, and patient responsibility and exertion. Grabbing this 360-degree point of view of the patient can in like manner wipe out monotonous and expensive testing, decrease bumbles in controlling and prescribing drugs, and even keep up a vital separation from preventable passings. In like manner, it is unquestionably essential that in the present human administration's condition, an indisputable predominant piece of the data made and along these lines available for uses no less than 75% of the data by a couple of appraisals is unstructured data. It ascends out of sources like the rapidly creating number of automated contraptions and sensors, messages, masters' and medicinal overseers' notes, lab tests, and untouchable sources outside the specialist's office.

REFERENCES

Blake, M. (2015). An Internet of Things for Healthcare. *IEEE Internet Computing*, *19*(4), 4–6. doi:10.1109/MIC.2015.89

Cai, S., Zhou, B., Liao, H., & Tan, C. (2017). Imaging Diagnosis of Chronic Encapsulated Intracerebral Hematoma, a Comparison of Computed Tomography (CT) and Magnetic Resonance Imaging (MRI) characteristics. *Polish Journal of Radiology / Polish Medical Society of Radiology*, *82*, 578–582. doi:10.12659/PJR.902417 PMID:29662588

Chalmers, I., Altman, D., McHaffie, H., Owens, N., & Cooke, R. (2013). Data sharing among data monitoring committees and responsibilities to patients and science. *Trials*, *14*(1), 102. doi:10.1186/1745-6215-14-102

Chung, H. (2017). Endoscopic Accessories Used for More Advanced Endoluminal Therapeutic Procedures. *Clinical Endoscopy*, *50*(3), 234–241. doi:10.5946/ce.2017.079

Cohen, E., Heiman, R., Carmi, M., Hadar, O., & Cohen, A. (2015). When physics meets signal processing: Image and video denoising based on Ising theory. *Signal Processing Image Communication*, *34*, 14–21. doi:10.1016/j.image.2015.02.007

Cresswell, K., & Sheikh, A. (2012). Electronic Health Record Technology. *Journal of the American Medical Association*, *307*(21). doi:10.1001/jama.2012.3520 PMID:22706825

Cruz-Cunha, M., Simoes, R., Varajão, J., & Miranda, I. (2014). Information Technology Supporting Healthcare and Social Care Services. *Journal of Information Technology Research*, *7*(1), 41–58. doi:10.4018/jitr.2014010104

Dalessandro, B., Perlich, C., & Raeder, T. (2014). Bigger is Better, but at What Cost? Estimating the Economic Value of Incremental Data Assets. *Big Data*, *2*(2), 87–96. doi:10.1089/big.2014.0010 PMID:27442302

Fatt, Q., & Ramadas, A. (2018). The Usefulness and Challenges of Big Data in Healthcare. *Journal of Health Communication, 03*(02). doi:10.4172/2472-1654.100131

Fife, C., & Eckert, K. (2017). Harnessing electronic healthcare data for wound care research: Standards for reporting observational registry data obtained directly from electronic health records. *Wound Repair and Regeneration, 25*(2), 192–209. doi:10.1111/wrr.12523 PMID:28370796

Fromenteze, T., Decroze, C., Abid, S., & Yurduseven, O. (2018). Sparsity-Driven Reconstruction Technique for Microwave/Millimeter-Wave Computational Imaging. *Sensors (Basel), 18*(5), 1536. doi:10.339018051536 PMID:29757241

Fusion of MRI and CT Images of Brain Tumor – Comprehensive Survey. (2018). *International Journal of Recent Trends in Engineering and Research, 4*(2), 12-17. doi:10.23883/ijrter.2018.4056.wy154

Gan, M., & Dai, H. (2014). Detecting and monitoring abrupt emergences and submergences of episodes over data streams. *Information Systems, 39*, 277–289. doi:10.1016/j.is.2012.05.009

Genetics: Genome made quickly from scratch. (2009). *Science News, 164*(24), 382-382. doi:10.1002cin.5591642416

Hoskins, M. (2014). Common Big Data Challenges and How to Overcome Them. *Big Data, 2*(3), 142–143. doi:10.1089/big.2014.0030 PMID:27442494

Juneja, P., & Kashyap, R. (2016). Optimal approach for CT image segmentation using improved energy-based method. *International Journal of Control Theory and Applications, 9*(41), 599–608.

Kashyap, R. (2019a). Security, Reliability, and Performance Assessment for Healthcare Biometrics. In D. Kisku, P. Gupta, & J. Sing (Eds.), Design and Implementation of Healthcare Biometric Systems (pp. 29-54). Hershey, PA: IGI Global. doi:10.4018/978-1-5225-7525-2.ch002

Kashyap, R. (2019b). Geospatial Big Data, Analytics, and IoT: Challenges, Applications, and Potential. In H. Das, R. Barik, H. Dubey & D. Sinha Roy (Eds.), Cloud Computing for Geospatial Big Data Analytics (pp. 191-213). Springer International Publishing.

Kashyap, R., & Gautam, P. (2015). Modified region based segmentation of medical images. *International Conference on Communication Networks (ICCN)*, 209–216. 10.1109/ICCN.2015.41

Kashyap, R., & Gautam, P. (2016). Fast level set method for segmentation of medical images. In *Proceedings of the International Conference on Informatics and Analytics (ICIA-16)*. ACM. 10.1145/2980258.2980302

Kashyap, R., & Gautam, P. (2017). Fast Medical Image Segmentation Using Energy-Based Method. *Biometrics, Concepts, Methodologies, Tools, and Applications, 3*(1), 1017–1042. doi:10.4018/978-1-5225-0983-7.ch040

Kashyap, R., Gautam, P., & Tiwari, V. (2018). Management and Monitoring Patterns and Future Scope. In Handbook of Research on Pattern Engineering System Development for Big Data Analytics. IGI Global. doi:10.4018/978-1-5225-3870-7.ch014

Kashyap, R., & Piersson, A. (2018a). *Impact of Big Data on Security. In Handbook of Research on Network Forensics and Analysis Techniques* (pp. 283–299). IGI Global. doi:10.4018/978-1-5225-4100-4.ch015

Kashyap, R., & Piersson, A. (2018b). Big Data Challenges and Solutions in the Medical Industries. In Handbook of Research on Pattern Engineering System Development for Big Data Analytics. IGI Global. doi:10.4018/978-1-5225-3870-7.ch001

Kashyap, R., & Tiwari, V. (2018). Active contours using global models for medical image segmentation. *International Journal of Computational Systems Engineering*, *4*(2/3), 195. doi:10.1504/IJCSYSE.2018.091404

Liu, W., Liang, W., & Xu, S. (2011). More information in imaging examination. *European Journal of Radiology*, *80*(2), 325. doi:10.1016/j.ejrad.2010.12.026 PMID:21255954

Manlhiot, C. (2018). Machine learning for predictive analytics in medicine: Real opportunity or overblown hype? *European Heart Journal Cardiovascular Imaging*, *19*(7), 727–728. doi:10.1093/ehjci/jey041 PMID:29538756

McPhail, G. (2017). Constructivism: Clearing up the confusion between a theory of learning and "constructing" knowledge. *Set: Research Information For Teachers*, (2), 30-22. doi:10.18296et.0081

Melin, P., & Sánchez, D. (2017). Multi-objective optimization for modular granular neural networks applied to pattern recognition. *Information Sciences*. doi:10.1016/j.ins.2017.09.031

Mi, H., Petitjean, C., Vera, P., & Ruan, S. (2015). Joint tumor growth prediction and tumor segmentation on therapeutic follow-up PET images. *Medical Image Analysis*, *23*(1), 84–91. doi:10.1016/j.media.2015.04.016 PMID:25988489

Miles-Tribble, V. (2017). Restorative justice as a public theology imperative. *Review & Expositor*, *114*(3), 366–379. doi:10.1177/0034637317721704

Mingle, D. (2017). Machine Learning Techniques on Microbiome -Based Diagnostics. *Advances In Biotechnology & Microbiology*, *6*(4). doi:10.19080/AIBM.2017.06.555695

Miyagi, T. (2009). Estimation of Inter-regional Trade Coefficients Using Neural Network Models. *Studies In Regional Science*, *39*(3), 519–538. doi:10.2457rs.39.519

Mutula, S. (2009). Ethical, Legal, and Social Issues in Medical Informatics. Hershey, PA: IGI Global.

Naimur Rahman, M., Esmailpour, A., & Zhao, J. (2016). Machine Learning with Big Data An Efficient Electricity Generation Forecasting System. *Big Data Research*, *5*, 9–15. doi:10.1016/j.bdr.2016.02.002

Nind, M. (2007). Supporting lifelong learning for people with profound and multiple learning difficulties. *Support for Learning*, *22*(3), 111–115. doi:10.1111/j.1467-9604.2007.00457.x

Palojoki, S., Pajunen, T., Saranto, K., & Lehtonen, L. (2016). Electronic Health Record-Related Safety Concerns: A Cross-Sectional Survey of Electronic Health Record Users. *JMIR Medical Informatics*, *4*(2), e13. doi:10.2196/medinform.5238 PMID:27154599

Phone, D. (2018). Proactive medicines management supports more patient-centric services. *International Journal of Integrated Care*, *18*(s1), 31. doi:10.5334/ijic.s1031

Recio, M. (2017). Practitioner's Corner • Data Protection Officer: The Key Figure to Ensure Data Protection and Accountability. *European Data Protection Law Review*, *3*(1), 114–118. doi:10.21552/edpl/2017/1/18

Rey-del-Castillo, P., & Cardeñosa, J. (2016). An Exercise in Exploring Big Data for Producing Reliable Statistical Information. *Big Data*, *4*(2), 120–128. doi:10.1089/big.2015.0045 PMID:27441716

Ruan, G., & Zhang, H. (2017). Closed-loop Big Data Analysis with Visualization and Scalable Computing. *Big Data Research*, *8*, 12–26. doi:10.1016/j.bdr.2017.01.002

Shukla, R., Gupta, R. K., & Kashyap, R. (2019). A multiphase pre-copy strategy for the virtual machine migration in cloud. In S. Satapathy, V. Bhateja, & S. Das (Eds.), *Smart Intelligent Computing and Applications. Smart Innovation, Systems and Technologies* (Vol. 104). Singapore: Springer. doi:10.1007/978-981-13-1921-1_43

Skiera, B., & Ringel, D. (2017). Using Big Search Data to Map Your Market: Marketing in a Digital Age. *IESE Insight*, (32), 31-37. doi:10.15581/002.art-2982

Tian, Y., & Peng, Y. (2011). Study on Communication of Massive 3D Spatial Data Based on ACE. *Geo-Information Science*, *12*(6), 819–827. doi:10.3724/SP.J.1047.2010.00819

Tiwari, S., Gupta, R. K., & Kashyap, R. (2019). To enhance web response time using agglomerative clustering technique for web navigation recommendation. In H. Behera, J. Nayak, B. Naik, & A. Abraham (Eds.), *Computational Intelligence in Data Mining. Advances in Intelligent Systems and Computing* (Vol. 711). Singapore: Springer. doi:10.1007/978-981-10-8055-5_59

Waoo, N., Kashyap, R., & Jaiswal, A. (2010). DNA nano array analysis using hierarchical quality threshold clustering. In *2010 2nd IEEE International Conference on Information Management and Engineering*. IEEE. 10.1109/ICIME.2010.5477579

Zhu, H., Lee, Y., & Rosenthal, A. (2016). Data Standards Challenges for Interoperable and Quality Data. *Journal Of Data And Information Quality*, *7*(1-2), 1–3. doi:10.1145/2903723

KEY TERMS AND DEFINITIONS

DM: Data mining is the way toward finding designs in broad informational indexes including techniques at the crossing point of machine learning, insights, and database systems. It is a necessary procedure where canny strategies are connected to extricate information patterns. It is an interdisciplinary subfield of PC science. The general objective of the information mining process is to remove data from an informational collection and change it into a logical structure for assist use. Aside from the crude investigation step, it includes database and information administration viewpoints, information pre-preparing, model and derivation contemplations, intriguing quality measurements, many-sided quality contemplations, post-handling of found structures, representation, and online updating data mining is the examination venture of the "learning disclosure in databases" process or KDD.

EHR: A personal electronic record or electronic medical record is the systematized accumulation of patient and populace electronically-put away wellbeing data in an advanced format. These records can be shared crosswise over various human services settings. Files are shared through system associated, endeavor broad data frameworks or other data systems and trades. EHRs may incorporate a scope of information, including socioeconomics, therapeutic history, solution and hypersensitivities, vaccination status, research facility test comes about radiology pictures, vital signs, individual measurements like age and weight, and charging information. EHR frameworks are intended to store information precisely and to catch the condition of a patient crosswise over time. It takes out the need to find a patient's past paper medicinal records and helps with guaranteeing information is precise and neat. It can lessen the danger of information replication as there is just a single modifiable document, which implies the record is more probable forward and diminishes the threat of lost printed material. Populace-based investigations of therapeutic records may likewise be encouraged by the across the board selection of EHRs and EMRs.

NLP: Natural language processing is a zone of software engineering, and computerized reasoning worried about the connections amongst PCs and human (characteristic) dialects, specifically how to program PCs to process a lot of regular dialect information productively. Difficulties in common idiom preparing as often as possible include discourse acknowledgment, normal dialect comprehension, and normal dialect age.

Compilation of References

Abdulhay, E., Arunkumar, N., Narasimhan, K., Vellaiappan, E., & Venkatraman, V. (2018). Gait and tremor investigation using machine learning techniques for the diagnosis of Parkinson disease. *Future Generation Computer Systems, 83*, 366–373. doi:10.1016/j.future.2018.02.009

Abiyev, R. H., & Abizade, S. (2016). Diagnosing Parkinson's Diseases Using Fuzzy Neural System. *Computational and Mathematical Methods in Medicine, 2016*, 1–9. doi:10.1155/2016/1267919 PMID:26881009

Ahmed, M., Shahjaman, M., Rana, M., Mollah, M., & Haque, N. (2017). Robustification of Naïve Bayes Classifier and Its Application for Microarray Gene Expression Data Analysis. *BioMed Research International*. PMID:28848763

Ahmed, S. S., Santosh, W., Kumar, S., & Christlet, H. T. (2009). Metabolic profiling of Parkinson's disease: Evidence of biomarker from gene expression analysis and rapid neural network detection. *Journal of Biomedical Science, 16*(63). PMID:19594911

Aich, S., Younga, K., Hui, K. L., Al-Absi, A. A., & Sain, M. (2018). A Nonlinear Decision Tree based Classification Approach to Predict the Parkinson's disease using Different Feature Sets of Voice Data. *International Conference on Advanced Communications Technology (ICACT)*, 638-642.

Ai, L., Wang, J., & Yao, R. (2011). Classification of parkinsonian and essential tremor using empirical mode decomposition and support vector machine. *Digital Signal Processing, 21*(4), 543–550. doi:10.1016/j.dsp.2011.01.010

Ain, Q., Jaffar, M. A., & Choi, T. (2014). Fuzzy anisotropic diffusion based segmentation and texture based ensemble classification of brain tumor. *Applied Soft Computing, 21*, 330–340. doi:10.1016/j.asoc.2014.03.019

Ajilchi, B., Kisely, S., Nejati, V., & Frederickson, J. (2018). Effects of intensive short-term dynamic psychotherapy on social cognition in major depression. *Journal of Mental Health (Abingdon, England)*, 1–5. doi:10.1080/09638237.2018.1466035 PMID:29792087

Akın, M. (2012). *Kanserli hücrelerin mikroarray gen ifadelerinin incelenmesi ve veri madenciliği yöntemleri kullanarak sınıflandırılması*. Gazi Üniversitesi, Fen Bilimleri Enstitüsü, Yüksek Lisans Tezi,Temmuz.

Akram, A., Christoffel, D., Rocher, A. B., Bouras, C., Kövari, E., Perl, D. P., ... Hof, P. R. (2008). Stereologic estimates of total spinophilin-immunoreactive spine number in area 9 and the CA1 field: Relationship with the progression of Alzheimer's disease. *Neurobiology of Aging, 29*(9), 1296–1307. doi:10.1016/j.neurobiolaging.2007.03.007 PMID:17420070

Aktan, E. (2018). Büyük Veri: Uygulama Alanları, Analitiği ve Güvenlik Boyutu. *Bilgi Yönetimi, 1*(1), 1–22.

Akyuz, G., & Kenis, O. (2014). Physical therapy modalities and rehabilitation techniques in the management of neuropathic pain. *American Journal of Physical Medicine & Rehabilitation, 93*(3), 253–259. doi:10.1097/PHM.0000000000000037 PMID:24322437

Alemami, Y., & Almazaydeh, L. (2014). Detecting of Parkinson Disease through Voice Signal Features. *The Journal of American Science*, 10.

Alhaddad, M. J., Kamel, M. I., Malibary, H. M., Alsaggaf, E. A., Thabit, K., Dahlwi, F., & Hadi, A. A. (2012). Diagnosis autism by fisher linear discriminant analysis FLDA via EEG. *International Journal of Bio-Science and Bio-Technology*, *4*(2), 45–54.

Alhussein, M. (2017). Monitoring Parkinson's Disease in Smart Cities. *IEEE Access: Practical Innovations, Open Solutions*, *5*, 19835–19841. doi:10.1109/ACCESS.2017.2748561

Al-Jarrah, O. Y., Yoo, P. D., Muhaidat, S., Karagiannidis, G. K., & Taha, K. (2015). Efficient machine learning for big data: A review. *Big Data Research*, *2*(3), 87–93. doi:10.1016/j.bdr.2015.04.001

Al-Mosaiwi, M., & Johnstone, T. (2018a). In an absolute state: Elevated use of absolutist words is a marker specific to anxiety, depression, and suicidal ideation. *Clinical Psychological Science*.

Al-Mosaiwi, M., & Johnstone, T. (2018b). Linguistic markers of moderate and absolute natural language. *Personality and Individual Differences*, *134*, 119–124. doi:10.1016/j.paid.2018.06.004 PMID:30393418

Alpaydın, E. (2013). *Yapay öğrenme, 2.* Baskı, Boğaziçi Üniversitesi Yayınevi.

Alpaydın, E. (2014). *Introduction to Machine Learning*. MIT Press.

Al-Shahi, R., Will, R., & Journal, C.-B. (2001). *Amount of research interest in rare and common neurological conditions: bibliometric study*. Retrieved from ncbi.nlm.nih.gov

Al-Shaikhli, S. D., Yang, M. Y., & Rosenhahn, B. (2014). Multi-region labeling and segmentation using a graph topology prior and atlas information in brain images. *Computerized Medical Imaging and Graphics*, *38*(8), 725–734. doi:10.1016/j.compmedimag.2014.06.008 PMID:24998760

Altarriba, J., & Morier, R. G. (2008). 10 Bilingualism: Language, Emotion, and Mental Health. The handbook of bilingualism, 8, 250.

Altındal, T. (2006). *Machine Learning Algorithms in Classification and Diagnostic Prediction of Cancers using Gene Expression Profilling* (Master Dissertation). Ulusal Tez Merkezi. (No. 181232)

American Psychiatric Association. (2011). Talk facts, Healthy Minds. *Healthy Minds Healthy Lives, 2.*

American Psychiatric Association. (2013). Diagnostic and Statistical Manual of Mental Disorders (DSM-5). American Psychiatric Publishing.

American Psychiatric Association. (2013). *Diagnostic and statistical manual of mental disorders (DSM-5®)*. American Psychiatric Pub.

Anderson, I. M., Shippen, C., Juhasz, G., Chase, D., Thomas, E., Downey, D., ... Deakin, J. W. (2011). State-dependent alteration in face emotion recognition in depression. *The British Journal of Psychiatry*, *198*(4), 302–308. doi:10.1192/bjp.bp.110.078139 PMID:21263011

Andrews, G., Basu, A., Cuijpers, P., Craske, M. G., McEvoy, P., English, C. L., & Newby, J. M. (2018). Computer therapy for the anxiety and depression disorders is effective, acceptable and practical health care: An updated meta-analysis. *Journal of Anxiety Disorders*, *55*, 70–78. doi:10.1016/j.janxdis.2018.01.001 PMID:29422409

Ang, K., Chin, Z., Wang, C., Guanand, C., & Zhang, H. (2012). Filterbank common spatial pattern algorithm on BCI competition IV Datasets2a and 2b. *Frontiers in Neuroscience*, *6*(39), 1–9. PMID:22479236

Angra, S., & Ahuja, S. (2017, March). Machine learning and its applications: a review. In *Big Data Analytics and Computational Intelligence (ICBDAC), 2017 International Conference on* (pp. 57-60). IEEE. 10.1109/ICBDACI.2017.8070809

Angst, J., Gamma, A., Rössler, W., Ajdacic, V., & Klein, D. N. (2009). Long-term depression versus episodic major depression: Results from the prospective Zurich study of a community sample. *Journal of Affective Disorders*, *115*(1-2), 112–121. doi:10.1016/j.jad.2008.09.023 PMID:18973954

Angulakshmi, M., & Priya, G. L. (2017). Automated brain tumour segmentation techniques- A review. *International Journal of Imaging Systems and Technology*, *27*(1), 66–77. doi:10.1002/ima.22211

Anita, S., & Aruna Priya, P. (2016). Early Prediction of Parkinson's Disease using Artificial Neural Network. *Indian Journal of Science and Technology*, *9*(36), 1–7. doi:10.17485/ijst/2016/v9i36/98401

Ansari, A., Atkeson, C. G., Choset, H., & Travers, M. (2015). *A Survey of Current Exoskeletons and Their Control Architectures and Algorithms* (Draft 4.0). Retrieved from www.cs.cmu.edu/~cga/exo/survey.pdf

Antoniou, E. E., Bongers, P., & Jansen, A. (2017). The mediating role of dichotomous thinking and emotional eating in the relationship between depression and BMI. *Eating Behaviors*, *26*, 55–60. doi:10.1016/j.eatbeh.2017.01.007 PMID:28135621

Apache Hive. (n.d.). Retrieved December 23, 2018, from https://hive.apache.org/

Apache Pig. (n.d.). Retrieved December 23, 2018, from https://pig.apache.org/

Argaman, O. (2010). Linguistic markers and emotional intensity. *Journal of Psycholinguistic Research*, *39*(2), 89–99. doi:10.100710936-009-9127-1 PMID:19644755

Aria, M., & Cuccurullo, C. (2017). bibliometrix : An R-tool for comprehensive science mapping analysis. *Journal of Informetrics*, *11*(4), 959–975. doi:10.1016/j.joi.2017.08.007

Arslan, A. K., Colak, C., & Sarihan, M. E. (2016). Different medical data mining approaches based prediction of ischemic stroke. *Computer Methods and Programs in Biomedicine*, *130*, 87–92. doi:10.1016/j.cmpb.2016.03.022 PMID:27208524

Artificial Intelligence. (n.d.). *Neural Networks*. Retrieved from https://www.tutorialspoint.com/artificial_intelligence/artificial_intelligence_neural_networks.htm

Aslam, A., Khan, E., & Beg, M. S. (2015). Improved Edge Detection Algorithm for Brain Tumor Segmentation. *Procedia Computer Science*, *58*, 430–437. doi:10.1016/j.procs.2015.08.057

Atalay, M., & Çelik, Ö. G. E. (2017). Artificial Intelligence and Machine Learning Applications in Big Data Analysis. *Mehmet Akif Ersoy University Journal of Social Sciences Institute*, *9*(22), 155–172.

Athmaja, S., Hanumanthappa, M., & Kavitha, V. (2017, March). A survey of machine learning algorithms for big data analytics. In *Innovations in Information, Embedded and Communication Systems (ICIIECS), 2017 International Conference on* (pp. 1-4). IEEE. 10.1109/ICIIECS.2017.8276028

Auerbach, R. P., Stanton, C. H., Proudfit, G. H., & Pizzagalli, D. A. (2015). Self-referential processing in depressed adolescents: A high-density event-related potential study. *Journal of Abnormal Psychology*, *124*(2), 233–245. doi:10.1037/abn0000023 PMID:25643205

Ayers, M. E. (2004). Neurofeedback for cerebral palsy. *Journal of Neurotherapy*, *8*(2), 93–94. doi:10.1300/J184v08n02_07

Bagroy, S., Kumaraguru, P., & De Choudhury, M. (2017). A social media based index of mental well-being in college campuses. *Proceedings of the 2017 CHI Conference on Human Factors in Computing Systems*. 10.1145/3025453.3025909

Baik, S. Y., Jeong, M., Kim, H. S., & Lee, S. H. (2018). ERP investigation of attentional disengagement from suicide-relevant information in patients with major depressive disorder. *Journal of Affective Disorders*, *225*, 357–364. doi:10.1016/j.jad.2017.08.046 PMID:28846957

Bailey, N. W., Hoy, K. E., Maller, J. J., Segrave, R. A., Thomson, R., Williams, N., ... Fitzgerald, P. B. (2014). An exploratory analysis of go/nogo event-related potentials in major depression and depression following traumatic brain injury. *Psychiatry Research: Neuroimaging*, *224*(3), 324–334. doi:10.1016/j.pscychresns.2014.09.008 PMID:25452196

Bailey, N., Freedman, G., Raj, K., Sullivan, C., Rogasch, N., Chung, S., ... Fitzgerald, P. (2018). Mindfulness meditators show altered distributions of early and late neural activity markers of attention in a response inhibition task. *bioRxiv*, 396259.

Baker, F., & Bor, W. (2008). Can music preference indicate mental health status in young people? *Australasian Psychiatry*, *16*(4), 284–288. doi:10.1080/10398560701879589 PMID:18608148

Baker, J. M. (2018). Gait Disorders. *The American Journal of Medicine*, *131*(6), 602–607. doi:10.1016/j.amjmed.2017.11.051 PMID:29288631

Balasupramanian, N., Ephrem, B. G., & Al-Barwani, I. S. (2017, July). User pattern based online fraud detection and prevention using big data analytics and self organizing maps. In *Intelligent Computing, Instrumentation and Control Technologies (ICICICT), 2017 International Conference on* (pp. 691-694). IEEE. 10.1109/ICICICT1.2017.8342647

Bandura, A. (1977). Self-efficacy: Toward a Unifying Theory of Behavioral Change. *Psychological Review*, *84*(2), 191–215. doi:10.1037/0033-295X.84.2.191 PMID:847061

Bandura, A. (1982). Self-efficacy mechanism in human agency. *The American Psychologist*, *37*(2), 122–147. doi:10.1037/0003-066X.37.2.122

Barrick, E. M., & Dillon, D. G. (2018). An ERP study of multidimensional source retrieval in depression. *Biological Psychology*, *132*, 176–191. doi:10.1016/j.biopsycho.2018.01.001 PMID:29305874

Barth, J., Munder, T., Gerger, H., Nüesch, E., Trelle, S., Znoj, H., ... Cuijpers, P. (2016). Comparative efficacy of seven psychotherapeutic interventions for patients with depression: A network meta-analysis. *Focus (San Francisco, Calif.)*, *14*(2), 229–243.

Batres-Mendoza, P., Ibarra-Manzano, M., Guerra-Hernandez, E., Almanza-Ojeda, D., Montoro-Sanjose, C., Romero-Troncoso, R., & Rostro-Gonzalez, H. (2017). Improving EEG-Based Motor Imagery Classification for Real-Time Applications Using the QSA Method. *Computational Intelligence and Neuroscience*, *2017*, 1–16. doi:10.1155/2017/9817305 PMID:29348744

Bauer, S., Wiest, R., Nolte, L., & Reyes, M. (2013). A survey of MRI-based medical image analysis for brain tumor studies. *Physics in Medicine and Biology*, *58*(13), R97–R129. doi:10.1088/0031-9155/58/13/R97 PMID:23743802

Bazazeh, D., & Shubair, R. (2016, December). Comparative study of machine learning algorithms for breast cancer detection and diagnosis. In *Electronic Devices, Systems and Applications (ICEDSA), 2016 5th International Conference on* (pp. 1-4). IEEE. 10.1109/ICEDSA.2016.7818560

BBCI. (n.d.). *BCI Competition IV*. Retrieved from http://www.bbci.de/competition/iv/#dataset1

Beck, A.T., Steer, R.A., & Brown, G.K. (1996). Beck depression inventory II. *San Antonio, 78*, 490-498.

Beck, Ward, & Mendelson. (1961). Beck depression inventory (bdi). *Archives of General Psychiatry*, *4*(6), 561–571. doi:10.1001/archpsyc.1961.01710120031004 PMID:13688369

Beck, A. T. (Ed.). (1979). *Cognitive therapy of depression.* Guilford Press.

Beck, A. T., & Alford, B. A. (2009). *Depression: Causes and treatment.* University of Pennsylvania Press.

Berger, T., Krieger, T., Sude, K., Meyer, B., & Maercker, A. (2018). Evaluating an e-mental health program ("deprexis") as adjunctive treatment tool in psychotherapy for depression: Results of a pragmatic randomized controlled trial. *Journal of Affective Disorders, 227*, 455–462. doi:10.1016/j.jad.2017.11.021 PMID:29154168

Bermejo, S., & Cabestany, J. (2000). Adaptive soft k-nearest-neighbour classifiers. *Pattern Recognition, 33*(12), 1999–2005. doi:10.1016/S0031-3203(99)00186-7

Bernick, J. P. (2015). The Role of Machine Learning in Drug Design and Delivery. *Journal of Develop Drugs, 4*(03), E143. doi:10.4172/2329-6631.1000e143

Berral García, J. L. (2016). A quick view on current techniques and machine learning algorithms for big data analytics. In *Proceedings of the 18th International Conference on Transparent Optical Networks (ICTON)* (pp. 1-4). Institute of Electrical and Electronics Engineers (IEEE). 10.1109/ICTON.2016.7550517

Bertolote, J. M., Fleischmann, A., De Leo, D., & Wasserman, D. (2004). Psychiatric diagnoses and suicide: Revisiting the evidence. *Crisis, 25*(4), 147–155. doi:10.1027/0227-5910.25.4.147 PMID:15580849

Bhande, S., & Raut, R. (2013). Parkinson Diagnosis using Neural Network: A Survey. *International Journal of Innovative Research in Science. Engineering and Technology, 2*(9), 4843–4846.

Bhardwa, S. (2017). *What do Student Mental Health Services Look Like Around the World.* Retrieved from https://www.timeshighereducation.com/student/blogs/what-do-student-mental-health-services-look-around-world

Bi, L., Fan, X. A., & Liu, Y. (2013). EEG-based brain-controlled mobile robots: A survey. *IEEE Transactions on Human-Machine Systems, 43*(2), 161–176. doi:10.1109/TSMCC.2012.2219046

Bina, R., Barak, A., Posmontier, B., Glasser, S., & Cinamon, T. (2018). Social workers' perceptions of barriers to interpersonal therapy implementation for treating postpartum depression in a primary care setting in Israel. *Health & Social Care in the Community, 26*(1), e75–e84. doi:10.1111/hsc.12479 PMID:28726342

Bingol, B., & Sheng, M. (2011). Deconstruction for reconstruction: The role of proteolysis in neural plasticity and disease. *Neuron, 69*(1), 22–32. doi:10.1016/j.neuron.2010.11.006 PMID:21220096

Bircan, H. (2004). Lojistik regresyon analizi: Tıp verileri üzerine bir uygulama. *Kocaeli Üniversitesi Sosyal Bilimler Enstitüsü Dergisi*, (8), 185-208.

Bishop, C. M. (2006). Pattern recognition and machine learning (information science and statistics). Academic Press.

Blake, M. (2015). An Internet of Things for Healthcare. *IEEE Internet Computing, 19*(4), 4–6. doi:10.1109/MIC.2015.89

Boele, F., Rooney, A., Grant, R., & Klein, M. (2015). Psychiatric symptoms in glioma patients: From diagnosis to management. *Neuropsychiatric Disease and Treatment, 1413.* doi:10.2147/ndt.s65874 PMID:26089669

Bohra, N., Srivastava, S., & Bhatia, M. S. (2015). Depression in women in Indian context. *Indian Journal of Psychiatry, 57*(6Suppl 2), S239. doi:10.4103/0019-5545.161485 PMID:26330641

Bonetti, L., Haumann, N. T., Vuust, P., Kliuchko, M., & Brattico, E. (2017). Risk of depression enhances auditory Pitch discrimination in the brain as indexed by the mismatch negativity. *Clinical Neurophysiology, 128*(10), 1923–1936. doi:10.1016/j.clinph.2017.07.004 PMID:28826023

Boschloo, L., Schoevers, R. A., Beekman, A. T., Smit, J. H., Van Hemert, A. M., & Penninx, B. W. (2014). The four-year course of major depressive disorder: The role of staging and risk factor determination. *Psychotherapy and Psychosomatics*, *83*(5), 279–288. doi:10.1159/000362563 PMID:25116639

Bosl, W., Tierney, A., Tager-Flusberg, H., & Nelson, C. (2011). EEG complexity as a biomarker for autism spectrum disorder risk. *BMC Medicine*, *9*(1), 18. doi:10.1186/1741-7015-9-18 PMID:21342500

Boutros, N. N., Galderisi, S., Pogarell, O., & Riggio, S. (2011). *Standard electroencephalography in clinical psychiatry: a practical handbook*. John Wiley & Sons. doi:10.1002/9780470974612

Boyd, R. L., & Pennebaker, J. W. (2017). Language-based personality: A new approach to personality in a digital world. *Current Opinion in Behavioral Sciences*, *18*, 63–68. doi:10.1016/j.cobeha.2017.07.017

Brain tumors: An Introduction. (2016). Retrieved from https://www.mayfieldclinic.com/PDF/PE-TumorIntro.pdf

Breiman, L. (2001). Random forests. *Machine Learning*, *45*(1), 5–32. doi:10.1023/A:1010933404324

Brenner, R. P. (1991). Utility of EEG in Delirium: Past Views and Current Practice. *International Psychogeriatrics*, *3*(2), 211–229. doi:10.1017/S1041610291000686 PMID:1811775

Brenninkmeijer, V., Lagerveld, S. E., Blonk, R. W., Schaufeli, W. B., & Wijngaards-de Meij, L. D. (2018). Predicting the effectiveness of work-focused CBT for common mental disorders: The influence of baseline self-efficacy, depression and anxiety. *Journal of Occupational Rehabilitation*, 1–11. PMID:29450678

Bridwell, D. A., Steele, V. R., Maurer, J. M., Kiehl, K. A., & Calhoun, V. D. (2015). The relationship between somatic and cognitive-affective depression symptoms and error-related ERPs. *Journal of Affective Disorders*, *172*, 89–95. doi:10.1016/j.jad.2014.09.054 PMID:25451400

Briggs, R., Tobin, K., Kenny, R. A., & Kennelly, S. P. (2018). What is the prevalence of untreated depression and death ideation in older people? Data from the Irish Longitudinal Study on Aging. *International Psychogeriatrics*, 1–9. PMID:29335038

Brockmeyer, T., Zimmermann, J., Kulessa, D., Hautzinger, M., Bents, H., Friederichs, H. C., ... Backenstrass, M. (2015). Me, myself, and I: Self-referent word use as an indicator of self-focused attention in relation to depression and anxiety. *Frontiers in Psychology*, *6*, 1564. doi:10.3389/fpsyg.2015.01564 PMID:26500601

Brodie, A., Smith, B., & Ray, J. (2018). The impact of rehabilitation on quality of life after hearing loss: A systematic review. *European Archives of Oto-Rhino-Laryngology*, *275*(10), 2435–2440. doi:10.100700405-018-5100-7 PMID:30159730

Brody, T., Harnad, S., & Carr, L. (2006). Earlier Web usage statistics as predictors of later citation impact. *Journal of the American Society for Information Science*, *57*(8), 1060–1072. doi:10.1002/asi.20373

Bruder, G. E., Kayser, J., Tenke, C. E., Leite, P., Schneier, F. R., Stewart, J. W., & Quitkin, F. M. (2002). Cognitive ERPs in depressive and anxiety disorders during tonal and phonetic oddball tasks. *Clinical EEG (Electroencephalography)*, *33*(3), 119–124. doi:10.1177/155005940203300308 PMID:12192661

Bruder, G. E., Kroppmann, C. J., Kayser, J., Stewart, J. W., McGrath, P. J., & Tenke, C. E. (2009). Reduced brain responses to novel sound in depression: P3 findings in a novelty oddball task. *Psychiatry Research*, *170*(2-3), 218–223. doi:10.1016/j.psychres.2008.10.023 PMID:19900720

Bruder, G. E., Tenke, C. E., Towey, J. P., Leite, P., Fong, R., Stewart, J. E., ... Quitkin, F. M. (1998). Brain ERPs of depressed patients to complex tones in an oddball task: Relation of reduced P3 asymmetry to physical anhedonia. *Psychophysiology*, *35*(1), 54–63. doi:10.1111/1469-8986.3510054 PMID:9499706

Bruder, G. E., Tenke, C. E., Warner, V., & Weissman, M. M. (2007). Grandchildren at high and low risk for depression differ in EEG measures of regional brain asymmetry. *Biological Psychiatry*, *62*(11), 1317–1323. doi:10.1016/j.biopsych.2006.12.006 PMID:17481594

Bunting-Perry, L. K. (2006). Palliative care in Parkinson's disease: Implications for neuroscience nursing. *The Journal of Neuroscience Nursing*, *38*(2), 106. doi:10.1097/01376517-200604000-00006 PMID:16681291

Burakgazi, Y. (2017). *Identification of Breast Cancer Sub-types by Using Machine Learning Techniques* (Master Dissertation). Ulusal Tez Merkezi. (No. 459190)

Burkhart, M. A., & Thomas, D. G. (1993). Event-related potential measures of attention in moderately depressed subjects. *Electroencephalography and Clinical Neurophysiology/Evoked Potentials Section, 88*(1), 42-50.

Cai, S., Zhou, B., Liao, H., & Tan, C. (2017). Imaging Diagnosis of Chronic Encapsulated Intracerebral Hematoma, a Comparison of Computed Tomography (CT) and Magnetic Resonance Imaging (MRI) characteristics. *Polish Journal of Radiology / Polish Medical Society of Radiology*, *82*, 578–582. doi:10.12659/PJR.902417 PMID:29662588

Caldas, R., Mundt, M., Potthast, W., Buarque de Lima Neto, F., & Markert, B. (2017). A systematic review of gait analysis methods based on inertial sensors and adaptive algorithms. *Gait & Posture*, *57*(February), 204–210. doi:10.1016/j.gaitpost.2017.06.019 PMID:28666178

Calero, D., Paul, S., Gesing, A., Alves, F., & Cordioli, J. A. (2018). A technical review and evaluation of implantable sensors for hearing devices. *Biomedical Engineering Online*, *17*(1), 1–26. doi:10.118612938-018-0454-z PMID:29433516

Caliskan, A., Badem, H., Baştürk, A., & Yüksel, M. E. (2017). Diagnosis of the Parkinson Disease by Using Deep Neural Network Classifier. *IU-JEEE*, *17*(2), 3311–3318.

Camastra, F., & Vinciarelli, A. (2008). *Machine Learning for Audio, Image and Video Analysis*. London: Springer. doi:10.1007/978-1-84800-007-0

Camfield, D. A., Burton, T. K., De Blasio, F. M., Barry, R. J., & Croft, R. J. (2018). ERP components associated with an indirect emotional stop signal task in healthy and depressed participants. *International Journal of Psychophysiology*, *124*, 12–25. doi:10.1016/j.ijpsycho.2017.12.008 PMID:29278691

Carlson, J. M., Foti, D., Harmon-Jones, E., & Proudfit, G. H. (2015). Midbrain volume predicts fMRI and ERP measures of reward reactivity. *Brain Structure & Function*, *220*(3), 1861–1866. doi:10.100700429-014-0725-9 PMID:24549705

Carnevale, L., Calabrò, R. S., Celesti, A., Leo, A., Fazio, M., Bramanti, P., & Villari, M. (2018). *Towards Improving Robotic-Assisted Gait Training: Can Big Data Analysis Help us? IEEE Internet of Things Journal.*

Carter, J. D., McIntosh, V. V., Jordan, J., Porter, R. J., Douglas, K., Frampton, C. M., & Joyce, P. R. (2018). Patient predictors of response to cognitive behaviour therapy and schema therapy for depression. *The Australian and New Zealand Journal of Psychiatry*. PMID:29325436

Castaneda, A. E., Tuulio-Henriksson, A., Marttunen, M., Suvisaari, J., & Lönnqvist, J. (2008). A review on cognitive impairments in depressive and anxiety disorders with a focus on young adults. *Journal of Affective Disorders*, *106*(1-2), 1–27. doi:10.1016/j.jad.2007.06.006 PMID:17707915

Cavazos-Rehg, P. A., Krauss, M., Sowles, S., Connolly, S., Rosas, C., Bharadwaj, M., & Bierut, L. (2016). A content analysis of depression-related tweets. *Computers in Human Behavior*, *54*, 351–357. doi:10.1016/j.chb.2015.08.023 PMID:26392678

Chakraborty, A., Chakraborty, A., & Mukherjee, B. (2016). Detection of Parkinson's Disease Using Fuzzy Inference System. In *Proceedings of Intelligent Systems Technologies and Applications* (pp. 79–90). Cham: Springer. doi:10.1007/978-3-319-23036-8_7

Chalmers, I., Altman, D., McHaffie, H., Owens, N., & Cooke, R. (2013). Data sharing among data monitoring committees and responsibilities to patients and science. *Trials*, *14*(1), 102. doi:10.1186/1745-6215-14-102

Chandra, G. R., & Rao, K. R. (2016). Tumor Detection In Brain Using Genetic Algorithm. *Procedia Computer Science*, *79*, 449–457. doi:10.1016/j.procs.2016.03.058

Chang, P. (2018). *What you need to Know About Depression*. Retrieved from https://virginiainfusiontherapies.com/what-you-need-to-know-about-depression/

Chapelle, O., Scholkopf, B., & Zien, A. (2009). Semi-supervised learning. IEEE Transactions on Neural Networks, 20(3), 542-542.

Chapuis, S., Ouchchane, L., Metz, O., Gerbaud, L., & Durif, F. (2005). Impact of the motor complications of Parkinson's disease on the quality of life. *Movement Disorders: Official Journal of the Movement Disorder Society, 20*(2), 224-230.

Charlson, F. J., Baxter, A. J., Cheng, H. G., Shidhaye, R., & Whiteford, H. A. (2016). The burden of mental, neurological, and substance use disorders in China and India: A systematic analysis of community representative epidemiological studies. *Lancet*, *388*(10042), 376–389. doi:10.1016/S0140-6736(16)30590-6 PMID:27209143

Chatterjee, J., Saxena, A., Vyas, G., & Mehra, A. (2017). An Efficient Real-Time Approach for Detection of Parkinson's Disease. In Intelligent Systems Design and Applications. ISDA 2017. Advances in Intelligent Systems and Computing. Springer.

Chawla, N. V., Bowyer, K. W., Hall, L. O., & Kegelmeyer, W. P. (2002). SMOTE: Synthetic minority over-sampling technique. *Journal of Artificial Intelligence Research*, *16*, 321–357. doi:10.1613/jair.953

Checkoway, H., & Nelson, L. M. (1999). Epidemiologic approaches to the study of Parkinson's disease etiology. *Epidemiology (Cambridge, Mass.)*, *10*(3), 327–336. doi:10.1097/00001648-199905000-00023 PMID:10230846

Chen, J., Zhang, Y., Wei, D., Wu, X., Fu, Q., Xu, F., ... Zhang, Z. (2015). Neurophysiological handover from MMN to P3a in first-episode and recurrent major depression. *Journal of Affective Disorders, 174*, 173-179.

Cheng, Y. (1995). Mean shift, mode seeking, and clustering. *IEEE Transactions on Pattern Analysis and Machine Intelligence*, *17*(8), 790–799. doi:10.1109/34.400568

Chen, H.-L., Huang, C.-C., Yu, X.-G., Xu, X., Sun, X., Wang, G., & Wang, S.-J. (2013). An efficient diagnosis system for detection of Parkinson's disease using fuzzy k-nearest neighbor approach. *Expert Systems with Applications*, *40*(1), 263–271. doi:10.1016/j.eswa.2012.07.014

Chen, J., Yang, L. Q., Zhang, Z. J., Ma, W. T., Xing-qu, W., Zhang, X. R., ... Hua, Z. (2013a). The association between the disruption of motor imagery and the number of depressive episodes of major depression. *Journal of Affective Disorders*, *150*(2), 337–343. doi:10.1016/j.jad.2013.04.015 PMID:23684121

Chen, P. H., Wang, R. L., Liou, D. J., & Shaw, J. S. (2013). Gait disorders in Parkinson's disease: Assessment and management. *International Journal of Gerontology*, *7*(4), 189–193. doi:10.1016/j.ijge.2013.03.005

Chen, S. W., Lin, S. H., Liao, L. D., Lai, H. Y., Pei, Y. C., Kuo, T. S., ... Chen, S. Y. (2011). Quantification and recognition of parkinsonian gait from monocular video imaging using kernel-based principal component analysis. *Biomedical Engineering Online*, *10*(1), 99. doi:10.1186/1475-925X-10-99 PMID:22074315

Chen, Y., Garcia, G., Huang, W., & Constantini, S. (2014). The involvement of secondary neuronal damage in the development of neuropsychiatric disorders following brain insults. *Frontiers in Neurology*, *5*, 22. doi:10.3389/fneur.2014.00022 PMID:24653712

Cherubini, A., Nisticó, R., Novellino, F., Salsone, M., Nigro, S., Donzuso, G., & Quattrone, A. (2014). Magnetic resonance support vector machine discriminates essential tremor with rest tremor from tremor-dominant Parkinson disease. *Movement Disorders*, *29*(9), 1216–1219. doi:10.1002/mds.25869 PMID:24729430

Cheung, A. H., Zuckerbrot, R. A., Jensen, P. S., Laraque, D., & Stein, R. E. (2018). Guidelines for adolescent depression in primary care (GLAD-PC): Part II. Treatment and ongoing management. *Pediatrics*, *141*(3). doi:10.1542/peds.2017-4082 PMID:29483201

Chiu, P. H., & Deldin, P. J. (2007). Neural evidence for enhanced error detection in major depressive disorder. *The American Journal of Psychiatry*, *164*(4), 608–616. doi:10.1176/ajp.2007.164.4.608 PMID:17403974

Choi, K. M., Jang, K. I., Huh, H. J., Baek, K. H., Kim, S. Y., Lee, S. M., ... Chae, J. H. (2015). The effects of 3 weeks of rTMS treatment on P200 amplitude in patients with depression. *Brain Stimulation: Basic, Translational, and Clinical Research in Neuromodulation*, *8*(2), 332. doi:10.1016/j.brs.2015.01.076

Christoffel, D. J., Golden, S. A., & Russo, S. J. (2011). Structural and synaptic plasticity in stress-related disorders. *Reviews in the Neurosciences*, *22*(5), 535–549. doi:10.1515/RNS.2011.044 PMID:21967517

Chung, C., & Pennebaker, J. W. (2007). The psychological functions of function words. *Social Communication, 1*, 343-359.

Chung, H. (2017). Endoscopic Accessories Used for More Advanced Endoluminal Therapeutic Procedures. *Clinical Endoscopy*, *50*(3), 234–241. doi:10.5946/ce.2017.079

Cipriani, A., Furukawa, T. A., Salanti, G., Chaimani, A., Atkinson, L. Z., Ogawa, Y., ... Egger, M. (2018). Comparative efficacy and acceptability of 21 antidepressant drugs for the acute treatment of adults with major depressive disorder: A systematic review and network meta-analysis. *Lancet*, *391*(10128), 1357–1366. doi:10.1016/S0140-6736(17)32802-7 PMID:29477251

Cisler, J. M., Olatunji, B. O., & Lohr, J. M. (2009). Disgust, fear, and anxiety disorders: A critical review. *Clinical Psychology Review*, *29*(1), 34–46. doi:10.1016/j.cpr.2008.09.007 PMID:18977061

Clement, S., Singh, S., & Psychiatry, T.-T. (2003). *Status of bipolar disorder research: bibliometric study*. Cambridge.org.

Clifford, F. R. (1999). *A Short History of Neurology*. Oxford, UK: Butterworth-Heinemann.

Coburn, K. L., Lauterbach, E. C., Boutros, N. N., Black, K. J., Arciniegas, D. B., & Coffey, C. E. (2006). The Value of Quantitative Electroencephalography in Clinical Psychiatry: A Report by the Committee on Research of the American Neuropsychiatric Association. *The Journal of Neuropsychiatry and Clinical Neurosciences*, *18*(4), 460–500. doi:10.1176/jnp.2006.18.4.460 PMID:17135374

Cohen, E., Heiman, R., Carmi, M., Hadar, O., & Cohen, A. (2015). When physics meets signal processing: Image and video denoising based on Ising theory. *Signal Processing Image Communication*, *34*, 14–21. doi:10.1016/j.image.2015.02.007

Colak, C., Karaman, E., & Turtay, M. G. (2015). Application of knowledge discovery process on the prediction of stroke. *Computer Methods and Programs in Biomedicine*, *119*(3), 181–185. doi:10.1016/j.cmpb.2015.03.002 PMID:25827533

Comaniciu, D., & Meer, P. (1999). Mean shift analysis and applications. *Paper presented at the Computer Vision, 1999. The Proceedings of the Seventh IEEE International Conference on.* 10.1109/ICCV.1999.790416

Comaniciu, D., & Meer, P. (2002). Mean shift: A robust approach toward feature space analysis. *IEEE Transactions on Pattern Analysis and Machine Intelligence, 24*(5), 603–619. doi:10.1109/34.1000236

Compare, A., Zarbo, C., Shonin, E., Van Gordon, W., & Marconi, C. (2014). Emotional regulation and depression: A potential mediator between heart and mind. *Cardiovascular Psychiatry and Neurology*. PMID:25050177

Cook, O'Brien, Berkovic, Murphy, Morokof, Fabinyi, … Himes. (2013). Prediction of seizure likelihood with a long-term, implanted seizure advisory system in patients with drug-resistant epilepsy: A first in- man study. *The Lancet Neurology, 12*(6), 563-571.

Cook, I. A., O'Hara, R., Uijtdehaage, S. H., Mandelkern, M., & Leuchter, A. F. (1998). Assessing the accuracy of topographic EEG mapping for determining local brain function. *Electroencephalography and Clinical Neurophysiology, 107*(6), 408–414. doi:10.1016/S0013-4694(98)00092-3 PMID:9922086

Corrigan, P. W., &Kleinlein, P. (2005). *The impact of mental illness stigma*. Academic Press.

Corrigan, P. W., &Kosyluk, K. A. (2014). *Mental illness stigma: Types, constructs, and vehicles for change*. Academic Press.

Corrigan, P. W., Druss, B. G., & Perlick, D. A. (2014). The impact of mental illness stigma on seeking and participating in mental health care. *Psychological Science in the Public Interest, 15*(2), 37–70. doi:10.1177/1529100614531398 PMID:26171956

Corrigan, P. W., & Watson, A. C. (2002). The paradox of self-stigma and mental illness. *Clinical Psychology: Science and Practice, 9*(1), 35–53. doi:10.1093/clipsy.9.1.35

Cover, T., & Hart, P. (1967). Nearest neighbor pattern classification. *IEEE Transactions on Information Theory, 13*(1), 21–27. doi:10.1109/TIT.1967.1053964

Cresswell, K., & Sheikh, A. (2012). Electronic Health Record Technology. *Journal of the American Medical Association, 307*(21). doi:10.1001/jama.2012.3520 PMID:22706825

Crippa, A., Salvatore, C., Perego, P., Forti, S., Nobile, M., Molteni, M., & Castiglioni, I. (2015). Use of machine learning to identify children with autism and their motor abnormalities. *Journal of Autism and Developmental Disorders, 45*(7), 2146–2156. doi:10.100710803-015-2379-8 PMID:25652603

Cruz-Cunha, M., Simoes, R., Varajão, J., & Miranda, I. (2014). Information Technology Supporting Healthcare and Social Care Services. *Journal of Information Technology Research, 7*(1), 41–58. doi:10.4018/jitr.2014010104

Cruz-Martín, A., Crespo, M., & Portera-Cailliau, C. (2010). Delayed stabilization of dendritic spines in fragile X mice. *The Journal of Neuroscience, 30*(23), 7793–7803. doi:10.1523/JNEUROSCI.0577-10.2010 PMID:20534828

Cuijpers, P., Cristea, I. A., Karyotaki, E., Reijnders, M., & Huibers, M. J. (2016). How effective are cognitive behavior therapies for major depression and anxiety disorders? A meta-analytic update of the evidence. *World Psychiatry; Official Journal of the World Psychiatric Association (WPA), 15*(3), 245–258. doi:10.1002/wps.20346 PMID:27717254

Dahab, Ghoniemy, Gamal, & Selim. (2012). Automated brain tumour detection and identification using image processing and probabilistic neural network techniques. *Int J Image Process Visual Commun.*

Dainer-Best, J., Trujillo, L. T., Schnyer, D. M., & Beevers, C. G. (2017). Sustained engagement of attention is associated with increased negative self-referent processing in major depressive disorder. *Biological Psychology, 129*, 231–241. doi:10.1016/j.biopsycho.2017.09.005 PMID:28893596

Dai, Q., & Feng, Z. (2011). Deficient interference inhibition for negative stimuli in depression: An event-related potential study. *Clinical Neurophysiology*, *122*(1), 52–61. doi:10.1016/j.clinph.2010.05.025 PMID:20605107

Dai, Q., & Feng, Z. (2012). More excited for negative facial expressions in depression: Evidence from an event-related potential study. *Clinical Neurophysiology*, *123*(11), 2172–2179. doi:10.1016/j.clinph.2012.04.018 PMID:22727714

Dai, Q., Wei, J., Shu, X., & Feng, Z. (2016). Negativity bias for sad faces in depression: An event-related potential study. *Clinical Neurophysiology*, *127*(12), 3552–3560. doi:10.1016/j.clinph.2016.10.003 PMID:27833064

Dalessandro, B., Perlich, C., & Raeder, T. (2014). Bigger is Better, but at What Cost? Estimating the Economic Value of Incremental Data Assets. *Big Data*, *2*(2), 87–96. doi:10.1089/big.2014.0010 PMID:27442302

Dariotis, J. K., Mirabal-Beltran, R., Cluxton-Keller, F., Gould, L. F., Greenberg, M. T., & Mendelson, T. (2016). A Qualitative Evaluation of Student Learning and Skills Use in a School-Based Mindfulness and Yoga Program. *Mindfulness*, *7*(1), 76–89. doi:10.100712671-015-0463-y PMID:26918064

Darnall, N., Donovan, C., Aktar, S., Tseng, H., Barthelmess, P., Cohen, P., & Lin, D. (2012). Application of machine learning and numerical analysis to classify tremor in patients affected with essential tremor or Parkinson's disease. *Gerontechnology (Valkenswaard)*, *10*(4), 208–219. doi:10.4017/gt.2012.10.4.002.00

Das, B., Krishnan, N. C., & Cook, D. J. (2013). Handling Class Overlap and Imbalance to Detect Prompt Situations in Smart Homes. *IEEE 13th Int. Conf. on Data Mining Workshops*, 266-273.

DaTSCAN. (2011). *European Medicines Society*. EMEA/H/C/000266.

Davidson, I., & Ravi, S. (2005). *Agglomerative hierarchical clustering with constraints: Theoretical and empirical results.* Paper presented at the European Conference on Principles of Data Mining and Knowledge Discovery. 10.1007/11564126_11

Davidson, R. J., Kabat-Zinn, J., Schumacher, J., Rosenkranz, M., Muller, D., Santorelli, S. F., ... Sheridan, J. F. (2003). Alterations in brain and immune function produced by mindfulness meditation. *Psychosomatic Medicine*, *65*(4), 564–570. doi:10.1097/01.PSY.0000077505.67574.E3 PMID:12883106

Davidson, R. J., & McEwen, B. S. (2012). Social influences on neuroplasticity: Stress and interventions to promote well-being. *Nature Neuroscience*, *15*(5), 689–695. doi:10.1038/nn.3093 PMID:22534579

De Bruijne, M. (2016). *Machine learning approaches in medical image analysis: From detection to diagnosis*. Academic Press.

De Choudhury, M., Gamon, M., Counts, S., & Horvitz, E. (2013). Predicting depression via social media. *ICWSM*, *13*, 1–10.

De Maesschalck, R., Estienne, F., Verdú-Andrés, J., Candolfi, A., Centner, V., Despagne, F., ... De Noord, O. E. (1999). The development of calibration models for spectroscopic data using principal component regression. *Internet Journal of Chemistry*, *2*(19), 1.

De Mauro, A., Greco, M., & Grimaldi, M. (2015, February). What is big data? A consensual definition and a review of key research topics. In AIP conference proceedings: Vol. 1644. *No. 1* (pp. 97–104). AIP. doi:10.1063/1.4907823

De Souza, J. W. M., Almeida, J. S., & Rebouças Filho, P. P. (2017). A New Approach for the Diagnosis of Parkinson's Disease Using a Similarity Feature Extractor. In Intelligent Systems Design and Applications. ISDA 2017. Advances in Intelligent Systems and Computing. Springer.

De, A., & Guo, C. (2015). An adaptive vector quantization approach for image segmentation based on SOM network. *Neurocomputing*, *149*, 48–58. doi:10.1016/j.neucom.2014.02.069

Deldin, P. J., Keller, J., Gergen, J. A., & Miller, G. A. (2000). Right-posterior face processing anomaly in depression. *Journal of Abnormal Psychology*, *109*(1), 116–121. doi:10.1037/0021-843X.109.1.116 PMID:10740942

Deldin, P. J., Naidu, S. K., Shestyuk, A. Y., & Casas, B. R. (2009). Neurophysiological indices of free recall memory biases in major depression: The impact of stimulus arousal and valence. *Cognition and Emotion*, *23*(5), 1002–1020. doi:10.1080/02699930802273573

Delle-Vigne, D., Wang, W., Kornreich, C., Verbanck, P., & Campanella, S. (2014). Emotional facial expression processing in depression: Data from behavioral and event-related potential studies. *Neurophysiologie Clinique. Clinical Neurophysiology*, *44*(2), 169–187. doi:10.1016/j.neucli.2014.03.003 PMID:24930940

Deng, W., Papavasileiou, I., Qiao, Z., Zhang, W., Lam, K. Y., & Song, H. (2018). Advances in Automation Technologies for Lower-extremity Neurorehabilitation: A Review and Future Challenges. *IEEE Reviews in Biomedical Engineering*, *11*, 289–305. doi:10.1109/RBME.2018.2830805 PMID:29994006

Dennis, T. A. (2010). Neurophysiological markers for child emotion regulation from the perspective of emotion–cognition integration: Current directions and future challenges. *Developmental Neuropsychology*, *35*(2), 212–230. doi:10.1080/87565640903526579 PMID:20390603

Dernovsek, M., Novak, T., & Sprah, L. (2010). PW01-09-Assessment of cognitive functioning within different emotional contexts in the group of euthymic bipolar patients. *European Psychiatry*, *25*, 1425. doi:10.1016/S0924-9338(10)71411-5

Deveney, C. M., & Deldin, P. J. (2004). Memory of faces: A slow wave ERP study of major depression. *Emotion (Washington, D.C.)*, *4*(3), 295–304. doi:10.1037/1528-3542.4.3.295 PMID:15456398

Deveney, C. M., & Deldin, P. J. (2006). A preliminary investigation of cognitive flexibility for emotional information in major depressive disorder and non-psychiatric controls. *Emotion (Washington, D.C.)*, *6*(3), 429–437. doi:10.1037/1528-3542.6.3.429 PMID:16938084

Dewaele, J. M. (2012). Multilingualism and emotions. The Encyclopedia of Applied Linguistics.

Dewaele, J. M. (2015). Bilingualism and multilingualism. *The international encyclopedia of language and social interaction*, 1-11.

Dewaele, J. M. (2010). *Emotions in multiple languages*. London: Palgrave. doi:10.1057/9780230289505

Diaz, I., & Boulanger, P. (2015). Atlas to patient registration with brain tumor based on a mesh-free method. *2015 37th Annual International Conference of the IEEE Engineering in Medicine and Biology Society (EMBC)*. doi:10.1109/embc.2015.7319004

Diner, B. C., Holcomb, P. J., & Dykman, R. A. (1985). P300 in major depressive disorder. *Psychiatry Research*, *15*(3), 175–184. doi:10.1016/0165-1781(85)90074-5 PMID:3862153

Dinov, I. D., Heavner, B., Tang, M., Glusman, G., Chard, K., Darcy, M., ... Foster, I. (2016). Predictive big data analytics: A study of Parkinson's disease using large, complex, heterogeneous, incongruent, multi-source and incomplete observations. *PLoS One*, *11*(8), e0157077. doi:10.1371/journal.pone.0157077 PMID:27494614

Diri, B. (n.d.). *Makine Öğrenmesine Giriş*. Retrieved from Lecture Notes Online Web site: https://www.ce.yildiz.edu.tr/personal/banud/file/2634/Makine+Ogrenmesi-ML-10.pdf

Disner, S. G., Beevers, C. G., Haigh, E. A., & Beck, A. T. (2011). Neural mechanisms of the cognitive model of depression. *Nature Reviews. Neuroscience*, *12*(8), 467–477. doi:10.1038/nrn3027 PMID:21731066

Domo. (n.d.). *Data Never Sleeps 6.0*. Retrieved January 1, 2019, from https://www.domo.com/learn/data-never-sleeps-6

Donkers, F. C., Nieuwenhuis, S., & Van Boxtel, G. J. (2005). Mediofrontal negativities in the absence of responding. *Brain Research. Cognitive Brain Research*, *25*(3), 777–787. doi:10.1016/j.cogbrainres.2005.09.007 PMID:16249075

Doyle, O. M., Greene, B. R., Murray, D. M., Marnane, L., Lightbody, G., & Boylan, G. B. (2007). The effect of frequency band on quantitative EEG measures in neonates with hypoxic-ischaemic encephalopathy. *Conference Proceedings; ... Annual International Conference of the IEEE Engineering in Medicine and Biology Society. IEEE Engineering in Medicine and Biology Society. Conference*, 717–721. doi:10.1109/IEMBS.2007.4352391 PMID:18002057

Drevets, W. C., Price, J. L., & Furey, M. L. (2008). Brain structural and functional abnormalities in mood disorders: Implications for neurocircuitry models of depression. *Brain Structure & Function*, *213*(1-2), 93–118. doi:10.100700429-008-0189-x PMID:18704495

Dubey, Y. K., Mushrif, M. M., & Mitra, K. (2016). Segmentation of brain MR images using rough set based intuitionistic fuzzy clustering. *Biocybernetics and Biomedical Engineering*, *36*(2), 413–426. doi:10.1016/j.bbe.2016.01.001

Dudani, S. (1967). The distance-weighted k-nearest-neighbor rule. *IEEE Transactions on Systems, Man, and Cybernetics*, *6*, 325–327.

Duman, R. S. (2014). Pathophysiology of depression and innovative treatments: Remodelling glutamatergic synaptic connections. *Dialogues in Clinical Neuroscience*, *16*(1), 11. PMID:24733968

Duman, R. S., & Monteggia, L. M. (2006). A neurotrophic model for stress-related mood disorders. *Biological Psychiatry*, *59*(12), 1116–1127. doi:10.1016/j.biopsych.2006.02.013 PMID:16631126

Dumitriu, D., Hao, J., Hara, Y., Kaufmann, J., Janssen, W. G., Lou, W., ... Morrison, J. H. (2010). Selective changes in thin spine density and morphology in monkey prefrontal cortex correlate with ageing-related cognitive impairment. *The Journal of Neuroscience*, *30*(22), 7507–7515. doi:10.1523/JNEUROSCI.6410-09.2010 PMID:20519525

Duncan, C. C., Barry, R. J., Connolly, J. F., Fischer, C., Michie, P. T., Näätänen, R., ... Van Petten, C. (2009). Event-related potentials in clinical research: Guidelines for eliciting, recording, and quantifying mismatch negativity, P300, and N400. *Clinical Neurophysiology*, *120*(11), 1883–1908. doi:10.1016/j.clinph.2009.07.045 PMID:19796989

Durieux, V., & Radiology, P. (2010). *Bibliometric indicators: quality measurements of scientific publication*. Retrieved from pubs.rsna.org

Eichstaedt, J. C., Smith, R. J., Merchant, R. M., Ungar, L. H., Crutchley, P., Preoţiuc-Pietro, D., ... Schwartz, H. A. (2018). Facebook language predicts depression in medical records. *Proceedings of the National Academy of Sciences of the United States of America*, *115*(44), 11203–11208. doi:10.1073/pnas.1802331115 PMID:30322910

Ejlerskov, P. (2015). *Immune gene prevents Parkinson's disease and dementia*. Retrieved from http://www.health.am/psy/more/prevents-parkinsons-disease-and-dementia/

Elble, R. J. (2017). *Tremor. In Neuro-Geriatrics* (pp. 311–326). Springer. doi:10.1007/978-3-319-56484-5_20

El-Dahshan, E. A., Mohsen, H. M., Revett, K., & Salem, A. M. (2014). Computer-aided diagnosis of human brain tumor through MRI: A survey and a new algorithm. *Expert Systems with Applications*, *41*(11), 5526–5545. doi:10.1016/j.eswa.2014.01.021

El-Gamal, F. E., Elmogy, M. M., Ghazal, M., Atwan, A., Casanova, M. F., Barnes, G. N., ... Khalil, A. (2018). A Novel Early Diagnosis System for Mild Cognitive Impairment Based on Local Region Analysis: A Pilot Study. *Frontiers in Human Neuroscience*, *11*, 643. doi:10.3389/fnhum.2017.00643 PMID:29375343

Elmannai, W., & Elleithy, K. (2017). Sensor-based assistive devices for visually-impaired people: Current status, challenges, and future directions. *Sensors (Switzerland)*, *17*(3), 565. doi:10.339017030565 PMID:28287451

Escolano, C., Aguilar, M., & Minguez, J. (2011). EEG-based upper alpha neurofeedback training improves working memory performance. *Proc. 33rd Annual International Conference of the IEEE*, 2327-2330 10.1109/IEMBS.2011.6090651

Escolano, C., Navarro-Gil, M., Garcia-Campayo, J., Congedo, M., De Ridder, D., & Minguez, J. (2014). A controlled study on the cognitive effect of alpha neurofeedback training in patients with major depression disorder. *Frontiers in Behavioral Neuroscience*, *8*, 296. doi:10.3389/fnbeh.2014.00296 PMID:25228864

Eskofier, B. M., Lee, S. I., Daneault, J.-F., Golabchi, F. N., Ferreira-Carvalho, G., Vergara-Diaz, G., . . . Kautz, T. (2016). *Recent machine learning advancements in sensor-based mobility analysis: deep learning for Parkinson's disease assessment.* Paper presented at the Engineering in Medicine and Biology Society (EMBC), 2016 IEEE 38th Annual International Conference of the. 10.1109/EMBC.2016.7590787

Evans, D. L., Charney, D. S., & Lewis, L. (2006). *The Physician's Guide to Depression & Bipolar Disorders*. McGraw-Hill Professional.

Factor, S., Feustel, P., Friedman, J., Comella, C., Goetz, C., Kurlan, R., ... Group, P. S. (2003). Longitudinal outcome of Parkinson's disease patients with psychosis. *Neurology*, *60*(11), 1756–1761. doi:10.1212/01.WNL.0000068010.82167.CF PMID:12796526

Fahn, S. (2011). Classification of movement disorders. *Movement Disorders*, *26*(6), 947–957. doi:10.1002/mds.23759 PMID:21626541

Fallgatter, A. J., Herrmann, M. J., Roemmler, J., Ehlis, A. C., Wagener, A., Heidrich, A., ... Lesch, K. P. (2004). Allelic variation of serotonin transporter function modulates the brain electrical response for error processing. *Neuropsychopharmacology*, *29*(8), 1506–1511. doi:10.1038j.npp.1300409 PMID:15187981

Farb, N., Anderson, A., Ravindran, A., Hawley, L., Irving, J., Mancuso, E., ... Segal, Z. V. (2018). Prevention of relapse/recurrence in major depressive disorder with either mindfulness-based cognitive therapy or cognitive therapy. *Journal of Consulting and Clinical Psychology*, *86*(2), 200–204. doi:10.1037/ccp0000266 PMID:29265831

Fatt, Q., & Ramadas, A. (2018). The Usefulness and Challenges of Big Data in Healthcare. *Journal of Health Communication*, *03*(02). doi:10.4172/2472-1654.100131

Feldmann, L., Piechaczek, C. E., Pehl, V., Bartling, J., Bakos, S., Schulte-Körne, G., & Greimel, E. (2018). State or trait? Auditory event-related potentials in adolescents with current and remitted major depression. *Neuropsychologia*, *113*, 95–103. doi:10.1016/j.neuropsychologia.2018.03.035 PMID:29604322

Feng, P. M., Ding, H., Chen, W., & Lin, H. (2013). Naive Bayes classifier with feature selection to identify phage virion proteins. *Computational and Mathematical Methods in Medicine*. PMID:23762187

Feng, R., Badgeley, M., Mocco, J., & Oermann, E. K. (2018). Deep learning guided stroke management: A review of clinical applications. *Journal of Neurointerventional Surgery*, *10*(4), 358–362. doi:10.1136/neurintsurg-2017-013355 PMID:28954325

Ferrari, A. J., Charlson, F. J., Norman, R. E., Patten, S. B., Freedman, G., Murray, C. J. L., ... Whiteford, H. A. (2013). Burden of Depressive Disorders by Country, Sex, Age, and Year: Findings from the Global Burden of Disease Study 2010. *PLoS Medicine*, *10*(11), e1001547. doi:10.1371/journal.pmed.1001547 PMID:24223526

Fife, C., & Eckert, K. (2017). Harnessing electronic healthcare data for wound care research: Standards for reporting observational registry data obtained directly from electronic health records. *Wound Repair and Regeneration*, *25*(2), 192–209. doi:10.1111/wrr.12523 PMID:28370796

Finberg, J. P. M., Schwartz, M., Jeries, R., Badarny, S., Nakhleh, M. K., Abu Daoud, E., ... Haick, H. (2018). Sensor Array for Detection of Early Stage Parkinson's Disease before Medication. *ACS Chemical Neuroscience*, *9*(11), 2548–2553. doi:10.1021/acschemneuro.8b00245 PMID:29989795

Fishbein, D., Miller, S., Herman-Stahl, M., Williams, J., Lavery, B., Markovitz, L., ... Johnson, M. (2016). Behavioral and psychophysiological effects of a yoga intervention on high-risk adolescents: A randomized control trial. *Journal of Child and Family Studies*, *25*(2), 518–529. doi:10.100710826-015-0231-6

Fleuriephysio. (2017). *10 Signs of Parkinson's Disease*. Retrieved from http://fleurieuphysiotherapy.com.au/10-signs-parkinsons-disease/

Fok, S., Schwartz, R., Ronkiewicz, M., Holmes, C., Zhang, J., Somers, T., ... Leuthardt, E. (2011). An EEG-based brain computer interface for rehabilitation and restoration of hand control following stroke using ipsilateral cortical physiology. *33rd Annual International Conf. of the IEEE EMBS*. 10.1109/IEMBS.2011.6091549

Force, R. B., Venables, N. C., & Sponheim, S. R. (2008). An auditory processing abnormality specific to liability for schizophrenia. *Schizophrenia Research*, *103*(1-3), 298–310. doi:10.1016/j.schres.2008.04.038 PMID:18571375

Fossati, P. (2018). Is major depression a cognitive disorder? *Revue Neurologique*, *174*(4), 212–215. doi:10.1016/j.neurol.2018.01.365 PMID:29618408

Foti, D., Olvet, D. M., Klein, D. N., & Hajcak, G. (2010). Reduced electrocortical response to threatening faces in major depressive disorder. *Depression and Anxiety*, *27*(9), 813–820. doi:10.1002/da.20712 PMID:20577985

Fox, H. C., Hong, K. A., & Sinha, R. (2008). Difficulties in emotion regulation and impulse control in recently abstinent alcoholics compared with social drinkers. *Addictive Behaviors*, *33*(2), 388–3948. doi:10.1016/j.addbeh.2007.10.002 PMID:18023295

Fradkin, D., & Muchnik, I. (2000). *Support Vector Machines for Classification*. DIMACS Series in Discrete Mathematics and Theoretical Computer Science.

Fried, E. I., Nesse, R. M., Guille, C., & Sen, S. (2015). The differential influence of life stress on individual symptoms of depression. *Acta Psychiatrica Scandinavica*, *131*(6), 465–471. doi:10.1111/acps.12395 PMID:25650176

Friedman, D., Cycowicz, Y. M., & Gaeta, H. (2001). The novelty P3: An event-related brain potential (ERP) sign of the brain's evaluation of novelty. *Neuroscience and Biobehavioral Reviews*, *25*(4), 355–373. doi:10.1016/S0149-7634(01)00019-7 PMID:11445140

Friedman, D., Simpson, G., & Hamberger, M. (1993). Age-related changes in scalp topography to novel and target stimuli. *Psychophysiology*, *30*(4), 383–396. doi:10.1111/j.1469-8986.1993.tb02060.x PMID:8327624

Frolov, A., Biryukova, E., Bobrov, P., Mokienko, O., Platonov, A., Pryanichnikov, V., & Chernikova, L. (2013). Principles of Neurorehabilitation Based on the Brain Computer Interface and Biologically Adequate Control of the Exoskeleton. *Human Physiology*, *39*(2), 196–208. doi:10.1134/S0362119713020035

Fromenteze, T., Decroze, C., Abid, S., & Yurduseven, O. (2018). Sparsity-Driven Reconstruction Technique for Microwave/Millimeter-Wave Computational Imaging. *Sensors (Basel)*, *18*(5), 1536. doi:10.339018051536 PMID:29757241

Furukawa, T. A., Efthimiou, O., Weitz, E. S., Cipriani, A., Keller, M. B., Kocsis, J. H., ... Schramm, E. (2018). Cognitive-Behavioral Analysis System of Psychotherapy, Drug, or Their Combination for Persistent Depressive Disorder: Personalizing the Treatment Choice Using Individual Participant Data Network Metaregression. *Psychotherapy and Psychosomatics*, *87*(3), 140–153. doi:10.1159/000489227 PMID:29847831

Fusion of MRI and CT Images of Brain Tumor – Comprehensive Survey. (2018). *International Journal of Recent Trends in Engineering and Research, 4*(2), 12-17. doi:10.23883/ijrter.2018.4056.wy154

Gandhi, T., Panigrahi, B. K., Bhatia, M., & Anand, S. (2010). Expert model for detection of epileptic activity in EEG signature. *Expert Systems with Applications*, *37*(4), 3513–3520. doi:10.1016/j.eswa.2009.10.036

Gandhi, V., Prasad, G., Coyle, D., Behera, L., & McGinnity, T. (2014). Quantum Neural Network-Based EEG Filtering for a Brain–Computer Interface. *IEEE Transactions on Neural Networks and Learning Systems*, *25*(2), 278–288. doi:10.1109/TNNLS.2013.2274436 PMID:24807028

Gandomi, A., & Haider, M. (2015). Beyond the hype: Big data concepts, methods, and analytics. *International Journal of Information Management*, *35*(2), 137–144. doi:10.1016/j.ijinfomgt.2014.10.007

Gan, M., & Dai, H. (2014). Detecting and monitoring abrupt emergences and submergences of episodes over data streams. *Information Systems*, *39*, 277–289. doi:10.1016/j.is.2012.05.009

Ganzalez-Ortega, D., Diaz-Pernas, F. J., & Martinez-Zarzuela, M. (2014). A Kinect-based system for cognition rehabilitation exercise monitoring. *Computer Methods and Programs in Biomedicine*, *113*(2), 620–631. doi:10.1016/j.cmpb.2013.10.014 PMID:24263055

García-Blanco, A., Salmerón, L., Perea, M., & Livianos, L. (2014). Attentional biases toward emotional images in the different episodes of bipolar disorder: An eye-tracking study. *Psychiatry Research*, *215*(3), 628–633. doi:10.1016/j.psychres.2013.12.039 PMID:24439518

Gartner I. T. Glossary. (n.d.) *Big data*. Retrieved December 12, 2018, from https://www.gartner.com/it-glossary/big-data

Genetics: Genome made quickly from scratch. (2009). *Science News, 164*(24), 382-382. doi:10.1002cin.5591642416

Ghosh, S., Dastidar, H. A., & Dadmehr, N. (2007). Mixedband wavelet-chaos-neural network methodology for epilepsy and epileptic seizure detection. *IEEE Transactions on Biomedical Engineering*, *54*(9), 1545–1551. doi:10.1109/TBME.2007.891945 PMID:17867346

Giese-Davis, J., Sephton, S. E., Abercrombie, H. C., Durán, R. E., & Spiegel, D. (2004). Repression and high anxiety are associated with aberrant diurnal cortisol rhythms in women with metastatic breast cancer. *Health Psychology*, *23*(6), 645–650. doi:10.1037/0278-6133.23.6.645 PMID:15546233

Gokul, S., Sivachitra, M., & Vijayachitra, S. (2013). *Parkinson's disease prediction using machine learning approaches.* Paper presented at the Advanced Computing (ICoAC), 2013 Fifth International Conference on. 10.1109/ICoAC.2013.6921958

Gollan, J. K., McCloskey, M., Hoxha, D., & Coccaro, E. F. (2010). How do depressed and healthy adults interpret nuanced facial expressions? *Journal of Abnormal Psychology*, *119*(4), 804–810. doi:10.1037/a0020234 PMID:20939654

Gomez-Pilar, J., & Corralejo, R. (2014). Assessment of neurofeedback training by means of motor imagery based-BCI for cognitive rehabilitation. *Proc Engineering in Medicine and Biology Society (EMBC), 36th Annual International Conference of the IEEE*, 3630-3633. 10.1109/EMBC.2014.6944409

Goode, L. (2016). *Messenger and WhatsApp Process 60 Billion Messages a Day, Three Times More than SMS.* Retrieved from https://www.theverge.com/2016/4/12/11415198/facebook-messenger-whatsapp-number-messages-vs-sms-f8-2016

Goodwin, F. K., & Jamison, K. R. (2007). *Manic-depressive illness: bipolar disorders and recurrent depression* (Vol. 1). Oxford University Press.

Gordon-King, K., Schweitzer, R. D., & Dimaggio, G. (2018). Metacognitive interpersonal therapy for personality disorders featuring emotional inhibition: A multiple baseline case series. *The Journal of Nervous and Mental Disease, 206*(4), 263–269. PMID:29377848

Gotink, R. A., Vernooij, M. W., Ikram, M. A., Niessen, W. J., Krestin, G. P., Hofman, A., ... Hunink, M. M. (2018). Meditation and yoga practice are associated with smaller right amygdala volume: The Rotterdam study. *Brain Imaging and Behavior*, 1–9. PMID:29417491

Grefkes, C., & Fink, G. R. (2011). Reorganization of cerebral network after stroke: New insights from neuroimaging with connectivity approaches. *Brain, 134*(5), 1264–1276. doi:10.1093/brain/awr033 PMID:21414995

Groves, P., Kayyali, B., Knott, D., & Van Kuiken, S. (2013). The 'big data'revolution in healthcare. *The McKinsey Quarterly, 2*(3).

Guo, P., Wang, J., Gao, X. Z., & Jarno, M. A. (2012). Epileptic EEG signal classification with marching pursuit based on harmony search method. *Conference Proceedings - IEEE International Conference on Systems, Man and Cybernetics*, 283-288.

Guo, L., Rivero, D., & Pazos, A. (2010). Daniel Rivero, and Alejandro Pazos. Epileptic seizure detection using multiwavelet transform based approximate entropy and artificial neural networks. *Journal of Neuroscience Methods, 193*(1), 156–163. doi:10.1016/j.jneumeth.2010.08.030 PMID:20817036

Gupta, D., Julka, A., Jain, S., Aggarwal, T., Khanna, A., Arunkumar, N., & de Albuquerque, V. H. C. (2018). Optimized Cuttlefish Algorithm for Diagnosis of Parkinson's Disease. *Cognitive Systems Research, 52*, 36–48. doi:10.1016/j.cogsys.2018.06.006

Gupta, D., Sundaram, S., Khanna, A., Hassanien, A. E., & de Albuquerque, V. H. C. (2018). Improved diagnosis of Parkinson's disease using optimized crow search algorithm. *Computers & Electrical Engineering, 68*, 412–424. doi:10.1016/j.compeleceng.2018.04.014

Guttfreund, D. G. (1990). Effects of language usage on the emotional experience of Spanish-English and English-Spanish bilinguals. *Journal of Consulting and Clinical Psychology, 58*(5), 604–607. doi:10.1037/0022-006X.58.5.604 PMID:2254507

Hadjahamadi, A. H., & Askari, T. J. (2012). A Detection Support System for Parkinson's Disease Diagnosis Using Classification and Regression Tree. *Journal of Mathematics and Computer Science, 4*(02), 257–263. doi:10.22436/jmcs.04.02.15

Hadjistavropoulos, H. D., Schneider, L. H., Edmonds, M., Karin, E., Nugent, M. N., Dirkse, D., ... Titov, N. (2017). Randomized controlled trial of internet-delivered cognitive behaviour therapy comparing standard weekly versus optional weekly therapist support. *Journal of Anxiety Disorders, 52*, 15–24. doi:10.1016/j.janxdis.2017.09.006 PMID:28964994

Hakulinen, C., Elovainio, M., Pulkki-Råback, L., Virtanen, M., Kivimäki, M., & Jokela, M. (2015). Personality and depressive symptoms: Individual participant meta-analysis of 10 cohort studies. *Depression and Anxiety, 32*(7), 461–470. doi:10.1002/da.22376 PMID:26014798

Hallett, M. (1991). Classification and treatment of tremor. *Journal of the American Medical Association, 266*(8), 1115–1117. doi:10.1001/jama.1991.03470080085035 PMID:1650852

Hammen, C. L. (2015). Stress and depression: Old questions, new approaches. *Current Opinion in Psychology, 4*, 80–85. doi:10.1016/j.copsyc.2014.12.024

Han, J., & Kamber, M. (2001). *Data Mining Concepts and Techniques* (2nd ed.). Morgan Kauffmann Publishers Inc.

Hanks, G., Blinderman, C. D., & Cherny, N. I. (2005). *Peer review in action: The contribution of referees to advancing reliable knowledge*. Academic Press.

Hansen, J. H. L., & Hasan, T. (2015). Speaker recognition by machines and humans: A tutorial review. *IEEE Signal Processing Magazine*, *32*(6), 74–99. doi:10.1109/MSP.2015.2462851

Hansenne, M., Pitchot, W., Moreno, A. G., Zaldua, I. U., & Ansseau, M. (1996). Suicidal behavior in depressive disorder: An event-related potential study. *Biological Psychiatry*, *40*(2), 116–122. doi:10.1016/0006-3223(95)00372-X PMID:8793043

Hardt, J. V., & Kamiya, J. (1978). Anxiety change through electroencephalographic alpha feedback seen only in high anxiety subjects. *Science*, *201*(4350), 79–81. doi:10.1126cience.663641 PMID:663641

Harerimana, G., Jang, B., Kim, J. W., & Park, H. K. (2018). Health Big Data Analytics: A Technology Survey. *IEEE Access: Practical Innovations, Open Solutions*, *6*, 65661–65678. doi:10.1109/ACCESS.2018.2878254

Hariharana, M., Polat, K., & Sindhu, R. (2014). A new hybrid intelligent system for accurate detection of Parkinson's disease. *Computer Methods and Programs in Biomedicine*, *113*(3), 904–913. doi:10.1016/j.cmpb.2014.01.004 PMID:24485390

Harrington, P. (2012). *Machine learning in Action* (Vol. 5). Greenwich, CT: Manning.

Harris, A., True, H., Hu, Z., Cho, J., Fell, N., & Sartipi, M. (2016, December). Fall recognition using wearable technologies and machine learning algorithms. In *Big Data (Big Data), 2016 IEEE International Conference on* (pp. 3974-3976). IEEE. 10.1109/BigData.2016.7841080

Hartigan, J. A., & Wong, M. A. (1979). Algorithm AS 136: A k-means clustering algorithm. *Journal of the Royal Statistical Society. Series C, Applied Statistics*, *28*(1), 100–108.

Harvey, J. A., Quinn, J. L., Liu, R., Aloyo, V. J., & Romano, A. G. (2004). Selective remodelling of rabbit frontal cortex: Relationship between 5-HT 2A receptor density and associative learning. *Psychopharmacology*, *172*(4), 435–442. doi:10.1007/00213-003-1687-4 PMID:14685644

Hasler, G., Drevets, W. C., Manji, H. K., & Charney, D. S. (2004). Discovering endophenotypes for major depression. *Neuropsychopharmacology*, *29*(10), 1765–1781. doi:10.1038j.npp.1300506 PMID:15213704

Hassanien, A.E. & Azar, A.T. (2015). *Brain Computer Interfaces: Current Trends and Applications* (Vol. 143). doi:10.1007/978-3-319-10978-7

Hassan, N. A., & Hijazi, R. (2018). *Open Source Intelligence Methods and Tools*. New York: Apress. doi:10.1007/978-1-4842-3213-2

Hausdorff, J. M., Lertratanakul, A., Cudkowicz, M. E., Peterson, A. L., Kaliton, D., & Goldberger, A. L. (2000). Gait Dynamics in Neuro-Degenerative Disease Data Base [Data set]. physionet.org. doi:10.13026/C27G6C

Havaei, M., Davy, A., Farley, D. W., Biard, A., Courville, A., Bengio, Y., ... Larochelle, H. (2016). Brain tumor segmentation with Deep neural networks. *Medical Image Analysis*, *35*, 18–31. doi:10.1016/j.media.2016.05.004 PMID:27310171

Hawkes, C. H., Del Tredici, K., & Braak, H. (2010). A timeline for Parkinson's disease. *Parkinsonism & Related Disorders*, *16*(2), 79–84. doi:10.1016/j.parkreldis.2009.08.007 PMID:19846332

Hayashi-Takagi, A., & Sawa, A. (2010). Disturbed synaptic connectivity in schizophrenia: Convergence of genetic risk factors during neurodevelopment. *Brain Research Bulletin*, *83*(3-4), 140–146. doi:10.1016/j.brainresbull.2010.04.007 PMID:20433911

Heinsfeld, A. S., Franco, A. R., Craddock, R. C., Buchweitz, A., & Meneguzzi, F. (2018). Identification of autism spectrum disorder using deep learning and the ABIDE dataset. *NeuroImage. Clinical*, *17*, 16–23. doi:10.1016/j.nicl.2017.08.017 PMID:29034163

Heller, W. (1993). Neuropsychological mechanisms of individual differences in emotion, personality, and arousal. *Neuropsychology*, *7*(4), 476–489. doi:10.1037/0894-4105.7.4.476

Herbert, C., Kissler, J., Junghöfer, M., Peyk, P., & Rockstroh, B. (2006). Processing of emotional adjectives: Evidence from startle EMG and ERPs. *Psychophysiology*, *43*(2), 197–206. doi:10.1111/j.1469-8986.2006.00385.x PMID:16712590

Heresco-Levy, U., & Javitt, D. (2018). *U.S. Patent Application No. 15/729,692*. Washington, DC: US Patent Office.

Hermens, D. F., Ward, P. B., Hodge, M. A. R., Kaur, M., Naismith, S. L., & Hickie, I. B. (2010). Impaired MMN/P3a complex in first-episode psychosis: Cognitive and psychosocial associations. *Progress in Neuro-Psychopharmacology & Biological Psychiatry*, *34*(6), 822–829. doi:10.1016/j.pnpbp.2010.03.019 PMID:20302901

Hinton. (1992). How Neural Networks Learn from Experience. *Scientific American, 267*(3), 144-151.

Holmes, A. J., & Pizzagalli, D. A. (2008). Spatiotemporal dynamics of error processing dysfunctions in major depressive disorder. *Archives of General Psychiatry*, *65*(2), 179–188. doi:10.1001/archgenpsychiatry.2007.19 PMID:18250256

Horrobin, D. F. (2001). Something rotten at the core of science? *Trends in Pharmacological Sciences*, *22*(2), 51–52.

Hoskins, M. (2014). Common Big Data Challenges and How to Overcome Them. *Big Data*, *2*(3), 142–143. doi:10.1089/big.2014.0030 PMID:27442494

Houston, R. J., Bauer, L. O., & Hesselbrock, V. M. (2003). Depression and familial risk for substance dependence: A P300 study of young women. *Psychiatry Research: Neuroimaging*, *124*(1), 49–62. doi:10.1016/S0925-4927(03)00074-X PMID:14511795

Hsieh, W. H., Lin, C. Y., Te, A. L. D., Lo, M. T., Wu, C. I., Chung, F. P., ... Hu, Y. F. (2017). A novel noninvasive surface ECG analysis using interlead QRS dispersion in arrhythmogenic right ventricular cardiomyopathy. *PLoS One*, *12*(8), e0182364. doi:10.1371/journal.pone.0182364 PMID:28771538

Huang, G.-B., Zhu, Q.-Y., & Siew, C.-K. (2004). Extreme Learning Machine: A New Learning Scheme of Feedforward Neural Networks. *Proc. Of IEEE Int. Joint Conf. on Neural Network*, *2*, 985-990.

Huang, G.-B., Zhu, Q.-Y., & Siew, C.-K. (2006). Extreme learning machine: Theory and applications. *Neurocomputing*, *70*(1-3), 489–501. doi:10.1016/j.neucom.2005.12.126

Huster, R. J., Enriquez-Geppert, S., Lavallee, C. F., Falkenstein, M., & Herrmann, C. S. (2013). Electroencephalography of response inhibition tasks: Functional networks and cognitive contributions. *International Journal of Psychophysiology*, *87*(3), 217–233. doi:10.1016/j.ijpsycho.2012.08.001 PMID:22906815

Hutcheson, J. A., & Kimberley, M. O. (1999). A pragmatic approach to characterising insect communities in New Zealand: Malaise trapped beetles. *New Zealand Journal of Ecology*, *23*(1), 69–79. doi:10.1016/S1474-4422(17)30299-5

IBM. (n.d.a). *What is big data? Bringing big data to the enterprise.* Retrieved May 5, 2018, from http://www-01.ibm.com/software/data/bigdata/

IBM. (n.d.b.). *What is MapReduce?* Retrieved December 22, 2018, from https://www.ibm.com/analytics/hadoop/mapreduce

Ibrahim, G., III. (2012). The most cited works in epilepsy: Trends in the "Citation Classics". Wiley Online Library.

Isensee, F., Kickingereder, P., Wick, W., Bendszus, M., & Maier-Hein, K. H. (2018). Brain Tumor Segmentation and Radiomics Survival Prediction: Contribution to the BRATS 2017 Challenge. Brainlesion: Glioma, Multiple Sclerosis, Stroke and Traumatic Brain Injuries Lecture Notes in Computer Science, 287-297. doi:10.1007/978-3-319-75238-9_25

Islam, M. S., Parvez, I., Deng, H., & Goswami, P. (2014) Performance Comparison of Heterogeneous Classifiers for Detection of Parkinson's Disease Using Voice Disorder (Dysphonia). *3rd International Conference on Informatics, Electronics & Vision*. 10.1109/ICIEV.2014.6850849

Iyer, K., & Khan, Z. A. (2012). Depression–A Review. *Research Journal of Recent Sciences, 1*(4), 79-87.

Jacobson, S. A., Leuchter, A. F., & Walter, D. O. (1993). Conventional and quantitative EEG in the diagnosis of delirium among the elderly. *Journal of Neurology, Neurosurgery, and Psychiatry*, *56*(2), 153–158. doi:10.1136/jnnp.56.2.153 PMID:8437004

Jagaroo, V., & Santangelo, S. L. (2017). Erratum to: Neurophenotypes. *Neurophenotypes*, *12*(193), 296.

James, C. D., Aimone, J. B., Miner, N. E., Vineyard, C. M., Rothganger, F. H., Carlson, K. D., & Plimpton, S. J. (2017). A historical survey of algorithms and hardware architectures for neural-inspired and neuromorphic computing applications. *Biologically Inspired Cognitive Architectures*, *19*, 49–54. doi:10.1016/j.bica.2016.11.002

Janghel, Shukla, Tiwari, & Kala. (2010). *Breast Cancer Diagnosis using Artificial Neural Network Models*. Academic Press.

Janghel, R. R., Shukla, A., & Tiwari, R. (2012). Hybrid computing based intelligent system for breast cancer diagnosis. *International Journal of Biomedical Engineering and Technology*, *10*(1), 1–18. doi:10.1504/IJBET.2012.049321

Janssen, P., Walther, C., & Lüdeke, M. (2012). *Cluster analysis to understand socio-ecological systems: a guideline*. Potsdam-Institut für Klimafolgenforschung.

Jarrold, W., Javitz, H. S., Krasnow, R., Peintner, B., Yeh, E., Swan, G. E., & Mehl, M. (2011). Depression and self-focused language in structured interviews with older men. *Psychological Reports*, *109*(2), 686–700. doi:10.2466/02.09.21.28.PR0.109.5.686-700 PMID:22238866

Jedud, I. (2018). *Interdisciplinary Approach to Emotion Detection from Text*. Academic Press.

Jennifer. (2013). Sleep Awake Disorder. In W. E. Craighead, D. J. Miklowitz, & L. W. Craighead (Eds.), Psychopathology: History, diagnosis, and empirical foundations. Academic Press.

Jensen, M. E., Pease, E. A., Lambert, K., Hickman, D. R., Robinson, O., McCoy, K. T., ... Ramirez, J. (2013). Championing person-first language: A call to psychiatric mental health nurses. *Journal of the American Psychiatric Nurses Association*, *19*(3), 146–151. doi:10.1177/1078390313489729 PMID:23698977

Jeon, H., Lee, W., Park, H., Lee, H. J., Kim, S. K., Kim, H. B., ... Park, K. S. (2017). High-accuracy automatic classification of Parkinsonian tremor severity using machine learning method. *Physiological Measurement*, *38*(11), 1980–1999. doi:10.1088/1361-6579/aa8e1f PMID:28933707

Ji, Z., Xia, Y., Sun, Q., Chen, Q., & Feng, D. (2014). Adaptive scale fuzzy local Gaussian mixture model for brain MR image segmentation. *Neurocomputing*, *134*, 60–69. doi:10.1016/j.neucom.2012.12.067

John, E. R. (2002). The Neurophysics of Consciousness. *Brain Research. Brain Research Reviews*, *39*(1), 1–28. doi:10.1016/S0165-0173(02)00142-X PMID:12086706

Jonkman, J., de Weerd, A. W., Portvliet, D. C., Veldhuizen, R. J., van Duijn, H., Rozeman, C. A., & Laman, M. (1992). Neurometrics in cerebral ischemia and uremic encephalopathy. *Brain Topography*, *4*(4), 277–284. doi:10.1007/BF01135565 PMID:1510871

Joo, J. H., Hwang, S., Abu, H., & Gallo, J. J. (2016). An innovative model of depression care delivery: Peer mentors in collaboration with a mental health professional to relieve depression in older adults. *The American Journal of Geriatric Psychiatry*, *24*(5), 407–416. doi:10.1016/j.jagp.2016.02.002 PMID:27066731

Joo, J. H., Hwang, S., Gallo, J. J., & Roter, D. L. (2018). The impact of peer mentor communication with older adults on depressive symptoms and working alliance: A pilot study. *Patient Education and Counseling*, *101*(4), 665–671. doi:10.1016/j.pec.2017.10.012 PMID:29128295

Joormann, J., Cooney, R. E., Henry, M. L., & Gotlib, I. H. (2012). Neural correlates of automatic mood regulation in girls at high risk for depression. *Journal of Abnormal Psychology*, *121*(1), 61–72. doi:10.1037/a0025294 PMID:21895344

Joormann, J., & Gotlib, I. H. (2006). Is this happiness I see? Biases in the identification of emotional facial expressions in depression and social phobia. *Journal of Abnormal Psychology*, *115*(4), 705–714. doi:10.1037/0021-843X.115.4.705 PMID:17100528

Joormann, J., & Gotlib, I. H. (2007). Selective attention to emotional faces following recovery from depression. *Journal of Abnormal Psychology*, *116*(1), 80–85. doi:10.1037/0021-843X.116.1.80 PMID:17324018

Joormann, J., & Gotlib, I. H. (2008). Updating the contents of working memory in depression: Interference from irrelevant negative material. *Journal of Abnormal Psychology*, *117*(1), 182–192. doi:10.1037/0021-843X.117.1.182 PMID:18266496

Joormann, J., & Stanton, C. H. (2016). Examining emotion regulation in depression: A review and future directions. *Behaviour Research and Therapy*, *86*, 35–49. doi:10.1016/j.brat.2016.07.007 PMID:27492851

Jordan, M. I., & Mitchell, T. M. (2015). Machine learning: Trends, perspectives, and prospects. *Science*, *349*(6245), 255–260. doi:10.1126cience.aaa8415 PMID:26185243

Joutsijoki, H., Haponen, M., Rasku, J., Aalto-Setälä, K., & Juhola, M. (2016). Machine learning approach to automated quality identification of human induced pluripotent stem cell colony images. *Computational and Mathematical Methods in Medicine*, *2016*, 1–15. doi:10.1155/2016/3091039 PMID:27493680

Juneja, P., & Kashyap, R. (2016). Optimal approach for CT image segmentation using improved energy-based method. *International Journal of Control Theory and Applications*, *9*(41), 599–608.

Kähkönen, S., Yamashita, H., Rytsälä, H., Suominen, K., Ahveninen, J., & Isometsä, E. (2007). Dysfunction in early auditory processing in major depressive disorder revealed by combined MEG and EEG. *Journal of psychiatry & neuroscience. JPN*, *32*(5), 316. PMID:17823647

Kalogerakou, S., Tsaltas, E., Anyfandi, E., Papakosta, V. M., Kontis, D., Angelopoulos, E., ... Zervas, I. M. (2018). Neuropsychological profile as a marker of major depressive disorder subtypes: contribution to treatment strategy formulation. *Dialogues in Clinical Neuroscience & Mental Health, 1.*

Kang, H. J., Voleti, B., Hajszan, T., Rajkowska, G., Stockmeier, C. A., Licznerski, P., ... Son, H. (2012). Decreased expression of synapse-related genes and loss of synapses in major depressive disorder. *Nature Medicine*, *18*(9), 1413–1417. doi:10.1038/nm.2886 PMID:22885997

Kannathal, N., & Min Lim Choo, U. (2005). Entropies for detection of epilepsy in EEG. *Computer Methods and Programs in Biomedicine*, *80*(3), 187–194. doi:10.1016/j.cmpb.2005.06.012 PMID:16219385

Kanungo, T., Mount, D. M., Netanyahu, N. S., Piatko, C. D., Silverman, R., & Wu, A. Y. (2002). An efficient k-means clustering algorithm: Analysis and implementation. *IEEE Transactions on Pattern Analysis and Machine Intelligence*, *24*(7), 881–892. doi:10.1109/TPAMI.2002.1017616

Karaaslan, F., Gonul, A. S., Oguz, A., Erdinc, E., & Esel, E. (2003). P300 changes in major depressive disorders with and without psychotic features. *Journal of Affective Disorders*, *73*(3), 283–287. doi:10.1016/S0165-0327(01)00477-3 PMID:12547298

Kartal, E. (2015). *Sınıflandırmaya Dayalı Makine Öğrenmesi Teknikleri ve Kardiyolojik Risk Değerlendirmesine İlişkin Bir Uygulama* (Doctoral Dissertation). Ulusal Tez Merkezi. (No.394514)

Kashyap, R. (2019a). Security, Reliability, and Performance Assessment for Healthcare Biometrics. In D. Kisku, P. Gupta, & J. Sing (Eds.), Design and Implementation of Healthcare Biometric Systems (pp. 29-54). Hershey, PA: IGI Global. doi:10.4018/978-1-5225-7525-2.ch002

Kashyap, R. (2019b). Geospatial Big Data, Analytics, and IoT: Challenges, Applications, and Potential. In H. Das, R. Barik, H. Dubey & D. Sinha Roy (Eds.), Cloud Computing for Geospatial Big Data Analytics (pp. 191-213). Springer International Publishing.

Kashyap, R., & Piersson, A. (2018b). Big Data Challenges and Solutions in the Medical Industries. In Handbook of Research on Pattern Engineering System Development for Big Data Analytics. IGI Global. doi:10.4018/978-1-5225-3870-7.ch001

Kashyap, R., Gautam, P., & Tiwari, V. (2018). Management and Monitoring Patterns and Future Scope. In Handbook of Research on Pattern Engineering System Development for Big Data Analytics. IGI Global. doi:10.4018/978-1-5225-3870-7.ch014

Kashyap, R., & Gautam, P. (2015). Modified region based segmentation of medical images. *International Conference on Communication Networks (ICCN)*, 209–216. 10.1109/ICCN.2015.41

Kashyap, R., & Gautam, P. (2016). Fast level set method for segmentation of medical images. In *Proceedings of the International Conference on Informatics and Analytics (ICIA-16)*. ACM. 10.1145/2980258.2980302

Kashyap, R., & Gautam, P. (2017). Fast Medical Image Segmentation Using Energy-Based Method. *Biometrics, Concepts, Methodologies, Tools, and Applications*, *3*(1), 1017–1042. doi:10.4018/978-1-5225-0983-7.ch040

Kashyap, R., & Piersson, A. (2018a). *Impact of Big Data on Security. In Handbook of Research on Network Forensics and Analysis Techniques* (pp. 283–299). IGI Global. doi:10.4018/978-1-5225-4100-4.ch015

Kashyap, R., & Tiwari, V. (2018). Active contours using global models for medical image segmentation. *International Journal of Computational Systems Engineering*, *4*(2/3), 195. doi:10.1504/IJCSYSE.2018.091404

Kaur, M., Battisti, R. A., Lagopoulos, J., Ward, P. B., Hickie, I. B., & Hermens, D. F. (2012). Neurophysiological biomarkers support bipolar-spectrum disorders within psychosis cluster. *Journal of psychiatry & neuroscience. JPN*, *37*(5), 313–321. doi:10.1503/jpn.110081 PMID:22469054

Kaur, M., Battisti, R. A., Ward, P. B., Ahmed, A., Hickie, I. B., & Hermens, D. F. (2011). MMN/P3a deficits in first episode psychosis: Comparing schizophrenia-spectrum and affective-spectrum subgroups. *Schizophrenia Research*, *130*(1-3), 203–209. doi:10.1016/j.schres.2011.03.025 PMID:21550211

Kaustio, O., Partanen, J., Valkonen-Korhonen, M., Viinamäki, H., & Lehtonen, J. (2002). Affective and psychotic symptoms relate to different types of P300 alteration in depressive disorder. *Journal of Affective Disorders*, *71*(1-3), 43–50. doi:10.1016/S0165-0327(01)00410-4 PMID:12167500

Kemmerer, D. (2015). *Cognitive neuroscience of language*. Psychology Press.

Kessler, R. C., & Bromet, E. J. (2013). The epidemiology of depression across cultures. *Annual Review of Public Health*, *34*(1), 119–138. doi:10.1146/annurev-publhealth-031912-114409 PMID:23514317

Khazaee, A., Ebrahimzadeh, A., & Babajani-Feremi, A. (2016). Application of advanced machine learning methods on resting-state fMRI network for identification of mild cognitive impairment and Alzheimer's disease. *Brain Imaging and Behavior*, *10*(3), 799–817. doi:10.100711682-015-9448-7 PMID:26363784

Khedher, L., Ramírez, J., Górriz, J. M., Brahim, A., & Segovia, F. (2015). Early diagnosis of Alzheimer′ s disease based on partial least squares, principal component analysis and support vector machine using segmented MRI images. *Neurocomputing*, *151*, 139–150. doi:10.1016/j.neucom.2014.09.072

Kiang, M., Farzan, F., Blumberger, D. M., Kutas, M., McKinnon, M. C., Kansal, V., ... Daskalakis, Z. J. (2017). Abnormal self-schema in semantic memory in major depressive disorder: Evidence from event-related brain potentials. *Biological Psychology*, *126*, 41–47. doi:10.1016/j.biopsycho.2017.04.003 PMID:28385626

Kiehl, K. A., & Liddle, P. F. (2001). An event-related functional magnetic resonance imaging study of an auditory oddball task in schizophrenia. *Schizophrenia Research*, *48*(2-3), 159–171. doi:10.1016/S0920-9964(00)00117-1 PMID:11295369

Kikkert, L. H., De Groot, M. H., van Campen, J. P., Beijnen, J. H., Hortobágyi, T., Vuillerme, N., & Lamoth, C. C. (2017). Gait dynamics to optimize fall risk assessment in geriatric patients admitted to an outpatient diagnostic clinic. *PLoS One*, *12*(6), e0178615. doi:10.1371/journal.pone.0178615 PMID:28575126

Kim, J., Shin, H. S., Shin, K., & Lee, M. (2009). Robust algorithm for arrhythmia classification in ECG using extreme learning machine. *Biomedical Engineering Online*, *8*(1), 31. doi:10.1186/1475-925X-8-31 PMID:19863819

Kircanski, K., Joormann, J., & Gotlib, I. H. (2012). Cognitive aspects of depression. *Wiley Interdisciplinary Reviews: Cognitive Science*, *3*(3), 301–313. doi:10.1002/wcs.1177 PMID:23240069

Kissler, J., Herbert, C., Winkler, I., & Junghofer, M. (2009). Emotion and attention in visual word processing—An ERP study. *Biological Psychology, 80*(1), 75-83.

Kızrak, A. (n.d.). *Yapay Sinir Ağı Nedir?* Retrieved January 9, 2018, from https://medium.com/deep-learning-turkiye/%C5%9Fu-kara-kutuyu-a%C3%A7alim-yapay-sinir-a%C4%9Flar%C4%B1-7b65c6a5264a

Klimesch, W. (1999). EEG alpha and theta oscillations reflect cognitive and memory performance: A review and analysis. *Brain Research. Brain Research Reviews*, *29*(2-3), 169–195. doi:10.1016/S0165-0173(98)00056-3 PMID:10209231

Knight, R. T. (1996). Contribution of human hippocampal region to novelty detection. *Nature*, *383*(6597), 256–259. doi:10.1038/383256a0 PMID:8805701

Kohonen, T. (1990). The self-organizing map. *Proceedings of the IEEE*, *78*(9), 1464–1480. doi:10.1109/5.58325

Kohonen, T. (2013). Essentials of the self-organizing map. *Neural Networks*, *37*, 52–65. doi:10.1016/j.neunet.2012.09.018 PMID:23067803

Koolschijn, P. C. M., van Haren, N. E., Lensvelt-Mulders, G. J., Hulshoff Pol, H. E., & Kahn, R. S. (2009). Brain volume abnormalities in major depressive disorder: A meta-analysis of magnetic resonance imaging studies. *Human Brain Mapping*, *30*(11), 3719–3735. doi:10.1002/hbm.20801 PMID:19441021

Korn, C. W., Sharot, T., Walter, H., Heekeren, H. R., & Dolan, R. J. (2014). Depression is related to an absence of optimistically biased belief updating about future life events. *Psychological Medicine*, *44*(3), 579–592. doi:10.1017/S0033291713001074 PMID:23672737

Koschorke, M., Evans-Lacko, S., Sartorius, N., & Thornicroft, G. (2017). Stigma in different cultures. In The Stigma of Mental Illness-End of the Story? (pp. 67-82). Springer. doi:10.1007/978-3-319-27839-1_4

Kotsiantis, S. B., Zaharakis, I., & Pintelas, P. (2007). Supervised machine learning: A review of classification techniques. *Emerging Artificial Intelligence Applications in Computer Engineering, 160*, 3-24.

Koza, J. R., Bennett, F. H., Andre, D., & Keane, M. A. (1996). Automated Design of Both the Topology and Sizing of Analog Electrical Circuits Using Genetic Programming. In J. S. Gero & F. Sudweeks (Eds.), *Artificial Intelligence in Design '96* (pp. 151–170). Dordrecht: Springer Netherlands. doi:10.1007/978-94-009-0279-4_9

Krawczyk, B., Galar, M., Jelen, L., & Herrera, F. (2016). Evolutionary undersampling boosting for imbalanced classification of breast cancer malignancy. *Applied Soft Computing*, *38*, 714–726. doi:10.1016/j.asoc.2015.08.060

Kriesel, D. (2005). A Brief Introduction to Neural Networks. Academic Press.

Kroemer, K., & Kroemer-Elbert, E. (2001). *Ergonomics: How to Design for Ease and Efficiency*. Englewood Cliffs, NJ: Prentice Hall.

Kubat, M., & Matwin, S. (1997). Addressing the curse of imbalanced training sets: one-sided selection. *Proc. Fourteenth International Conference on Machine Learning*, 179-186.

Kullmann, F., Hollerbach, S., Lock, G., Holstege, A., Dierks, T., & Scholmerich, J. (2001). Brain electrical activity mapping of EEG for the diagnosis of (sub)clinical hepatic encephalopathy in chronic liver disease. *European Journal of Gastroenterology & Hepatology*, *13*(5), 513–522. doi:10.1097/00042737-200105000-00009 PMID:11396530

Kumar, S., & Singh, M. (2019). Big data analytics for healthcare industry: Impact, applications, and tools. *Big Data Mining and Analytics*, *2*(1), 48–57. doi:10.26599/BDMA.2018.9020031

Lahmiri, S., Dawson, D. A., & Shmuel, A. (2018). Performance of machine learning methods in diagnosing Parkinson's disease based on dysphonia measures. *Biomedical Engineering Letters*, *8*(1), 29–39. doi:10.100713534-017-0051-2 PMID:30603188

Lannin, D. G., Vogel, D. L., Brenner, R. E., Abraham, W. T., & Heath, P. J. (2016). Does self-stigma reduce the probability of seeking mental health information? *Journal of Counseling Psychology*, *63*(3), 351–358. doi:10.1037/cou0000108 PMID:26323042

Lecardeur, L., Briand, C., Prouteau, A., Lalonde, P., Nicole, L., Lesage, A., & Stip, E. (2009). Preserved awareness of their cognitive deficits in patients with schizophrenia: Convergent validity of the SSTICS. *Schizophrenia Research*, *107*(2-3), 303–306. doi:10.1016/j.schres.2008.09.003 PMID:18835134

LeCun, Y., Bengio, Y., & Hinton, G. (2015). Deep Learning. *Nature*, *521*(7553), 436–444. doi:10.1038/nature14539 PMID:26017442

Lee, E. J., Kim, Y. H., Kim, N., & Kang, D. W. (2017). Deep into the brain: Artificial intelligence in stroke imaging. *Journal of Stroke*, *19*(3), 277–285. doi:10.5853/jos.2017.02054 PMID:29037014

Legg, T. J. (2018). Is neurofeedback effective for treating ADHD. *Medical News Today*. Retrieved from https://www.medicalnewstoday.com/articles/315261.php

Lejoyeux, M., & Lehert, P. (2010). Alcohol-use disorders and depression: Results from individual patient data meta-analysis of the acamprosate-controlled studies. *Alcohol and Alcoholism (Oxford, Oxfordshire)*, *46*(1), 61–67. doi:10.1093/alcalc/agq077 PMID:21118900

Lemmens, L. H., van Bronswijk, S. C., Peeters, F., Arntz, A., Hollon, S. D., & Huibers, M. J. (2018). Long-term outcomes of acute treatment with cognitive therapy v. interpersonal psychotherapy for adult depression: Follow-up of a randomized controlled trial. *Psychological Medicine*, 1–9. PMID:29792234

LeMoult, J., & Gotlib, I. H. (2018). Depression: A cognitive perspective. *Clinical Psychology Review*. doi:10.1016/j.cpr.2018.06.008 PMID:29961601

LeMoult, J., Kircanski, K., Prasad, G., & Gotlib, I. H. (2017). Negative self-referential processing predicts the recurrence of major depressive episodes. *Clinical Psychological Science*, *5*(1), 174–181. doi:10.1177/2167702616654898 PMID:28286705

LeMoult, J., Yoon, K. L., & Joormann, J. (2012). Affective priming in major depressive disorder. *Frontiers in Integrative Neuroscience*, *6*, 76. doi:10.3389/fnint.2012.00076 PMID:23060758

Lennon, S., & Stokes, M. (2009). *Pocket book of Neurologcial physciotherapy*. Elsevier Publication.

Leung, K. M. (2007). *Naive Bayesian classifier*. Polytechnic University Department of Computer Science/Finance and Risk Engineering.

Leuthardt, E., Schalk, G., Wolpaw, J., Ojemann, J., & Moran, D. (2004). A brain–computer interface using electrocorticographic signals in humans. *Journal of Neural Engineering*, *1*(2), 63–71. doi:10.1088/1741-2560/1/2/001 PMID:15876624

Levens, S. M., & Gotlib, I. H. (2009). Impaired selection of relevant positive information in depression. *Depression and Anxiety*, *26*(5), 403–410. doi:10.1002/da.20565 PMID:19347861

Levens, S. M., & Gotlib, I. H. (2010). Updating positive and negative stimuli in working memory in depression. *Journal of Experimental Psychology. General*, *139*(4), 654–664. doi:10.1037/a0020283 PMID:21038984

Levens, S. M., & Phelps, E. A. (2008). Emotion processing effects on interference resolution in working memory. *Emotion (Washington, D.C.)*, *8*(2), 267–280. doi:10.1037/1528-3542.8.2.267 PMID:18410200

Levine, D., Richards, J., & Whittle, M. W. (2012). *Whittle's Gait Analysis-E-Book*. Elsevier Health Sciences.

Li & Li. (2013). Online Finger Gesture Recognition Using Surface Electromyography Signals. *Journal of Signal and Information Processing, 4*(2).

Li, B. J., Friston, K., Mody, M., Wang, H. N., Lu, H. B., & Hu, D. W. (2018). A brain network model for depression: From symptom understanding to disease intervention. *CNS Neuroscience & Therapeutics*, *24*(11), 1004–1019. doi:10.1111/cns.12998 PMID:29931740

Li, D.-C., Liu, C.-W., & Hu, S. C. (2010). A learning method for the class imbalance problem with medical data sets. *Computers in Biology and Medicine*, *40*(5), 509–518. doi:10.1016/j.compbiomed.2010.03.005 PMID:20347072

Li, J., Ritter, A., & Hovy, E. (2014). Weakly supervised user profile extraction from Twitter. *Proceedings of ACL*. 10.3115/v1/P14-1016

Likas, A., Vlassis, N., & Verbeek, J. J. (2003). The global k-means clustering algorithm. *Pattern Recognition*, *36*(2), 451–461. doi:10.1016/S0031-3203(02)00060-2

Lin, G., Wang, W., Kang, C., & Wang, C. (2012). Multispectral MR images segmentation based on fuzzy knowledge and modified seeded region growing. *Magnetic Resonance Imaging*, *30*(2), 230–246. doi:10.1016/j.mri.2011.09.008 PMID:22133286

Lin, L. Y., Sidani, J. E., Shensa, A., Radovic, A., Miller, E., Colditz, J. B., ... Primack, B. A. (2016). Association between Social Media use and Depression among U.S. young adults. *Depression and Anxiety*, *33*(4), 323–331. doi:10.1002/da.22466 PMID:26783723

Lisak, R. P., Truong, D. D., Carroll, W. M., & Bhidayasiri, R. (Eds.). (2016). *International Neurology*. John Wiley & Sons. doi:10.1002/9781118777329

Little, M. A., McSharry, P. E., Roberts, S. J., Costello, D. A., & Moroz, I. M. (2007). Exploiting nonlinear recurrence and fractal scaling properties for voice disorder detection. *Biomedical Engineering Online*, *6*(1), 23. doi:10.1186/1475-925X-6-23 PMID:17594480

Liu, S., Liu, S., Cai, W., Pujol, S., Kikinis, R., & Feng, D. (2014, April). Early diagnosis of Alzheimer's disease with deep learning. In *Biomedical Imaging (ISBI), 2014 IEEE 11th International Symposium on* (pp. 1015-1018). IEEE. 10.1109/ISBI.2014.6868045

Liu, R. J., & Aghajanian, G. K. (2008). Stress blunts serotonin-and hypocretin-evoked EPSCs in prefrontal cortex: Role of corticosterone-mediated apical dendritic atrophy. *Proceedings of the National Academy of Sciences of the United States of America*, *105*(1), 359–364. doi:10.1073/pnas.0706679105 PMID:18172209

Liu, S., Shen, Z., McKeown, M. J., Leung, C., & Miao, C. (2014, July). A fuzzy logic based parkinson's disease risk predictor. In *Proceedings of IEEE International Conference on Fuzzy Systems* (pp. 1624-1631). IEEE. 10.1109/FUZZ-IEEE.2014.6891613

Liu, W. H., Huang, J., Wang, L. Z., Gong, Q. Y., & Chan, R. C. (2012). Facial perception bias in patients with major depression. *Psychiatry Research*, *197*(3), 217–220. doi:10.1016/j.psychres.2011.09.021 PMID:22357354

Liu, W., Liang, W., & Xu, S. (2011). More information in imaging examination. *European Journal of Radiology*, *80*(2), 325. doi:10.1016/j.ejrad.2010.12.026 PMID:21255954

Liu, Y., Spulber, G., Lehtimäki, K. K., Könönen, M., Hallikainen, I., Gröhn, H., ... Soininen, H. (2011). Diffusion tensor imaging and tract-based spatial statistics in Alzheimer's disease and mild cognitive impairment. *Neurobiology of Aging*, *32*(9), 1558–1571. doi:10.1016/j.neurobiolaging.2009.10.006 PMID:19913331

Li, Y., Lenaghan, S. C., & Zhang, M. (2012). A data-driven predictive approach for drug delivery using machine learning techniques. *PLoS One*, *7*(2), e31724. doi:10.1371/journal.pone.0031724 PMID:22384063

Lledó, L. D., Badesa, F. J., Almonacid, M., Cano-Izquierdo, J. M., Sabater-Navarro, J. M., Fernández, E., & Garcia-Aracil, N. (2015). Supervised and dynamic neuro-fuzzy systems to classify physiological responses in robot-assisted neurorehabilitation. *PLoS One*, *10*(5), e0127777. doi:10.1371/journal.pone.0127777 PMID:26001214

Lloyd, S., Mohseni, M., & Rebentrost, P. (2013). *Quantum algorithms for supervised and unsupervised machine learning*. arXiv preprint arXiv:1307.0411

Lo, C. L., & Tseng, H. T. (2017). Predicting rehabilitation treatment helpfulness to stroke patients: A supervised learning approach. *Artificial Intelligence Review*, *6*(2), 1. doi:10.5430/air.v6n2p1

Lohaugen, G. C., Beneventi, H., & Andersen, G. L. (2014). Do children with cerebral palsy benefit from computerized working memory training – Study protocol for a randomized controlled trail. *BioMed Central*, *15*(269), 2–9.

Long, B., & Koyfman, A. (2018). Secondary Gains: Advances in Neurotrauma Management. *Emergency Medicine Clinics of North America*, *36*(1), 107–133. doi:10.1016/j.emc.2017.08.007 PMID:29132572

Lorenzetti, V., Allen, N. B., Whittle, S., & Yücel, M. (2010). Amygdala volumes in a sample of current depressed and remitted depressed patients and healthy controls. *Journal of Affective Disorders*, *120*(1-3), 112–119. doi:10.1016/j.jad.2009.04.021 PMID:19464062

Lorraine, V. K., & Anthony, E. L. (2015). Parkinson's disease. *Lancet*, *386*(9996), 896–912. doi:10.1016/S0140-6736(14)61393-3 PMID:25904081

Lotte, F., Congedo, M., Lsecuyer, A., Lamarche, F., & Arnaldi, B. (2007). A Review of Classification Algorithms for EEG-based Brain-Computer Interfaces. *Journal of Neural Engineering*, *4*(2), 1–13. doi:10.1088/1741-2560/4/2/R01 PMID:17409472

Louis, E. D. (2014). Re-thinking the biology of essential tremor: from models to morphology. *Parkinsonism & Related Disorders, 20*, S88-S93. Retrieved from https://www.techleer.com/articles/203-machine-learning-algorithm-backbone-of-emerging-technologies/ files/74/203-machine-learning-algorithm-backbone-of-emerging-technologies.html

Louis, D. N., Ohgaki, H., Wiestler, O. D., Cavenee, W. K., Burger, P. C., Jouvet, A., ... Kleihues, P. (2007). The 2007 WHO Classification of Tumours of the Central Nervous System. *Acta Neuropathologica*, *114*(2), 97–109. doi:10.100700401-007-0243-4 PMID:17618441

Lowe, B., Kroenke, K., Herzog, W., & Grafe, K. (2004). Measuring depression outcome with a brief self-report instrument: Sensitivity to change of the Patient Health Questionnaire (PHQ-9). *Journal of Affective Disorders*, *81*(1), 61–66. doi:10.1016/S0165-0327(03)00198-8 PMID:15183601

Lubar, J. F. (1997). Neocortical Dynamics: Implications for Understanding the Role of Neurofeedback and Related Techniques for the Enhancement of Attention. *Applied Psychophysiology and Biofeedback*, *22*(2), 111–126. doi:10.1023/A:1026276228832 PMID:9341967

Luck, S. J. (2014). *An introduction to the event-related potential technique*. MIT Press.

Luck, S. J., & Kappenman, E. S. (Eds.). (2011). *The Oxford handbook of event-related potential components*. Oxford University Press.

Luu, P., Tucker, D. M., & Makeig, S. (2004). Frontal midline theta and the error-related negativity: Neurophysiological mechanisms of action regulation. *Clinical Neurophysiology*, *115*(8), 1821–1835. doi:10.1016/j.clinph.2004.03.031 PMID:15261861

Machine Learning Algorithms Mindmap. (2015). Retrieved from https://jixta.wordpress.com/2015/07/17/machine-learning-algorithms-mindmap/

MacQueen, G., & Frodl, T. (2011). The hippocampus in major depression: Evidence for the convergence of the bench and bedside in psychiatric research? *Molecular Psychiatry*, *16*(3), 252–264. doi:10.1038/mp.2010.80 PMID:20661246

Madsen, K. H., Krohne, L. G., Cai, X. L., Wang, Y., & Chan, R. C. (2018). Perspectives on Machine Learning for Classification of Schizotypy Using fMRI Data. *Schizophrenia Bulletin*, *44*(suppl_2), S480–S490. doi:10.1093chbulby026 PMID:29554367

Maity, N. G., & Das, S. (2017, March). Machine learning for improved diagnosis and prognosis in healthcare. In *Aerospace Conference, 2017 IEEE* (pp. 1-9). IEEE. 10.1109/AERO.2017.7943950

Manlhiot, C. (2018). Machine learning for predictive analytics in medicine: Real opportunity or overblown hype? *European Heart Journal Cardiovascular Imaging*, *19*(7), 727–728. doi:10.1093/ehjci/jey041 PMID:29538756

Mannini, A., Trojaniello, D., Cereatti, A., & Sabatini, A. M. (2016). A machine learning framework for gait classification using inertial sensors: Application to elderly, post-stroke and huntington's disease patients. *Sensors (Basel)*, *16*(1), 134. doi:10.339016010134 PMID:26805847

Mao, W., Wang, Y., & Wang, D. (2005). Cognitive impairment in major depressive disorder revealed by event-related potential N270. *Clinical EEG and Neuroscience*, *36*(1), 9–14. doi:10.1177/155005940503600104 PMID:15683192

Marjama-Lyons, J., & Koller, W. (2000). Tremor-predominant Parkinson's disease. *Drugs & Aging*, *16*(4), 273–278. doi:10.2165/00002512-200016040-00003 PMID:10874522

Mathur, N., Mathur, S., & Mathur, D. (2016). A Novel Approach to Improve Sobel Edge Detector. *Procedia Computer Science*, *93*, 431–438. doi:10.1016/j.procs.2016.07.230

Mathworks. (n.d.). *What is Machine Learning?* Retrieved May 6, 2018, from https://www.mathworks.com/discovery/machine-learning.html

MATLAB User's Guide: R2016a Documentation. (2016). Natick, MA: MathWorks Inc.

Matsushima, A., Yoshida, K., Genno, H., & Ikeda, S. I. (2017). Principal component analysis for ataxic gait using a triaxial accelerometer *Journal of Neuroengineering and Rehabilitation*, *14*(1), 37. doi:10.118612984-017-0249-7 PMID:28464831

Mayberg, H. S. (1997). Limbic-cortical dysregulation: A proposed model of depression. *The Journal of Neuropsychiatry and Clinical Neurosciences*, *9*, 471–481. PubMed

Mayberg, H. S. (2009). Targeted electrode-based modulation of neural circuits for depression. *The Journal of Clinical Investigation*, *119*(4), 717–725. doi:10.1172/JCI38454 PMID:19339763

McCabe, R., Garside, R., Backhouse, A., & Xanthopoulou, P. (2018). Effectiveness of brief psychological interventions for suicidal presentations: A systematic review. *BMC Psychiatry*, *18*(1), 120. doi:10.118612888-018-1663-5 PMID:29724203

McDermott, B., O'Halloran, M., Porter, E., & Santorelli, A. (2018). Brain haemorrhage detection using a SVM classifier with electrical impedance tomography measurement frames. *PLoS One*, *13*(7), e0200469. doi:10.1371/journal.pone.0200469 PMID:30001401

McEwen, B. S. (2012). The ever-changing brain: Cellular and molecular mechanisms for the effects of stressful experiences. *Developmental Neurobiology*, *72*(6), 878–890. doi:10.1002/dneu.20968 PMID:21898852

McFarquhar, T., Luyten, P., & Fonagy, P. (2018). Changes in interpersonal problems in the psychotherapeutic treatment of depression as measured by the Inventory of Interpersonal Problems: A systematic review and meta-analysis. *Journal of Affective Disorders*, *226*, 108–123. doi:10.1016/j.jad.2017.09.036 PMID:28968563

McPhail, G. (2017). Constructivism: Clearing up the confusion between a theory of learning and "constructing" knowledge. *Set: Research Information For Teachers*, (2), 30-22. doi:10.18296et.0081

Medications, F. (2016). *Causes of Parkinson's Disease*. Retrieved from https://www.atrainceu.com/course-module-short-view/1874200-080_antiparkinson-strategies-module-03

Megan, A. (2011). Feeling bad on Facebook: Depression disclosures by college students on a social networking site. *Depression and Anxiety*, *28*(6), 447–455. doi:10.1002/da.20805 PMID:21400639

Mehl, M. R., Raison, C. L., Pace, T. W., Arevalo, J. M., & Cole, S. W. (2017). Natural language indicators of differential gene regulation in the human immune system. *Proceedings of the National Academy of Sciences of the United States of America*, *114*(47), 12554–12559. doi:10.1073/pnas.1707373114 PMID:29109260

Mei, P. A., Carneiro, C. D., Fraser, S. J., Min, L. L., & Reis, F. (2015). Analysis of neoplastic lesions in magnetic resonance imaging using self-organizing maps. *Journal of the Neurological Sciences*, *359*(1-2), 78–83. doi:10.1016/j.jns.2015.10.032 PMID:26671090

Melin, P., & Sánchez, D. (2017). Multi-objective optimization for modular granular neural networks applied to pattern recognition. *Information Sciences*. doi:10.1016/j.ins.2017.09.031

Mendlewicz, L., Linkowski, P., Bazelmans, C., & Philippot, P. (2005). Decoding emotional facial expressions in depressed and anorexic patients. *Journal of Affective Disorders*, *89*(1-3), 195–199. doi:10.1016/j.jad.2005.07.010 PMID:16256204

Mi, H., Petitjean, C., Vera, P., & Ruan, S. (2015). Joint tumor growth prediction and tumor segmentation on therapeutic follow-up PET images. *Medical Image Analysis*, *23*(1), 84–91. doi:10.1016/j.media.2015.04.016 PMID:25988489

Milanov, I. (2001). Electromyographic differentiation of tremors. *Clinical Neurophysiology*, *112*(9), 1626–1632. doi:10.1016/S1388-2457(01)00629-0 PMID:11514245

Milders, M., Bell, S., Platt, J., Serrano, R., & Runcie, O. (2010). Stable expression recognition abnormalities in unipolar depression. *Psychiatry Research*, *179*(1), 38–42. doi:10.1016/j.psychres.2009.05.015 PMID:20478626

Miles-Tribble, V. (2017). Restorative justice as a public theology imperative. *Review & Expositor*, *114*(3), 366–379. doi:10.1177/0034637317721704

Millán, J., Renkens, F., Mouriño, J., & Gerstner, W. (2003). Non-Invasive Brain-Actuated Control of a Mobile Robot. *Proceedings of the 18th International Joint Conference on Artificial Intelligence.*

Mingle, D. (2017). Machine Learning Techniques on Microbiome -Based Diagnostics. *Advances In Biotechnology & Microbiology*, *6*(4). doi:10.19080/AIBM.2017.06.555695

Miranda, E., Irwansyah, E., Amelga, A. Y., Maribondang, M. M., & Salim, M. (2016). Detection of cardiovascular disease risk's level for adults using naive Bayes classifier. *Healthcare Informatics Research*, *22*(3), 196–205. doi:10.4258/hir.2016.22.3.196 PMID:27525161

Mitchell, T. M. (1997). Machine learning. Burr Ridge, IL: McGraw Hill.

Mitchell, T. M. (2006). *The discipline of machine learning* (Vol. 9). Pittsburgh, PA: Carnegie Mellon University, School of Computer Science, Machine Learning Department.

Miyagi, T. (2009). Estimation of Inter-regional Trade Coefficients Using Neural Network Models. *Studies In Regional Science*, *39*(3), 519–538. doi:10.2457rs.39.519

Mnih, V., Badia, A. P., Mirza, M., Graves, A., Lillicrap, T., Harley, T., . . . Kavukcuoglu, K. (2016). *Asynchronous methods for deep reinforcement learning.* Paper presented at the International conference on machine learning.

Mohamed, G. S. (2016). Parkinson's Disease Diagnosis: Detecting the Effect of Attributes Selection and Discretization of Parkinson's Disease Dataset on the Performance of Classifier Algorithms. *Open Access Library Journal*, *3*, 1–11.

More, A. (2016). *Survey of resampling techniques for improving classification performance in unbalanced datasets.* Cornel University Library.

Morgan, C., Mason, E., Newby, J. M., Mahoney, A. E., Hobbs, M. J., McAloon, J., & Andrews, G. (2017). The effectiveness of unguided internet cognitive behavioural therapy for mixed anxiety and depression. *Internet Interventions*, *10*, 47–53. doi:10.1016/j.invent.2017.10.003 PMID:30135752

Morphological Image Processing. (n.d.). Retrieved from https://www.cs.auckland.ac.nz/courses/compsci773s1c/lectures/ImageProcessing-html/topic4.htm

Mouradian, M. M. (Ed.). (2001). *Parkinson's Disease: Methods and Protocols* (Vol. 62). Springer Science & Business Media. doi:10.1385/1592591426

Mumtaz, W., Ali, S. S. A., Yasin, M. A. M., & Malik, A. S. (2018). A machine learning framework involving EEG-based functional connectivity to diagnose major depressive disorder (MDD). *Medical & Biological Engineering & Computing*, *56*(2), 233–246. doi:10.100711517-017-1685-z PMID:28702811

Murphy, K. P. (2006). *Naive Bayes classifiers, Technical Report.* Available: http://www.cs.ubc.ca/murphyk/ Teaching/CS 340 - Fall 06 /reading/NB.pdf

Mutula, S. (2009). Ethical, Legal, and Social Issues in Medical Informatics. Hershey, PA: IGI Global.

Mu, Z., Chang, Y., Xu, J., Pang, X., Zhang, H., Liu, X., ... Wan, Y. (2016). Pre-attentive dysfunction of musical processing in major depressive disorder: A mismatch negativity study. *Journal of Affective Disorders, 194*, 50–56. doi:10.1016/j.jad.2016.01.028 PMID:26802507

Näätänen, R., & Kreegipuu, K. (2011). The Mismatch negativity (MMN). In S. Kappenman & S. J. Luck (Eds.), The Oxford Handbook of Event-Related Potential Components (pp. 143-158). Oxford University Press.

Näätänen, R., Kujala, T., Kreegipuu, K., Carlson, S., Escera, C., Baldeweg, T., & Ponton, C. (2011). The mismatch negativity: An index of cognitive decline in neuropsychiatric and neurological diseases and in ageing. *Brain, 134*(12), 3435–3453. doi:10.1093/brain/awr064 PMID:21624926

Naimur Rahman, M., Esmailpour, A., & Zhao, J. (2016). Machine Learning with Big Data An Efficient Electricity Generation Forecasting System. *Big Data Research, 5*, 9–15. doi:10.1016/j.bdr.2016.02.002

Naismith, S. L., Mowszowski, L., Ward, P. B., Diamond, K., Paradise, M., Kaur, M., ... Hermens, D. F. (2012). Reduced temporal mismatch negativity in late-life depression: An event-related potential index of cognitive deficit and functional disability? *Journal of Affective Disorders, 138*(1-2), 71–78. doi:10.1016/j.jad.2011.12.028 PMID:22301116

Nan, C., Wang, G., Wang, H., Wang, X., Liu, Z., Xiao, L., ... Wu, S. (2018). The P300 component decreases in a bimodal oddball task in individuals with depression: An event-related potentials study. *Clinical Neurophysiology, 129*(12), 2525–2533. doi:10.1016/j.clinph.2018.09.012 PMID:30366168

Nasehi, S., & Pourghassem, H. (2011). Epileptic seizure onset detection algorithm using dynamic cascade feed-forward neural networks. *2011 International Conference on Intelligent Computation and Bio-Medical Instrumentation (ICBMI)*, 196–199. 10.1109/ICBMI.2011.59

National Institute of Mental Health. (2015). Retrieved from https://www.nih.gov/about-nih/what-we-do/nih-almanac/national-institute-mental-health-nimh

Nguyen, T.-N., Lars, G., & Zeno, S-T. (2010). Cost-Sensitive Learning Methods for Imbalanced Data. *Int. Joint Conference on Neural Networks.*

Nicolas-Alonso, L., Corralejo, R., Gomez-Pilar, J., Álvarez, D., & Hornero, R. (2015). Adaptive Stacked Generalization for Multiclass Motor Imagery-Based Brain Computer Interfaces. *IEEE Transactions on Neural Systems and Rehabilitation Engineering, 23*(4), 702–712. doi:10.1109/TNSRE.2015.2398573 PMID:25680208

Nidal, K., & Malik, A. S. (2017). *EEG/ERP Analysis method and applications.* Boca Raton, FL: CRC Press.

Nigam, V. P., & Graupe, D. (2004). A neural-network-based detection of epilepsy. *Neurological Research, 26*(1), 55–60. doi:10.1179/016164104773026534 PMID:14977058

Nilashi, M., Ibrahim, O., & Ahani, A. (2016). Accuracy improvement for predicting Parkinson's disease progression. *Scientific Reports, 6*(1), 34181. doi:10.1038rep34181 PMID:27686748

Nilashi, M., Ibrahim, O., Ahmadi, H., Shahmoradi, L., & Farahmand, M. (2018). A hybrid intelligent system for the prediction of Parkinson's Disease progression using machine learning techniques. *Biocybernetics and Biomedical Engineering, 38*(1), 1–15. doi:10.1016/j.bbe.2017.09.002

Nimeesha, K.M., & Gowda, R.M. (2013). Brain tumour segmentation using Kmeans and fuzzy c-means clustering algorithm. *Int J Comput Sci Inf Technol Res Excell*, 60–65.

Nind, M. (2007). Supporting lifelong learning for people with profound and multiple learning difficulties. *Support for Learning*, *22*(3), 111–115. doi:10.1111/j.1467-9604.2007.00457.x

Nukala, B. T., Nakano, T., Rodriguez, A., Tsay, J., Lopez, J., Nguyen, T. Q., ... Lie, D. Y. (2016). Real-time classification of patients with balance disorders vs. normal subjects using a low-cost small wireless wearable gait sensor. *Biosensors*, *6*(4), 58. doi:10.3390/bios6040058 PMID:27916817

Nyer, M., Roberg, R., Nauphal, M., & Streeter, C. C. (2019). Yoga as a Treatment for Depression. In *The Massachusetts General Hospital Guide to Depression* (pp. 223–231). Cham: Humana Press. doi:10.1007/978-3-319-97241-1_17

O'Leary, D. E. (2013). Artificial intelligence and big data. *IEEE Intelligent Systems*, *28*(2), 96–99. doi:10.1109/MIS.2013.39 PMID:25505373

O'Sullivan, P. (2005). Diagnosis and classification of chronic low back pain disorders: Maladaptive movement and motor control impairment as underlying mechanism. *Manual Therapy*, *10*(4), 242–255. doi:10.1016/j.math.2005.07.001 PMID:16154380

Ogura, C., Nageishi, Y., Omura, F., Fukao, K., Ohta, H., Kishimoto, A., & Matsubayashi, M. (1993). N200 component of event-related potentials in depression. *Biological Psychiatry*, *33*(10), 720–726. doi:10.1016/0006-3223(93)90122-T PMID:8353167

Olanrewaju, R. F., Sahari, N. S., Musa, A. A., & Hakiem, N. (2014). Application of Neural Networks in Early Detection and Diagnosis of Parkinson's Disease. *Proc. of Int. Conf. on Cyber and IT service Mang. (CITSM)*, 78-82.

Ollila, P., Knekt, P., Heinonen, E., & Lindfors, O. (2016). Patients' pre-treatment interpersonal problems as predictors of therapeutic alliance in long-term psychodynamic psychotherapy. *Psychiatry Research*, *241*, 110–117. doi:10.1016/j.psychres.2016.04.093 PMID:27173654

Olofsson, J. K., Nordin, S., Sequeira, H., & Polich, J. (2008). Affective picture processing: An integrative review of ERP findings. *Biological Psychology*, *77*(3), 247–265. doi:10.1016/j.biopsycho.2007.11.006 PMID:18164800

Onose, G., Grozea, C., Anghelescu, A., Daia, C., Sinescu, C., Ciurea, A., ... Popescu, F. (2012). On the feasibility of using motor imagery EEG-based brain-computer interface in chronic tetraplegics for assistive robotic arm control: A clinical test and long-term post-trial follow-up. *Spinal Cord*, *50*(8), 599–608. doi:10.1038c.2012.14 PMID:22410845

Ornelas-Vences, C., Sanchez-Fernandez, L. P., Sanchez-Perez, L. A., Garza-Rodriguez, A., & Villegas-Bastida, A. (2017). Fuzzy inference model evaluating turn for Parkinson's disease patients. *Computers in Biology and Medicine*, *89*, 379–388. doi:10.1016/j.compbiomed.2017.08.026 PMID:28866303

Otte, C., Gold, S. M., Penninx, B. W., Pariante, C. M., Etkin, A., Fava, M., ... Schatzberg, A. F. (2016). Major depressive disorder. *Nature Reviews. Disease Primers*, *2*, 16065. doi:10.1038/nrdp.2016.65 PMID:27629598

Oussous, A., Benjelloun, F. Z., Lahcen, A. A., & Belfkih, S. (2018). Big Data technologies: A survey. *Journal of King Saud University-Computer and Information Sciences*, *30*(4), 431–448. doi:10.1016/j.jksuci.2017.06.001

Özköse, H., Arı, E. S., & Gencer, C. (2015). Yesterday, today and tomorrow of big data. *Procedia: Social and Behavioral Sciences*, *195*, 1042–1050. doi:10.1016/j.sbspro.2015.06.147

Pagani, G., Cekic, M., & Guo, Y. (2008). "Thinking about not thinking": Neural correlates of conceptual processing during Zen meditation. *PLoS One*, *3*(9), e3083. doi:10.1371/journal.pone.0003083 PMID:18769538

Pahwa, R. (Ed.). (2013). *Handbook of Parkinson's Disease*. London: CRC Press. doi:10.3109/9781841849096

Palojoki, S., Pajunen, T., Saranto, K., & Lehtonen, L. (2016). Electronic Health Record-Related Safety Concerns: A Cross-Sectional Survey of Electronic Health Record Users. *JMIR Medical Informatics*, *4*(2), e13. doi:10.2196/medinform.5238 PMID:27154599

Pandav, S. (2014). Brain tumor extraction using marker controlled watershed segmentation. *Int J Eng Res Technol.*

Pang, X., Xu, J., Chang, Y., Tang, D., Zheng, Y., Liu, Y., & Sun, Y. (2014). Mismatch negativity of sad syllables is absent in patients with major depressive disorder. *PLoS One*, *9*(3), e91995. doi:10.1371/journal.pone.0091995 PMID:24658084

Parisi, L., RaviChandran, N., & Manaog, M. L. (2018). Feature-driven machine learning to improve early diagnosis of Parkinson's disease. *Expert Systems with Applications*, *110*, 182–190. doi:10.1016/j.eswa.2018.06.003

Park, E., Chang, H. J., & Nam, H. S. (2017). Use of Machine Learning Classifiers and Sensor Data to Detect Neurological Deficit in Stroke Patients. *Journal of Medical Internet Research*, *19*(4), e120. doi:10.2196/jmir.7092 PMID:28420599

Patel, J. A., & Sharma, P. (2014, August). Big data for better health planning. In *2014 International Conference on Advances in Engineering and Technology Research (ICAETR)* (pp. 1-5). Unnao: IEEE.

Patel, Z. M. (2017). The evidence for olfactory training in treating patients with olfactory loss. *Current Opinion in Otolaryngology & Head & Neck Surgery*, *25*(1), 43–46. doi:10.1097/MOO.0000000000000328 PMID:27841770

Pause, B. M., Raack, N., Sojka, B., Göder, R., Aldenhoff, J. B., & Ferstl, R. (2003). Convergent and divergent effects of odors and emotions in depression. *Psychophysiology*, *40*(2), 209–225. doi:10.1111/1469-8986.00023 PMID:12820862

Pavlenko, A. (2005). *Emotions and multilingualism*. Cambridge, UK: Cambridge University Press.

Pavlenko, A. (2006). *Bilingual minds: Emotional experience, expression, and representation*. New York: Multilingual Matters. doi:10.21832/9781853598746

Pearl, R. L., Forgeard, M. J., Rifkin, L., Beard, C., & Björgvinsson, T. (2017). Internalized stigma of mental illness: Changes and associations with treatment outcomes. *Stigma and Health*, *2*(1), 2–15. doi:10.1037ah0000036

Pedrosa, T. Í., Vasconcelos, F. F., Medeiros, L., & Silva, L. D. (2018). Machine Learning Application to Quantify the Tremor Level for Parkinson's Disease Patients. *Procedia Computer Science*, *138*, 215–220. doi:10.1016/j.procs.2018.10.031

Pennebaker, J. W., & Graybeal, A. (2001). Patterns of natural language use: Disclosure, personality, and social integration. *Current Directions in Psychological Science*, *10*(3), 90–93. doi:10.1111/1467-8721.00123

Pennebaker, J. W., Mehl, M. R., & Niederhoffer, K. G. (2003). Psychological aspects of natural language use: Our words, our selves. *Annual Review of Psychology*, *54*(1), 547–577. doi:10.1146/annurev.psych.54.101601.145041 PMID:12185209

Pennebaker, J. W., & Stone, L. D. (2003). Words of wisdom: Language use over the life span. *Journal of Personality and Social Psychology*, *85*(2), 291–301. doi:10.1037/0022-3514.85.2.291 PMID:12916571

Penninx, B. W., Nolen, W. A., Lamers, F., Zitman, F. G., Smit, J. H., Spinhoven, P., ... Verhaak, P. (2011). Two-year course of depressive and anxiety disorders: Results from the Netherlands Study of Depression and Anxiety (NESDA). *Journal of Affective Disorders*, *133*(1-2), 76–85. doi:10.1016/j.jad.2011.03.027 PMID:21496929

Penniston, E. G., & Kulkosky, P. J. (1989). Alpha-theta brainwave training and betaendorphin levels in alcoholics. *Alcoholism, Clinical and Experimental Research*, *13*(2), 271–279. doi:10.1111/j.1530-0277.1989.tb00325.x PMID:2524976

Penniston, E., & Kulkosky, P. (1991). Alpha-theta brainwave neurofeedback for Vietnam veterans with combat related post-traumatic stress disorder. *Medical Psychotherapy*, *4*, 47–60.

Penzes, P., & VanLeeuwen, J. E. (2011). Impaired regulation of synaptic actin cytoskeleton in Alzheimer's disease. *Brain Research. Brain Research Reviews*, *67*(1-2), 184–192. doi:10.1016/j.brainresrev.2011.01.003 PMID:21276817

Pereira, S., Pinto, A., Alves, V., & Silva, C. A. (2016). Brain Tumor Segmentation Using Convolutional Neural Networks in MRI Images. *IEEE Transactions on Medical Imaging*, *35*(5), 1240–1251. doi:10.1109/TMI.2016.2538465 PMID:26960222

PET/MRI Scan. (n.d.). Retrieved from https://stanfordhealthcare.org/medical-tests/p/pet-mri-scan.html

Pezoulas, V. C., Zervakis, M., Pologiorgi, I., Seferlis, S., Tsalikis, G. M., Zarifis, G., & Giakos, G. C. (2017). A tissue classification approach for brain tumor segmentation using MRI. *2017 IEEE International Conference on Imaging Systems and Techniques (IST)*. 10.1109/IST.2017.8261542

Phaf, R. H., & Kan, K. J. (2007). The automaticity of emotional Stroop: A meta-analysis. *Journal of Behavior Therapy and Experimental Psychiatry*, *38*(2), 184–199. doi:10.1016/j.jbtep.2006.10.008 PMID:17112461

Phone, D. (2018). Proactive medicines management supports more patient-centric services. *International Journal of Integrated Care*, *18*(s1), 31. doi:10.5334/ijic.s1031

Picillo, M., Moccia, M., Spina, E., Barone, P., & Pellecchia, M. T. (2015). Biomarkers of Parkinson's disease: Recent insights, current challenges, and future prospects. *Journal of Parkinsonism and Restless Legs Syndrome*, *6*, 1–13.

Piech, C. (n.d.). *K-Means.* Retrieved from Lecture Notes from Web site http://stanford.edu/~cpiech/cs221/handouts/kmeans.html

Pihlaja, S., Stenberg, J. H., Joutsenniemi, K., Mehik, H., Ritola, V., & Joffe, G. (2018). Therapeutic alliance in guided internet therapy programs for depression and anxiety disorders–a systematic review. *Internet Interventions, 11*, 1-10.

Pinkham, A. E. (2014). Social cognition in schizophrenia. *The Journal of Clinical Psychiatry*, *75*(suppl 2), 14–19. doi:10.4088/JCP.13065su1.04 PMID:24919166

Pizzagalli, D. A. (2014). Depression, stress, and anhedonia: Toward a synthesis and integrated model. *Annual Review of Clinical Psychology*, *10*(1), 393–423. doi:10.1146/annurev-clinpsy-050212-185606 PMID:24471371

Polat, K. (2012). Classification of Parkinson's disease using feature weighting method on the basis of fuzzy C-means clustering. *International Journal of Systems Science*, *43*(4), 597–609. doi:10.1080/00207721.2011.581395

Polat, K., & Güneş, S. (2007). Classification of epileptiform EEG using a hybrid system based on decision tree classifier and fast Fourier transform. *Applied Mathematics and Computation*, *187*(2), 1017–1026. doi:10.1016/j.amc.2006.09.022

Polich, J. (2007). Updating P300: An integrative theory of P3a and P3b. *Clinical Neurophysiology*, *118*(10), 2128–2148. doi:10.1016/j.clinph.2007.04.019 PMID:17573239

Polich, J., & Criado, J. R. (2006). Neuropsychology and neuropharmacology of P3a and P3b. *International Journal of Psychophysiology*, *60*(2), 172–185. doi:10.1016/j.ijpsycho.2005.12.012 PMID:16510201

Pope, A. T., & Palsson, O. S. (2001). *Helping video games "Rewire our minds."* Retrieved from https://ntrs.nasa.gov/archive/nasa/casi.ntrs.nasa.gov/20040086464.pdf

Praveena, M. A., & Bharathi, B. (2017, February). A survey paper on big data analytics. In *Information Communication and Embedded Systems (ICICES), 2017 International Conference on* (pp. 1-9). IEEE. 10.1109/ICICES.2017.8070723

Prinsloo, S., Novy, D., Driver, L., Lyle, R., Ramondetta, L., Eng, C., ... Cohen, L. (2017). Randomized controlled trial of neurofeedback on chemotherapy-induced peripheral neuropathy: A pilot study. *Cancer*, *123*(11), 1989–1997. doi:10.1002/cncr.30649 PMID:28257146

Proudfit, G. H., Bress, J. N., Foti, D., Kujawa, A., & Klein, D. N. (2015). Depression and event-related potentials: Emotional disengagement and reward insensitivity. *Current Opinion in Psychology, 4*, 110–113. doi:10.1016/j.copsyc.2014.12.018 PMID:26462292

Qiao, Z., Yu, Y., Wang, L., Yang, X., Qiu, X., Zhang, C., ... Liu, J. (2013). Impaired pre-attentive change detection in major depressive disorder patients revealed by auditory mismatch negativity. *Psychiatry Research: Neuroimaging, 211*(1), 78–84. doi:10.1016/j.pscychresns.2012.07.006 PMID:23149029

Qin, L., Ding, L., & He, B. (2005). Motor imagery classification by means of source analysis for brain–computer interface applications. *Journal of Neural Engineering, 2*(4), 65–72. doi:10.1088/1741-2560/2/4/001 PMID:16317229

Qiu, J., Wu, Q., Ding, G., Xu, Y., & Feng, S. (2016). A survey of machine learning for big data processing. *EURASIP Journal on Advances in Signal Processing, 2016*(1), 67. doi:10.118613634-016-0355-x

Radloff, L. S. (1977). The CES-D scale: A self-report depression scale for research in the general population. *Applied Psychological Measurement, 1*(3), 385–401. doi:10.1177/014662167700100306

Raes, F., Hermans, D., & Williams, J. M. G. (2006). Negative bias in the perception of others' facial emotional expressions in major depression: The role of depressive rumination. *The Journal of Nervous and Mental Disease, 194*(10), 796–799. doi:10.1097/01.nmd.0000240187.80270.bb PMID:17041294

Raghupathi, W., & Raghupathi, V. (2014). Big data analytics in healthcare: promise and potential. *Health Information Science and Systems, 2*(1), 3.

Rahul Kala, R. R. (2011). Diagnosis of breast cancer by modular evolutionary neural networks. *International Journal of Biomedical Engineering and Technology, 7*(2), 194. doi:10.1504/IJBET.2011.043179

Rajendra Acharya, U., Vinitha Sree, S., & Swapna, G. (2013). Roshan Joy Martis, and Jasjit S. Suri. Automated EEG analysis of epilepsy: A review. *Knowledge-Based Systems, 45*, 147–165. doi:10.1016/j.knosys.2013.02.014

Rajkowska, G., Miguel-Hidalgo, J. J., & Wei, J. (1999). Morphometric evidencenfor neuronal and glial prefrontal cell pathology in major depression. *Biological Psychiatry, 45*, 1085–1098. doi:10.1016/S0006-3223(99)00041-4 PMID:10331101

Ralph, G. (2001). Andrzejak, Klaus Lehnertz, Florian Mormann, Christoph Rieke, Peter David, and Christian E. Elger. Indications of nonlinear deterministic and nite-dimensional structures in time series of brain electrical activity: Dependence on recording region and brain state. *Physical Review. E, 64*(6), 061907. doi:10.1103/PhysRevE.64.061907

Ramadan, R. A., & Vasilakos, A. V. (2017). Brain computer interface: control signals review. *Neurocomputing, 223*, 26–44. doi:10.1016/j.neucom.2016.10.024

Ramirez-Esparza, N., Chung, C. K., Kacewicz, E., & Pennebaker, J. W. (2008, March). *The Psychology of Word Use in Depression Forums in English and in Spanish: Texting Two Text Analytic Approaches.* ICWSM.

Rapinesi, C., Bersani, F. S., Kotzalidis, G. D., Imperatori, C., Del Casale, A., Di Pietro, S., ... Angeletti, G. (2015). Maintenance deep transcranial magnetic stimulation sessions are associated with reduced depressive relapses in patients with unipolar or bipolar depression. *Frontiers in Neurology, 6*, 16. doi:10.3389/fneur.2015.00016 PMID:25709596

Reali, F., Soriano, T., & Rodríguez, D. (2016). How we think about depression: The role of linguistic framing. *Revista Latinoamericana de Psicología, 48*(2), 127–136. doi:10.1016/j.rlp.2015.09.004

Recio, M. (2017). Practitioner's Corner • Data Protection Officer: The Key Figure to Ensure Data Protection and Accountability. *European Data Protection Law Review, 3*(1), 114–118. doi:10.21552/edpl/2017/1/18

Reece & Danforth. (2016). *Instagram photos reveal predictive markers of depression.* Academic Press.

Reece, A.G., Reagan, A.J., Lix, K.L.M., Dodds, P.S., Danforth, C.M., & Langer, E.J. (2016). *Forecasting the Onset and Course of Mental Illness with Twitter Data*. Academic Press.

Reimer, P. (2010). *Clinical MR imaging: A practical approach*. Heidelberg, Germany: Springer. doi:10.1007/978-3-540-74504-4

Rey-del-Castillo, P., & Cardeñosa, J. (2016). An Exercise in Exploring Big Data for Producing Reliable Statistical Information. *Big Data*, *4*(2), 120–128. doi:10.1089/big.2015.0045 PMID:27441716

Reynolds, D. A., & Rose, R. C. (1995). Robust text-independent speaker identification using Gaussian mixture speaker models. *IEEE Transactions on Speech and Audio Processing*, *3*(1), 72–83. doi:10.1109/89.365379

Rice, S., Gleeson, J., Davey, C., Hetrick, S., Parker, A., Lederman, R., ... Russon, P. (2018). Moderated online social therapy for depression relapse prevention in young people: Pilot study of a 'next generation'online intervention. *Early Intervention in Psychiatry*, *12*(4), 613–625. doi:10.1111/eip.12354 PMID:27311581

Rice, S., Robinson, J., Bendall, S., Hetrick, S., Cox, G., Bailey, E., ... Alvarez-Jimenez, M. (2016). Online and social media suicide prevention interventions for young people: A focus on implementation and moderation. *Journal of the Canadian Academy of Child and Adolescent Psychiatry*, *25*(2), 80. PMID:27274743

Richards, V. (2018). The importance of language in mental health care. *The Lancet. Psychiatry*, *5*(6), 460–461. doi:10.1016/S2215-0366(18)30042-7 PMID:29482994

Rivero. (2009). Classification of EEG Signals Using Relative Wavelet Energy and Artificial Neural Networks. Academic Press.

Robert, C. (2014). Machine Learning, a Probabilistic Perspective. *Chance*, *27*(2), 62–63. doi:10.1080/09332480.2014.914768

Rodrıguez-Martın, D., Sama, A., Pérez-López, C., Catala, A., Moreno Arostegui, J. M., Cabestany, J., ... Rodríguez-Molinero, A. (2017). Home detection of freezing of gait using support vector machines through a single waist-worn triaxial accelerometer. *PLoS One*, *12*(2), e0171764. doi:10.1371/journal.pone.0171764 PMID:28199357

Rokach, L., & Maimon, O. (2005). Clustering methods. In *Data mining and knowledge discovery handbook* (pp. 321–352). Boston, MA: Springer. doi:10.1007/0-387-25465-X_15

Rosenfeld, J. P., Baehr, E., Baehr, R., Gotlib, I. H., & Ranganath, C. (1996). Ranganath. (1996). Preliminary evidence that daily changes in frontal alpha asymmetry correlate with changes in affect in therapy sessions. *International Journal of Psychophysiology*, *23*(1-2), 137–141. doi:10.1016/0167-8760(96)00037-2 PMID:8880374

Rottenberg, J. (2005). Mood and emotion in major depression. *Current Directions in Psychological Science*, *14*(3), 167–170. doi:10.1111/j.0963-7214.2005.00354.x

Ruan, G., & Zhang, H. (2017). Closed-loop Big Data Analysis with Visualization and Scalable Computing. *Big Data Research*, *8*, 12–26. doi:10.1016/j.bdr.2017.01.002

Ruan, Y., Xue, X., Liu, H., Tan, J., & Li, X. (2017). Quantum algorithm for k-nearest neighbors classification based on the metric of hamming distance. *International Journal of Theoretical Physics*, *56*(11), 3496–3507. doi:10.100710773-017-3514-4

Ruchsow, M., Herrnberger, B., Beschoner, P., Grön, G., Spitzer, M., & Kiefer, M. (2006). Error processing in major depressive disorder: Evidence from event-related potentials. *Journal of Psychiatric Research*, *40*(1), 37–46. doi:10.1016/j.jpsychires.2005.02.002 PMID:15882872

Rude, S., Gortner, E. M., & Pennebaker, J. (2004). Language use of depressed and depression-vulnerable college students. *Cognition and Emotion*, *18*(8), 1121–1133. doi:10.1080/02699930441000030

Rüsch, N., Zlati, A., Black, G., & Thornicroft, G. (2014). Does the stigma of mental illness contribute to suicidality? *The British Journal of Psychiatry*, *205*(4), 257–259. doi:10.1192/bjp.bp.114.145755 PMID:25274313

Russom, P. (2011). Big data analytics. *TDWI Best Practices Report, 19*(4), 1-34.

Saad, N. M., Abu-Bakar, S. A., Muda, S., & Mokji, M. (2011). Segmentation of brain lesions in diffusion-weighted MRI using thresholding technique. *2011 IEEE International Conference on Signal and Image Processing Applications (ICSIPA)*. 10.1109/ICSIPA.2011.6144092

Saberioon, M., Císař, P., Labbé, L., Souček, P., Pelissier, P., & Kerneis, T. (2018). Comparative Performance Analysis of Support Vector Machine, Random Forest, Logistic Regression and k-Nearest Neighbours in Rainbow Trout (Oncorhynchus Mykiss) Classification Using Image-Based Features. *Sensors (Basel)*, *18*(4), 1027. doi:10.339018041027 PMID:29596375

Sachdeva, J., Kumar, V., Gupta, I., Khandelwal, N., & Ahuja, C. K. (2016). A package-SFERCB-"Segmentation, feature extraction, reduction and classification analysis by both SVM and ANN for brain tumors. *Applied Soft Computing*, *47*, 151–167. doi:10.1016/j.asoc.2016.05.020

Sadati, N., Mohseni, H. R., & Maghsoudi, A. (2006). Epileptic Seizure Detection Using Neural Fuzzy Networks. *2006 IEEE International Conference on Fuzzy Systems*, 596-600. 10.1109/FUZZY.2006.1681772

Sadeque, F., Xu, D., & Bethard, S. (2017, September). Uarizona at the CLEF erisk 2017 pilot task: Linear and recurrent models for early depression detection. In *CEUR workshop proceedings* (Vol. 1866). NIH Public Access.

Saeed, S. A., Antonacci, D. J., & Bloch, R. M. (2010). Exercise, yoga, and meditation for depressive and anxiety disorders. *American Family Physician*, *81*(8). PMID:20387774

Sagiroglu, Ş., & Sinanc, D. (2013, May). Big data: A review. In *Collaboration Technologies and Systems (CTS), 2013 International Conference on* (pp. 42-47). Academic Press. 10.1109/CTS.2013.6567202

Sağıroğlu, Ş. (2017). *Büyük Veri ve Açık Veri Analitiği: Yöntemler ve Uygulamalar* (Ş. Sağıroğlu & O. Koç, Eds.). Ankara: Grafiker Yayınları.

Sahu, S. K., Jacintha, M. M., & Singh, A. P. (2017, May). Comparative study of tools for big data analytics: An analytical study. In *Computing, Communication and Automation (ICCCA), 2017 International Conference on* (pp. 37-41). IEEE.

Saikia, A., Mazumdar, S., Sahai, N., Paul, S., Bhatia, D., Verma, S., & Rohilla, P. K. (2016). Recent advancements in prosthetic hand technology. *Journal of Medical Engineering & Technology*, *40*(5), 255–264. doi:10.3109/03091902.2016.1167971 PMID:27098838

Samara, Z., Evers, E. A., Peeters, F., Uylings, H. B., Rajkowska, G., Ramaekers, J. G., & Stiers, P. (2018). Orbital and medial prefrontal cortex functional connectivity of major depression vulnerability and disease. *Biological Psychiatry: Cognitive Neuroscience and Neuroimaging*, *3*(4), 348–357. PMID:29628067

Sambo, F., Trifoglio, E., Di Camillo, B., Toffolo, G. M., & Cobelli, C. (2012). Bag of Naïve Bayes: Biomarker selection and classification from genome-wide SNP data. *BMC Bioinformatics*, *13*(14Suppl 14), S2. doi:10.1186/1471-2105-13-S14-S2 PMID:23095127

Sang, H., & Tan, D. (2018). Internalizing behavior disorders symptoms reduction by a social skills training program among Chinese students: A randomized controlled trial. *NeuroQuantology: An Interdisciplinary Journal of Neuroscience and Quantum Physics*, *16*(5). doi:10.14704/nq.2018.16.5.1312

Sansone, R. A., & Sansone, L. A. (2009). Dysthymic disorder: Forlorn and overlooked? *Psychiatry (Edgmont)*, *6*(5), 46. PMID:19724735

Sapolsky, R. M. (2000). Glucocorticoids and hippocampal atrophy in neuropsychiatric disorders. *Archives of General Psychiatry*, *57*(10), 925–935. doi:10.1001/archpsyc.57.10.925 PMID:11015810

Saritha, K., & Abraham, S. (2017, July). Prediction with partitioning: Big data analytics using regression techniques. In *Networks & Advances in Computational Technologies (NetACT), 2017 International Conference on* (pp. 208-214). IEEE.

Sarkar, S. D., Goswami, S., Agarwal, A., & Aktar, J. (2014). A novel feature selection technique for text classification using Naive Bayes. *International Scholarly Research Notices*.

Sass, S. M., Heller, W., Stewart, J. L., Silton, R. L., Edgar, J. C., Fisher, J. E., & Miller, G. A. (2010). Time course of attentional bias in anxiety: Emotion and gender specificity. *Psychophysiology*, *47*(2), 247–259. doi:10.1111/j.1469-8986.2009.00926.x PMID:19863758

Savitz, J., & Drevets, W. C. (2009). Bipolar and major depressive disorder: Neuroimaging the developmental-degenerative divide. *Neuroscience and Biobehavioral Reviews*, *33*(5), 699–771. doi:10.1016/j.neubiorev.2009.01.004 PMID:19428491

Saxena, A., Prasad, M., Gupta, A., Bharill, N., Patel, O. P., Tiwari, A., ... Lin, C. T. (2017). A review of clustering techniques and developments. *Neurocomputing*, *267*, 664–681. doi:10.1016/j.neucom.2017.06.053

Sayad, S. (n.d.a). *Logistic Regression*. Retrieved May 9, 2018, from, http://www.saedsayad.com/logistic_regression.htm

Sayad, S. (n.d.b). *Self Organizing Map*. Retrieved May 7, 2018, from, http://www.saedsayad.com/clustering_som.htm

Scharnowski, F., & Weiskopt, N. (2015). Cognitive enhancement through real-time fMRI neurofeedback. *Current Opinion in Behavioral Sciences*, *4*(1), 122–127. doi:10.1016/j.cobeha.2015.05.001

Schindlbeck, K. A., & Eidelberg, D. (2018). Network imaging biomarkers: Insights and clinical applications in Parkinson's disease. *Lancet Neurology*, *17*(7), 629–640. doi:10.1016/S1474-4422(18)30169-8 PMID:29914708

Schnaas, F. J. (2003). Handbook of depression. *The Journal of Clinical Psychiatry*, *64*(12), 1523–1524. doi:10.4088/JCP.v64n1218c

Schnyer, D. M., Clasen, P. C., Gonzalez, C., & Beevers, C. G. (2017). Evaluating the diagnostic utility of applying a machine learning algorithm to diffusion tensor MRI measures in individuals with major depressive disorder. *Psychiatry Research: Neuroimaging*, *264*, 1–9. doi:10.1016/j.pscychresns.2017.03.003 PMID:28388468

Schomerus, G., Stolzenburg, S., Freitag, S., Speerforck, S., Janowitz, D., Evans-Lacko, S., ... Schmidt, S. (2018). Stigma as a barrier to recognizing personal mental illness and seeking help: A prospective study among untreated persons with mental illness. *European Archives of Psychiatry and Clinical Neuroscience*, 1–11. PMID:29679153

Schrijvers, D., De Bruijn, E. R., Maas, Y. J., Vancoillie, P., Hulstijn, W., & Sabbe, B. G. (2009). Action monitoring and depressive symptom reduction in major depressive disorder. *International Journal of Psychophysiology*, *71*(3), 218–224. doi:10.1016/j.ijpsycho.2008.09.005 PMID:18926863

Schultz, T., Wand, M., Hueber, T., Krusienski, D. J., Herff, C., & Brumberg, J. S. (2017). Biosignal-Based Spoken Communication: A Survey. *IEEE/ACM Transactions on Audio Speech and Language Processing*, *25*(12), 2257–2271. doi:10.1109/TASLP.2017.2752365

Scott, G. G., O'Donnell, P. J., Leuthold, H., & Sereno, S. C. (2009). Early emotion word processing: Evidence from event-related potentials. *Biological Psychology*, *80*(1), 95–104. doi:10.1016/j.biopsycho.2008.03.010 PMID:18440691

Seetha, J., & Raja, S. S. (2018). Brain Tumor Classification Using Convolutional Neural Networks. *Biomedical & Pharmacology Journal, 11*(3), 1457–1461. doi:10.13005/bpj/1511

Segal, Z. V., Williams, M., & Teasdale, J. (2018). *Mindfulness-based cognitive therapy for depression*. Guilford Publications.

Seixas, F. L., Zadrozny, B., Laks, J., Conci, A., & Saade, D. C. M. (2014). A Bayesian network decision model for supporting the diagnosis of dementia, Alzheimer' s disease and mild cognitive impairment. *Computers in Biology and Medicine, 51*, 140–158. doi:10.1016/j.compbiomed.2014.04.010 PMID:24946259

Selvan & Srinivasan. (1999). Removal of ocular artifacts from EEG using an efficient neural network based adaptive filtering technique. *IEEE Signal Processing Letters, 6*(12), 330-332.

Shah, P. J., Ebmeier, K. P., Glabus, M. F., & Goodwin, G. M. (1998). Cortical grey matter reductions associated with treatment-resistant chronic unipolar depression: Controlled magnetic resonance imaging study. *The British Journal of Psychiatry, 172*(6), 527–532. doi:10.1192/bjp.172.6.527 PMID:9828995

Shansky, R. M., & Morrison, J. H. (2009). Stress-induced dendritic remodeling in the medial prefrontal cortex: Effects of circuit, hormones and rest. *Brain Research, 1293*, 108–113. doi:10.1016/j.brainres.2009.03.062 PMID:19361488

Sharma, A., & Giri, R. N. (2014). Automatic Recognition of Parkinson Disease via Artificial Neural Network and Support Vector Machine. *IJITEE, 4*, 35–41.

Sharma, S., Moon, C. S., Khogali, A., Haidous, A., Chabenne, A., Ojo, C., ... Ebadi, M. (2013). Biomarkers in Parkinson's disease (recent update). *Neurochemistry International, 63*(3), 201–229. doi:10.1016/j.neuint.2013.06.005 PMID:23791710

Shen, G., Ding, Y., Lan, T., Chen, H., & Qin, Z. (2018). Brain Tumor Segmentation Using Concurrent Fully Convolutional Networks and Conditional Random Fields. *Proceedings of the 3rd International Conference on Multimedia and Image Processing - ICMIP 2018*. 10.1145/3195588.3195590

Shen, C. P., Chen, C. C., Hsieh, S. L., Chen, W. H., Chen, J. M., Chen, C. M., ... Chiu, M. J. (2013). High-performance seizure detection system using a wavelet-approximate entropy-fSVM cascade with clinical validation. *Clinical EEG and Neuroscience, 44*(4), 247–256. doi:10.1177/1550059413483451 PMID:23610456

Shestyuk, A. Y., & Deldin, P. J. (2010). Automatic and strategic representation of the self in major depression: trait and state abnormalities. *The American Journal of Psychiatry, 167*(5), 536–544. doi:10.1176/appi.ajp.2009.06091444 PMID:20360316

Shirakawa, T., Sugiyama, N., Sato, H., Sakurai, K., & Sato, E. (2017). Gait analysis and machine learning classification on healthy subjects in normal walking. *International Journal of Parallel Emergent and Distributed Systems, 32*(2), 185–194. doi:10.1080/17445760.2015.1044007

Shi, Y. (2011). Brain storm optimization algorithm. In *Proceedings of International Conference in Swarm Intelligence* (pp. 303-309). Springer.

Shorten, C. (2018). *Machine Learning vs. Deep Learning*. Retrieved July 20, 2018, from https://towardsdatascience.com/machine-learning-vs-deep-learning-62137a1c9842

Shouval, R., Bondi, O., Mishan, H., Shimoni, A., Unger, R., & Nagler, A. (2014). Application of machine learning algorithms for clinical predictive modeling: A data-mining approach in SCT. *Bone Marrow Transplantation, 49*(3), 332–337. doi:10.1038/bmt.2013.146 PMID:24096823

Shrivastava, P., Shukla, A., Vepakomma, P., Bhansali, N., & Verma, K. (2017). A survey of nature-inspired algorithms for feature selection to identify Parkinson's disease. *Computer Methods and Programs in Biomedicine, 139*, 171–179. doi:10.1016/j.cmpb.2016.07.029 PMID:28187888

Shukla, R., Gupta, R. K., & Kashyap, R. (2019). A multiphase pre-copy strategy for the virtual machine migration in cloud. In S. Satapathy, V. Bhateja, & S. Das (Eds.), *Smart Intelligent Computing and Applications. Smart Innovation, Systems and Technologies* (Vol. 104). Singapore: Springer. doi:10.1007/978-981-13-1921-1_43

Siddiquee, A. B., Mazumder, M., Hoque, E., & Kamruzzaman, S. M. (2010). *A Constructive Algorithm for Feedforward Neural Networks for Medical Diagnostic Reasoning*. Academic Press.

Simon, N. M., McNamara, K., Chow, C. W., Maser, R. S., Papakostas, G. I., Pollack, M. H., ... Wong, K. K. (2008). A detailed examination of cytokine abnormalities in Major Depressive Disorder. *European Neuropsychopharmacology, 18*(3), 230–233. doi:10.1016/j.euroneuro.2007.06.004 PMID:17681762

Singh, D., & Reddy, C. K. (2015). A survey on platforms for big data analytics. *Journal of Big Data, 2*(1), 8.

Singh, R., Pal, B. C., & Jabr, R. A. (2010). Statistical representation of distribution system loads using Gaussian mixture model. *IEEE Transactions on Power Systems, 25*(1), 29–37. doi:10.1109/TPWRS.2009.2030271

Sitaram, R., Zhang, H., Guan, C., Thulasidas, M., Hoshi, Y., Ishikawa, A., ... Birbaumer, N. (2007). Temporal classification of multichannel near-infrared spectroscopy signals of motor imagery for developing a brain–computer interface. *NeuroImage, 34*(4), 1416–1427. doi:10.1016/j.neuroimage.2006.11.005 PMID:17196832

Siuly, L., Li, Y., & Wen, P. (2011). EEG signal classification based on simple random sampling technique with least square support vector machine. *International Journal of Biomedical Engineering and Technology, 7*(4), 390–409. doi:10.1504/IJBET.2011.044417

Siuly, S., & Zhang, Y. (2016). Medical big data: Neurological diseases diagnosis through medical data analysis. *Data Science and Engineering, 1*(2), 54–64. doi:10.100741019-016-0011-3

Skiera, B., & Ringel, D. (2017). Using Big Search Data to Map Your Market: Marketing in a Digital Age. *IESE Insight*, (32), 31-37. doi:10.15581/002.art-2982

Smith, K. M., & Caplan, D. N. (2018). Communication impairment in Parkinson's disease: Impact of motor and cognitive symptoms on speech and language. *Brain and Language, 185*, 38–46. doi:10.1016/j.bandl.2018.08.002 PMID:30092448

Smulders, K., Dale, M. L., Carlson-Kuhta, P., Nutt, J. G., & Horak, F. B. (2016). Pharmacological treatment in Parkinson's disease: Effects on gait. *Parkinsonism & Related Disorders, 31*, 3–13. doi:10.1016/j.parkreldis.2016.07.006 PMID:27461783

Sokolova, M., & Lapalme, G. (2009). A systematic analysis of performance measures for classification tasks. *Information Processing & Management, 45*(4), 427–437. doi:10.1016/j.ipm.2009.03.002

Song, Y., & Liò, P. (2010). A new approach for epileptic seizure detection: Sample entropy based feature extraction and extreme learning machine. *Journal of Biomedical Science and Engineering, 03*(06), 556–567. doi:10.4236/jbise.2010.36078

Sonu, S. R., Prakash, V., Ranjan, R., & Saritha, K. (2017, August). Prediction of Parkinson's disease using data mining. In *2017 International Conference on Energy, Communication, Data Analytics and Soft Computing (ICECDS)* (pp. 1082-1085). IEEE. 10.1109/ICECDS.2017.8389605

Specht. (1990). Probabilistic neural networks. *Neural Networks, 3*(1), 109-118.

Speed, B. C., Nelson, B. D., Auerbach, R. P., Klein, D. N., & Hajcak, G. (2016). Depression risk and electrocortical reactivity during self-referential emotional processing in 8 to 14 year-old girls. *Journal of Abnormal Psychology, 125*(5), 607–619. doi:10.1037/abn0000173 PMID:27175985

Spijker, J. A. N., De Graaf, R., Bijl, R. V., Beekman, A. T., Ormel, J., & Nolen, W. A. (2002). Duration of major depressive episodes in the general population: Results from The Netherlands Mental Health Survey and Incidence Study (NEMESIS). *The British Journal of Psychiatry*, *181*(3), 208–213. doi:10.1192/bjp.181.3.208 PMID:12204924

Srinivasan, V., Eswaran, C., & Sriraam, N. (2005). Artificial neural network based epileptic detection using time-domain and frequency-domain features. *Journal of Medical Systems*, *29*(6), 647–660. doi:10.100710916-005-6133-1 PMID:16235818

Stafford, M. (2018). Psychotic depression: How to diagnose this often undetected—and hidden—condition. *The Brown University Child and Adolescent Behavior Letter*, *34*(4), 1–7. doi:10.1002/cbl.30284

Statista. (n.d.). *Number of monthly active Facebook users worldwide as of 4th quarter 2018 (in millions)*. Retrieved from https://www.statista.com/statistics/264810/number-of-monthly-active-facebook-users-worldwide/

Steinbach, M., Karypis, G., & Kumar, V. (2000). *A comparison of document clustering techniques*. Paper presented at the KDD workshop on text mining.

Stein, R., & Oĝuztöreli, M. (1976). Tremor and other oscillations in neuromuscular systems. *Biological Cybernetics*, *22*(3), 147–157. doi:10.1007/BF00365525 PMID:1276248

Sternberg, S. (1969). The discovery of processing stages: Extensions of Donders' method. *Acta Psychologica*, *30*, 276–315. doi:10.1016/0001-6918(69)90055-9

Stirman, S. W., & Pennebaker, J. W. (2001). Word use in the poetry of suicidal and non-suicidal poets. *Psychosomatic Medicine*, *63*(4), 517–522. doi:10.1097/00006842-200107000-00001 PMID:11485104

Streeter, C. C., Gerbarg, P. L., Whitfield, T. H., Owen, L., Johnston, J., Silveri, M. M., ... Hernon, A. M. (2017). Treatment of major depressive disorder with Iyengar yoga and coherent breathing: A randomized controlled dosing study. *Journal of Alternative and Complementary Medicine (New York, N.Y.)*, *23*(3), 201–207. doi:10.1089/acm.2016.0140 PMID:28296480

Stuart, A. (1979). A new depression scale designed to be sensitive to change. *The British Journal of Psychiatry*, *134*(4), 382–389. doi:10.1192/bjp.134.4.382 PMID:444788

Suarez-Escobar, M., & Rendon-Velez, E. (2018). An overview of robotic/mechanical devices for post-stroke thumb rehabilitation. *Disability and Rehabilitation. Assistive Technology*, *13*(7), 683–703. doi:10.1080/17483107.2018.1425746 PMID:29334274

Subasi, A. (2007). EEG signal classification using wavelet feature extraction and a mixture of expert model. *Expert Systems with Applications*, *32*(4), 1084–1093. doi:10.1016/j.eswa.2006.02.005

Subbanna, N. K., & Arbel, T. (2012). Probabilistic Gabor and Markov random fields, segmentation of brain tumours in MRI volumes. *Proceedings of the MICCAI-BRATS*.

Subbanna, N., Precup, D., & Arbel, T. (2014). Iterative Multilevel MRF Leveraging Context and Voxel Information for Brain Tumour Segmentation in MRI. *2014 IEEE Conference on Computer Vision and Pattern Recognition*. 10.1109/CVPR.2014.53

Sudharani, K., Sarma, T., & Prasad, K. S. (2016). Advanced Morphological Technique for Automatic Brain Tumor Detection and Evaluation of Statistical Parameters. *Procedia Technology*, *24*, 1374–1387. doi:10.1016/j.protcy.2016.05.153

Suhara, Y., Xu, Y., & Pentland, A. S. (2017). *DeepMood: Forecasting Depressed Mood Based on Self-Reported Histories via Recurrent Neural Networks*. Retrieved from http://papers.www2017.com.au.s3-website-ap-southeast-2.amazonaws.com/proceedings/p715.pdf

Sun, Z. (2017). *Big Data Analytics and Artificial Intelligence*. UNITECH Research Committee Seminar, No. 7, PNG University of Technology.

Sun, J., & Reddy, C. K. (2013, August). Big data analytics for healthcare. In *Proceedings of the 19th ACM SIGKDD international conference on Knowledge discovery and data mining* (pp. 1525-1525). ACM.

Sun, Z., Sun, L., & Strang, K. (2018). Big data analytics services for enhancing business intelligence. *Journal of Computer Information Systems*, *58*(2), 162–169. doi:10.1080/08874417.2016.1220239

Surathi, P., Jhunjhunwala, K., Yadav, R., & Pal, P. K. (2016). Research in Parkinson's disease in India: A review. *Annals of Indian Academy of Neurology*, *19*(1), 9. doi:10.4103/0972-2327.167713 PMID:27011622

Ta, V. D., Liu, C. M., & Nkabinde, G. W. (2016, July). Big data stream computing in healthcare real-time analytics. In *Cloud Computing and Big Data Analysis (ICCCBDA), 2016 IEEE International Conference on* (pp. 37-42). IEEE.

Takei, Y., Kumano, S., Hattori, S., Uehara, T., Kawakubo, Y., Kasai, K., ... Mikuni, M. (2009). Preattentive dysfunction in major depression: A magnetoencephalography study using auditory mismatch negativity. *Psychophysiology*, *46*(1), 52–61. doi:10.1111/j.1469-8986.2008.00748.x PMID:19055502

Tang, J. X., Deng, C., & Huang, G.-B. (2016). Extreme Learning Machine for Multilayer Perceptron. *IEEE Transactions on Neural Networks and Learning Systems*, *24*(4), 809–821. doi:10.1109/TNNLS.2015.2424995 PMID:25966483

Tarai, S., Bit, A., dos Reis, H. J., Palotás, A., Rizvanov, A., & Bissoyi, A. (2016). Stratifying Heterogeneous Dimension of Neurodegenerative Diseases: Intervention for Stipulating Epigenetic Factors to Combat Oxidative Stress in Human Brain. *BioNanoScience*, *6*(4), 411–422. doi:10.100712668-016-0240-y

Tarai, S., Mukherjee, R., Qurratul, Q. A., Singh, B. K., & Bit, A. (2018). Use of Prosocial Word Enhances the Processing of Language: Frequency Domain Analysis of Human EEG. *Journal of Psycholinguistic Research*, 1–17. PMID:30043323

Tas, F. (2014). An analysis of the most-cited research papers on oncology: Which journals have they been published in? *Tumour Biology*, *35*(5), 4645–4649. doi:10.100713277-014-1608-7 PMID:24414487

Tausczik, Y. R., & Pennebaker, J. W. (2010). The psychological meaning of words: LIWC and computerized text analysis methods. *Journal of Language and Social Psychology*, *29*(1), 24–54. doi:10.1177/0261927X09351676

Taylor, W. D., MacFall, J. R., Gerig, G., & Krishnan, R. R. (2007). Structural integrity of the uncinate fasciculus in geriatric depression: Relationship with age of onset. *Neuropsychiatric Disease and Treatment*, *3*(5), 669. PMID:19300596

Tesio, L., & Gamba, C. (1995). Rehabilitation: the Cinderella of neurological research? A bibliometric study. Springer.

The Telegraph India. (2018). *Silent tormentor of students: depression*. Retrieved from https://www.telegraphindia.com/states/jharkhand/silent-tormentor-of-students-depression/cid/1373651

Thomas, K. M., & Duke, M. (2007). Depressed writing: Cognitive distortions in the works of depressed and nondepressed poets and writers. *Psychology of Aesthetics, Creativity, and the Arts*, *1*(4), 204–218. doi:10.1037/1931-3896.1.4.204

Thompson, R., & Spencer, W. (1966). Habituation: A model phenomenon for the study of neuronal substrates of behavior. *Psychological Review*, *73*(1), 16–43. doi:10.1037/h0022681 PMID:5324565

Thornicroft, G. (2006). *Shunned: discrimination against people with mental illness* (Vol. 399). Oxford, UK: Oxford University Press.

Tian, Y., & Peng, Y. (2011). Study on Communication of Massive 3D Spatial Data Based on ACE. *Geo-Information Science*, *12*(6), 819–827. doi:10.3724/SP.J.1047.2010.00819

Tirumala, S. S., Shahamiri, S. R., Garhwal, A. S., & Wang, R. (2017). Speaker identification features extraction methods: A systematic review. *Expert Systems with Applications*, *90*, 250–271. doi:10.1016/j.eswa.2017.08.015

Tiwari, S., Gupta, R. K., & Kashyap, R. (2019). To enhance web response time using agglomerative clustering technique for web navigation recommendation. In H. Behera, J. Nayak, B. Naik, & A. Abraham (Eds.), *Computational Intelligence in Data Mining. Advances in Intelligent Systems and Computing* (Vol. 711). Singapore: Springer. doi:10.1007/978-981-10-8055-5_59

Tomek, I. (1976). Two modifications of CNN. *IEEE Transactions on Systems, Man, and Cybernetics*, 769–772.

Tondo, L., Visioli, C., Preti, A., & Baldessarini, R. J. (2014). Bipolar disorders following initial depression: Modeling predictive clinical factors. *Journal of Affective Disorders*, *167*, 44–49. doi:10.1016/j.jad.2014.05.043 PMID:25082113

Tran, N. T., Baggio, S., Dawson, A., O'Moore, É., Williams, B., Bedell, P., ... Wolff, H. (2018). Words matter: A call for humanizing and respectful language to describe people who experience incarceration. *BMC International Health and Human Rights*, *18*(1), 41. doi:10.118612914-018-0180-4 PMID:30445949

Tran, T. N., Drab, K., & Daszykowski, M. (2013). Revised DBSCAN algorithm to cluster data with dense adjacent clusters. *Chemometrics and Intelligent Laboratory Systems*, *120*, 92–96. doi:10.1016/j.chemolab.2012.11.006

Trevino, A. (n.d.). *Introduction to K-means Clustering*. Retrieved from https://www.datascience.com/blog/k-means-clustering

Trifu, R. N., Nemeş, B., Bodea-Haţegan, C., & Cozman, D. (2017). Linguistic indicators of language in major depressive disorder (MDD). An evidence-based research. *Journal of Evidence-Based Psychotherapies*, *17*(1), 105–128. doi:10.24193/jebp.2017.1.7

Trivedi, M. H., Rush, A. J., Wisniewski, S. R., Nierenberg, A. A., Warden, D., Ritz, L., ... Shores-Wilson, K. (2006). Evaluation of outcomes with citalopram for depression using measurement-based care in STAR* D: Implications for clinical practice. *The American Journal of Psychiatry*, *163*(1), 28–40. doi:10.1176/appi.ajp.163.1.28 PMID:16390886

Troy, A. S., Wilhelm, F. H., Shallcross, A. J., & Mauss, I. B. (2010). Seeing the silver lining: Cognitive reappraisal ability moderates the relationship between stress and depressive symptoms. *Emotion (Washington, D.C.)*, *10*(6), 783–795. doi:10.1037/a0020262 PMID:21058843

Tutorialspoint.com. (n.d.). *Genetic Algorithms Tutorial*. Retrieved from https://www.tutorialspoint.com/genetic_algorithms/

Ueoka, Y., Tomotake, M., Tanaka, T., Kaneda, Y., Taniguchi, K., Nakataki, M., ... Ohmori, T. (2011). Quality of life and cognitive dysfunction in people with schizophrenia. *Progress in Neuro-Psychopharmacology & Biological Psychiatry*, *35*(1), 53–59. doi:10.1016/j.pnpbp.2010.08.018 PMID:20804809

Umadevi, S., & Marseline, K. J. (2017, July). A survey on data mining classification algorithms. In *Signal Processing and Communication (ICSPC), 2017 International Conference on* (pp. 264-268). IEEE. 10.1109/CSPC.2017.8305851

Understanding Brain Tumors. (1999). Retrieved from https://www.brainandlife.org/siteassets/about-us/about-brain--life/understanding-brain-tumors.pdf

Üstün, T. B., Ayuso-Mateos, J. L., Chatterji, S., Mathers, C., & Murray, C. J. L. (2000). Global burden of depressive disorders in the year. *The British Journal of Psychiatry*, *2004*(184), 386–392. PMID:15123501

Uzun, E. (2016). *Supervised ve Unsupervised Learning*. Retrieved January 01, 2018, from, https://www.e-adys.com/makine_ogrenmesi/hangisini-secmeliyim-supervised-ve-unsupervised-learning/

van Bronswijk, S. C., Lemmens, L. H., Keefe, J. R., Huibers, M. J., DeRubeis, R. J., & Peeters, F. P. (2018). A prognostic index for long-term outcome after successful acute phase cognitive therapy and interpersonal psychotherapy for major depressive disorder. *Depression and Anxiety*. doi:10.1002/da.22868 PMID:30516871

van der Sanden, R. L., Pryor, J. B., Stutterheim, S. E., Kok, G., & Bos, A. E. (2016). Stigma by association and family burden among family members of people with mental illness: The mediating role of coping. *Social Psychiatry and Psychiatric Epidemiology*, *51*(9), 1233–1245. doi:10.100700127-016-1256-x PMID:27357819

Venema, V., Ament, F., & Simmer, C. (2006). A stochastic iterative amplitude adjusted fourier transform algorithm with improved accuracy. *Nonlinear Processes in Geophysics*, *13*(3), 321–328. doi:10.5194/npg-13-321-2006

Verma, J. P., Agrawal, S., Patel, B., & Patel, A. (2016). Big data analytics: Challenges and applications for text, audio, video, and social media data. *International Journal on Soft Computing, Artificial Intelligence and Applications, 5*(1).

Verma, H., Agrawal, R., & Sharan, A. (2016). An improved intuitionistic fuzzy c-means clustering algorithm incorporating local information for brain image segmentation. *Applied Soft Computing*, *46*, 543–557. doi:10.1016/j.asoc.2015.12.022

Verma, S. K., Bharti, P., & Singh, T. (2018). Does stigma always have negative consequences? *Journal of Community & Applied Social Psychology*, *28*(6), 495–507. doi:10.1002/casp.2382

Vernon, D. J. (2005). Can neurofeedback training enhance performance? An evaluation of the evidence with implications for future research. *Applied Psychophysiology and Biofeedback*, *30*(4), 347–364. doi:10.100710484-005-8421-4 PMID:16385423

Vijay, V., Kavitha, A., & Rebecca, S. R. (2016). Automated Brain Tumor Segmentation and Detection in MRI Using Enhanced Darwinian Particle Swarm Optimization (EDPSO). *Procedia Computer Science*, *92*, 475–480. doi:10.1016/j.procs.2016.07.370

Viji, K. S., & Jayakumari, J. (2013). Modified texture based region growing segmentation of MR brain images. *2013 IEEE Conference On Information And Communication Technologies*. 10.1109/CICT.2013.6558183

Vlasveld, R. (2013). *Introduction to One-class Support Vector Machines*. Retrieved from http://rvlasveld.github.io/blog/2013/07/12/introduction-to-one-class-support-vector-machines/

Vyškovský, R., Schwarz, D., Janoušová, E., & Kašpárek, T. (2016). Random subspace ensemble artificial neural networks for first-episode Schizophrenia classification. In *Computer Science and Information Systems (FedCSIS), 2016 Federated Conference on* (pp. 317-321). IEEE.

Wacker, J., Dillon, D. G., & Pizzagalli, D. A. (2009). The role of the nucleus accumbens and rostral anterior cingulate cortex in anhedonia: Integration of resting EEG, fMRI, and volumetric techniques. *NeuroImage*, *46*(1), 327–337. doi:10.1016/j.neuroimage.2009.01.058 PMID:19457367

Wairagkar, M. (2014). Motor Imagery based Brain Computer Interface (BCI) using Artificial Neural Network Classifiers. *Proceedings of the British Conference of Undergraduate Research.*

Walker, J. E., Shea, T. M., & Bauer, A. M. (2016). *Generalization and the Effects of Consequences*. Retrieved from www.education.com

Wang, W.-T., Wu, Y.-L., Tang, C.-Y., & Hor, M.-K. (2015). *Adaptive density-based spatial clustering of applications with noise (DBSCAN) according to data.* Paper presented at the Machine Learning and Cybernetics (ICMLC), 2015 International Conference on.

Wang, S., Chaovalitwongse, W., & Babuska, R. (2012). Machine learning algorithms in bipedal robot control. *IEEE Transactions on Systems, Man and Cybernetics. Part C, Applications and Reviews*, *42*(5), 728–743. doi:10.1109/TSMCC.2012.2186565

Wang, Y., Kung, L., & Byrd, T. A. (2018). Big data analytics: Understanding its capabilities and potential benefits for healthcare organizations. *Technological Forecasting and Social Change*, *126*, 3–13. doi:10.1016/j.techfore.2015.12.019

Waoo, N., Kashyap, R., & Jaiswal, A. (2010). DNA nano array analysis using hierarchical quality threshold clustering. In *2010 2nd IEEE International Conference on Information Management and Engineering*. IEEE. 10.1109/ICIME.2010.5477579

Ward, J. S., & Barker, A. (2013). *Undefined by data: a survey of big data definitions.* arXiv preprint arXiv:1309.5821

Weinberg, A., Perlman, G., Kotov, R., & Hajcak, G. (2016). Depression and reduced neural response to emotional images: Distinction from anxiety, and importance of symptom dimensions and age of onset. *Journal of Abnormal Psychology*, *125*(1), 26–39. doi:10.1037/abn0000118 PMID:26726817

Weishaar, M. E., & Beck, A. T. (1992). Hopelessness and suicide. *International Review of Psychiatry (Abingdon, England)*, *4*(2), 177–184. doi:10.3109/09540269209066315

Weitz, E., Kleiboer, A., van Straten, A., & Cuijpers, P. (2018). The effects of psychotherapy for depression on anxiety symptoms: A meta-analysis. *Psychological Medicine*, 1–13. PMID:29361995

Wilcox, S. K. (2010). Extending palliative care to patients with Parkinson's disease. *British Journal of Hospital Medicine, 71*(1), 26-30.

Winstein, C. J., Stein, J., Arena, R., Bates, B., Cherney, L. R., Cramer, S. C., … Zorowitz, R. D. (2016). Guidelines for Adult Stroke Rehabilitation and Recovery: A Guideline for Healthcare Professionals from the American Heart Association/American Stroke Association. *Stroke*, *47*. doi:10.1161/STR.0000000000000098

Winterburn, J. L., Voineskos, A. N., Devenyi, G. A., Plitman, E., de la Fuente-Sandoval, C., Bhagwat, N., ... Chakravarty, M. M. (2017). Can we accurately classify schizophrenia patients from healthy controls using magnetic resonance imaging and machine learning? A multi-method and multi-dataset study. *Schizophrenia Research*. doi:10.1016/j.schres.2017.11.038 PMID:29274736

Winthorst, W. H., Roest, A. M., Bos, E. H., Meesters, Y., Penninx, B. W., Nolen, W. A., & de Jonge, P. (2017). Seasonal affective disorder and non-seasonal affective disorders: results from the NESDA study. *BJPsych Open, 3*(4), 196-203.

Wolfson, J., Bandyopadhyay, S., Elidrisi, M., Vazquez-Benitez, G., Musgrove, D., Adomavicius, G., . . . O'Connor, P. (2014). *A Naive Bayes machine learning approach to risk prediction using censored, time-to-event data.* arXiv preprint arXiv:1404.2124

Wongrakpanich, S., Petchlorlian, A., & Rosenzweig, A. (2016). Sensorineural Organs Dysfunction and Cognitive Decline: A Review Article. *Aging and Disease*, *7*(6), 763. doi:10.14336/AD.2016.0515 PMID:28053826

Woods, H. C., & Scott, H. (2016). #Sleepyteens: Social media use in adolescence is associated with poor sleep quality, anxiety, depression and low self-esteem. *Journal of Adolescence*, *51*, 41–49. doi:10.1016/j.adolescence.2016.05.008 PMID:27294324

Woolley, C. S., Gould, E., Frankfurt, M., & McEwen, B. S. (1990). Naturally occurring fluctuation in dendritic spine density on adult hippocampal pyramidal neurons. *The Journal of Neuroscience*, *10*(12), 4035–4039. doi:10.1523/JNEUROSCI.10-12-04035.1990 PMID:2269895

World Health Organization. (2017). *Depression and other common mental disorders: global health estimates.* WHO.

World Health Organization. (2017a). *Depression and Other Common Mental Disorders*. Retrieved from https://apps.who.int/iris/bitstream/handle/10665/254610/WHO-MSD-MER-2017.2-eng.pdf;jsessionid=1529C9707E98EA8E0BAA603CF50A1927?sequence=1

World Health Organization. (2017b). *Depression in India Let's talk*. Retrieved from http://www.searo.who.int/india/depression_in_india.pdf

World Health Organization. (2018). *Depression*. Retrieved from https://www.who.int/news-room/fact-sheets/detail/depression

World Health Organization. (n.d.). *Suicide Data*. Retrieved from https://www.who.int/mental_health/prevention/suicide/suicideprevent/en/

Wu, J., & Wu, B. (2015). The novel quantitative technique for assessment of gait symmetry using advanced statistical learning algorithm. *BioMed Research International*. PMID:25705672

Wu, J., & Xu, H. (2016). An advanced scheme of compressed sensing of acceleration data for telemonintoring of human gait. *Biomedical Engineering Online*, *15*(1), 27. doi:10.118612938-016-0142-9 PMID:26946302

Wu, T., Hallett, M., & Chan, P. (2015). Motor automaticity in Parkinson's disease. *Neurobiology of Disease*, *82*, 226–234. doi:10.1016/j.nbd.2015.06.014 PMID:26102020

Wu, X., Zhu, X., Wu, G. Q., & Ding, W. (2014). Data mining with big data. *IEEE Transactions on Knowledge and Data Engineering*, *26*(1), 97–107. doi:10.1109/TKDE.2013.109

Wu, Z., Zhong, X., Peng, Q., Chen, B., Mai, N., & Ning, Y. (2017). Negative bias in expression-related mismatch negativity (MMN) in remitted late-life depression: An event-related potential study. *Journal of Psychiatric Research*, *95*, 224–230. doi:10.1016/j.jpsychires.2017.08.019 PMID:28892767

Wyczesany, M., Ligeza, T. S., & Grzybowski, S. J. (2015). Effective connectivity during visual processing is affected by emotional state. *Brain Imaging and Behavior*, *9*(4), 717–728. doi:10.100711682-014-9326-8 PMID:25339066

Xu, K., Yue, H., Guo, L., Guo, Y., & Fang, Y. (2015, June). Privacy-preserving machine learning algorithms for big data systems. In *Distributed Computing Systems (ICDCS), 2015 IEEE 35th International Conference on* (pp. 318-327). IEEE. 10.1109/ICDCS.2015.40

Xu, H., Hunt, M., Foreman, K. B., Zhao, J., & Merryweather, A. (2018). Gait alterations on irregular surface in people with Parkinson's disease. *Clinical Biomechanics (Bristol, Avon)*, *57*, 93–98. doi:10.1016/j.clinbiomech.2018.06.013 PMID:29966960

Yadav, G., & Mutha, P. K. (2016). Deep Breathing Practice9 Facilitates Retention of Newly Learned Motor Skills. *Scientific Reports*, *6*(1), 37069. doi:10.1038rep37069 PMID:27841345

Yahyaouı, A. (2017). *Göğüs Hastalıklarının Teşhis Edilmesinde Makine Öğrenmesi Algoritmalarının Kullanılması* (Doctoral Dissertation). Ulusal Tez Merkezi. (No. 462917)

Yang, G., Deng, J., Pang, G., Zhang, H., Li, J., Deng, B., ... Xie, H. (2018). An IoT-Enabled Stroke Rehabilitation System Based on Smart Wearable Armband and Machine Learning. *IEEE Journal of Translational Engineering in Health and Medicine*, *6*, 1–10. doi:10.1109/JTEHM.2018.2879085 PMID:29805919

Yang, Z., & Gao, D. (2013). Classification for Imbalanced and Overlapping Classes Using Outlier Detection and Sampling Techniques. *Applied Mathematics & Information Sciences*, *7*(1), 375–381. doi:10.12785/amis/071L50

Yeung, N., Botvinick, M. M., & Cohen, J. D. (2004). The neural basis of error detection: Conflict monitoring and the error-related negativity. *Psychological Review, 111*(4), 931–959. doi:10.1037/0033-295X.111.4.931 PMID:15482068

Yoo, C., Ramirez, L., & Liuzzi, J. (2014). Big data analysis using modern statistical and machine learning methods in medicine. *International Neurourology Journal, 18*(2), 50. doi:10.5213/inj.2014.18.2.50 PMID:24987556

Yoon, K. L., Joormann, J., & Gotlib, I. H. (2009). Judging the intensity of facial expressions of emotion: Depression-related biases in the processing of positive affect. *Journal of Abnormal Psychology, 118*(1), 223–228. doi:10.1037/a0014658 PMID:19222328

Yu, H., & Kim, S. (2012). SVM tutorial—classification, regression and ranking. In *Handbook of Natural computing* (pp. 479–506). Berlin: Springer. doi:10.1007/978-3-540-92910-9_15

Yule, G. (2016). *The study of language*. Cambridge University Press.

Yusof, N. F. A., Lin, C., & Guerin, F. (2017). Analysing the causes of depressed mood from depression vulnerable individuals. In *Proceedings of the International Workshop on Digital Disease Detection using Social Media 2017 (DDDSM-2017)* (pp. 9-17). Academic Press.

Zarkogianni, K., Athanasiou, M., Thanopoulou, A. C., & Nikita, K. S. (2017). Comparison of machine learning approaches towards assessing the risk of developing Cardiovascular disease as a long term diabetes complication. *IEEE Journal of Biomedical and Health Informatics, 2194*(c). PMID:29990007

Zeng, W., Liu, F., Wang, Q., Wang, Y., Ma, L., & Zhang, Y. (2016). Parkinson's disease classification using gait analysis via deterministic learning. *Neuroscience Letters, 633*, 268–278. doi:10.1016/j.neulet.2016.09.043 PMID:27693437

Zhai, J., Wang, X., Zhang, S., & Hou, S. (2018). Tolerance rough fuzzy decision tree. *Information Sciences, 465*, 425–438. doi:10.1016/j.ins.2018.07.006

Zhang, A., Wang, K. J., & Mao, Z. H. (2018, August). Design and Realization of Alzheimer. In *2018 IEEE 6th International Conference on Future Internet of Things and Cloud (FiCloud)* (pp. 141-148). IEEE.

Zhang, H., Chin, Z., Ang, K., Guan, C., & Wang, C. (2011). Optimum Spatio-Spectral Filtering Network for Brain–Computer Interface. *IEEE Transactions on Neural Networks, 22*(1), 52–63. doi:10.1109/TNN.2010.2084099 PMID:21216696

Zhao, C. Y., Zhang, X. G., & Guo, Q. (2012). The application of machine-learning on lower limb motion analysis in human exoskeleton system. Lecture Notes in Computer Science, 7621, 600–611. doi:10.1007/978-3-642-34103-8_61

Zhao, X., Wu, Y., Song, G., Li, Z., Fan, Y., & Zhang, Y. (2016). Brain Tumor Segmentation Using a Fully Convolutional Neural Network with Conditional Random Fields. Brainlesion: Glioma, Multiple Sclerosis, Stroke and Traumatic Brain Injuries Lecture Notes in Computer Science, 75-87. doi:10.1007/978-3-319-55524-9_8

Zhao, Q., Tang, Y., Chen, S., Lyu, Y., Curtin, A., Wang, J., ... Tong, S. (2015). Early perceptual anomaly of negative facial expression in depression: An event-related potential study. *Neurophysiologie Clinique. Clinical Neurophysiology, 45*(6), 435–443. doi:10.1016/j.neucli.2015.09.011 PMID:26602972

Zhao, Z., Yang, L., Chen, D., & Luo, Y. (2013). A human ECG identification system based on ensemble empirical mode decomposition. *Sensors (Basel), 13*(5), 6832–6864. doi:10.3390130506832 PMID:23698274

Zhou, W., & Gotman, J. (2004). Removal of EMG and ECG artifacts from EEG based on wavelet transform and ICA. *26th Annual International Conference of the IEEE Engineering in Medicine and Biology Society, 1*, 392-395.

Zhou, L., Pan, S., Wang, J., & Vasilakos, A. V. (2017). Machine learning on big data: Opportunities and challenges. *Neurocomputing, 237*, 350–361. doi:10.1016/j.neucom.2017.01.026

Zhu, H., Lee, Y., & Rosenthal, A. (2016). Data Standards Challenges for Interoperable and Quality Data. *Journal Of Data And Information Quality*, *7*(1-2), 1–3. doi:10.1145/2903723

Zimmermann, J., Wolf, M., Bock, A., Peham, D., & Benecke, C. (2013). The way we refer to ourselves reflects how we relate to others: Associations between first-person pronoun use and interpersonal problems. *Journal of Research in Personality*, *47*(3), 218–225. doi:10.1016/j.jrp.2013.01.008

Zuo, W. L., Wang, Z. Y., Liu, T., & Chen, H. L. (2013). Effective detection of Parkinson's disease using an adaptive fuzzy k-nearest neighbor approach. *Biomedical Signal Processing and Control*, *8*(4), 364–373. doi:10.1016/j.bspc.2013.02.006

About the Contributors

Sudip Paul is currently Assistant Professor in Department of Biomedical Engineering, North-Eastern Hill University, Shillong, India. It is Central University located in the northeast part of the country. He received his Ph.D degree from Indian Institute of Technology (Banaras Hindu University), Varanasi with specialization in Electrophysiology and brain signal analysis. He was selected as Post Doc Fellow under Biotechnology Overseas Associateship for the Scientists working in North Eastern States of India: 2017-18 supported by DBT, Government of India. He has many credentials in his credit out of which his First Prize in Sushruta Innovation Award 2011 sponsored by Department of Science and Technology, Govt. of India and also he also organized many workshops and conferences out of which most significant are the 29th Annual meeting of the SNCI, India and IRBO/APRC Associate School 2017. Dr. Sudip published more than 90 International journal and conference papers and also filled four patents. He is member of APSN, ISN, IBRO, SNCI, SfN, IEEE. He received many awards specially WFN travelling fellowship, Young Investigator Award, IBRO Travel Awardee and ISN Travel Awardee.

* * *

Paramasivam Alagumariappan completed his M.E. at Karpaga Vinayaga College of Engineering and Technology in the field of Power Electronics and Drives a. At present, he is a Ph.D. Research Scholar at the Department of Instrumentation Engineering, Madras Institute of Technology Campus, Anna University, Chennai. He is a student member of Bernoulli Society for Mathematical Statistics and Probability and ASTM, and has authored 6 research papers in journals and conferences.

Sateesh Reddy Avutu is Asst professor in the Department of Electronics and Communication Engineering in Vikas College of Engineering and Technology, Nunna, Vijayawada. He has nearly 7 years of teaching experience. At present he was pursuing Ph.D in Biomedical Engineering department, North Eastern Hill University, Shillong. He is a recipient Visvesvaraya fellowship. He is member of the Institution Engineers (India).

Ebru Aydindag Bayrak is currently Ph.D student of Department of Engineering Sciences, Faculty of Engineering, the University of İstanbul Cerrahpaşa. She was received Bsc degree from Department of Mathematics, Faculty of Science and Literature, Çanakkale Onsekiz Mart University at 2012 and also she was graduated pedagogical formation from Faculty of Education from there. Then, she received her MSc degree from Institue of Science, İstanbul University about Fractal Analysis of Active Fault Data in the San Andreas and the North Anatolian Fault Zones. Her poster presentation about Fractal Analysis of Active Fault Data in North Anatolian Fault Zone won first poster prize in meeting of Active Tectonic Research Group at 2015. Also she was graduated Department of Business Administration (BBA degree) from İstanbul University at 2016. In Ph.D studies she has working on machine learning techniques for the prediction of cancer. She continues to work on academic studies in conferences, journals and symposiums for both national and international.

Dinesh Bhatia pursued his PhD in Biomechanics and Rehabilitation Engineering from MNNIT, Allahabad, India in 2010 with Bachelor's (2002) and Master's degree (2004) in Biomedical Engineering from Mumbai University. He completed his MBA from IMT Ghaziabad in 2007. He is currently working as Associate Professor and Head, Department of Biomedical Engineering, North Eastern Hill University (NEHU), Shillong, Meghalaya, India since August 2013. Previously, he was employed as an Assistant Professor (Sr. Grade) at the Department of Biomedical Engineering, Deenbandhu Chhotu Ram University of Science and Technology, Murthal (Sonepat), Haryana (State Government University), India from July 2006 to July 2013. He was selected for the "Young Scientist Award (BOYSCAST)" in (2011-12) by Government of India to pursue research in osteoarthritis (OA) for one year at Adaptive Neural Systems Laboratory, Biomedical Engineering Department, Florida International University, Miami, Florida, USA. He is also the recipient of "INAE fellowship award" in 2011 by Indian National Academy of Engineering. He was selected as one of the twelve young Biomedical scientists by the ICMR, Govt. of India to pursue research fellowship (2014-15) in the field of sensory prosthetics at University of Glasgow, Scotland, UK. He has attended Biomechanics and human Gait training at Munich, Germany in March, 2017 and training of use of rTMS, EEG and EMG in disabled children in Ivanovo, Russia in September, 2017. He has several research papers in reputed journals, conference, seminars and symposia with teaching and research experience of more than fourteen (14) years. He is invited panel member of many professional bodies, editorial boards, committees, societies and forums. He is currently having several funded projects from Government of India on physically challenged, disabled and paralyzed persons. He authored a book titled "Medical Informatics" published (2015) by PHI and "Current aspects in Stroke Rehabilitation" (2016) by ABS Publishers. His research focuses on understanding muscle mechanics, joint kinematics and dynamics involved in performing locomotion and routine tasks and undermining it effects during an injury or disease. His interest areas are medical instrumentation, biomechanics and rehabilitation engineering, medical informatics, signal and image processing, marketing and international business.

Saroj Biswas obtained his Bachelor of Technology degree in Computer Science and Engineering from Jalpaiguri Govt. Engineering College. He obtained his Master of Technology degree in Computer Science & Engineering from National Institute of Technical Teachers' Training and Research, Kolkata in 2008 and Ph.D. degree in Computer Science and Engineering from National Institute of Technology Silchar in 2015. He has been working as an Assistant Professor in Computer Science & Engineering Department, NIT Silchar since 3rd May, 2010. His research interest includes Machine learning, Artificial Intelligence, Pattern Recognition and Data Mining. Four M. Tech students have completed their dissertation under him and two students are presently carrying out their M. Tech dissertation. Five Ph.D. scholars are presently doing their Ph. D. work under him. He presently runs one DEITY sponsored R&D Project. He has published total 18 international journals in various reputed publication house worldwide including ELSEVIER, SPRINGER, WORLD SCIENTICFIC, IGI GLOBAL, INDERSCIENCE etc.

Debashree Devi is currently a research scholar at the department of Computer Science and Engineering, in National Institute of technology Silchar. She has completed her B.Tech degree from Gandhi Institute of Engineering and Technology, Orissa in the year 2011. She has achieved her M.Tech degree from Assam Don Bosco University with the specialization in Artificial Intelligence (AI) in the year 2013. She has published 7 international conference and journal papers, and 3 edited book chapters. Her area of research includes data mining, artificial intelligence, pattern recognition, cloud computing and machine intelligence. She has worked as organizing member in a number of workshops and the 6th International conference on Advanced Computing, Networking, and Informatics (ICACNI 2018), organized by Department of CSE, NIT Silchar. She has also acted as chair of ACM Student Chapter, NIT Silchar, for a tenure of 1 year from January, 2018- December, 2018. Ms. Debashree Devi has been a reviewer of international conference (FSDM 2018), journals IJOSSP (IGI Global), Neurocomputing (Elsevier), and book chapter (IGI Global).

Divya Govindaraju is currently pursuing her PhD in Madras Institute of Technology, Anna University,Chennai. She received her Bachelor of Engineering (B.E.) degree in Instrumentation and Control Engineering from PSG College of Technology (Affiliated to Anna University), Coimbatore. She has also received her Master of Engineering (M.E) degree in Applied Electronics from PSG College of Technology (Affiliated to Anna University), Coimbatore. Her research interest includes biomedical instrumentation, multivariate analysis using spectroscopy, signal processing and machine learning.

Meena Gupta has a Masters of physiotherapy in neurology and pursuing PhD in biomedical engineering. published more than 12 research paper in good impact factor journals. Have more than 10 years experience in the field of disabilities.

Masaraf Hussain is currently working as an Assistant Professor in the Department of Neurology, North Eastern Indira Gandhi Regional Institute of Health and Medical Science, Shillong. He completed his MBBS from NSCB Medical College, Jabalpur, India in 1998 and MD (Medicine) in 2002 from NSCB Medical College, Jabalpur. He also completed his DM in Neurology from Guwahati Medical College, Assam in 2012. He has several research papers in reputed journals in the field of Neurology.

Mohammad Shahid Husain is a Research professional and Faculty member with thirteen years of teaching & research experience. He is currently working as Assistant Professor in College of Applied Sciences, Ministry of Higher Education, Oman. He has done his M.Tech. in Information Technology (spl: Intelligent System) from the Indian Institute of Information Technology, Allahabad (www.iiita.ac.in), India, which is one among the premier research Institute of India. He has done his PhD in Computer Science & Engineering from Integral University, Lucknow (www.iul.ac.in), India. His area of interest are Artificial Intelligence, Information Retrieval, Natural Language Processing, Data Mining, Web mining, Sentiment Analysis and Computer Networks & Security. Dr. Mohd. Shahid Husain has published 2 books, 4 book chapters & more than 30 research papers in Journals/conferences of international repute. He was involved with many sponsored projects as PI/Co-PI. Currently he is involved in ongoing project sponsored by CAS, MoHE. He is also contributing his knowledge and experience as member of Editorial Board/Advisory committee and TPC in various international Journals/Conferences of repute. Dr. Mohd Shahid Husain is active member of different professional bodies including ACM, IEEE young professionals, IEEE-TCII, ISTE, CSTA, IACSIT. Dr. Mohd Shahid Husain qualified UGC-NET (National Eligibility Test) in June 2014 and GATE (Graduate Aptitude Test in Engineering) in 2008.

Rekh Janghel is serving as an Assistant Professor in Department of Information Technology at National Institute of Technology Raipur. He did Ph.D. from Indian Institute of Information Technology and Management Gwalior in 2013 and M.Tech from National Institute of Technology, Raipur (C.G.) in 2007 and B.Tech from Rungta College of Engineering and Technology, Bhilai (C.G) in 2005. He secured first position in his post-graduation from NIT Raipur. He has published more than 30 research papers in international and national journals and conferences. He also published two book chapters in reputed publication. His areas of research include Deep Learning, Machine Learning, biomedical Healthcare System, expert systems, neural networks, hybrid computing and soft computing. He has guided various research projects in UG and PG level.

Ramgopal Kashyap's areas of interest are image processing, pattern recognition, and machine learning. He has published many research papers in international journals, and conferences like Springer, Inder-science, Elsevier, ACM, and IGI-Global indexed by Science Citation Index (SCI) and Scopus (Elsevier) and many book chapters. He has Reviewed Research Papers in the Science Citation Index Expanded, Springer Journals and Editorial Board Member and conferences programme committee member of the IEEE, Springer international conferences and journals held in countries: Czech Republic, Switzerland, UAE, Australia, Hungary, Poland, Taiwan, Denmark, India, USA, UK, Austria, and Turkey. He has written many book chapters published by IGI Global, USA.

Pinar Kirci is currently an Associate Professor in the Department of Engineering Sciences, Faculty of Engineering, Istanbul University-Cerrahpaşa. She received her Bsc degree from Department of Mathematics-Computer, Faculty of Science and Literature, Beykent University in 2002. Then, she received her MSc degree from Department of Computer Engineering in Istanbul University in 2005 about fiber optical networks. She received her Ph.D degree from Department of Computer Engineering in Istanbul University in 20011 about multiplexing in fiber optical networks. Lately, she has worked on wireless sensor networks.

Subrota Mazumdar is a B.Tech student in school of computer engineering, KIIT University.

Puspanjali Mohapatra is currently working as an Assistant Professor in the Department of Computer Science & Engineering at IIIT Bhubaneswar, Odisha, India. She did her Masters in Computer Science in the year 2002 from Utkal University, Bhubaneswar, MBA in Systems, IT & HR from BPUT Rourkela in the year 2009 and Ph.D. in Computer Science in the year 2017 from SOA University, Bhubaneswar, Odisha, India. She has more than 16 years of experience in teaching and research. She is having around thirty publications in reputed journals and conferences. Her major areas of research are Time Series Data Mining, Bioinformatics, Evolutionary and Soft Computing Techniques.

Gururaj Nagarajan is currently employed as Senior Business Development Analyst. He completed his Bachelor of Engineering (B.E.) in Instrumentation and Control Engineering from PSG college of Technology (Affiliated to Anna University),Coimbatore. He also completed his Masters (M.S. in Research) in Software Engineering from Birla Institute of Technology and Science (BITS), Pilani, Rajasthan. His field of interest is Data Science, AI/ML, IoT and IT Business Development/Sales. He has varied work experience with Global Telecom leaders having worked at multiple geographies. Overall, he has a strong technical and business work experience in the field of Information Technology (IT).

Swati Pattnaik is a final year Btech in Information Technology student at IIIT BBSR. Her current research interest lies in the field of soft computing.

Sudip Paul is currently Visiting Research Fellow at School of Computer Science and Software Engineering, The University of Western Australia, Perth. He was one of the most precious fellowship awardee (Biotechnology Overseas Associateship for the Scientists working in North Eastern States of India: 2017-18 supported by Department of Department of Biotechnology, Government of India). Apart from this affiliation, he is also as an Assistant Professor in Department of Biomedical Engineering, School of Technology, North-Eastern Hill University (NEHU), Shillong, India. It is a Central University located in the northeast part of the country. He received his Ph.D degree from Indian Institute of Technology (Banaras Hindu University), Varanasi with specialization in Electrophysiology and brain signal analysis. He has many credentials in his credit out of which his First Prize in Sushruta Innovation Award 2011 sponsored by Department of Science and Technology, Govt. of India and also he also organized many workshops and conferences out of which most significant are the 29th Annual meeting of the Society for Neurochemistry, India and IRBO/APRC Associate School 2017. Dr. Sudip published more than 90 International journal and conference papers and also filled four patents. Recently he completed three book projects and two are ongoing as editor. Dr. Sudip is a member of different Societies and professional bodies, including APSN, ISN, IBRO, SNCI, SfN, IEEE and many more since 2009, 2010, and 2011 onwards. He received many awards specially World federation of Neurology (WFN) travelling fellowship, Young Investigator Award, IBRO Travel Awardee and ISN Travel Awardee. Dr. Sudip also contributed his knowledge in different international journals as editorial board members. He has presented his research accomplishments in USA, Greece, France, South Africa and Australia.

Biswajit Purkayastha is currently working in National Institute of Technology, Silchar, India as an Associate Professor in CSE department. He has achieved his B. Tech. in Electronics and Telecommunication Engineering from College of Engineering, Kakinada under Jawaharlal Nehru Technological University, Hyderabad, and M. Tech. in Computer Engineering from IIT, Kharagpur and Ph.D. from Computer Science Department of Assam University on Soft Computing. His area of research includes Data structure, Design and analysis of algorithm, computer organization and architecture, microprocessor, and introduction to computing.

Surendra Rahamatkar's areas of interest are image processing and machine learning. He has published many research papers in international journals and conferences like Springer, Inderscience, Elsevier, ACM, and IGI-Global indexed by Science Citation Index (SCI) and Scopus (Elsevier) and many book chapters. He has Reviewed Research Papers in the Science Citation Index Expanded, Springer Journals.

Yogesh Kumar Rathore received M. Tech. degree in Computer Science Engineering from Chhattisgarh Swami Vivekanand Technical University, Bhilai, India in the year 2010.He has 13 years experience of working, as a Asst. Prof. (Department of Computer Science Engineering) at different institutes of Chhattisgarh state. Currently he is a Ph.D. scholar at Department of Information Technology, National

Institute of Technology, Raipur. His interests include pattern recognition, image processing, Deep Learning, machine learning, and artificial intelligence.

S. Ravikumar is an Assistant Professor of Library and Information Science in North-Eastern Hill University, Shillong, India. Dr. Ravi's research and scholarly expertise are in the Scientometric, Information Visualisation, and Social Network Analysis.

Angana Saikia is currently pursuing her PhD in the Department of Biomedical Engineering, NEHU, Shillong. Previously she was working as a Senior Research Fellow (SRF) Department of Biomedical Engineering, NEHU, Shillong. She completed her B.E in Applied Electronics and Instrumentation from Guwahati University, Assam, in 2011 and her M-Tech in Bioelectronics from Tezpur Central University, Assam, India in 2014. Presently she is pursuing her PhD from Department of Biomedical Engineering, NEHU, Shillong. She is specialized in Electrophysiology, Neurorehabilitation, Biomedical Signal Processing and Instrumentation. .Recently she wrote a book on "Overview of Parkinson's disease and its Relevance" published by LAP LAMBERT Academic Publishing, Germany.

Sanjay Saxena is the assistant professor in the department of computer science & engineering, IIIT Bhubaneswar, India. His research area lies in the field of medical image processing, computer vision, high-performance computing.

Moksha Singh is an assistant professor in the Department of Humanities and Social Sciences at National Institute of Technology Raipur, India. Her two major areas of research concern human rights and children's rights. She holds PhD degree from Indian Institute of Technology Kanpur, India.

Shashikanta Tarai is currently serving as Assistant Professor, Department of Humanities and Social Sciences, NIT Raipur, India. For the last ten years, he has been involved in teaching and research related to English language, linguistics, neurolinguistics, and psycholinguistics. From 2011-2014, he worked as a post-doctoral fellow at CBCS, University of Allahabad. He was awarded Ph.D. from IIT Madras in 2012.

Gautam Tatiparti received B.Tech. degree from Pragati Engineering College, Surampalem. and M. Tech. degree in Information Technology from the National Institute of Technology, Raipur, Chhattisgarh, India. His research areas of interest include artificial intelligence, machine learning, and soft computing.

Index

A

Absolutist Words 221, 223-224
ADHD 19, 22, 25
Alzheimer's Disease Neuroimaging Initiative (ADNI) 277, 291
Anxiety 19, 62, 130, 167, 169, 176, 179, 181, 200, 202, 205, 216-221, 224-227, 230, 232, 234
Artificial intelligence 26-27, 53-54, 97, 136, 217, 253-255, 258, 262, 264, 274, 278, 281
Artificial neural networks 54, 145, 153, 161, 258, 263-265, 281, 312
Attention 13-14, 19-20, 22, 25, 39, 112-115, 166, 169, 172, 174, 176-177, 181, 219-222, 226

B

bibliometric 1-3
Big Data 205, 252-262, 274, 278, 281, 291, 297, 308, 310-311
Big Data Analytics 252, 254-255, 257-262, 278, 281, 291
Big Data Samples 252, 255, 291
Bi-Multilingual 216, 225-226
Bradykinesia 62-63, 95, 109, 113-114, 131-132
Brain disorders 242
Brain Tumor 39-41, 43, 46, 48-51, 54-56, 297

C

Central Nervous System 8, 10-11, 26, 62, 95, 97, 146-147
Classification 20, 26-28, 30, 33-34, 41, 43, 51, 53-56, 69, 88, 95-100, 106, 109-111, 115-118, 128, 134, 138, 145-146, 148, 152-153, 162, 170, 205-207, 210-211, 241-243, 245, 248-249, 254, 262-263, 265-266, 268, 270, 274-281
Classifiers 85, 96-98, 106, 109-111, 115, 117-118, 120-121, 145, 153, 158-160, 242-243, 274-275, 280
Clustering 33, 49-52, 54, 137, 139-143, 145, 205, 262-263, 269-271, 275, 280
co-citation 1, 9-10
cognition 14-15, 22, 27, 33, 97, 179, 217, 221, 223, 233
cognitive impairment 108-109, 174, 274, 277, 281
co-word 1

D

Data Imbalance 63-64, 67, 69, 78, 82, 86, 90-91, 95
Data Mining 33, 63, 67, 254, 258, 261, 275-276, 279, 306, 320
Data processing 51, 117, 254-255, 281
Depression 13-14, 20, 62, 114, 165-181, 199-203, 205-209, 213, 216-227, 230, 232-235, 276, 281
Depressive disorder 165-169, 172, 175-178, 181, 201, 218-219, 276
Devices 26-29, 32-35, 44, 242, 257, 260, 274, 278-279, 294, 300-302, 304, 309
Disability 21, 27, 31, 62-63, 108-109, 113-114, 200, 217
Disease diagnosis 260
Dopamine 61-64, 91, 95, 109, 113-114, 124, 128, 132-133

E

Early Detection 61, 63-64, 68-69, 86, 88, 90-91, 96, 110-111, 200, 217-218, 274
EEG 13-15, 18, 20-22, 30, 32, 152-153, 155, 161, 165, 167-173, 180, 241-246, 248, 260, 276, 280
EHR 296, 299, 302, 321
electroencephalogram 15, 18, 25, 30, 168, 241, 260, 276, 280
Electroencephalography 13, 15, 152-153, 280
Electromyography 112, 132, 146, 148

Emotions 62, 165, 181, 206, 208-209, 217, 222-223, 225, 231, 234
epilepsy 1-2, 152-153, 169, 280-281
Event-related potentials 165, 168
Extreme Learning Machine 61, 69, 95, 274

F

Freezing of gait 109, 115
Function Words 216, 222, 224, 232-234
Functionality 27, 45
Fuzzy Classifier 96-98, 106

G

Gait Disorder 108, 112-115

H

Health Information Technology 302
healthcare system 252, 259-260, 281

I

Intellectual structure 1
Intelligent big data analytics 252, 258, 281
Internet of Things 274, 301

K

k-NN 241, 243-244, 246-249

L

Linguistic Behavior 216, 221, 234
Linguistic Marker 233

M

Machine Learning 26, 33, 41, 54, 81, 85, 96-97, 103, 106, 117, 128, 136, 138-139, 141, 145-146, 148, 152, 205-206, 209, 213, 242-243, 252, 254-255, 258, 260-263, 268-269, 274-281, 291, 295, 302-306, 308, 311-314, 316, 320
Machine Learning Methods 209, 252, 255, 262-263, 274-277, 279-281, 291, 295
Machine Learning System 136, 252, 262, 281
Magnetic Resonance Imaging 44, 167, 178, 260, 275, 293
Mapping 1, 53, 78, 137, 145, 263, 269, 271-272, 275-276, 296
Mental State 199, 201, 205, 208, 211-212, 219, 223-224, 245, 247
Motor Imagery 15, 241-246, 248-249

N

Naive Bayes 110, 115, 117, 145, 206, 263, 266, 274-277, 279-280
Neurodegenerative Disorder 61-62, 108-109, 131
Neurofeedback 13-16, 18-20, 22, 25
Neurological Disorder 2-3, 8, 11, 26-27, 29, 43, 108-109, 152, 281, 291
Non-Invasive 39, 56, 96-97, 112-113, 168, 242

O

One-Class SVM 61, 69, 72, 95
Overlapping Cases 63-64, 69, 74, 78, 82, 86, 90-91, 95

P

Parkinson’s disease (PD) 61-62, 108-109, 128, 131, 274-275
Parkinsonian Tremor 113, 136
Parkinsonism 28, 62, 95, 111
Principal Component Analysis 56, 98, 110, 116, 206-207, 272-275, 278

S

Segmentation 39, 41, 46-49, 51-56, 269, 278, 292, 309
seizure detection 152-153, 161, 280
Smart Devices 257
SMR 19, 21, 25
Social Media 199, 201-202, 205-208, 213, 219, 222, 253-254, 260
Speech Analysis 96-97, 106
Support Vector Machine 51, 103-104, 109-111, 115, 117, 128, 145, 206-207, 264, 274-280

T

Technology 22, 27-28, 31, 34-35, 91, 113, 136, 148, 182, 235, 257-258, 278, 302
Tomek-Link 69, 73-74, 91, 95
Tremor 28, 62-63, 109, 113, 128-132, 134, 136, 145-146, 148
Twitter 199, 201, 203, 205-207, 213, 260

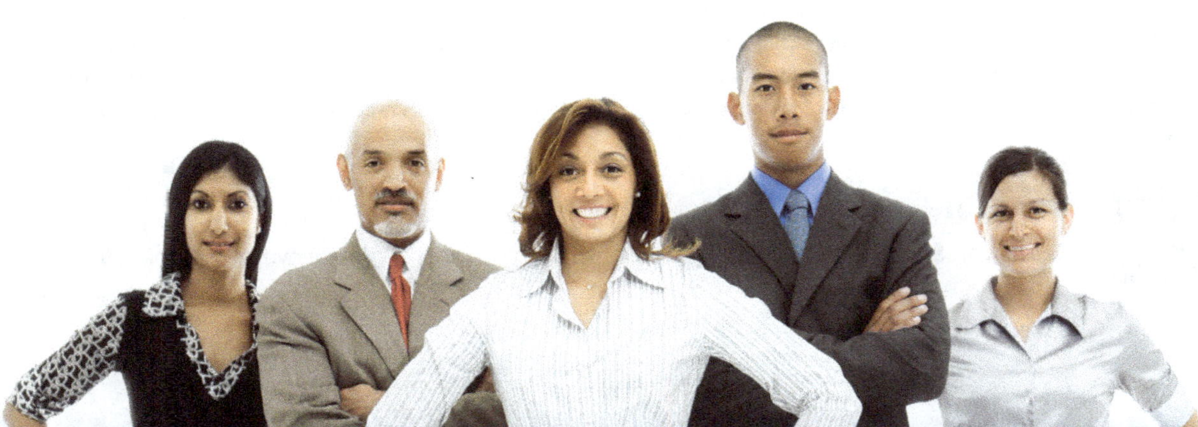

www.ingramcontent.com/pod-product-compliance
Lightning Source LLC
LaVergne TN
LVHW060302011026
849161LV00011B/2756